PHARMACEUTICAL CARE PRACTICE

THE PATIENT-CENTERED APPROACH TO MEDICATION MANAGEMENT SERVICES

third edition

PHARMACEUTICAL CARE PRACTICE

THE PATIENT-CENTERED APPROACH TO MEDICATION MANAGEMENT SERVICES

Robert J. Cipolle, PharmD
Professor Emeritus

Linda M. Strand, PharmD, PhD, DSc (Hon)
Professor Emerita

Peter C. Morley, PhD
Professor (Retired)

University of Minnesota
Minneapolis, Minnesota

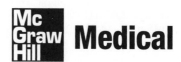

New York   Chicago   San Francisco   Lisbon   London   Madrid   Mexico City
Milan   New Delhi   San Juan   Seoul   Singapore   Sydney   Toronto

The **McGraw·Hill** Companies

Pharmaceutical Care Practice: The Patient-centered Approach to Medication Management Services, Third Edition

3 4 5 6 7 8 9 0 DOC/DOC 17 16 15 14 13

ISBN 978-0-07-175638-9
MHID 0-07-175638-8

This book was set in Adobe Garamond by Thomson Digital.
The editors were Michael Weitz and Christie Naglieri.
The production supervisor was Sherri Souffrance.
Project management was provided by Aakriti Kathuria, Thomson Digital.
The designer was Eve Siegel; the cover designer was Ashley Lau.
RR Donnelley was printer and binder.

This book is printed on acid-free paper.

Library of Congress Cataloging-in-Publication Data

Cipolle, Robert J.
  Pharmaceutical care practice / Robert J. Cipolle, Linda M. Strand,
Peter C. Morley.—3rd ed.
     p. ; cm.
  Rev. ed. of : Pharmaceutical care practice / Robert J. Cipolle, Linda
M. Strand, Peter C. Morley. 2nd ed. c2004.
  Includes bibliographical references and index.
  ISBN-13: 978-0-07-175638-9 (softcover : alk. paper)
  ISBN-10: 0-07-175638-8 (softcover : alk. paper)
  I. Cipolle, Robert J. II. Strand, Linda M. III. Morley, Peter C.
Pharmaceutical care practice. IV. Title.
  [DNLM: 1. Pharmaceutical Services. 2. Professional Practice. 3. Drug
Therapy. QV 21]
  615'.1068—dc23
                                                    2011037335

McGraw-Hill books are available at special quantity discounts to use as premiums and sales promotions, or for use in corporate training programs. To contact a representative please e-mail us at bulksales@mcgraw-hill.com.

Our families have always played a significant role
in our work. That has become even more apparent in recent years as
we have lost members of our families and found others. Therefore,
we write this volume in memory of those we have lost:

Bette Cipolle	*1964–1985*
Norm Cipolle	*1925–2010*
Norma Gassman	*1930–2008*
Clarence Morley	*1917–1996*
Joan Morley	*1920–2010*

And, we dedicate this volume to those who have
helped us to find our way; our children:

Christina and Anthony
Karesa, Cheryl, and Georgia

Contents

Contributors

Anna Birna Almarsdóttir, PhD
Professor
Faculty of Pharmaceutical Sciences
University of Iceland
Reykjavik, Iceland

Lynne M. Bye, DipPharm, PG DipHlthMngt
Senior Tutor
School of Pharmacy
Faculty of Medical and Health Sciences
The University of Auckland, New Zealand
Chair
Pharmacy Advisory Group
Waitemata District Health Board
Auckland, New Zealand

Andreas Niclas Föerster, PharmD
Clinical Assistant Professor
Professional Education
University of Minnesota
College of Pharmacy
Senior Pharmacist
Adler Apotheke Velbert, Germany

Johan J. de Gier, PharmD, PhD
Professor
Department of Pharmacotherapy and Pharmaceutical Care
Faculty of Mathematics and Natural Sciences
University of Groningen
Groningen, The Netherlands

Dr. Paul F. Grassby, BSc, PhD, MRPharmS
Deputy Head of Pharmacy
School of Pharmacy
University of East Anglia, Norwich
Norfolk, United Kingdom

Brian J. Isetts, PhD, BCPS
Professor
Department of Pharmaceutical Care & Health Systems
University of Minnesota College of Pharmacy
Minneapolis, Minnesota

Nadir M. Kheir, PhD, FNZCP, MPS
Assistant Professor
Coordinator of Continuing Professional Pharmacy Development
College of Pharmacy
Qatar University
Doha, Qatar

Eunyoung Kim, PharmD, BCPS, PhD
Assistant Professor
College of Pharmacy
Chungnam National University
Daejoeon, South Korea

Manuel J. Machuca, PhD, PharmD
Community Pharmacist
Clinical Pharmacist at a Unit for Drug-Therapy Optimization
Seville, Spain

Geoff March, BPharm, PhD
Quality Use of Medicine and Pharmacy Research Centre
Sansom Institute for Health Research
University of South Australia
Adelaide, South Australia

Barbara Gobis Ogle, BSc(Pharm), ACPR, MScPhm
Pharmacist Consultant
North Vancouver
British Columbia, Canada

Djenane Ramalho de Oliveira, BSc, RPh, MSc, PhD
Professor
Social Pharmacy Department
College of Pharmacy, Universidade
Federal de Minas Gerais
Belo Horizonte, Brazil

Researcher and MTM Pharmacist Specialist
Medication Therapy Management Department
Fairview Pharmacy Services
Minneapolis, Minnesota

Adjunct Faculty
Department of Pharmaceutical Care & Health Systems
College of Pharmacy, University of Minnesota
Minneapolis, Minnesota

Jochen Pfeifer, PharmD, MRPharmS
Clinical Assistant Professor
Professional Education
University of Minnesota, College of Pharmacy
Owner and Head Pharmacist
Adler Apotheke Velbert, Germany

Geeta Pradeep, MPharm
Research Scholar
School of Medical Sciences
Discipline of Pharmacy
College of Science, Engineering and Health
Royal Melbourne Institute of Technology
Victoria, Australia

Siting Zhou, PhD
Research Analyst
HealthCore, Inc.
Wilmington, Delaware

Preface

Medication management services are a response to a problem. Although the term is relatively new, the problem is not. The problem of medication-related morbidity and mortality has been with us as long as drug therapy has been in use; however, the problem has grown to such a magnitude that something now must be done to address it.

Consider the following scenario:

The next time you are driving down the road and an ambulance goes by with its sirens loudly screaming and its lights brightly flashing—stop and think what *you* might have done to prevent the victim inside from needing that trip to the hospital. Ask yourself: was there some aspect of his drug therapy that I could have changed in order to prevent the need for that ambulance ride? Probably! Likely!!

In fact, it is very likely that the patient in the ambulance is on the way to a drug-related hospitalization. One in four hospitalizations is due to a drug therapy problem[1]. What we find even more interesting is that the vast majority of these drug-related hospitalizations are preventable.[1–4] Do the math. One out of every six admissions to a hospital is caused by a preventable drug therapy problem. The most common classes of drugs associated with drug-related hospitalizations are cardiovascular agents, anticoagulants, hypoglycemic agents, and anti-inflammatory agents.

In the ambulatory setting, the stories are similar.[5] Over 27% of adverse drug events in elderly patients are preventable. In 2006, the drugs most commonly involved include cardiovascular agents, diuretics, analgesics, hypoglycemics, and anticoagulants. That same year, a report describing the over 700,000 patients brought to the emergency department because of a drug-related problem described the drugs most commonly involved.[6] The list will sound familiar: warfarin, insulin, nonsteroidal anti-inflammatory drugs, and digoxin.[7,8] None of these drug products is new. There is little about their pharmacology that we do not know. In fact, we can measure concentrations and calculate individualized doses of three of the drugs most commonly involved in emergency department visits. These three drugs (warfarin, insulin, and digoxin) have a narrow, but known therapeutic index, yet they are involved in one-third of the emergency departments' adverse drug events in the United States. A large part of the public health burden of adverse drug events is attributable to "older drugs, used poorly." How much longer are we going to continue to use these very effective drugs "poorly"?

In the patients over 65 years of age, we spend over $201 billion per year due to adverse drug events (50% of which are preventable).[9] Over 40% of these patients are readmitted to hospital within 1 year.[10,11] This is a substantial opportunity for practitioners who have the skills and knowledge to bring order and a rational approach to the use of medications throughout our health care systems. The impact that we can have on the health of our patients, our friends, and even our families is enormous.

The problem, its causes and its solutions, are multidimensional so it has been difficult to identify a solution that can make a significant difference to the patient and/or the health care system. In fact, little that has been done over the past three decades has improved the situation. In 1991 (2 decades ago), a group from Utah published their findings of 52 hospitalizations due to adverse drug events.[12] These events more than doubled the patient's hospital stay. Similarly, most emergency hospitalizations for adverse drug events in older adults are caused by a few commonly used medications (warfarin, insulins, oral antiplatelet agents, and oral hypoglycemic agents).[13] We are old enough to remember the first set of results from the Boston Collaborative Drug Surveillance program over 35 years ago.[14] The drugs most often involved in adverse outcomes back then were the same as those being reported today.

It is clear that we need a new practitioner who can apply new practice standards that allow them to contribute meaningfully to appropriate, effective, safe, and convenient drug therapy for all patients. Pharmaceutical care practice standards can create a continuum of high-quality care for patients from research through practice because these standards bring rational solutions to managing the benefits and risks of medication use.[15]

We remain convinced that medication management services offer a rational solution to this problem. Behind these services is a lengthy history of research, education, and practice, which show that medication management services are a valuable solution to the suffering and pain caused by the inappropriate use of medications. The patient-centered approach, combined with an orderly, logical, rational decision-making process assessing the indication, effectiveness, safety, and adherence of all of a patient's drug therapies has a measurable positive impact on the outcomes of drug therapy.

It is time to make a change. Indeed, positive change is long overdue! This change requires a community of practitioners to stop watching ambulances scurry by and take seriously the philosophy of pharmaceutical care practice, thus accepting the responsibility for the outcomes of drug therapies—good or bad—and to identify, resolve, and prevent drug therapy problems. Only by individual practitioners seeing and providing care for one patient at a time will we finally have the positive impact on overall outcomes of drug therapy that our patients expect and deserve.

This book is written for the purpose of facilitating this change. The book describes medication management services and explains their evolution. The book describes how a practitioner delivers the service and it provides a vision of how these services "fit" into the evolving health care structures. This is accomplished by bringing together medication management services and the professional practice that serves as its foundation, pharmaceutical care practice. The book is organized in the following manner.

Chapter 1 provides an overview of medication management services; what they are, how they developed, why they are needed, the value of the services and how the services are delivered in practice.

Chapter 2 establishes the professional practice of pharmaceutical care as the foundation for medication management services. Chapter 3 explains why the philosophy of pharmaceutical care practice is necessary and why it plays such a significant role in a patient care practice.

Chapter 4 explains the centrality of patient-centeredness to medication management services. Although the term patient-centeredness is used frequently today, we describe the specific meaning it has to a patient's medication experience and adherence behavior.

Chapters 5 through 8 provide a detailed description of how to provide medication management services in a patient-centered manner through the professional practice of pharmaceutical care. Pharmaceutical care is the ethical, clinical, and legal foundation for the delivery of comprehensive medication management services. This section starts with understanding how a patient's medication experience can change our way of thinking about adherence and why the medication experience must be the starting point for any quality medication management service. A quality service includes a comprehensive assessment, a personalized care plan, and timely follow-up evaluations. Chapter 9 explains how this patient care process is best documented.

Chapter 10 describes the skills and knowledge required to prepare qualified practitioners who are able to deliver a patient-centered medication management service.

Chapter 11 changes the focus from the individual practitioner providing pharmaceutical care to how medication management services can be established and managed within the health care system.

Chapter 12 consists of contributed authors from around the world who discuss pharmaceutical care practice and the development of medication management services in each of their geographic areas. The authors explain the local origin of the services and the current adoption level for these services. In addition, there is a discussion of how these services can be disseminated on a large scale in the future, given the cultural, political, and social structures in place.

This book is written for health care practitioners and those involved in the many aspects of our health care systems. The purpose of the book is to provide the basic information necessary to establish, support, deliver and maintain medication management services. Within the context of medication management services drug therapy can be experienced as intended and can achieve the goals of therapy essential to the highest level of optimal clinical outcomes, and directly contribute to improving the patient's quality of life. These goals are well within our reach, now we need both individual and collective resolve to move forward and seize every opportunity to develop and implement medication management services. Patients deserve no less!

Robert J. Cipolle, PharmD
Linda M. Strand, PharmD, PhD, DSc (Hon)
Peter C. Morley, PhD

REFERENCES

1. Samoy LJ, Zed PJ, Wilbur K, Balen RM, Abu-Laban RB, Roberts M. Drug-related hospitalizations in a tertiary care internal medicine service of a Canadian hospital: a prospective study. *Pharmacotherapy.* 2006;26(11):1578–1586.

2. Patel KJ, Kedia MS, Bajpai D, Mehta SS, Kshirsagar NA, Gogtay NJ. Evaluation of the prevalence and economic burden of adverse drug reactions presenting to the medical emergency department of a tertiary referral centre: a prospective study. *Br J Clin Pharmacol.* 2007;7:8.

3. Howard RL, Avery AJ, Slavenburg S, et al. Which drugs casue preventable admissions to hospital? A systematic review. *Br J Clin Pharmacol.* 2007;63(2):136–147.

4. Leendertse AJ, Egberts AC, Stoker LJ, van den Bemt PM. Frequency of and risk factors for preventable medication-related hospital admissions in the Netherlands. *Arch Intern Med.* 2008;168(17):1890–1896.

5. Gandhi TK, Weingart SN, Borus J, et al. Adverse drug events in ambulatory care. *N Engl J Med.* 2003;348(16):1556–1564.

6. Budnitz DS, Shehab N, Kegler SR, Richards CL. Medication use leading to emergency department visits for adverse drug events in older adults. *Ann Intern Med.* 2007;147(11):755–765.

7. Zhang M, Holman CDJ, Price SD, Sanfilippo FM, Preen DB, Bulsara MK. Comorbidity and repeat admission to hospital for adverse drug reactions in older adults: retrospective cohort study. *Br Med J.* 2009;338: a2752. doi:10.1136/bmj.a2752.

8. Zhang M, Holman CDJ, Preen DB, Brameld K. Repeat adverse drug reactions causing hospitalization in older Australians: a population-based longitudinal study 1980-2003. *Br J Clin Pharmacol.* 2006;63(2):163–170.

9. Clark TR. *Startling Statistics About Seniors and Medication Use.* Alexandria: American Society of Consultant Pharmacists; 2008.

10. Davies EC, Green CF, Mottram DR, Rowe PH, Pirmohamed M. Emergency readmissions to hospital due to adverse drug reactions within 1 year of the index admission. *Br J Clin Pharmacol.* 2010;70(5):749–755.

11. Jencks SF, Williams MV, Coleman EA. Rehospitalizations among patients in the Medicare fee-for-service program. *N Engl J Med.* 2009;360(14):1418–1428.

12. Classen DC, Pestotnik SL, Evans RS, Burke JP. Computerized surveillance of adverse drug events in hospital patients. *JAMA.* 1991;266(20):2847–2851.

13. Budnitz DS, Lovegrove MC, Shehab N, Richards CL. Emergency hospitalizations for adverse drug events in older Americans. *N Engl J Med.* 2011;365(21):2002–2012.

14. Miller RR. Hospital admissions due to adverse drug reactions: a report from the Boston Collaborative Drug Surveillance Program. *Arch Intern Med.* 1974;134(2):219–223.

15. Cipolle CL, Cipolle RJ, Strand LM. Consistent standards in medication use: the need to care for patients from research to practice. *J Am Pharm Assoc.* 2006;46(2):205–212.

Acknowledgments

The practice of pharmaceutical care as described here has been under development since 1978. It would be virtually impossible to thank all of the individuals who have helped to create the ideas described in this volume. There have been practitioner colleagues, physicians, professional students, graduate students, faculty, as well as thousands of patients who have contributed significantly to the development of this practice. There have been those who have supported our research financially and those who have constructively disagreed with us. We owe a tremendous amount of gratitude to all of them.

This text could not have been prepared without the efforts of Karen E. McCauley, who has stuck with us through three editions and 15 years of work. We also wish to acknowledge the constructive critique and practical ideas provided by Victoria Losinski, PharmD, PhD, and Christina Cipolle, PharmD.

The authors want to recognize the support, contributions, and friendship of Mike Frakes, PharmD. Dr. Frakes has led the efforts to develop and continually improve the computerized documentation system (Assurance System) that supports pharmaceutical care practitioners. All of the clinical evidence describing the impact of pharmaceutical care in this text was made possible through his work and the work of practitioners across the United States. These practitioners provide the evidence of the value of this practice on a daily basis.

We are forever indebted to Dean Emeritus Lawrence C. Weaver, PhD, of the College of Pharmacy at the University of Minnesota, who was the greatest mentor any group with ideas could ever have. His moral support, wonderful vision, and constant enthusiasm have kept us focused for over three decades.

We would also like to acknowledge the effort put forward by our international authors. Chapter 12 represents the work of several of our colleagues who provide us with a global view of the "world of pharmaceutical care practice." This volume would have been incomplete without this work and the time and effort put into it has been extraordinary. Thank you very much.

And, finally, we have been working to develop this practice for the majority of our careers. It has been challenging since change is never easy or comfortable. However, the opportunity to positively impact the lives of patients has been a privilege. We cannot imagine a better career and for this we are eternally grateful.

About the Authors

Robert J. Cipolle Dr. Cipolle is a pharmacist and educator. He received his Bachelor of Pharmacy Degree (Honors) from the College of Pharmacy at the University of Illinois Medical Center, and the Doctor of Pharmacy Degree from the University of Minnesota College of Pharmacy. He has held faculty and administrative positions at the University of Minnesota that included Department Chair, Associate Dean for Academic Affairs, and Dean of the College of Pharmacy. Dr. Cipolle has practiced in the areas of clinical pharmacokinetics, ambulatory care, and long-term care. He has developed educational programs for pharmacy students, residents, fellows, and graduate students in therapeutic drug monitoring, specialty areas of pharmacotherapy and pharmaceutical care. Dr. Cipolle joined Dr. Strand in 1978 to begin the work that eventually resulted in the development of the practice of pharmaceutical care and a documentation system to support practitioners.

Dr. Cipolle was one of the first clinical pharmacists to be recognized as a fellow by both the American College of Clinical Pharmacy (FCCP—1985) and the American Society of Health System Pharmacists (FASHP—1991). He has received a number of awards to recognize his contribution to pharmacy practice. These include the Hallie Bruce Award from the Minnesota Society of Hospital Pharmacists, and the Larry and Dee Weaver Medal for sustained contributions to the University of Minnesota College of Pharmacy.

Dr. Cipolle held the position of Professor and Director of the Peters Institute of Pharmaceutical Care in the College of Pharmacy at the University of Minnesota in Minneapolis, Minnesota, from 1992 to 2011. He presently holds the position of Professor Emeritus at the University of Minnesota and is a founder and member of the Board of Directors for Medication Management Systems, Inc.

Linda M. Strand Dr. Strand is a pharmacist and an educator. She received her Bachelor of Science Degree, Doctor of Pharmacy Degree, and Doctor of Philosophy Degree in Pharmacy Administration from the University of Minnesota. In 2001, Dr. Strand was presented an honorary Doctor of Science Degree from Robert Gordon University in Aberdeen, Scotland.

Dr. Strand held faculty positions in the colleges of pharmacy at the University of Utah and the University of Florida before returning to the University of Minnesota. Throughout her career, she practiced in community, hospital, and clinical pharmacy settings. Dr. Strand has taught the practice of pharmaceutical care at the professional student level as well as the graduate level.

Dr. Strand began working with the ideas that eventually became the practice of pharmaceutical care in 1978. She began working with Dr. Cipolle at that time and in 1983 Dr. Peter Morley joined the research team. In 1990, her work was integrated with the work of Dr. Charles D. Hepler in the landmark paper entitled "Opportunities and Responsibilities in Pharmaceutical Care." Since then she has worked to further develop and teach the practice of pharmaceutical care. Dr. Strand received the Remington Medal in 1997 from the American Pharmacists Association. This medal is the highest recognition given to an individual working in the profession of pharmacy.

Dr. Strand's work is internationally recognized. She has lectured throughout the world and conducted pharmaceutical care training programs for practitioners from over 12 nations.

Dr. Strand held the position of Distinguished Professor in the College of Pharmacy at the University of Minnesota from 2001 to 2009. She presently holds the position of Professor Emerita at the University of Minnesota and is Vice President of Professional Services at Medication Management Systems. Dr. Strand is also a founder and member of the Board of Directors for Medication Management Systems, Inc.

Peter C. Morley Dr. Morley is a medical anthropologist and an educator. He received his Bachelor of Arts Degree (Honors) in politics, sociology, and anthropology and the Master of Arts Degree in Political Science from Simon Fraser University in British Columbia, Canada. He continued his education at Stirling University in Stirling, Scotland, where he received the Doctor of Philosophy Degree in Anthropology.

Dr. Morley held faculty positions at Stirling University in Scotland and Memorial University Medical School of Newfoundland, Canada, the School of Nursing and College of Pharmacy at the University of Utah, the College of Pharmacy at the University of Florida and the College of Pharmacy at the University of Minnesota. He served as the Director of the Transcultural Nursing program while at the University of Utah. Dr. Morley's work has taken him to many countries and involved him in many different cultures around the world.

Dr. Morley has advised over 100 graduate students from every discipline in the health and social sciences. He has been elected a fellow of the Royal Anthropological Institute of Great Britain and a fellow of the Society for Applied Anthropology of the United States.

Dr. Morley joined the research team of Drs. Cipolle and Strand in 1983 and has been working to further develop and teach the practice of pharmaceutical care since then. His work focuses on the ethical, and sociocultural aspects of pharmaceutical care practice. He has been instrumental in making the patient's perspective central to the practice of pharmaceutical care and understanding the process of change and development in a health profession.

Dr. Morley held the position of Professor in the College of Pharmacy at the University of Minnesota from 1990 to 2008 when he retired from the University. He is a founder of Medication Management Systems, Inc.

DISCLOSURE

In 2006 the University of Minnesota, Office of Business Development facilitated the formation of the company Medication Management Systems, Inc. This company was cofounded by Drs. Cipolle, Strand, and Morley. They all share ownership in the company. In addition, Drs. Cipolle and Strand serve on the Board of Directors of the company.

The goal of this company is to make the intellectual property developed by Drs. Cipolle, Strand, and Morley (practice software, practice instruments, management, and marketing support of comprehensive medication management services) available to practitioners all over the world.

The software program licensed to Medication Management Systems, Inc. (The Assurance System) was used to generate the data reported throughout this text. The data resulted from the pharmaceutical care provided by pharmacists across the United States in ambulatory practice settings of all types.

PHARMACEUTICAL CARE PRACTICE

THE PATIENT-CENTERED APPROACH TO MEDICATION MANAGEMENT SERVICES

Medication Management Services

♀ KEY CONCEPTS

1 Medication management services are the experienced, measurable events when pharmaceutical care is practiced.

2 Two distinct approaches to medication management services have emerged: the prescription-focused and the patient-centered approaches. This book is about the patient-centered approach.

3 The need for medication management services results from more complex therapies, increase in the number of medications prescribed and the cost of new medications, as well as the lack of a structured, systematic decision making process for drug selection and dosing.

4 Solutions to address the high level of drug-related morbidity and mortality have been in place at the policy and institutional levels with some success. However, it is the intervention at the patient-specific level that impacts decisions made on a daily basis for an individual patient. Medication management services "fit" at the patient-specific level of improving medication use.

5 Medication management services should be available to all patients who need them. Access should not be limited until we understand more about who will benefit most from the service.

6 The value of medication management services has been established, documented, published, and reproduced in many practice settings around the world.

7 Medication management services are being delivered in the ambulatory and institutional settings. They are recognized in the medical home and accountable care environments, and can function anywhere patients and qualified practitioners come together.

MEDICATION MANAGEMENT SERVICES EMERGE: A DEFINITION

Medication management services are relatively new to those in and out of the health care professions. The first use of the term on a broad scale in the United States was in 2006 when the Federal Government implemented a new drug benefit (Part D) within the federal insurance program of Medicare, which now includes a drug benefit for the elderly population. As part of this benefit a new service was required to help patients to manage these "covered" medications and this new service was called medication therapy management. This phrase was taken from terminology used in the British Health System where it referred to managing treatment options and was called therapy management. When the term was imported to the United States and applied to the management of medications taken by the beneficiaries of the Medicare program, it became medication therapy management.

A clear definition of the term medication therapy management did not accompany the introduction of the benefit to the elderly. This may explain why so many different definitions of the concept have arisen, each with a slightly different emphasis, depending on the organization defining the term. Generally speaking, however, there are two different approaches being taken to medication therapy management: the prescription-focused approach and the patient-centered approach. Each of these will be described in detail later in this chapter; however, first we will define patient-centered medication management because it will be the focus of this book. We should also clarify at this point that we will be using the term medication therapy management to refer only to the program defined by the Federal Government in Part D of the Medicare Program, and we will be using medication management services to refer to the patient-centered services described in this book.

There are now a number of consistent definitions for patient-centered, medication management services, and we rely on these for our definition as they come from the medical and political forces in the marketplace today. These include (1) the definition from the Patient Centered Primary Care Collaborative (PCPCC), the national organization in the United States, which represents over 500 stakeholder organizations, which is leading the health care reform movement toward primary care services delivered in the context of the "medical home,"[1] (2) the definition offered by the American Medical Association as part of the Clinical Procedural Terminology codes, which were granted so payment for medication management services could occur,[2] and (3) the definition offered by the Minnesota State Legislature in 2006 when legislation was passed to allow for medication management services to be delivered to Medicaid patients by pharmacists and reimbursed by the state government.[3]

All of these definitions are consistent with the definition used throughout this book:

> Medication management services are the professional activities needed to meet the standard of care which ensures each patient's medications (whether they are prescription, nonprescription, alternative, traditional, vitamins, or nutritional supplements) are individually assessed to determine that each medication is appropriate

for the medical condition being treated, that the medication is being effective and achieving the goals established, that the medication is safe for the patient in the presence of the co-morbidities and other medications the patient may be taking, and the patient is able and willing to take the medications as intended. This assessment is completed in a systematic and comprehensive manner.

In addition to the comprehensive assessment of the patient's drug-related needs, medication management services include an individualized care plan that utilizes the patient's medication experience and preferences to determine desired goals of therapy with the patient, as well as appropriate follow-up to evaluate actual patient outcomes that result from the care plan. This all occurs because the patient understands, agrees with, and actively participates in the treatment regimen, thus optimizing each patient's medication experience and clinical outcomes. Medication management services must be delivered and documented in a manner that adds unique value to the care of the patient and integrates easily with the medical team caring for the patient.

These interventions must be grounded in the philosophy and ethics of the professional practice of pharmaceutical care and delivered according to the standards of practice for the patient care process prescribed by the practice.

The Medication Management Task Force, which is part of the PCPCC (www.pcpcc.net), provided even more guidance in the Resource Document on Comprehensive Medication Management Services of 2010.[1] This document outlines the 10 steps that need to be completed each time these services are delivered in order to qualify as comprehensive medication management. This is a critical development in the widespread dissemination of these services as the largest organized physician groups in the United States endorse these 10 steps. Members of the PCPCC include more than 500 organizations, all active stakeholders in the health care system. In addition to all of the major professional physician organizations, membership includes patient advocacy groups, pharmaceutical companies, nurse and pharmacy professional organizations, health information technology companies, and many others. With the publication of the resource document described above, PCPCC recognized and endorsed comprehensive medication management services as necessary when delivering integrated, coordinated, and comprehensive primary care services. Table 1-1 describes the 10 steps.

If we take one-step back, medication management services are the activities a "nonprofessional" sees when a "professional" is applying his knowledge and skills to execute his professional responsibilities. So the services are what patients, administrators, and payers relate to when they discuss what this practitioner does to deliver medication management services. For example, what we "observe" at the dentist are the services he performs for us—cleaning, drilling, filling, etc.—but what the dentist sees and does is very different—it

Table 1-1 Ten steps to achieve comprehensive medication management

1.	Identify patients who have not achieved clinical goals of therapy.
2.	Understand the patient's personal medication experience/history and preferences/beliefs.
3.	Identify actual use patterns of all medications including over-the-counter, bioactive supplements, and prescribed medications.
4.	Assess each medication (in the following order) for appropriateness, effectiveness, safety (including drug interactions), and adherence, focused on achievement of the clinical goals for each therapy.
5.	Identify all drug therapy problems (the gap between current therapy and that needed to achieve optimal clinical outcomes).
6.	Develop a care plan addressing recommended steps, including therapeutic changes needed to achieve optimal outcomes.
7.	Patient agrees with and understands care plan, which is communicated to the prescriber/provider for his or her consent/support.
8.	Document all steps and current clinical status versus goals of therapy.
9.	Follow-up evaluations with the patient are critical to determine effects of changes, reassess actual outcomes, and recommend further therapeutic changes to achieve desired clinical goals/outcomes, other team members and personalized (patient unique) goals of therapy are understood by all team members.
10.	Comprehensive medical management is a reiterative process—care is coordinated with personalized (patient unique) goals of therapy are understood by all team members.

is his professional practice, his decision-making process, his professional techniques. It is the same activity described at two different levels—the professional practice of the practitioner and the services experienced by the others in the health care system. In this case, the professional practice is pharmaceutical care and the services delivered are medication management services.

KEY CLINICAL CONCEPTS

Medication management services are the identifiable events in practice surrounding the professional responsibility of managing a patient's medications.

Therefore, medication management services are the activities which are recognized by nonpractitioners as evidence that care is being provided; it is what is recognized as valuable by a payer, and are deemed necessary to achieve success if you are an administrator. Medication management services are the components of a professional practice that can be standardized, measured, evaluated, and reproduced so that accountability and reward for these services can occur. They are, in essence, the nonprofessional's way of thinking about what professionals do when they care for patients so that payment and accountability for the services can occur.

However, services that involve decisions that can result in both life-saving and life-threatening consequences cannot be provided without a clearly defined professional mandate and ethical framework that is the foundation for these activities. This mandate requires the use of knowledge that is evidence-based and is delivered by a practitioner who is qualified to make the decisions implicit in taking this responsibility. Therefore, medication management services can be provided responsibly only when the practitioner delivering these services is engaged in a professional practice. The professional practice that is at the foundation of ethical, quality medication management services is pharmaceutical care practice.

So to put it simply, pharmaceutical care is the professional practice of the practitioner providing medication management services to patients within a health system. This volume will describe both medication management services and the professional practice of pharmaceutical care. However, before this discussion takes place, it is useful to step back and consider the different interpretations of medication management services occurring today. This will also help to place patient-centered services and pharmaceutical care into the proper context.

APPROACHES TO MEDICATION MANAGEMENT SERVICES

There is still significant confusion at present about what are and what are not, medication management services.

KEY CLINICAL CONCEPTS

There are two different approaches to delivering medication management services emerging in practice: (1) the prescription-focused approach, and (2) the patient-centered approach.

Although these two approaches are not entirely different from each other, for explanatory purposes, we will focus on the major differences between them. Although this book will focus entirely on the patient-centered approach, it will be useful to understand both approaches.

The Prescription-focused Approach

The first approach represents those activities that are performed at the time of dispensing the drug product to the patient. These activities include generic substitution, drug formulary reconciliation, the provision of drug information, disease education focused around the drug product, population-based clinical rules for the use of the drug product, and some drug-specific monitoring. These interventions are performed where and when the prescription is received, or they are provided as the result of prescription claims data analysis. In the latter case, the patient's name is "queued-up" for the pharmacist to act upon when the prescription request is completed. As these activities are executed at the site and time of the dispensing process, they are mostly delivered face-to-face and are usually episodic in that the activities are performed only once for a patient. The activities involved are varied, and they are performed at the discretion of the pharmacist or are specified by the health plan or payer. Usually a list of acceptable interventions is provided and the appropriate ones are performed when and if the pharmacist sees fit. The specific activities performed are dependent on the "available time" of the pharmacist and the patient at the moment of dispensing, and usually involve a limited amount of documentation at the end of the encounter. In summary, these activities begin with the prescription and are almost exclusively focused on a specific drug product.

There are a number of advantages and challenges to performing activities in this manner. The greatest advantage at this time is that payers recognize this delivery structure and compensate for these activities. In addition, limited training of the pharmacist is required. As these activities are at the discretion of the pharmacist, only those that are most comfortable for the pharmacist and can be delivered with confidence are the ones that are offered. This is seen as an advantage to those wanting a quick and easy approach to providing these services.

Performing these activities also present a number of challenges. Perhaps the greatest challenge for patients and prescribers is that a standard service, which is delivered by all pharmacists in a similar manner, does not occur. This confuses both patients and prescribers and provides a challenge for payers as they try to understand and determine the value of a wide range of interventions. In addition, the activities can be disruptive to the dispensing process and they have the potential to make the dispensing process more inefficient and less accurate because of the disruption.

Also, the episodic nature of these activities is inconsistent with the standards and expectations of other patient care providers and team members. And because prescribers are not allowed to refer patients to a specific pharmacy, recruiting patients into a practice quickly becomes an issue. Other challenges include the fact that these activities have limited impact on the patient and therefore have less economic value than is necessary to support a financially viable practice. Payment for the service is relatively low compared to other health care professionals, and it is difficult to establish a patient care practice this way.

Perhaps the most threatening challenge to the prescription-focused approach is the conflict of interest that exists in this structure—if the prescription-focused activities result in an increase in the use of prescription or nonprescription products, then the pharmacist profits financially from the decision. This is an issue because it is considered unacceptable for physicians to make decisions about a patient's medications (write a prescription) and then profit from the sale of the product. This is the reason why physicians are prohibited from owning pharmacies in the United States as well as many other countries. This economic and ethical conflict of interest will have to be managed carefully for prescription-focused services to persist. Pharmacists will have to separate the dispensing business and functions from the patient care business and process for this approach to be successful. Significant work needs to occur to make prescription-focused medication management services a viable option for the pharmacist.

The Patient-centered Approach

The second approach, and the one that will be described in detail in this book, is illustrated in Figure 1-1, and will be referred to as the patient-centered approach.

This approach delivers medication management services completely separate from the dispensing process. This approach includes a specially trained practitioner who is usually a pharmacist working in a clinic setting, a patient's home, in a space separate from the dispensing area in a retail pharmacy, in a mental health facility, or, as a consultant to physician group practices or assisted living facilities for elderly or disabled. This approach also includes the patient. The practitioner works face-to-face, or telephonically, usually on an appointment basis, in a systematic manner to deliver a consistent service, and applies specific standards of care to each patient encounter. This service is longitudinal and is based on the professional practice of pharmaceutical care.

This patient-centered service starts with understanding each patient's medication experience: their concerns, preferences, beliefs, and behaviors associated with their medications. The service engages the patient from the initial assessment of his drug-related needs to the identification of drug

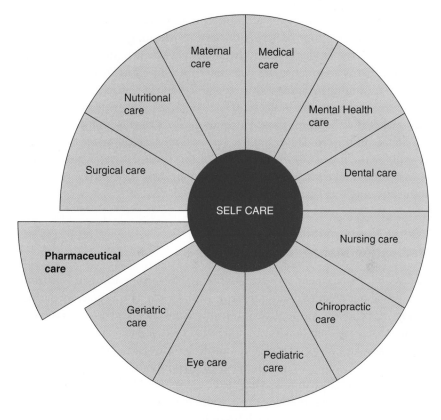

Figure 1-1   The patient-centered approach.

therapy problems, from establishing goals of therapy through to developing the care plan, and to completing a follow-up evaluation to determine the actual outcomes experienced by the patient. There are a number of advantages and challenges to this approach as well.

One advantage is that patient-centered services are delivered in a manner that is consistent with, and can be easily integrated into, the delivery of care by a medical team. It is easy for a prescriber to refer patients to these practitioners. The patient-centered practice is consistent in terminology and standards with medicine, nursing, dentistry, and veterinary medicine. When medication management services are provided in this patient-centered manner, the practitioner can demand a high enough level of reimbursement to financially sustain a practice. These services report a consistently positive return on investment (ROI) because documentation is extensive enough to measure outcomes and economic impact.

A number of challenges to this approach are also apparent. The training of practitioners in the practice of pharmaceutical care is not yet the focus of most colleges of pharmacy. In addition, this approach requires that pharmacists have dedicated time to deliver the service. Meaningful documentation is required, and the service is relatively new so payers are hesitant to reimburse at a level that is commensurate with the time and effort involved. In addition, the economic benefits of this service are largely realized on the medical side of the health system budget rather than on the drug side of the budget. This makes it difficult for those trying to decrease the costs of medications.

Details of how to deliver patient-centered medication management services will be the subject of the remainder of this book. However, the question of who should take responsibility for providing these services is a very interesting one, and one that needs to be considered.

Taking Responsibility for Medication Management Services

Medication management is the responsibility of everyone involved in making decisions about a patient's drug therapy. And, to a certain degree, medication management now occurs in patient care practices on a daily basis. It is certainly the case that prescribers have the training and experience to manage medications in their area of generalist or specialist knowledge. However, it is logical that with the increasing complexity and number of medications being used, they will want to seek assistance in managing medications outside of their usual scope of care, or when patients are taking medications that put them at particular risk, or when the patient is unable to reach his or her intended goals of therapy.

The practitioner who provides medication management services is not there to replace the physician, the dispensing pharmacist, or any other health care practitioner. Medication management services are meant to complement existing patient care practices to make drug therapy more effective and safe. The responsibilities associated with drug therapy have become so numerous and complex that the need for a practitioner with this focus has become urgent. The practitioner who provides medication management services is essentially a new patient care provider within the health care system. It would appear that this practitioner is likely to be the pharmacist who receives additional training to provide these services.

Drug therapy has long been the focus of the pharmacist. Dispensing the medications has been the primary responsibility for most pharmacists for the past six decades; however, since the 1960s pharmacists have been expanding their responsibilities to the patient care arena. With the expansion of the education for pharmacists moving from 2 formal years in the 1950s to 6, 7, or 8, depending on the specific program, in 2012, pharmacists receive more formal education on the use of medications than any other health care provider. The education of the pharmacist in the United States and around the world is moving toward a Doctor of Pharmacy level degree with a minimum of 5 and in some cases as many as 8 years of preparation in the understanding and use of medications. Although pharmacy curricula, since 2000 (in the United States), have focused on the preparation of practitioners capable of delivering these services, additional training is often necessary to focus the service on the whole patient and all of the patient's medications, using the philosophy and patient care process of pharmaceutical care practice. With this training, pharmacists can contribute essential and new knowledge to the care of patients; however, the ability to do this has been limited by the lack of recognition and payment for these services. This is now changing with the acceptance of medication management services as a necessary component for optimal patient care.

Medication management services introduce a new standard for the use of medications in society. These standards ensure that all medications are the most appropriate, the most effective available, the safest possible, and convenient enough for a specific patient to take as intended. There are many variables that affect these decisions. These variables include specific information about the patient, the patient's particular medical conditions, and the drug therapy being used to treat the conditions. Because the sciences around the use of medications has expanded so dramatically in the past three decades, a sophisticated level of knowledge is now necessary to make the decisions in a systematic, comprehensive, and consistent manner, which defines a new standard for medication use.

Practicing to this standard requires extensive knowledge in the areas of pharmacology, pharmacokinetics, biopharmaceutics, pharmacotherapeutics, toxicology, and physical chemistry, in addition to knowledge of pathophysiology and patient behavior. And, although any health care provider who has command of the knowledge, expertise, and experience required to make systematic, comprehensive decisions about drug therapy can provide medication management services, it is the pharmacist who appears to be the most logical practitioner to contribute to this new standard.

It is not our intention to say who can and who cannot provide this service. There is overlap in the knowledge possessed and the activities performed by all patient care providers, whether they are physicians, physician assistants, nurses, nurse practitioners, or other clinical personnel. However, to add unique value to patient care, each patient care provider must have specific knowledge for which he or she is responsible. The physician identifies, resolves, and prevents medical problems; the nurse, nursing care problems; and in the case of medication management services, this responsibility involves the identification, resolution, and prevention of drug therapy problems. Pharmacists are now being prepared to execute these responsibilities in order to optimize the care patients receive.

We will refer to the person providing medication management services as the practitioner or clinician, and it can safely be assumed that we are referring to a specially trained pharmacist who has demonstrated the ability to deliver quality medication management services. However, a nurse or a physician who has undergone similar academic and clinical preparation would also qualify.

THE NEED FOR MEDICATION MANAGEMENT SERVICES

Not long ago there was considerable debate about *whether* medication management services were necessary to provide quality patient care. This debate has changed recently to focus not on whether they are necessary, because the data supporting this position are very convincing, but how these services can be delivered on a broad scale so more patients can benefit on a daily basis. In spite of this change in focus we would like to describe, in an abbreviated manner, why medication management services are necessary for the comprehensive, integrated, and coordinated care of patients. This discussion will look at the need for medication management services from two perspectives: (1) how medications themselves have changed, as have their daily use, and (2) how the level of drug-related morbidity and mortality associated with the use of these medications has increased to an unacceptable level. These arguments should convince even the most skeptical that patients deserve better management of their medications.

Changes in Medications and How They Are Used

Medications themselves, as well as the manner in which we use medications, have undergone significant changes in the past decades. These changes include (a) increased complexity and specificity of the products themselves as well as how they are monitored, (b) increases in the number and types of practitioners with prescribing rights, as well as an increase in the number of prescriptions being written, (c) increased costs of new medications, and (d) the continued lack of a structured, systematic decision-making process for drug selection, dosing, and monitoring of medication use. All of these factors together contribute to the need for a more evidence-based, patient-centered approach to managing a patient's medications.

Medications become more complex in their structure and more specific in their function as science evolves. They have become more specific in terms of their "sites of action" in patient-specific receptor characteristics, as well as more specific in their "mechanism of action" due to more advanced knowledge about the pathophysiology of diseases such as AIDS, rheumatoid arthritis, and diabetes. This increase in complexity and specificity changes the way these medications must be dosed, monitored, and used in combination with other medications. These medications interact with others in unique ways and the characteristics of the side effects are more complex. Even the manner in which a patient's goals of therapy are established is different from previous generations of drug therapy. Therefore, monitoring today's medications for effectiveness and safety requires more time, more skill, and more knowledge than ever before. Drug therapy is becoming very sophisticated from a medical science perspective, and we have to be sure that we have practitioners who are prepared to optimize these medications so patients can achieve maximum benefit and minimal risk from these scientific advances.

Along with the progress in the complexity and specificity of medications has come a dramatic increase in the number and type of practitioners with pre-scribing privileges who can utilize these medications. In addition to allopathic and osteopathic physicians, dentists, nurses, physician assistants, chiroprac-tors, podiatrists, psychiatrists, ophthalmologists, and now pharmacists, under collaborative practice agreements, can all initiate drug therapy, change doses, and monitor medication use in patients. In fact, patients over 65 in the United States see an average of 13 different practitioners who prescribe medications, often without the full knowledge of what other practitioners are prescribing.[4] These same patients have an average of eight comorbidities and are taking an average of 15 different medications. The potential for something to go wrong for these patients is very high. In fact, 60% of these patients have a drug therapy problem that must be fixed immediately in order to prevent costly and painful consequences. Certainly, multiple prescribers, multiple comorbidities, and multiple medications contribute to this very complex picture.[5]

Retail prescriptions dispensed in the United States alone, has reached a total eye-catching 3.99 billion. Prescriptions dispensed under Medicare Part D amount to 871 million, or 22% of the total.[6] The number of prescriptions written (per patient) annually has increased from 6 to 18 over the past three decades. Although this would not be harmful in and of itself, we know that 25% of those prescriptions are inappropriate, ineffective, unsafe, or cannot be taken by the patient as intended. This level of risk and complications with prescriptions must be addressed.

As people age they take more prescription drugs. And, because the popu-lation is aging, more and more medications are being used by patients. Even allowing for attrition as people die, the elderly population in the United States is projected to double by the year 2030. Medications are becoming a larger and more significant variable in peoples' lives because of the increase in the chronic illnesses experienced by people who are living longer. In 1999, 82% of aging Medicare beneficiaries had one or more chronic condition, and 65% had multiple chronic conditions. Twenty-four percent had four or more chronic conditions. Per capita Medicare expenditures increase with the number and types of chronic conditions from $211 among beneficiaries without a chronic condition to $13,973 for those with four or more chronic diseases. On average, patients 65 and older with two or more chronic conditions see seven different physicians per year.[7]

All of these sophisticated changes in the medications being used, the increase in the number of practitioners who are prescribing, and the increase in the number of prescriptions written as a result in the increase in chronic illness have all contributed to the continual increase in the cost of medications. When we look at spending in major therapy areas such as diabetes, we find that spending grew by $1.9 billion in 2010 of which $1.3 billion was for human insulin and its synthetic analogues. The most recent data available show that in 2010 spending on medications "exceeds $307 billion," more than $200 billion on prescription medication and another $100 billion on nonprescription products in the United States alone.[6] A single patient's out-of-pocket expense for medications can reach hundreds of thousands of dollars annually in the United States. Whether it is the patient himself who is paying the bill, as is common in the United States, or the government, as is the case in most other health care systems, these are costs that cannot be sustained.

KEY CLINICAL CONCEPTS

Increased medication complexity, the increased use, and increased costs of medications are three important factors in explaining the need for medication management services. Another significant factor is the continued lack of a rational, systematic, and comprehensive decision-making process for drug selection, dosing, and monitoring being taught in schools of medicine and applied in practice.

Although the lack of a systematic decision making process is not broadly studied or recognized, it is a major contributor to drug-related morbidity and mortality. Early research into how prescribers make decisions and what influences a prescriber's decision about which medication to use, how much to use, and how long to use it, reveals the arbitrary nature of these decisions. Much of this work resulted from allegations that the pharmaceutical industry was having "undo" influence on prescriber decisions through "perks" and benefits that included everything from free pens and free trips to salary supplementation through speaking engagements and clinical research. Although these concerns have led to significant changes in what is and is not allowed by the pharmaceutical industry, little was revealed about how decision-making might be improved.

In 1983, Strand initiated what became a career of research that suggested at the time that prescribers were inconsistent in their selection of medications and dosing guidelines.[8] The inconsistency in decision making was so pronounced that it was not possible to reproduce the same decision for the selection of a drug product, or the dosing of a medication for the same patient, within a matter of weeks. Further research into the literature and medical practice revealed the absence of a logical, systematic, and comprehensive decision-making process being taught to or practiced by prescribers. This comes as a tremendous surprise to most, especially because so much care is taken to teach physicians and nurses how to diagnose medical and nursing problems systematically and consistently. It would appear that when the diagnostic process is complete and the treatment modality is selected (e.g., surgery, radiation, or pharmacology), the decision-making process becomes arbitrary and less structured. Most prescribers of medications learn their pharmacology in practice from those who learned it from practitioners who came before them, in the "see one, do one, teach one" tradition. So, it is not surprising that the same behaviors, be they good or bad, are passed down from one generation of practitioner to the next and limited reflection on the process occurs.

These results revealed the need for a rational, systematic, and comprehensive approach to the selection, dosing, monitoring, and evaluation of outcomes around the use of medications. Strand et al. suggested this should be the unique contribution that pharmacists make to the care of patients.[9] And, for the next three decades Strand and colleagues worked to define the most logical and accurate way to select medications, dose drug therapy, and monitor patient outcomes.[7,10,11]

Further research by Strand and colleagues revealed that the only systematic decision-making process available is the relatively straightforward approach of problem solving. Therefore, it was necessary to develop a taxonomy for all of the drug therapy problems that could possibly exist in practice so that practitioners could be taught to identify, resolve, and prevent a finite set of problems. After significant clinical work to define the categories, seven discrete drug therapy problems were defined that are mutually exclusive and all inclusive.[9] These categories, which represent the rational thought process to making decisions about drug therapy, are listed in Table 1-2.

In addition to the taxonomy of drug therapy problems, Strand and colleagues defined the set of common causes of each of the drug therapy problem categories. These problem categories, their causes, and the process for identifying, resolving, and preventing them will be discussed in Chapter 5.

When the drug therapy problems were categorized, it then became possible to define the problem-solving process that could lead to their identification, resolution, and most importantly, prevention of these problems. This research culminated in the Pharmacotherapy Workup.[10] This Workup parallels the workup of the differential diagnosis for physicians. It is the essence of the practice of pharmaceutical care and is the decision-making process that allows practitioners to fulfill their professional responsibilities.

Table 1-2 Seven categories of drug therapy problems

1.	The patient requires drug therapy for an indication that would benefit from medications but presently is not being treated with a medication.
2.	The patient does not have a legitimate indication for a medication, which is being taken, and the medication should be discontinued.
3.	The patient is taking a medication that is not able to be effective for the medical condition being treated.
4.	The patient is not taking enough of the medication to be therapeutically effective.
5.	The patient is experiencing an adverse event as a result of the medication so the medication should be discontinued.
6.	The patient is taking too much of the medication and it is causing a toxic effect.
7.	The patient is not able and/or willing to take the medication as intended.

These tools made it possible for a practitioner to intervene in a patient's drug therapy with predictable outcomes. This was new and provided the basis for developing both the professional practice of pharmaceutical care and the new set of services, now known as medication management services.

With these new developments; a taxonomy of drug therapy problems, a rational decision-making process, the Pharmacotherapy Workup, and a new professional practice, it became possible to manage a patient's medications in a manner that could significantly impact the level of drug-related morbidity and mortality that is documented around the world. Let's consider this problem in more detail.

Increased Levels of Drug-related Morbidity and Mortality

Deeply embedded in the ongoing discussion on health care costs and the need for reform are the specific costs associated with drug-related morbidity and mortality. Such costs are quite staggering and complex. Early work by Johnson and Bootman presented an alarming account of the high costs of drug-related morbidity and mortality.[12–14] They argued that these costs could reach $136 billion and this figure represents 1997 dollars! Howard and colleagues concluded "preventable drug-related admissions were associated with prescribing problems (30.6%), adherence problems (33.3%), and monitoring problems (22.2%)."[15] Of particular interest in the United States is that in emergency departments, one-third of adverse drug events found in persons over 65 were caused by warfarin, insulin, and digoxin.[15] These are medications we have used for over six decades, with well-understood pharmacology, dosing guidelines, and monitoring parameters.

Outside the United States similar problems are documented. One very useful study was conducted in Germany by Renee Stark and colleagues. Here, they posited that approximately 2 million adults would have an adverse drug reaction in 2007 and the health care costs associated with them would be 816 million Euros.[16] Furthermore, approximately 58% of these costs came from hospitalization, 11% from emergency room visits, and 21% were found to be in the area of long-term care.[17] Overall the costs of adverse drug events in the ambulatory context were found to be alarming.

Field et al. carried out a 1-year retrospective cohort study among Medicare patients. In this study, 1210 older patients were experiencing an adverse drug event. Among other findings they reported that for "all adverse drug events, the increase in post event costs over the pre-event period was $1310."[18] This was found to be "greater than those experiencing an adverse drug event than the comparison group after controlling for age, sex, co-morbidity, number of scheduled medications, and having been hospitalized during the pre-event period". Of particular interest is that "for preventable adverse drug events, the adjusted increase was $1988." Upon examination, the rates of adverse drug events "would have annual costs related to adverse drug events in the ambulatory setting of $65,631, with $27,365 of this associated with preventable events."

When we attempt to put all of the pieces of the puzzle together we find some unsettling figures. Here we are assisted by a compilation prepared by the American Society of Consultant Pharmacists For example, they cite Kongkaew et al. who conclude that 10.7% of hospital admissions in older adults can be attributed to adverse drug reactions.[19] This report also cites Gurwitz et al. and highlights the following:

> if the findings of the present study are generalized to the population of all Medicare enrollees, then more than 1,900,000 adverse events – more than a quarter of which are preventable – occur each year among 38 million Medicare enrollees; furthermore, estimates based on our study suggest that there are in excess of 180,000 life threatening or fatal adverse drug events per year, of which more than 50% may be preventable.[20]

For all the reform efforts that are being put into place, the problem of drug-related morbidity and mortality is growing. It is alarming to find that more than $200 billion is added to the United States health care costs through adverse drug reactions and other medication-related problems. Additionally, these figures are equally staggering: 37% of preventable medication errors occur due to dosing errors, 11% occur due to drug allergies or drug interactions, 22% occur during admission to the hospital, 66% during "transitions in care," and a significant 12% take place during discharge. Dispensing errors can be seen as a large piece of a problem where we find almost 100 "undetected dispensing errors" that can occur on a daily basis.[20]

The above facts and figures are by no means exhaustive. On the contrary, they only "scratch the surface" of what has to be seen as a major health care problem. Given the centrality of pharmaceuticals in care, and the rapidly escalating cost, a comprehensive reckoning of the benefits, risks, and costs of prescription drugs must take place at the national level.[21] More to the point, discussion must occur concerning the remedy for this growing crisis. It is our unrelenting position that pharmaceutical care, within the administrative context of medication management services, takes us a long way to the solution. Indeed, our experience has provided us with great confidence that pharmaceutical care intervention can and does work.

We give the last word in this section to Johnson and Bootman who have developed a probability-pathway model that estimates "the degree to which pharmaceutical care could minimize negative therapeutic outcomes."[12] Their work remain very important and most encouraging:

> According to the model, with the reductions in negative therapeutic outcomes that would result if all ambulatory care pharmacy settings provided pharmaceutical care, nearly 84% of patients would achieve optimal therapeutic outcomes due to drug therapy. According to our previous estimate, if pharmacists were available to provide only a dispensing function in typical ambulatory care settings, less than 60% of patients receiving medication would have no problems. Thus, the provision of pharmaceutical care would lead to an increase in optimal therapeutic outcomes of more than 40%.[12]

There are not too many other health innovations that could be expected to improve outcomes by more than 40%.

Much has been said about both the level of drug-related morbidity and mortality in the world as well as the extreme costs associated with this problem. The government, the medical community, as well as the pharmacy community have all documented the problem to the point where it is broadly accepted by those in the health care industry that drug-related morbidity and mortality is so high that it must be addressed in a timely manner.

ATTEMPTS TO REDUCE DRUG-RELATED MORBIDITY AND MORTALITY

Efforts to better manage medications have been extensive and ongoing for as long as drug therapy has been available. It is not our intention to describe all of them in detail; however, it is useful to step back and reflect on the many solutions that have been offered so we can understand the challenges that must be overcome if medication management services are going to accomplish more than previous efforts.

KEY CLINICAL CONCEPTS

Medications are managed at three different levels. Efforts are being made at (1) the policy or system level, (2) the institutional level, and (3) the patient-specific level.

Figure 1-2 illustrates these levels as well as the different solutions offered at each level. All three are described below. This material is summarized in order to understand what has historically worked and not worked, and to see where medication management services might "fit" with the previous efforts.

Solutions Offered at the Policy or System Levels

At the system level, governments pass laws, regulations, and policies to try to manage the use of medications. The controlled substances designations,

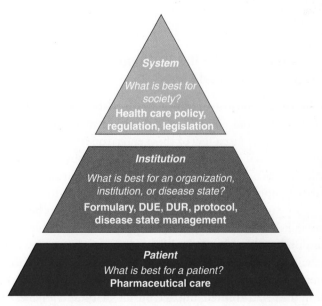

Figure 1-2 Levels of managing medications.

the need for a prescription, the control over who can prescribe, and the application process for a new drug product are all examples of how we manage medication use at the system level. Although much progress has been made at this level in the United States and around the world, there are still significant challenges to controlling medications at this level. For example, a number of medications are still available around the world without a prescription and/or the oversight of a physician, a nurse, or a pharmacist. And, fraudulent medication formulations are appearing at increasing rates around the world.

The relatively recent decision by the United States government to allow direct-to-consumer advertising by the pharmaceutical industry is another example of how policy at the system level can contribute to drug-related morbidity and mortality. The impact of these advertisements on the patients' willingness to take medications is not yet known; however, patients in practice voice grave concerns over taking medications that cause all of the side effects listed in these televised scripts. Magazines, talk shows, friends, and now the Internet all offer "advice" on the use of medications, much of which we are finding is unreferenced, of questionable help, and at the very least, confusing. Some of it is simply wrong.

Any country's inability to control the illicit use of drugs speaks to our limited success of managing medications at the system level. In addition, the expanded demand for cheaper generic medications has introduced the highest level of counterfeit medications ever seen. It is difficult to control medication use at the system level.

Solutions Applied at the Institutional, Practice, or Professional Levels

Efforts at this level involve organizational approaches, practitioner approaches at the practice level, and efforts directed toward managing a population of patients. Let us review just a few of these endeavors.

Hospitals, as well as managed care organizations, have attempted to manage their drug costs and the use of drug therapy, through Pharmacy and Therapeutics Committees, also known as P&T Committees. The method most commonly used by these decision-making bodies has been the formulary system. The formulary is a list of drug products available for use in the institution, prepared by the committee members, after reviewing the drug products based on their therapeutic characteristics. This process limited the available alternatives, emphasized cost issues, tried to avoid therapeutic duplication, and had limited impact on all of these variables. However, the pharmaceutical industry and its pricing structure, to say nothing of the marginally legal "rebates," has had so much influence on the decision-making of these groups that the formulary is now known to represent cost accounting decisions, and not drug use decisions. Perhaps the most significant contribution resulting from the formulary has been to expand the use of generic products instead of brand name products. Generic use has now reached 60% to 70% of prescribed medications.

More recently the decision-making bodies in managed care organizations, hospitals, and physician group practices have focused on developing protocols and national practice guidelines for drug therapy use by physicians and other health care professionals who prescribe drug therapy. Protocol development is based on the "best-practice" standards available in the literature or developed by a group of practitioners. The protocols are meant to represent guidelines used for decision-making in situations where drug therapy is indicated. This process successfully brought to our attention the need to standardize the decisions concerning drug therapy. However, although they can be helpful as a starting place, the protocol makes it difficult to manage patient-specific variations. In addition, practitioners in this country are not entirely comfortable with decision rules for drug therapy. This may be the case as few of the educational programs for prescribers teach a rational, systematic decision process for drug therapy selection, dosing, and monitoring. Therefore the protocol, by definition, interferes with, and does not complement, the practitioners' individual decision-making processes.

Pharmacists in management positions in hospitals, managed care organizations, and nursing homes have implemented drug use evaluations (DUEs) and drug utilization reviews (DURs) to influence drug use in their respective organizations. These evaluations are usually done retrospectively in response to a problem of prescribing identified in the institution. The DURs and DUEs provide a framework for critically evaluating the use of drugs. However, the results lack timeliness and have quite limited impact. These activities have been part of the clinical pharmacy movement that influenced drug use in hospitals through the development of specialty clinics (e.g., warfarin dosing, diabetes education, refill clinics) and clinical services (e.g., pharmacokinetic dosing services, total parenteral nutrition services). The clinical pharmacy service movement had significant impact on those patients receiving the services. However, after 30 years of development, only a very small percentage of patients receive limited assistance from these services, and this is almost exclusively in hospital settings.

All of the approaches just described have been ongoing for the past two to three decades, and yet, as recently as 2010, the National Institute of Medicine indicated that a significant change in the level of drug-related morbidity and mortality has yet to occur, in spite of all of these efforts.[22]

We are certain that there are many different reasons why the approaches described above have had a limited impact on the use of drug therapy. However, one reasonable explanation may be that these approaches have primarily been developed and implemented on a population, political, or economic basis, and not on a patient-specific basis of caring for an individual patient. The patient-specific level is where the practitioner and the patient interact and where drug-taking behavior is determined and acted upon on a daily basis.

Solutions Delivered at the Patient-specific Level

The health care delivery system can cause a number of problems for patients and prescribers. For example, formulary restrictions make it difficult to gain access to a particular medication or a medication may not be available to the patient at all. Also, the manufacturer, or the pharmacy, can have a shortage of supply so the product is not available in a timely manner, but most issues surrounding medication use develop because of decisions made by the specific patient and prescriber.

Pharmaceutical companies have tried to influence decisions made by individual practitioners through their "detailing" processes. It is debatable as to whether this impact is positive or negative, but it is certainly a vehicle for prescribers to obtain important information about a medication and this is a positive outcome. Also, physicians continually seek input into decisions about a patient's drug therapy through medical conferences, practitioner interactions, and continuing education.

It is more difficult for patients to obtain unbiased, informed input into their decisions about drug therapy. The health care system in general has kept patients quite uninformed about medications. Prescribers seldom involve patients in the decisions and prescribers seldom engage the patient in the development of the care plan that is implemented by the prescriber. And yet, patients decide every day, sometimes two or three times per day, to take a medication or not, and how to take the medication.

So relatively little effort has been directed toward managing drug therapy at the patient-specific level. This level of intervention has been left to the physician in terms of prescribing medications and to patients in terms of taking medications. The high level of nonadherence and the significant level of drug therapy problems indicate that we have failed to manage medications well at the patient-specific level. Medication management services change this. These services are implemented on a patient-specific basis for the purpose of helping individual patients make better decisions on a daily basis. This is where medication management services "fit" into our efforts to control the use of medications in the health care system.

PATIENTS WHO BENEFIT MOST FROM MEDICATION MANAGEMENT SERVICES

One of the first questions asked about medication management services is, which patients will benefit most from medication management services? Presumably this is such a common question because it is assumed that we cannot afford to deliver the service to every patient taking medications. Perhaps before this assumption is accepted as fact, we should consider the converse—can we afford NOT to provide these services to every patient taking medications? Consider how expensive it is to pay for medications that are inappropriate, ineffective, unsafe, and inconvenient for the patient. Because these problems exist at such high frequency, we may want to re-think the assumptions underlying this question.

This question of who will benefit most is difficult to answer at this early stage in the development of medication management services, for a number of reasons. First, there is a lack of sufficient data to draw a conclusion and make informed decisions about who should and who should not receive the service. Second, there is significant pressure from administrators to be cost-effective in adding new services, so the error is naturally toward providing fewer services. Finally, there are demands of starting and expanding a new health care service that go against this administrative bias. All three issues will be discussed below.

What the Data Reveal

Unfortunately, the data collected in practice to date are not very helpful in defining which patient populations will benefit most from medication management services. The prevalence of drug therapy problems, when comprehensively assessed, is so high that it is difficult to predict who will benefit and who will not benefit.

KEY CLINICAL CONCEPTS

One out of two ambulatory patients filling a prescription (regardless of specific patient, disease, and medications) has a drug therapy problem that is of enough concern that it needs to be addressed. With statistics this high, it is difficult to arrive at a demographic group that would not benefit from medication management services.

As all patients, all medical conditions, and all medications can contribute to a drug therapy problem, it is logical to assume that it takes an assessment of a specific patient's drug-related needs to determine the level of need. As with all health care professional services, an assessment of needs must be done to determine what work needs to occur. This is true with the physician making a diagnosis, the dentist determining what dental needs a patient has and even the veterinarian. This does not have to take a significant amount of time and it can be done almost anywhere. Far too much time is being spent on determining who does *not* need medication management services. Perhaps our time would be better spent evaluating which patients might logically need the service and learn from the experience so we can make better decisions in the future.

Establishing which patients are most in need of medication management services will require the service be provided on a broader basis to more patients for a longer period of time. So, we may not know for some time, which patients benefit most from the service. However, if we look at the largest database of documented patients receiving comprehensive medication management services to date, we can get an idea of which variables are most revealing. This is the database generated from the Assurance System software. To date, over 150,000 patients have been seen during over half a million encounters by hundreds of practitioners throughout the United States, Puerto Rico, and Canada. Although averages are not very useful in health care, we are often asked to describe the typical or the "average" patient who receives medication management services. From the data, the average patient is a female who is 66 years old and has six active medical conditions being managed with nine medications (three of which do not require a prescription). She will have two drug therapy problems identified at her initial assessment and will have two additional drug therapy problems at some time over the course of her care. Over the first 90 days of care, $435 in health care costs will be saved through the provision of medication management services (see Chapter 7).

The Assurance System database (www.medsmanagement.com) lets us search for patients in whom a hospitalization was avoided by the identification and resolution of a serious drug therapy problem. These patients were mostly female (63%) with an average age of 60 (median age of 61 years). They were taking an average of 13 medications (varied from 1 to 43 medications) to treat or prevent an average of nine different medical conditions. The vast majority of their drug therapy problems (82%) were caused by underdosing, adverse drug reactions, and noncompliance resulting from the patient not understanding how to take her medication properly. Average health care savings were $4211 per patient. Their drug therapy problems involved commonly used medications such as inhalers for asthma and chronic obstructive pulmonary disease, insulin and oral antidiabetic agents, furosemide, warfarin, nonsteroidal anti-inflammatory drugs, angiotensin-converting enzyme inhibitors/angiotensin II receptor blockers, and oral prednisone. These data support the numerous worldwide reports of medication-related hospitalizations that have not improved over the past 40 years.[18,19,23,24]

Although these data do not provide us with an accurate predictive model yet, we are collecting the information that will soon allow us to identify those patients most in need. Until this information is widely known, we should make every effort to provide as much care to as many patients as possible. Only after we have sufficient data will we know how to deliver this service most effectively.

The Business Demands

The cost of adding a new service is a concern when the costs of current health care services are growing every year. It is the sign of a vigilant manager who questions the addition of new services. From his perspective, it is necessary to insist on data to demonstrate the value of any service being delivered, especially a new service that is unfamiliar to most and not yet routinely reimbursed. The natural reaction is to limit the scope, and therefore the cost of the new service. For these reasons, criteria have been applied to patient data to select out those patients who "seem to benefit most from the service." These criteria can include the number of medications being taken, the number of chronic diseases being treated, and the amount of money spent on medications. Others are using the presence of patients in case management or disease management programs or those being reviewed in a prior authorization program, to trigger inclusion in the medication management service.

Although these criteria serve a purpose in defining where a new service should begin, it would be unethical to withhold a necessary service from a patient, especially when the patient can benefit tremendously from that service. This discussion needs to continue. More data are needed before a clear picture will evolve.

Initiating This Service in Practice

Every new patient care practice is started with a single patient. Therefore, a practitioner cannot hope to take care of everyone in a physician's practice on the first day. Any logical approach can be taken in terms of determining who needs medication management services (number of medications, type of medical condition, cost of care or cost of medications), but perhaps the best way to start is by asking prescribers which patients need the service most.

Patients who (a) have not reached their therapeutic goal, (b) are taking very complex dosage regimens, (c) have newly diagnosed medical conditions, (d) have questions or concerns about their medications, and/or (e) demand more time discussing the use of their medications than physicians can provides are all very logical places to start to provide medication management services. Physicians, nurse practitioners, and physician assistants are all good sources of patients who can benefit from the service.

It is imperative to collect data on the medication management services provided so that the decision of who needs the service most can be answered as quickly and effectively as possible in your practice. Because medication management services are new and recently reimbursed, it may take 2 years to build a full-time practice so it is necessary to take care of as many patients as possible, as quickly as possible. It must be remembered that a practitioner must see sufficient patients to become very proficient at the practice and to maintain a financially viable practice. Be cautious not to limit the service to such an extent that a service cannot be supported in terms of numbers of patients or payment levels or the service will not be available in the long term.

THE VALUE OF MEDICATION MANAGEMENT SERVICES

Medication management services result in measurable, reproducible value to the patient, other patient care providers, the payer, and the health care system in general. Here we discuss how the value of the service is measured and what the results have shown.

KEY CLINICAL CONCEPTS

Medication management services have been shown to decrease medical costs, improve clinical outcomes, and have significant impact on the appropriateness, effectiveness, safety, and compliance with medications.

The value of this service is experienced in a number of ways for a number of stakeholders. First, and hopefully, most importantly, the patient benefits not only from improved outcomes but from having an individual who focuses on questions, concerns, and needs around the use of medications. The patient benefits directly from the increased individualized attention to medications and the role they play in his or her daily life. Physicians benefit when someone with pharmacotherapeutic expertise is able to help manage complex drug therapies and the treatment selection process, enabling them to be more efficient, see more patients, and spend more time providing medical care.[25]

In general, health plans, employers, and payers benefit tremendously when they pay only for medications that are safe, appropriate, and effective for the patient and are used as intended. Keeping patients out of the hospital is one of the most cost-effective outcomes, and providing comprehensive medication management to complex patients is one way to accomplish this.[1]

The Clinical Value to the Patient

Early results from a high-risk Medicaid population involving 1651 patients who were seen during 4453 encounters demonstrate very positive results. Patients, who had an average age of 48 and averaged 9 medical conditions and 13 medications, experienced an average of 7 drug therapy problems per patient. The percentage of medical conditions at goal changed from 54% at baseline to 80% with the service, and an average savings of $1594 per patient and $2,729,424 in total cost savings were realized as a result of identifying and resolving drug therapy problems.[25]

A Medicare group of 706 patients (average age 70) was found to have an average of 18 medications and 11 medical conditions. These patients were eligible to receive Part D MTM services, but were actually offered comprehensive medication management services. Approximately 28% of these patients were found to have 10 or more drug therapy problems! As these drug therapy problems were identified and resolved, significant improvements in clinical parameters ($P < 0.0005$) in cholesterol and blood pressure control were documented with an average cost savings of over $1750 per participant. Approximately 97% of the savings are related to nonpharmacy costs such as reductions in hospital, long-term care, and provider cost, approximately $2.2 million of this group.[1]

Perhaps the measure of most interest to the greatest number of people is the economic value of the service to the health care system.

The Economic Value to the Health Care System

Another way to measure value is through the calculation of ROI, or how much value the service adds compared to the cost of delivering the service. ROI data are frequently difficult to obtain and vary significantly, depending on the patient population being evaluated. However, the ROI of medication management services has been established. The data from the delivery of this service are positive, with a demonstrated ROI of as high as 12:1 and an average of 3:1 to 5:1. ROI reflects an ability to decrease hospital admissions, physician visits, and emergency room admissions and reduce the use of unnecessary and inappropriate medications. This is a conservative estimate as practitioners express concern about overestimating the impact of their interventions.

The Asheville Project began in 1996. This project involved community pharmacy based practitioners who were specially trained to address issues in patients with diabetes. This project was later expanded to include cardiovascular health, asthma, and depression, and is continuing today. Direct mean medical costs decreased between $1200 and $1872 per patient per year, compared to the baseline, for each of the first 5 years, with a 4:1 ROI. Interestingly, Asheville is ranked in the top five communities by the Dartmouth Atlas for high medical outcomes and low cost of medical services. Asheville Project results were successfully replicated in the *Diabetes Ten City Challenge*, which implemented services in over 50 employers in 10 sites across the country.[26–29]

A randomized controlled trial in Minnesota delivered comprehensive medication management services and demonstrated a 12:1 ROI when the service was delivered by qualified providers (trained clinical pharmacists) in a commercial insurance population resulting in a $3768 (31.5%) decrease in costs per patient in one year. Clinical goals of therapy improved from a baseline of 76% to 90% with an average of 2.2 drug therapy problems identified and resolved per patient.[25]

The service has been shown to have value both clinically and economically. Patients, other health care providers, health system administrators, and payers have all recognized the unique contribution that better medication management makes to all the other services being provided. Now it is necessary to consider where these services can be accessed for patients who will benefit from the service. Some of these settings already have services established, whereas others are just getting started.

STRUCTURES FOR DELIVERING MEDICATION MANAGEMENT SERVICES

KEY CLINICAL CONCEPTS

Medication management services are being provided in a number of different practice settings. They are being delivered to patients in ambulatory clinics and in institutional settings.

The service is being delivered face-to-face and offered telephonically. A number of these delivery systems will be described below.

Although medication management services are, and will be, offered in a number of different patient care settings, the professional practice must remain the same across all practice settings. As with all professional practices in health care (medicine, nursing, dentistry, and veterinary medicine), the practice process and standards associated with the practice will remain the same in all settings, only the delivery technique changes. In fact, to be evidence-based, patient-centered, and accountable, there will be one professional practice of pharmaceutical care used throughout the world to provide medication management services. This will result in consistent, comprehensive medication management services provided worldwide. The standards of practice for pharmaceutical care will define what needs to be done regardless of practice setting or cultural context. These standards can be found in Appendix 1 and apply to all practice settings. It is clear that in order to be taken seriously as a patient care provider by other health care professionals all practitioners must be held to the same practice standards, which need to be transparent to the patient and other care providers. These standards, and how to meet them, will be discussed in detail in Chapters 6 to 8.

The Ambulatory Care Setting

The delivery of patient care services by pharmacists in ambulatory clinics is not new. In fact, this may represent the clinical service that most closely approximates the delivery of medication management to patients. For decades, clinical pharmacists have been employed by family practice clinics and utilized by health care providers to help patients to not only better manage their medications but teach physicians the best practices of medication selection, dosing, and monitoring.[30]

In most of the early examples, the pharmacist was employed by the clinic (and/or college of pharmacy) and was assigned to a patient population in the clinic. Direct reimbursement for the clinical pharmacist's work was never achieved on a broad scale and these examples did not include a consistent definition of the professional practice that served as the ethical and clinical foundation for the services delivered. This meant that there was not a consistent standard of care delivered across practitioners, patients, or practice settings. Medication management services are meant to utilize the best of the clinical services that have been provided in the ambulatory clinics for many years and introduce a professional practice, a standard of care, and a reimbursement mechanism to those clinical services so financially viable practices can be realized.

A number of changes have made this possible. Forty-six of the 50 states in the United States and 7 provinces in Canada allow for collaborative practice agreements between pharmacists and prescribers. These agreements provide the pharmacist the right to select medications, establish and changes doses of medications, and discontinue medications on behalf of the prescriber if done in a manner consistent with the agreement. This legislation has made it possible for pharmacists providing medication management services to increase the efficiency of physicians and nurses. The pharmacist is able to work with the patient to achieve goals faster and more often, provide answers to questions and concerns, and ultimately, to improve adherence by eliminating legitimate reasons for the patients not taking their medications as intended.

Medication management services are being provided in family practice, internal medicine, and general medicine clinics. A number of these have been described in the literature.[5,29–36]

Medication Management Services in the Medical Home and the Accountable Care Organization

The concept of the medical home has existed in the United States since the 1960s. However, the use of the medical home to describe the integrated, comprehensive management of a patient's medical needs in the primary care setting on a large scale is relatively new in the United States. And, the concept of the Accountable Care Organization (ACO) is a completely new concept in the United States. For this reason, basic information about both will be described below. However, as the focus here is on medication management services, we refer you to other more comprehensive resources to understand the medical home[1,37] and the ACO[38] in more detail.

The medical community in the United States, as represented by and articulated by the PCPCC (www.pcpcc.net) is calling for "a personal medical home for each patient, ensuring access to comprehensive, integrated care through an ongoing relationship." In addition, this "medical home" would provide "a basket of acute, chronic, and preventive medical care services for each patient, and would serve as a repository of patients' health-related information."[39] The primary concepts that must be fulfilled by the medical home have been defined by the PCPCC,[1] the National Committee for Quality Assurance (36), and the Commonwealth Fund.[40]

The ACO is still a new concept in the United States as they will not become active entities until 2012. It is a concept developed through federal legislation for the purpose of controlling costs, specifically for Medicare patients because a large portion of the U.S. population (e.g., "baby boomers") will soon become eligible for Medicare benefits.

An ACO is a network of doctors and hospitals that shares responsibility for providing care to patients. In the new law, an ACO would agree to manage all of the health care needs of a minimum of 5000 Medicare beneficiaries for at least 3 years. ACOs would make providers jointly accountable for the health of their patients, giving them strong incentives to cooperate and save money by avoiding unnecessary tests and procedures. For ACOs to work they will have to seamlessly share information. Those that save money while also meeting quality targets would keep a portion of the savings. But some providers could also be at risk for losing money. Primary care doctors who are part of an ACO would be required to tell their patients. Although physicians will likely want to refer patients to hospitals and specialists within the ACO network, patients would still be free to see doctors of their choice outside the network without paying more. ACOs also will be under pressure to provide high-quality care because if they do not meet standards, they will not get to share in any savings—and could lose their contracts.

Because the ACO is at risk for the care of a population, the administrators will be looking for services that can save money. Medication management is such a service and it is anticipated that these services will be in high demand by ACO administrators in the near future. In this setting the pharmacist providing medication management services may be employed by the ACO or contract with the ACO for these services.

The demand for medication management services is likely to grow tremendously as both the medical home and the ACO become common structures for delivering care to patients throughout the United States.

Medication Management Services in Community Pharmacy Settings

Pharmacists have been trying to deliver patient care services in the community pharmacy setting for many years. However, payment for these services on a large scale has never materialized. In fact, fees for dispensing prescriptions have continuously decreased and in many cases are now below what it costs to fill the prescription. Therefore, pharmacists have had to fill more and more prescriptions in order to make the business profitable. This has constantly interfered with the pharmacist's ability to take the time needed to provide quality patient care in this setting.

If services are offered in the community pharmacy setting, they are usually prescription-focused services (described earlier in this chapter). The services are usually focused on the prescription being filled and are one-time events. Limited payment is available for some of these services.

There are a small number of exceptions to this, however. A limited number of chain pharmacies in the United States have created a separate management "track" for pharmacists who want to provide patient-centered medication management services. When this occurs, pharmacists are assigned to a particular pharmacy for at least 1 day a week. Appointments will be set up with the pharmacist for that day and care is provided completely separate from the dispensing process. One pharmacist may service as many as four different pharmacies during a week. This schedule is maintained until there are more appointments than time allows and a second day of the week is added at that site.

In addition to the limited amount of time available to community pharmacists, there is a conflict of interest that needs to be managed. When a pharmacist is making decisions about a patient's medications, it introduces an ethical conflict for those who benefit directly from the sale of the product. In addition, neither patients nor physicians expect clinical services to be provided in a commercial, retail setting, so perceptions will have to change before this becomes a common setting for medication management services.

Medication Management Services in the Inpatient Setting

Although clinical pharmacy services have been provided to patients receiving care in the inpatient setting for decades, there is little comprehensive medication management being delivered as direct patient care in the inpatient setting. Most clinical pharmacy services are defined for a specific activity (individualizing dosing for digoxin, aminoglycosides, anticoagulants, or parenteral nutrition), or activities are performed for an entire team (rounding, drug information, etc.), but seldom are pharmacists signed on to a particular patient's care and manage all of the medications comprehensively during the hospital stay. This could easily be done if a pharmacist were assigned to each admitting team and given responsibility for a patient's care throughout the length of stay.

The recent threat of refusal of payment for re-hospitalization of Medicare patients within 30 days of discharge for certain diagnoses has given rise to pharmacists being assigned to discharged patients for follow-up to keep these patients out of the hospital. Imagine the benefit if they were assigned when the patients were admitted before many of the medication changes and difficulties with medications arise. In addition to trying to slow down hospital readmissions due to medications, a tremendous amount of attention is now being placed on adherence of patients to medication regimens in order to stop hospitalizations in the first place. Because hospitalizations are so expensive, it now appears that pharmacists who wish to provide medication management services have still another focus for their efforts.

Medication Management Services in Long-term Care, Assisted Living, Mental Health and Rehabilitation Facilities

Although pharmacists have been require by law to provide 30-day reviews in long-term care facilities in the U.S. since 1983, there is no significant evidence that medication management services are being provided in these facilities on a large scale. And, there is debate occurring as to the differences between the 30-day reviews and medication management services. The federal government is proposing regulations that would require that patients who qualify for Medicare Part D services receive them in the nursing home where they reside. This introduces a number of questions about the value of the 30-day review compared to medication management services, which plan would be expected to provide the medication management service, and how payment would be structured.

The situation is not as complicated in mental health facilities where pharmacists have been active clinically for a number of years. A practice that is delivered as part of a care team and is integrated well with other patient care providers is described in detail by the Canadian Collaborative.[41]

In all the situations described above, medication management services have to be provided as a team effort. It is becoming increasingly clear that individuals will no longer provide services in an isolated environment separate from where and how the patient receives other health care services. For this reason, we devote significant space in the next chapter to what it means to provide care in the primary care setting, alongside other patient care providers, integrating medication management services with the medical care a patient receives.

SUMMARY

Medication management services are now recognized and accepted as necessary to assure that patients are taking medications that are appropriate for them, effective, safe, and convenient enough to be taken as intended. These services, although relatively new to the health care system, result when pharmaceutical care is practiced, which has been evolving for the past 20 years. These services have been shown to be necessary, they have been demonstrated to be valuable, and they are now being delivered in all types of practice settings. Now it is necessary to better understand the professional practice of pharmaceutical care that is at the core of all patient-centered medication management services.

REFERENCES

1. PCPCC. In: McInnis T, Strand LM, Webb CE, eds. *The Patient Centered Medical Home: Integrating Comprhensive Medication Management to Optimize Patient Outcomes.* Patient-Centered Primary Care Collaborative; 2010.
2. Abraham M, Ahlman JT, Boudreau AJ, Connelly JL. *CPT 2011 CPT/Current Procedural Terminology.* Chicago, IL: American Medical Association; 2011.
3. *Minnesota Statute 256B.0625 Subd. 13h;* 2005. Available at: https://www.revisor.mn.gov/statutes/?id=256B.0625.
4. Anderson GF. The future of Medicare: recognizing the need for chronic care coordination. In: *Special Committee on Aging.* U.S. Senate Hearing Publications; 2007:19–20.
5. Strand LM, Cipolle RJ, Morley PC, Frakes MJ. The impact of pharmaceutical care practice on the practitioner and the patient in the ambulatory practice setting: twenty-five years of experience. *Curr Pharm Des.* 2004;10(31):3987–4001.
6. IMS Institute For Health Care Informatics. *The use of medicines in the United States: review of 2010.* 2011.
7. Cipolle RJ, Strand LM, Morley PC. *Pharmaceutical Care Practice: The Clinician's Guide.* 2nd ed. New York, NY: McGraw-Hill; 2004.
8. Strand LM. Decision analysis of physician prescribing in the treatment of essential hypertension. In: *Department of Social and Administrative Pharmacy.* Minneapolis, MN: University of Minnesota; 1978.
9. Strand LM, Morley PC, Cipolle RJ, Ramsey R, Lamsam GD. Drug-related problems: their structure and function. *DICP: Ann Pharmacother.* 1990;24(11):1093–1097.
10. Strand LM, Cipolle RJ, Morley PC. Documenting the clinical pharmacist's activities: back to basics. *Drug Intell Clin Pharm.* 1988;22(1):63–67.
11. Cipolle RJ, Strand LM, Morley PC. *Pharmaceutical Care Practice.* New York, NY: McGraw-Hill; 1998.
12. Johnson JA, Bootman JL. Drug-related morbidity and mortality. A cost-of-illness model. *Arch Intern Med.* 1995;155(18):1949–1956.
13. Johnson JA, Bootman JL. Drug-related morbidity and mortality and the economic impact of pharmaceutical care. *Am J Health System Pharm.* 1997;54(5):554–558.
14. Ernst FR, Grizzle AJ. Drug-related morbidity and mortality: updating the cost-of-illness model. *J Am Pharma Assoc.* 2001;41(2):192–199.
15. Howard RL, Avery AJ, Slavenburg, et al. *Which drugs cause preventable admissions to hospital? A systematic review.* Br J Clin Pharmacol. 2007;63(2):136–147.
16. Stark RG, John J, Leidl R. Health care use and costs of adverse drug events emerging from outpatient treatment in Germany: a modelling approach. *BMC Health Serv Res.* 2011;11:9.
17. Budnitz DS, Pollock DA, Weidenbach KN, Mendelsohn AB, Schroeder TJ, Annest JL. National surveillance of emergency department visits for outpatient adverse drug events. *JAMA.* 2006;296(15):1858–1866.
18. Field TS, Gilman BH, Subramanian S, Fuller JC, Bates DW, Gurwitz JH. The costs associated with adverse drug events among older adults in the ambulatory setting. *Med Care.* 2005;43(12):1171–1176.
19. Kongkaew C, Noyce PR, Ashcroft DM. Hospital admissions associated with adverse drug reactions: a systematic review of prospective observational studies. *Ann Pharmacother.* 2008;42(7):1017–1025.
20. Gurwitz JH, Field TS, Harrold LR, et al. Incidence and preventability of adverse drug events among older persons in the ambulatory setting. *JAMA.* 2003;289(9):1107–1116.

21. Bobb A, Gleason K, Husch M, Feinglass J, Yarnold PR, Noskin GA. The epidemiology of prescribing errors: the potential impact of computerized prescriber order entry. *Arch Intern Med.* 2004;164(7):785–792.
22. Shaw G. To err is still human: medication errors are a persistent challenge. *Anesthesiology News.* 2011:37.
23. Budnitz DS, Shehab N, Kegler SR, Richards CL. Medication use leading to emergency department visits for adverse drug events in older adults. *Ann Intern Med.* 2007;147(11):755–765.
24. Beijer HJ, de Blaey CJ. Hospitalisations caused by adverse drug reactions (ADR): a meta-analysis of observational studies. *Pharm World Sci.* 2002;24(2):46–54.
25. Isetts BJ, Schondelmeyer SW, Artz MB, et al. Clinical and economic outcomes of medication therapy management services: the Minnesota experience. *J Am Pharm Assoc.* 2008;48(2):203–211.
26. Cranor CW, Bunting BA, Christensen DB. The Asheville Project: long-term clinical and economic outcomes of a community pharmacy diabetes care program. *J Am Pharm Assoc.* 2003;43(2):173–184.
27. Cranor CW, Christensen DB. The Asheville Project: factors associated with outcomes of a community pharmacy diabetes care program. *J Am Pharm Assoc.* 2003;43(2):160–172.
28. Cranor CW, Christensen DB. The Asheville Project: short-term outcomes of a community pharmacy diabetes care program. *J Am Pharm Assoc.* 2003;43(2):149–159.
29. Fera T, Bluml BM, Ellis WM. Diabetes Ten City Challenge: final economic and clinical results. *J Am Pharm Assoc.* 2009;49(3):383–391.
30. Ramalho de Oliveira D, Brummel AR, Miller DB. Medication therapy management: 10 years of experience in a large integrated health care system. *J Manag Care Pharm.* 2010;16(3):185–195.
31. Barnett MJ, Frank J, Wehring H, et al. Analysis of pharmacist-provided medication therapy management (MTM) services in community pharmacies over 7 years. *J Manag Care Pharm.* 2009;15(1):18–31.
32. Alvarez-Risco A, van Mil JW. Pharmaceutical care in community pharmacies: practice and research in Peru. *Ann Pharmacother.* 2007;41(12):2032–2037.
33. Group TL. Medication therapy management services: a critical review (Executive Summary). *J Am Pharm Assoc.* 2005;45(5):580–587.
34. Harris IM, Westberg SM, Frakes MJ, Van Vooren JS. Outcomes of medication therapy review in a family medicine clinic. *J Am Pharm Assoc.* 2009;49(5):623–627.
35. Isetts BJ. *Evaluating Effectiveness of the Minnesota Medication Therapy Management Care Program.* St. Paul, MN: DHS; 2009.
36. Smith M, Giuliano MR, Starkowski MP. In Connecticut: improving patient medication management in primary care. *Health Aff.* 2011;30(4):646–654.
37. Carrier E, Gourevitch MN, Shah NR. Medical homes: challenges in translating theory into practice. *Med Care.* 2009;47(7):714–722.
38. Berwick DM. Launching accountable care organizations: the proposed rule for the Medicare Shared Savings Program. *N Engl J Med.* 2011;364(16):e32.
39. Martin JC, Avant RF, Bowman MA, et al. The Future of Family Medicine: a collaborative project of the family medicine community. *Ann Fam Med.* 2004;2(suppl 1):S3–S32.
40. Commonweath-Fund, www.commonwealthfund.org.
41. Craven MA Bland R. Better practices in collaborative health care: an analysis of the evidence base. Can J Psychiatry. 2006;51(6 suppl 1):7S-72S.

chapter two

Pharmaceutical Care as the Professional Practice for Patient-Centered Medication Management Services

---

♀ KEY CONCEPTS

1 Pharmaceutical care is a professional patient care practice, which, when provided as an organized service, is experienced, documented, evaluated, and paid for as medication management services.

2 Whenever expert knowledge is required to solve a specific set of problems, a "professional" is brought in to intervene in another individual's life by making decisions and taking actions. A professional practice is necessary to function as the ethical reference point, the clinical framework, and the basis for legal definitions and defenses in the health care professions.

3 All professional patient care practices, whether it be medicine, nursing, or dentistry, consist of three major components; a philosophy of practice, a patient care process, and a practice management system. Pharmaceutical care has all three components defined.

4 Pharmaceutical care uses the common vocabulary of medicine, nursing, and other patient care practices. This is necessary to integrate pharmaceutical care with these services.

5 The philosophy of pharmaceutical care practice consists of (a) a description of the social need for the practice, (b) a clear statement of individual practitioner responsibilities to meet this social need, (c) the expectation to be patient-centered, and (d) the requirement to function within the caring paradigm. A philosophy of practice is expected when working with medicine and nursing and is practiced by all health care professionals.

6 The patient care process, which must be consistent with the patient care processes of the other health care providers, consists of (a) an assessment of the patient's drug-related needs, (b) a care plan to meet the specific needs of the patient,

and (c) a follow-up evaluation to determine the impact of the decisions made and actions taken.

7   The practice management system includes all of the resources required to bring the service to the patient. Physical space, the appointment system, documentation, reporting, evaluation, payment for the service, and much more are included in the management of a service.

8   Pharmaceutical care practice evolved from clinical pharmacy as a direct patient care practice with specific standards of practice consistent with other health care providers.

9   Pharmaceutical care is a generalist practice. A generalist practice is necessary to structure specialist practices because they are defined relative to the generalist practice (they use the same patient care process).

10   As pharmaceutical care is a generalist practice, it is consistent with the concepts of primary health care generally and the medical home specifically.

THE NEED FOR A PROFESSIONAL PRACTICE

It is most common for a professional practice to develop first and for the services that result from that practice to be defined after the practice has been implemented and recognized as legitimate in the health care system. This is not the case with medication management services. Although the professional practice of pharmaceutical care was introduced and endorsed by the profession of pharmacy as early as 1990, by the time medication management services were introduced in 2006, the practice had been extensively talked about but only minimally developed in practice by practitioners. Perhaps this helps to explain the current confusion and lack of consensus around medication management services today.

The professional practice of a patient care profession (such as medicine, nursing, dentistry, veterinarian medicine) serves as the ethical reference point, the clinical framework for applying evidence and conducting research, and the basis for legal definitions and defenses. So a professional practice is necessary whenever a professional intervenes in another person's life. This is most relevant for the health care professions.

Ever since the functions of the physician and the pharmacist separated into different professions in the 1800s, pharmacists have not been responsible for providing direct patient care. In fact, pharmacy is the only profession included in the health science professions (medicine, nursing, dentistry, and veterinarian medicine), which does not have (take) direct patient care responsibilities. Pharmacy has developed "differently" in this respect. Although clinical pharmacy services are delivered in the "environment" of the patient and the pharmacist functions very "close" to the physician, it is the physician or the nurse who still assumes ultimate responsibility for the decisions or recommendations made by the pharmacist, in most situations.

As will be described later in the text, direct patient care involves three very distinct responsibilities: (1) assessing each individual patient's needs, in a comprehensive manner, to determine what a professional must do to return the patient to a state of health; (2) organizing all the available resources into a treatment plan, which will meet the needs of the individual patient; and (3) following up with the patient in order to be held accountable for the decisions made and the results achieved. Unless all three activities are performed to a consistent standard for each patient, direct care to a patient has not occurred. So, the majority of pharmacists was not applying a professional patient care practice in the same manner and to the same standard as the other health professionals when medication management services became a reality.

As pharmacists had not consistently been taught a professional practice, it is especially difficult to communicate the need for one, the importance of it, and the role that it plays in defining education, research, and practice standards. For these reasons, we will start at the beginning and explain what a professional patient care practice is and how it functions.

Characteristics of All Professional Practices

The professional practice described in this text, universally known as pharmaceutical care practice, was developed to meet the standards and to be consistent with the professional practices of medicine, nursing, dentistry, and veterinarian medicine. In fact, it was developed only after extensive study and observation of medical and nursing practice from educational, research, and practice perspectives. The terminology for the practice was selected carefully so that those practicing pharmaceutical care can easily integrate with those practicing medicine and nursing. This practice was developed to survive the "fads" and "fancies" that come and go, wax and wane, change and go away. It was developed to withstand economic pressures and changes in social norms and expectations. It should be a practice that serves the patient and the practitioner well for many decades to come.

However, because it is a *new* professional practice, new to practition-ers, new to patients, and new to the health care system, we believe that it is necessary to begin with the basic question, "What is a professional practice?" This question is especially challenging as other health care practices (e.g., medicine, dentistry, nursing, and veterinary medicine) have existed for such a long time and have changed in relatively small ways that we tend to take for granted what a health care practice is and how it functions. We are also likely to assume that the internal logic and processes of practices (such as medicine, nursing, and dentistry) have been clearly defined and systemati-cally studied. This has not been the case. However, over time, these profes-sions have evolved with a reasonably well-understood conceptualization of what it means to "practice" their responsibilities. Thus, almost every physi-cian, for example, tacitly understands her roles, responsibilities, and the rules that define practice. Pharmacy is presently coming to terms with definitional developments as these shape practice.

KEY CLINICAL CONCEPTS

A professional practice is the application of knowledge which is guided by a philosophy and purpose to the resolution of specific problems. This special knowledge held by a practitioner is applied according to a standard that is accepted by professional review. Moreover, practice is the experiences a practitioner encounters during the process of caring for a patient.

All health care professionals bring their knowledge and expertise to patients in the form of a *practice*. Indeed, in common use, "practice" refers to what those with knowledge actually do or can potentially do. At best there is a tacit understanding that the application of specific forms of knowledge to daily actions constitutes practice. Also, there is the confusing, but frequent, reference to practice as "place" or context—where the action occurs. In short, practice is a concept that all too frequently appears vague, confusing, and somewhat taken-for-granted.

Practice is more than simply a list of activities—no matter how impor-tant these may be to those conducting them. Most importantly, "practices are not just agents' activities but also the configuration of the world within which those activities are significant."[1] Within the context of pharmacy, the concept of practice has taken on the oversimplified meaning of "doing." That is to say, practice is generally taken to mean whatever activities pharmacists engage in at any given time. This view is simply too narrow.

Here, our purpose is to broaden the conceptualization of practice and provide it with a deeper meaning than that found in common use. Practices are more than the application of knowledge to some ill-defined end. Practices contain a strong commitment to providing good. Thus, for our present purpose, practicing pharmaceutical care means to apply knowledge to promote the well-being of others. In this sense, practice clearly contains a strong ethical component that defines purpose and end. Morality is to be seen as inescapably an integral part of all practices. Any practice must have a clear, recognizable understanding of its internal goods, goods shared by all members of the community participating in the practice. There must be a common understanding of, and commitment to, a moral purpose that sets it apart from the more general, discursive, moral frameworks that define goods external to the practice. For MacIntyre, virtues have a key role to play in sustaining practices. He contends that:

> Every practice requires a certain kind of relationship between those who participate in it. Now the virtues are those goods by reference to which, whether we like it or not, we define our relationship to those people with whom we share the kind of purposes and standards which inform practices.[2]

When we place this within the context of pharmaceutical care, we contend that its practice requires a shared understanding of, and commitment to, those values and virtues that promote group solidarity (practitioners), circumscribed by a commonly held philosophy that defines rules, roles, responsibilities, and purpose. Moreover, as MacIntyre makes quite clear, practices consist of whole systems of meanings, and are not to be seen as confined to those skills and technical interventions which tend to dominate as defining characteristics of this concept. Thus, he observes, "brick-laying is not a practice; architecture is. Planting turnips is not a practice, farming is."[3]

Practices must also be sustained over time. In a real sense, this means that the foundations that support them must be solid and provide ongoing reference points for practitioners. Practices build traditions and become socially visible. They act as the source of practitioner identity and prepare nascent members for future growth and development. Like culture, practices exist before any particular individual, and "acculturate" future members into the group.

Furthermore, they "are identifiable as patterns of ongoing engagement with the world, but these patterns exist only through their repetition or continuation." These patterns "are sustained only through the establishment and enforcement of 'norms'" and standards.[1] Thus, practices depend not on the autonomous (often idiosyncratic) actions of practitioners, but on whether they "understand and respond to one another as capable of acting in accordance with norms." It is important to recognize that central to the very notion of a practice is the idea that "practices are understood by their practitioners *as* enforced."[1] The norms that sustain practice must be held in common by all practitioners.

Pharmaceutical care embraces norms and expectations of performance that must be accepted by all who claim to practice it. This is not to suggest an authoritarian presence, but rather to define standards of practice, and thereby provide a rationale for all those electing to commit to the practice itself. A complete set of the standards of practice for pharmaceutical care practice is in Appendix 1 of this book.

In light of the above discussion, pharmaceutical care practice is defined by its foundational philosophy, dedicated to a patient care process with all its attendant responsibilities, and is an acceptance of accountability for all practitioner interventions. Moreover, pharmaceutical care practice provides a visible, consistent *identity* for its practitioners. Public scrutiny will reveal practitioners who hold specific responsibilities *in common*. The identity of such a practitioner will be clear and meaningful to patients and other health care providers alike.

Components of a Professional Practice

It might be helpful at this point to review the difference between practice and service; in this case, pharmaceutical care practice from medication management services. As described above, pharmaceutical care practice is the specific application of scientific knowledge and clinical experience to the needs of a patient in a very specific manner to achieve a very specific end. When these individual, patient-specific activities are organized and integrated into the health care system and a delivery system is developed, which allows the practitioner to "practice" his profession repeatedly, on a daily basis, complete with an appointment process, defined care process, reimbursement system, and everything else needed to "practice," then a service is being provided. So, what is seen from the practitioner's perspective is his practice, what is seen from the patient's side, is the service being delivered.

KEY CLINICAL CONCEPTS

All patient care practices consist of three primary components: (1) the philosophy of practice, which is the ethical foundation for the practice and prescribes appropriate professional behavior; (2) the patient care process, which organizes the knowledge and decisions that need to be made and the actions that need to be taken; and (3) the practice management system, which allows the services to be delivered in an organizational structure that assures quality, accountability, and payment in order to sustain the long-term viability of the practice.

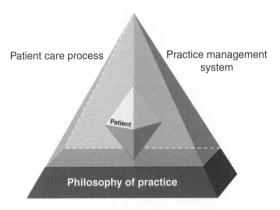

Patient care process

Practice management system

Patient

Philosophy of practice

Figure 2-1 The components of a patient-centered practice.

Figure 2-1 illustrates the relationship of the three components to each other.

The philosophy of practice is the base or anchor for a practice. It is the moral compass so that the patient care process and the practice management system can constantly push against it and determine what is appropriate and consistent with that philosophy. The philosophy of practice is different from the other components in that it is quite stable, it does not change on a day-to-day basis, and it only changes or evolves slowly, over time.

We can see from the figure that the patient care process determines the type of management system needed to support its activities on a daily basis. The patient care process represents the work that must be accomplished and the practice management system must facilitate that work every day.

Each of the components of a professional practice serves a slightly different purpose. The philosophy of practice is prescriptive in that it informs the practitioner of what is and is not acceptable behavior; it outlines the responsibilities of the practitioner, and it claims a social purpose for the profession. In addition, it prescribes the working paradigm so everyone knows what is expected of the practitioner. The patient care process, on the other hand, describes the work that occurs between one practitioner and one patient. It sets the standard for the care process so that patients and practitioners know what to expect. The patient care process provides the practitioner with a decision-making process that is explicit, comprehensive, systematic, and effective each time it is applied in practice. This is most important in the case of health care where the practitioner is making decisions that impact another person and the impact can be dramatic (life-saving or life-ending). To intervene without a philosophy of practice and a patient care process would be unethical and very unprofessional. The standards of care for pharmaceutical care practice are described in Chapters 6, 7, and 8 and in Appendix 1.

The practice management system is defined not at the practitioner and patient level, but at the health care system level. The practice management system organizes what the practitioner does on a patient-specific, individual level, into a set of services that contribute value and are worthy of payment. The practice management system provides the support needed by the practitioner to provide services to as many patients as possible in the course of the day. This support can be personnel, space, equipment, billing, and documentation, to name just a few of the necessary resources to make a professional practice financially viable and long lasting. The practice management system is what makes it possible to deliver quality in education management services.

PHARMACEUTICAL CARE AS A PROFESSIONAL PRACTICE

Definition   Pharmaceutical care is a practice in which the practitioner takes responsibility for a patient's drug-related needs, and is held accountable for this commitment.[4] In the course of this practice, responsible drug therapy is provided for the purpose of achieving positive patient outcomes.[4,5]

Each of the practice components will be described in detail in their own chapters in this textbook. However, it is useful to see all of the components summarized together before the pieces are dissected and discussed. This practice should become the focus of the curricula in colleges of pharmacy, and it will become the organizing force for practice research in the years to come. As it will define how pharmacists provide care in the future, it needs to be understood by all stakeholders in providing medication management services. Following is an abstracted description of the practice.

The Philosophy of Practice

KEY CLINICAL CONCEPTS

The philosophy of pharmaceutical care consists of four key elements: a description of the social need for the practice, a clear statement of individual practitioner responsibilities to meet this social need, the expectation to be patient-centered, and the requirement to function within the caring paradigm.

At its most global level, it begins with a statement of social need to reduce drug-related morbidity and mortality. The philosophy continues by describing how this social need is met only when fulfilling individual practitioner responsibilities on a patient-specific basis, so these responsibilities are spelled out in detail for the practitioner. The philosophy continues by prescribing how these responsibilities should be performed; namely, in a patient-centered context, using a caring paradigm. These four constructs—social need, practitioner responsibilities, patient-centered context, and the caring paradigm—work together to prescribe appropriate behavior when engaged in pharmaceutical care practice. Unless this philosophy is internalized by its practitioners, it is difficult to deliver care at a standard that can be defended ethically, clinically, and legally.

Statement of Social Need

Professions exist for the sole purpose of meeting a social need. Professionals are expensive to prepare, demand autonomy, insist on regulating themselves, and are closed to those not meeting the requirements for inclusion. However, in return for this privileged role in society, the profession must contribute meaningfully to solving a set of problems better than anyone else in society. Pharmaceutical care was developed to optimize the use of medications and minimize the drug-related morbidity and mortality associated with medication use. This statement of social need moves from a slogan that can be repeated mindlessly to a meaningful raison d'être only when a profession's practitioners prepare themselves appropriately and fulfill their responsibilities on a patient-specific basis.

Description of the Practitioner Responsibilities

As stated earlier, all professionals must be able to identify a set of problems more effectively than others to earn the role of professional. This is certainly true in the practice of pharmaceutical care. Most simply stated, the practitioner's responsibilities in pharmaceutical care practice are to identify, resolve, and prevent drug therapy problems. This problem solving occurs during the patient care process, specifically as the practitioner assesses the patient's drug-related needs.

Each and every patient deserves to be taking medication that is appropriate for the medical condition being treated. Patients have a right to have all of their medical conditions treated with medications that work and they have a right to be prescribed only those medications that are necessary for them. Patients deserve to be taking only the most effective medications and to be taking them in therapeutic doses that can be effective for the specific medical condition being treated. In addition, patients have a right to be on medication that will not cause adverse effects and will be given in doses that are safe for the patient. Finally patients need to be able to take the medication as indicated so adherence to the regimen produces the intended results. So, in summary, the responsibilities of the pharmaceutical care practitioner are to ensure that all of the medications being taken by the patient are appropriate, effective, safe, and able to be taken as intended.

Expectation to be Patient-centered

These responsibilities have to be carried out in a very specific manner to benefit the patient. The practitioner must fulfill his responsibilities in a patient-centered manner. There has been significant discourse about the meaning of patient-centeredness but most practitioners agree that it is difficult to grasp this concept. The easiest way to describe this approach is that the patient comes first; the patient's needs determine all that you do and the patient is at the center of all decision making, actions taken and results interpreted. No aspect of the care that is delivered is done without including the patient, without letting the individual needs and preferences of the patient dictate what occurs when the practitioner's responsibilities are executed. This is a very different mindset than traditionally used in medicine. It translates into the pharmacist working for the patient, not the physician; the pharmacist responding to the patient's needs, not the expectations of the employer or manager; the pharmacist "finishing" when the patient meets their therapeutic goals, not when time runs out or interest wanes. The best way to characterize patient-centeredness in pharmaceutical care practice is by reiterating the obvious, "drugs don't have doses - people have doses."[6]

Decisions about the future health care system are focused on patient-centeredness as a primary stimulus for change. A professional practice without patient-centeredness as a key element to its philosophy has no role in the future. The patient will be the "driver" of health care in so many different ways so patient-centered will be how pharmaceutical care is delivered.

Need to Function in the Caring Paradigm

Much has been written about the concept of caring. In one way it is the simplest of concepts and in another way it is complex. The paradigm certainly includes the feelings and actions associated with compassion, understanding, human tenderness, respect, and even devotion. In pharmaceutical care it means doing all that one can to decrease the suffering of others through the use of medications. To care for someone in pharmaceutical care practice means we take the time and the energy to understand each individual patient's medication experience so we can optimize future experiences with drug therapy. It means understanding the necessity for a therapeutic relationship that involves trust and mutual respect and a commitment to take responsibility and be held accountable for all that we do.

Caring is basic to all patient care professions but it must be acted upon, in a prescribed manner, meeting established standards, to be considered professional caring. So unless we do the individual assessments of need, unless we mobilize all the resources needed to meet those needs, and unless we follow-up to determine what happens to our patient—we simply don't care. This concept is captured best in the phrase, "If you do not follow-up, you do not care." It should come as no surprise that the patient care process is simply a reflection of the caring process: assessment, care planning, and follow-up.

The Patient Care Process

KEY CLINICAL CONCEPTS

The three major steps in the patient care process are (1) the *assessment* of the patient, his or her medical problems, and drug therapies leading to drug therapy problem identification, (2) *care plan* development, and (3) follow-up *evaluations*.

These steps are all highly dependent upon each other. The completion of all steps is necessary to practice pharmaceutical care and to have a positive impact on your patient's medication experience. The process is continuous and occurs over multiple patient visits. Your initial assessment, drug therapy problem identification, and care planning occur at your first encounter with each patient, and follow-up evaluations and additional adjustments to drug therapy occur at subsequent patient encounters. However, before we explore the three steps, it is necessary to discuss the basic foundation of the patient care process, the piece of the patient care process that occurs in the mind of the practitioner and cannot be seen in practice. This is the decision-making process that is specific to the practice and is the trademark of the pharmaceutical care practitioner.

The Foundation of the Patient Care Process: The Pharmacotherapy Workup

All patient care practitioners, be they physicians, nurses, dentists, or pharmaceutical care practitioners, need a structured, rational thought process for making clinical decisions. What makes a practitioner qualified to do his or her work is the application of a unique knowledge base and set of clinical skills using a systematic thought process to assess the needs of a patient, identify and resolve problems, and prevent problems from occurring. In the case of the pharmaceutical care practitioner, this unique knowledge base is focused on pharmacology, pharmacotherapy, and pharmaceutical care practice, in which the practitioner identifies, resolves, and prevents drug therapy problems. The systematic thought process used in this practice is the Pharmacotherapy Workup.

> **Definition**   The Pharmacotherapy Workup is a rational decision-making process used in pharmaceutical care practice to identify, resolve, and prevent drug therapy problems, establish goals of therapy, select interventions and evaluate outcomes. It is a description of the thought processes, hypotheses, decisions, and patient problems that occur during practice.

The Pharmacotherapy Workup is the cognitive work occurring in the mind of the practitioner while caring for the patient. In contrast, the patient care process, is what the patient experiences when he or she receives pharmaceutical care. This process is a series of interactions between patient and pharmaceutical care practitioner. The patient care process is where the practitioner's unique knowledge and clinical skills are applied to solve health care problems for patients.

The Steps of the Patient Care Process

The best way to think about pharmaceutical care practice is in terms of the work that occurs between the patient and the practitioner. This work is described as the patient care process. The three steps of the patient care process are illustrated in Figure 2-2, and the activities and responsibilities of each step are summarized in Table 2-1. The three steps in the patient care process are described in detail in Chapters 6 to 8.

Because the identification, statement of cause, prioritization, resolution, and prevention of drug therapy problems represent the unique contribution of the pharmaceutical care practitioner, a separate chapter has been devoted to this portion of the assessment (refer to Chapter 5).

Remember that the patient care process describes the interaction between the patient and the practitioner. It is that portion of practice that is actually *seen* and *experienced* by both patients and practitioners. All practitioners use the same patient care process and structured decision-making process regardless of the patient's characteristics, the patient's medical conditions, the specific drug therapy being used, or the practitioner's expertise.

Table 2-1 integrates both the cognitive (Pharmacotherapy Workup) and physical work (the patient care process) of the pharmaceutical care practitioner. Each of these steps will be briefly presented here to describe the entire patient care process.

Assessment

The purpose of the assessment is threefold: (1) to understand the patient and the patient's medication experience well enough to make rational

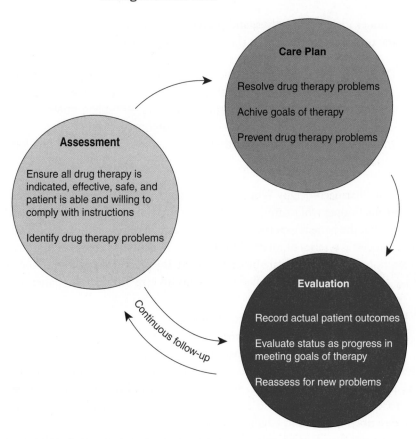

Figure 2-2 The patient care process.

drug therapy decisions with and for him or her; (2) to determine if the patient's drug therapy is appropriate, effective, and safe, and if the patient is compliant with his or her medications; and (3) to identify drug therapy problems.

The information required to make clinical decisions with your patient includes *patient data* (demographic information, medication experience), *disease data* (current medical conditions, medical history, nutritional status, review of systems), and *drug data* (current medications, past medication use, social drug use, immunizations, allergies, and alerts).

The three major activities that occur during the assessment are as follows:

1. Gathering information from the patient, and the patient's health records
2. Eliciting the patient's medication experience
3. Making clinical decisions about the patient's medications and identifying drug therapy problems.

Table 2-1 Activities and responsibilities in the patient care process

	Activities	Responsibilities
ASSESSMENT	Meet the patient Elicit relevant information from the patient Make rational drug therapy decisions using the Pharmacotherapy Workup	Establish the therapeutic relationship Determine who your patient is as an individual by learning about the reason for the encounter, the patient's demographics, medication experience, and other clinical information Determine whether the patient's drug-related needs are being met (indication, effectiveness, safety, adherence), identify drug therapy problems

CARE PLAN	Establish goals of therapy
	Select appropriate interventions to:
	  resolve drug therapy problems
	  achieve goals of therapy
	  prevent drug therapy problems
	  schedule follow-up evaluation
		Negotiate and agree upon endpoints and time frame for pharmacotherapies with the patient and other providers
		Consider therapeutic alternatives
		Select patient-specific pharmacotherapies
		Consider nondrug interventions
		Education of the patient

FOLLOW-UP EVALUATION	Elicit clinical and/or laboratory evidence of actual patient outcomes, compare them to the goals of therapy to determine effectiveness of drug therapy Elicit clinical and/or laboratory evidence of adverse effects to determine safety of drug therapy Document clinical status of each condition being managed with drug therapy Reassess patient for any new drug therapy problems Schedule the next follow-up evaluation	Evaluate effectiveness of pharmacotherapy Evaluate safety of pharmacotherapy Determine patient adherence Make a judgment as to the clinical status of the patient's conditions being managed with drug therapies Identify any new drug therapy problems and their cause Provide continuous care

The assessment begins by getting to know your patient by discussing the patient's *medication experience.* The medication experience is a new and important concept in health care (refer to Chapter 4 for a detailed description of the patient's medication experience). Patients relate to the impact that taking medications have on their everyday lives as their medication experience. The medication experience is the patient's personal approach to taking medication. It is the sum of all the events in a patient's life that involve medication use. The medication experience is the patient's beliefs, perceptions, understandings, attitudes, and behaviors about drug therapy. It is these factors that will most directly influence the patient's decisions about whether to take a medication or not, how much of the medication to take, and how to take the medication. Patients come with their own medication experience. Our responsibility is to understand it and positively influence it.

Therefore, the more you know about the patient's medication experience, the more likely you are to have a lasting and positive influence on it. The medication experience includes more technical aspects as well; the patient's current medications, social drug use, immunizations, allergies, alerts, and medication history. It is usually easier to deal with the technical aspects of the medication experience; however, your ability to influence these dimensions depends upon how well you understand the patient's personal approach to taking medication. Take the time and learn the skills to effectively elicit the patient's description of his or her medication experience—it will always be worth your effort. The quality of the care you can provide depends upon it.

The pharmaceutical care practitioner has a responsibility to understand the patient's medication experience because it directly impacts the decisions a patient makes about his or her drug therapy. Although physicians, nurses, and pharmaceutical care practitioners can make suggestions to a patient, it is the patient who ultimately decides what he or she will do about taking the medication.

The major decisions that the pharmaceutical care practitioner makes during the assessment include (1) whether the patient's drug-related needs are being met at this time, and (2) whether the patient is experiencing drug therapy problems. Therefore, an understanding of drug therapy problems is important. (See Chapter 5 for details.)

Definition Drug therapy problems are undesirable events or risks experienced by the patient that involve or are suspected to involve drug therapy, that inhibit or delay him or her from achieving the desired goals of therapy, and require professional judgment to resolve.

These problems are identified during the assessment process, so that they can be resolved through individualized changes in the patient's drug therapy regimens. Drug therapy problems are identified by assessing sociological, pathophysiological, and pharmacological information of the patient, disease, and drug therapy collected during the assessment step. The synthesis and application of this knowledge occurs in a logical, systematic manner using the Pharmacotherapy Workup. (See chapter 6 for details.)

The process used to identify whether or not the patient is experiencing a drug therapy problem requires a continuous assessment of four logical questions:

1. Does the patient have a clinical indication for each of his or her drug therapies, and is each of the patient's indications being treated with drug therapy?
2. Are these drug therapies effective for the patient's medical condition?
3. Are the drug therapies as safe as possible?
4. Is the patient able and willing to take the medication as intended?

When clinicians apply knowledge of patient, diseases, and drugs to this set of inquires, they can make clinical decisions as to whether or not a drug therapy problem exists. If the patient is experiencing a drug therapy problem, it can be classified into one of the seven categories described in Table 2-2.

Once categorized, it is then necessary to identify the cause for each drug therapy problem. Knowing the cause of the problem leads to the best solution for the patient. These three components are necessary to be able to adequately

Table 2-2   Categories of drug therapy problems

Drug therapy problem	Description of the drug therapy problem
Unnecessary drug therapy	The drug therapy is unnecessary because the patient does not have a clinical indication at this time.
Needs additional drug therapy	Additional drug therapy is required to treat or prevent a medical condition.
Ineffective drug	The drug product is not effective at producing the desired response for this patient.
Dosage too low	The dosage is too low to produce the desired response for this patient.
Adverse drug reaction	The drug is causing an adverse drug reaction.
Dosage too high	The dosage it too high resulting in undesirable effects.
Adherence	The patient is not able or not willing to take the drug regimen as instructed.

describe the patient's drug therapy problem. This process includes identifying the medical condition involved in the problem, the drug therapy associated with the problem, and the cause of the problem.

When multiple drug therapy problems are present, they need to be prioritized to determine which should be addressed first. The order of priority of drug therapy problems is based on the patient's views regarding which one is causing the most concern, the preferences he or she has toward addressing the problem(s), and the clinical severity of the problem(s).

The result of the assessment of a patient's drug-related needs is the description and prioritization of the drug therapy problem(s) to be resolved through specific interventions in the care plan. The identification and resolution of drug therapy problems represents the unique contribution made to the patient's care by the pharmaceutical care practitioner.

Care Plan Development

The purpose of the care plan is to organize all of the work agreed upon by the practitioner and the patient to achieve the goals of therapy. This requires interventions to resolve drug therapy problems, to meet these goals, and to prevent new drug therapy problems from developing, thereby optimizing the patient's medication experience. These are described in detail in Chapter 7.

Care plans are developed primarily to help the patient achieve the established goals of therapy for each of his or her medical conditions or illnesses. Constructing care plans is done in collaboration with the patient and, when appropriate, other health care practitioners providing care to the patient.

Care plans are organized by medical condition, and a separate care plan is constructed for each condition or illness. Constructing a care plan involves three steps: establishing goals of therapy, selecting appropriate individualized interventions, and scheduling the next follow-up evaluation. If a patient has multiple medical conditions, the care plans will have to be integrated and a single care plan presented to the patient.

The first and most important step in the care planning process is to establish goals of therapy for each medical condition. Goals of therapy consist of a parameter, a value, and a time frame. Throughout the text, goals of therapy are used to describe the future desired endpoints. The goals of therapy guide all subsequent decisions, actions, interventions, and patient education. Therefore, goals of therapy must be explicitly stated, consistent with the patient's preferences and desires, clinically sound, and observable or measurable in a stated time frame. Perhaps most importantly, the goals of therapy must be understood and agreed upon by practitioner and patient.

Each care plan contains a plan of action to be taken on behalf of the patient. The specific actions are called *interventions.*

Care plans contain interventions designed to

- resolve drug therapy problems
- achieve the stated goals of therapy
- prevent new drug therapy problems from developing.

The first interventions in a care plan should be those intended to resolve identified drug therapy problems. Resolving drug therapy problems takes precedence within the care planning process because goals of therapy cannot be achieved until and unless the patient's drug therapy problems are successfully resolved. Most common interventions are to initiate new drug therapy, discontinue drug therapy, increase dosages, decrease dosages, provide patient-specific education, or refer the patient to another health care practitioner with the expertise needed to solve the patient's health problem.

A second type of intervention in care plan development ensures that the patient achieves the goals of therapy. Interventions to achieve goals of therapy most often include changes in drug therapy regimens and individualized patient instructions. These interventions include relevant patient education or instructions as to the optimal use of medications, related technology, and/or diet and exercise to increase the probability of success with the medication regimen.

Interventions made to prevent the development of drug therapy problems are necessary to complete a care plan. These interventions are especially important for patients who have a higher than normal probability of developing a drug therapy problem due to some identified risk factor(s).

The final step in every care plan is to schedule the follow-up evaluation to determine the outcomes of drug therapy. During the follow-up evaluation, the results of care plan actions are judged as to their positive or negative impact on the patient. Therefore, the decision regarding when to schedule the next follow-up evaluation needs to incorporate the timing of the expected positive outcomes, achievement of the goals of therapy, and the probable timing of any negative outcomes including side effects and/or adverse reactions from the medication. If there are multiple care plans, the schedules for the follow-up evaluations must be coordinated.

The patient and the practitioner always negotiate the components of the care plan including goals of therapy, interventions, and the schedule for the next evaluation.

Follow-up Evaluation

The purpose of the follow-up evaluation is to determine the actual outcomes of drug therapy for the patient, compare these results with the intended goals of therapy, determine the effectiveness and safety of pharmacotherapy, evaluate patient adherence, and establish the current status of the patient's medical conditions being managed with drug therapy. These are described in detail in Chapter 8.

It should be noted that the term "outcomes" in pharmaceutical care practice is used to describe the actual clinical result and should not be confused with the goals of therapy or general concepts of outcomes that are vaguely defined.

The evaluation step is where clinical experience and new knowledge are gained. In fact, most learning occurs during follow-up evaluations. The follow-up evaluation is the step in the process when the practitioner sees which medications and doses were most effective or caused the most harm.

In a well-conducted follow-up evaluation, the practitioner evaluates the patient's response to drug therapies in terms of effectiveness, safety, and adherence and also determines if any new problems have developed.

The specific activities performed at a follow-up evaluation are described as follows:

- Observe or measure the positive results the patient has experienced from drug therapies (*effectiveness*).
- Observe or measure any undesirable effects the patient has experienced that were caused by a drug therapy (*safety*).
- Determine the actual dosage of medication the patient is taking that is producing the results observed (*adherence*).
- Make a clinical judgment of the status of the patient's medical condition or illness being managed with drug therapy (*outcomes*).
- Reassess the patient to determine if he or she developed any new drug therapy problems.

The practitioner must gather data to evaluate the effectiveness of the drug therapies. These data often include the improvement or reduction of the signs or symptoms of the patient's medical condition or illness.

Effectiveness is also evaluated using data to demonstrate the extent to which abnormal laboratory test results have returned to within the desired or normal range. The practitioner must also gather data to evaluate the safety of the drug therapies instituted in the care plan. Safety data include the evaluation of unintended pharmacological effects (side effects) of the patient's drug therapy. Evaluation of safety data also includes whether laboratory tests have become dangerously abnormal due to the drug therapy. Because both effectiveness and safety are evaluated based upon the drug dosages that the patient has actually taken, it is important to determine patient compliance at each follow-up evaluation.

A clinical judgment is made as to the outcome status of each medical condition being treated with drug therapies. At each evaluation the status might be resolved, stable, improved, partially improved, unimproved, worsened, or failed. Each term has a specific meaning in practice and contains two items of important information: the patient's present condition and what was done to the drug therapy in response to the patient's condition. This clinical judgment is recorded and compared to the status at each subsequent evaluation to determine if the individualized drug therapies are helping the patient to meet the desired goals of therapy.

At each follow-up evaluation, the practitioner must also determine if the patient has developed any new drug therapy problems or illnesses since the last encounter. If so, the patient care process will begin all over again.

An important goal of completing the patient care process is to establish a meaningful, therapeutic relationship with the patient. This relationship is different from any other relationship you might develop with an individual. It involves a high level of trust, respect, and sharing. Without this relationship, the patient care process cannot be completed well and the quality of care will be compromised. It takes time to develop such a relationship and it is able to grow with each encounter. It is very difficult to provide pharmaceutical care without such a relationship. The therapeutic relationship is discussed in detail in Chapter 4.

The Practice Management System

The key to a successful practice is to add new patients continually so the practice can become financially viable, and survive over the long term. Providing care to a large number of patients requires an efficient and effective structure and the appropriate resources to be successful. To accomplish this, a practice management system that facilitates the work that must be done—in this case, provide pharmaceutical care, must be developed. This is described in detail in Chapter 11.

KEY CLINICAL CONCEPTS

A practice management system includes all the resources required to provide a service to patients in an effective and efficient manner.

The practice management system will involve the following major categories of information about the practice:

- a clear mission for the practice (a clear description of the service provided), this mission then defines the environment and culture in which the service will be provided.

- recognition of all the resources required to deliver the service (it includes physical, financial, and human resources, and it includes tangible and intangible aspects of these resources).
- development of methods for evaluation of the practice. In the short term this represents evaluation processes that measure the practitioner's ability to manage the patient, and in the long term, the ability of the practitioner, or in some situations a manager, to manage the practice. Both aspects will contribute to the outcomes described above.
- identification of ways to reward the practitioner and financially support the longevity of the practice (reimbursement mechanisms). This represents the value of the service to the patient in the short term and to society in the long term.

The practice management system is invisible when one practitioner cares for one patient. It becomes crucial when a practitioner must see 10 to 20 patients a day to earn the revenue needed to continue in practice. There are a number of issues associated with managing a practice: some of them clinical, some legal, and many of them business-related. Usually the clinician is not the best person to manage the practice and care should be taken to identify the most qualified individuals when practices are established.

The Language and Vocabulary of Practice

We have introduced a number of new terms related to the professional practice into the pharmacist's vocabulary. We want to take just a moment to emphasize the importance of vocabulary in patient care practice. The French philosopher Paul Ricœur concluded that the most significant factor that connects us to the social world is language. Language constructs our realities, and shapes our sense of who we are.[7]

All health care professions, over time, have generated a descriptive language for their roles and responsibilities, and they continuously introduce technical vocabularies that serve to define and delineate specific tasks and interventions.[8] These frequently function to specifically identify who is carrying out these acts. Thus, we find that physicians customarily establish "diagnoses," nurses perform "physical assessments," and pharmacists practicing pharmaceutical care conduct "assessments of drug-related needs."

On the surface much of this is self-evident. However, as pharmaceutical care practice develops, its language/vocabulary describing unique purpose and function, process, and action(s) taken must also evolve and represent these to others. This cannot be overemphasized for it is through language/vocabulary that we will communicate what we do, for whom, and how we do it. In short, we communicate our identity as practitioners, our responsibilities, and our particular unique knowledge base, through our language. Therefore, pharmacists must learn the new language of pharmaceutical care practice and use it consistently.

Our language/vocabulary will communicate our practice, its meaning and value, to all other health care professionals, patients, third-party payers, potential clients, university colleagues, and other members of the general public. Furthermore, the language we use is a form of empowerment.[9] It is essential that pharmaceutical care practitioners learn to "speak with authority" on those matters that lie within his or her area of expertise. To engage in clinical discourse with other health care practitioners requires that pharmacists speak-like-clinicians, and articulate their expert recommendations with a technical clarity that conveys meaning. There is no room for obfuscation in clinical exchange. Language is also about legitimacy and recognition. Other practitioners will listen to and respect those who present authoritative knowledge and information in competent, coherent language. This is certainly the case when any unique body of knowledge, sometimes seemingly wrapped in highly technical disciplinary-bound "jargon," is communicated to "outsiders."

To facilitate a "beginning," we have constructed a glossary at the end of this book that provides a point of departure in our attempt to build and communicate the essence of pharmaceutical care practice to other practitioners and to patients. We have included those terms most directly related to pharmaceutical care practice. We encourage readers/practitioners/students/patients to build upon this vocabulary as they focus on the importance of linguistic competency in practice.

This special emphasis on language is made here because as we mentioned earlier, the pharmacy profession developed differently from medicine and nursing. Its focus has been the drug product and not the patient for most of its existence. The profession has developed its own vocabulary in its isolation from other direct patient care providers, and this now is causing a significant amount of confusion for all involved. Pharmacists must be cognizant of these differences as they move into positions of direct patient care. Misunderstandings about vocabulary can have dire consequences when a patient's health is the subject of the confusion. For this reason, we will take a moment to illustrate how key terms are used differently in pharmacy and the rest of the medical world. It should be obvious that pharmacists will have to "give up" their meanings and adopt the common definitions for terms as used by other health care providers if they want to participate on a team of health care practitioners.

Some of the terms that have developed different meanings for pharmacists than for the other patient care providers include practice, care, standards of practice, counseling, generalist, specialist, and many more examples are available. A few of these will be discussed to illustrate the point.

For all other patient care providers, one's practice includes the specific type of care that is delivered and the type of patients who receive that care. For example, a physician might describe his practice in the following manner: I provide pediatric care to patients between the ages of 6 months and 16 years. I see approximately 20 patients a day in my practice, which includes two other physicians, a nurse practitioner, and two nursing assistants. Pharmacists, on the other hand, are used to describing their practice by the physical building in which they work. "I am in retail practice, long term care practice, or hospital practice."

Pharmacists usually include all the activities they perform (even dispensing-related functions) in their meaning of caring for a patient. This is a very different meaning than that used in the practice of medicine. To care for a patient, three activities have to be performed in their entirety for each patient: (1) an assessment of their individual needs, (2) an individualized care plan that brings all the necessary resources together must be developed for the patient, and (3) follow-up with the patient must occur to determine the actual outcomes that result from the decisions made by the practitioner. This is what is meant when someone says they have provided care to patients. These three activities are not optional, one is not provided without the other, and, the content of the activities are defined by the patient's needs, not the practitioner's time availability, personal preference, or a manager's wishes.

Standards of practice traditionally have had a different meaning in the pharmacy profession. Standards have routinely been determined by surveying what pharmacists are presently doing and then the professional organizations turn these common activities into the standards of practice. These standards of practice are optional and can be chosen to reflect personal preferences, time availability, and comfort with the activity.

In patient care practice, these standards are defined by performance at 100% when care is delivered comprehensively and optimally to a patient. These standards of care are consistent across patients, independent of disease or drug therapy, and are transparent to both patient and other practitioners. Patient care standards are not optional, negotiable, or based on individual preferences. Patient care must be evidence based, thoroughly and expertly performed and all practitioners must be accountable for their decisions and actions. This requires a very concise and comprehensive definition of the standards of care within a professional practice. These have been developed for pharmaceutical care and will be discussed in detail in the chapters to follow.

Counseling is a word used by the pharmacy profession to describe the "patient care" activities performed by pharmacists at the time of dispensing a prescription. For many years pharmacists sought payment for performing "counseling" activities. These activities included giving patients directions for taking the medication as prescribed, cautioning the patient about potential side effects and/or answering questions patients have about their medications. Medicine uses the word "counseling" to mean something very different. First, counseling is done only by licensed clinical practitioners in medical practice. For example, social workers, psychologists, psychiatrists, ministers, and crisis interventionists would all have a clinical license to "counsel" patients. So, imagine the confusion when pharmacists constantly talk about "counseling" patients in a retail pharmacy setting.

Another concept that is frequently confused is that of a generalist and specialist practitioner. In medicine, specialists developed to address more complex problems than can be managed by the generalist. In pharmacy, "specialists" were developed more as content experts and didn't evolve relative to the care provided by generalist practitioners since there were no generalists. Generalists and specialists use the same philosophy and patient care process, which is why specialists evolve to solve more complex problems relative to the generalist and specialists evolve after the generalists. Pharmaceutical care was developed as a generalist practice and the meaning of this will be described in the next section.

There are many other words that are used differently, and this will interfere with the smooth integration of the pharmacist into the medical team where patient care is the common goal. This point is made so strongly here because the practice of pharmaceutical care was developed using the vocabulary and meanings of the patient care professions and not the vocabulary of the pharmacy profession.

KEY CLINICAL CONCEPTS

The words used to describe pharmaceutical care are chosen carefully and their definitions are very specific to their use in practice. This, among other things, is why it is very easy to integrate the practice of pharmaceutical care with the practice of medicine or nursing or any of the other patient care professions. Without a common language, little care can be delivered and many negative consequences are possible.

PHARMACEUTICAL CARE AS A GENERALIST PRACTICE

The practice of pharmaceutical care has been developed as a generalist practice. This is significant because clinical pharmacy practice developed as a specialty practice. Although this has occurred, it is not the way medicine functions and in order to be successful in patient care, pharmacists will need a generalist practice on which to build its specialist practices. This practice will be pharmaceutical care practice. Both the definition of a generalist practice and the need for a generalist practitioner are described here.

Generalist Practitioner Defined

Definition A generalist practitioner is one who provides continuing, comprehensive, and coordinated care to a population undifferentiated by gender, disease, drug treatment category, or organ system (adapted from American Boards of Family Practice and Internal Medicine).[10,11]

The European Academy of Teachers in General Practice developed a standard definition for general practice (and Family Medicine). In doing so, they describe 11 characteristics of a general practice, the first characteristic being:

"the point of first medical contact within the health care system, providing open and unlimited access to its users, dealing with all health problems regardless of the age, sex, or any other characteristic of the person concerned."

Other characteristics within this comprehensive definition of general practice include: coordinating care with other professionals, being patient-centered, establishing a relationship over time, providing longitudinal care, using a specific decision-making process based on the prevalence and incidence of illness in the community, managing simultaneously both acute and chronic health problems, early management of risk factors, promoting health and well-being within the community, and dealing with health problems in their physical, psychological, sociocultural, and existential dimensions.[11]

KEY CLINICAL CONCEPTS

The pharmaceutical care practitioner assesses all of a patient's medications, medical conditions, and outcome parameters, not just those chosen by disease state, drug action, or quantity of medications consumed. The generalist identifies, resolves, and prevents drug therapy problems up to a level of complexity defined by the standard of care for practice.

Although disease state management became popular as an approach to patient care, and one commonly taken by clinical pharmacists in practice, it has recently been shown to have less value than originally predicted. Treating a single disease in patients with an average of five to eight comorbidities has limited utility, especially as it applies to medications. Selecting out certain disease states because of familiarity and confidence, or personal interest, is not consistent with the patient-centered philosophy of pharmaceutical care practice. It is necessary to make an assessment of all of a patient's drug-related needs and apply the same standard of care across all diseases and all medications. Once a basic standard of pharmaceutical care is assured, then specialists can solve problems that the generalist is not capable of solving.

Patient care specialists in health care disciplines are defined relative to the generalist. Therefore, only when pharmaceutical care is practiced widely, and practitioners become familiar with the practice process, can specialists develop practice areas. The generalist and the specialist must have the same philosophy of practice, use the same patient care process, have a common vocabulary, and refer patients back and forth between themselves for the practice to work efficiently and cost effectively. In pharmaceutical care, the complexity of the drug therapy problem will dictate whether the patient's pharmacotherapy is best managed by a generalist or by a specialist, so both must be identifying and resolving drug therapy problems.

The generalist practice described here is applicable in all patient care practice settings, including ambulatory, long-term care, hospital, and clinic settings. The practice of pharmaceutical care does not change depending upon setting because the practice can accommodate all types of patients and medical conditions, as well as all types of drug therapies.

The data indicate that over half of all patients have drug therapy problems that must be solved. Problems of inappropriateness, ineffectiveness, and unsafe medications as well as the lack of adherence all occur at a high frequency. Young patients, old patients, patients with all types of medical conditions on all types of medications, even those patients who are not taking medications but need them, experience drug therapy problems. Therefore, for the foreseeable future, efforts should be directed at preparing generalist practitioners who are able to provide pharmaceutical care.

PHARMACEUTICAL CARE AS PRIMARY HEALTH CARE

As pharmaceutical care was developed as a generalist practice, it is ready for integration into primary care practice. Primary care has always been an important part of medical care in countries other than the United States. In the United States specialty practice has been the primary delivery structure for the past four decades. This is about to change since the Health Care Reform Act of 2010 reintroduces primary care in the form of the Medical Home as the structure for the future. The Medical Home concept takes primary care to the next level. However, first, let's understand what is meant by primary care so it becomes clear how pharmaceutical care can be easily integrated into both primary care and the Medical Home.

Primary Care Defined

The distinguished physician and bioethicist Eric Cassell identifies primary care medicine "as the capstone of twentieth century medicine," and "the foundation for twenty-first century doctoring."[12] Primary care is rapidly emerging as the dominant form of medical practice within the context of managed care. Indeed, as Cassell contends, primary care has emerged as a "sophisticated generalism" that is "propelled by the mismatch between the high-technology medicine at which we excel and the health care needs of large groups of the population—for example, the poor, chronically ill, aged, and disabled."[12]

Historically, primary health care has been afflicted with ambiguity and has taken on several different meanings. One of the earliest definitions (1920) focused on organizing medical services into primary health centers and teaching hospitals.[13] This organizational framework—"definition-by-location"— was used to organize medical services until 1978 when an international conference (Alma-Ata) moved the emphasis from medical to health services. This was a significant change as it broadened the concept, and somewhat subverted medical hegemony as the "defining" force.

This broader, more sociocultural, ecological framework also contained explicit acknowledgment of the political nature of all health matters. Indeed, what is essentially an anthropological conceptualization challenged the biomedical model and the professional dominance of the medical profession. Finally a radical humanistic approach to health that opened all areas of health care to critical scrutiny was being offered. So primary health care was transformed into a more collaborative effort with numerous health professions participating in the provision of services.

After 1979, discourse on primary care appeared in the form of two distinct views. The first was developed by the World Health Organization (WHO), which focused on operationalizing an "approach" to primary care.[14] This particular approach encompassed a broad range of interests: health education, environmental sanitation, prevention, drugs, nutrition, and traditional medicine. The WHO approach was most commonly accepted in less developed or modernizing countries.

The second view of primary health care was more focused on a constellation of health activities and/or emphasized temporality or a basic "level of service," usually at the point of first contact.[15] These services might include responsive care for episodic illness, continuing care for chronic illness, health screening and monitoring, preventive services, appropriate health education, and integration with care in acute and long-term institutions.[16] This view of primary care was most commonly accepted in developed countries such as the United States.

Practitioners have been differentiated over time as primary, secondary, or tertiary, based on the variety of problems encountered. Primary care practitioners are seen as those encountering greater variety among the most common diagnoses (50% of all visits), whereas the secondary and tertiary practitioners see more variety among the rare diagnoses.[13] In addition, a larger percentage of primary health care visits are prevention related and involve more patients who are continuing in care than are coming into the health care system for the first time.[13]

Regardless of the view taken, either the "approach" of the WHO, or the alternatives emphasizing "levels of service," there are common core elements to primary care. These may be summarized thus:

- services that are comprehensive, continuous, coordinated, accessible, and acceptable
- strategies for serving the vulnerable
- first contact care (gate keeping function)
- "de facto" care for most people's problems, most of the time
- care provided by multiple practitioners
- emphasis on health *not* medicine
- proliferation of generalist practitioners

Developed countries such as the United States will have to undergo a significant conceptual shift to move beyond specialized medicine to the concepts of primary health care. Subtle shifts from specialized medicine to a more "generalist" practice of primary care are reflected in the change in focus from illness to health, and from cure to prevention and care. Also, important shifts in content must occur. We should expect to see movement from an emphasis on specific problems to one on comprehensive care, episodic care to continuous care, and treatment to health promotion. We can also expect the increased emergence of teams whose members are drawn from a number of professions. Solo practice is already a thing of the past. These changes are beginning to take shape in the United States.

Primary health care is "based on the centrality of the patient rather than on an organ system or a disease, as is the case with specialism." Moreover:

It is addressed to both the sick and the well. It understands functional impairment and disease to be processes that enter into the patient's life story, so that its interventions are chosen with the development of that story in mind. Because of this, it is as well suited to prevention as to treatment, to children as to adults, and especially to the care of the chronically ill, who make up the largest number of sick in our society.[12]

Cassell concludes:

Primary care medicine can best be provided by generalists who are specifically trained to meet the broad, as well as the intellectually and technically exacting, demands implied in the definition of the term.[12]

Hibbard and Nutting also offer a valuable description of primary care, which serves to "situate" pharmaceutical care in this context.

...primary care is distinguished by being 'front-line' or 'first contact' care, person-centered (rather than disease or organ system-centered), and comprehensive in scope, rather than being limited to illness episodes or by the organ systems or disease process involved. Primary care is distinguished from other levels of care by the scope, character, and integration of the services provided. Primary care practitioners deal with ambulatory patients at the initial interface of the individual with the health care system. Patients present with a variety of illnesses, ailments, and concerns that represent early stages of disease that are not easily classified by organ system or diagnostic label. Often patients have multiple problems, and a rational approach to one problem may make another worse. Primary care thus provides an integrating function, balancing the multiple requirements of the patients problem(s), using information developed from many sources, and developing a strategy to help each individual achieve the highest level of function possible.[17]

This definitional framework leads us to conclude that in all conceptualizations of primary health care the patient's needs dictate the services required. Therefore, primary care is not the same as specialized services such as disease management, pharmacokinetic services, or drug utilization review. In addition, we can conclude that practitioner selected services, or those specified by health care plans such as formulary control, adverse drug reaction (ADR) reporting, and generic/therapeutic substitution are not necessarily a subset of primary health care because, to be a subset of a patient's care plan the *whole* must exist.

KEY CLINICAL CONCEPTS

Pharmaceutical care, in theory and practice, is primary health care.

Indeed, the basic focus of primary health care and pharmaceutical care are the same. These include

- patient-centeredness
- addresses both acute and chronic conditions
- emphasizes prevention
- documentation systems continuously record patient need and care provided
- accessible, frontline, first contact
- continuous and systematic care
- integration of care
- accountability
- emphasis on ambulatory patients
- includes educational/health promotional intervention

These concepts apply to the primary care practice environment and are consistent with the new concept of the medical home.

Medication Management Services in the Medical Home

These defining characteristics of primary care have also become the principles of the Medical Home concept, according to the Patient-Centered Primary Care Collaborative (PCPCC). The Task Force on Medication Management Services of the PCPCC has taken the concepts of primary care as expressed as the principles of the Medical Home and applied them to the practice of pharmaceutical care.[18] Table 2-3 demonstrates how well the practice of pharmaceutical care accommodates and integrates with the principles of the medical home. Certainly this service is ready to facilitate the work that needs to be done in this practice context.

All that remains in describing the professional practice of pharmaceutical care is to speak to its origins.

ORIGINS OF PHARMACEUTICAL CARE PRACTICE

Pharmaceutical care practice developed out of the need to re-professionalize pharmacy, much the same way as nursing re-professionalized itself during the 1980s and 1990s. Although the science around the use of medications was expanding exponentially, the efforts to apply this knowledge in practice, as a practice, were not working in either the clinical pharmacy or the clinical pharmacology paradigms. In an effort to get this knowledge to more patients in a more effective manner with more efficient systems, pharmaceutical care was born.

Table 2-3 Contribution of medication management to medical home principles[18]

Medical home principle	Medication management contribution
Personal relationship with physician or other practitioner	The therapeutic relationship is established and the patient's medication experience is revealed and used to improve care.
Team approach	The rational decision-making process for drug therapy is utilized and the assessment, care plan, and follow-up of drug therapy is integrated with the team's efforts.
Comprehensive whole/person approach	All of a patient's medications (regardless of source) are coordinated and evaluated to ensure they are appropriate, effective, safe, and convenient.
Coordination and integration of care	The intended therapeutic goals, which are made measurable and individualized to the patient, serve to coordinate and integrate the patient's care with other team members.
Quality and safety are hallmarks	Drug therapy problems are identified, resolved, and prevented in a systematic and comprehensive manner so everyone is working most effectively to realize appropriate, effective, safe, and convenient drug therapy for the patient.
Expanded access to care	Physicians are extended, made more efficient and more effective through the optimal management of a patient's medications.
Added value is recognized	Clinical outcomes are improved, return-on-investment is positive, acceptance by patients is high, and physician support the practice.

Pharmaceutical Care as the New Paradigm

Pharmaceutical care was first used to describe the care that a given patient requires and receives, which assures safe and rational drug usage. Although the term has been used a number of times since its introduction, elaboration was not substantially forthcoming until Brodie et al.[19] suggested that pharmaceutical care includes the determination of the drug needs for a given individual and the provision not only of required drugs but also of the services necessary (before, during, and after treatment) to ensure optimally safe and effective therapy. Brodie's conceptualization includes the idea of a feedback mechanism as a means of facilitating continuity of care by those who provide it. Thus, Brodie's work contributed to furthering the cause of safe and effective drug use and paved the way toward heightened consciousness and greater public/professional discourse. The changes that occurred subsequent to his work focused primarily on controlling the availability and distribution of the drug product, and not specifically on patient need within identifiable clinical parameters.

In 1988 Hepler,[20] in a more philosophical vein, described pharmaceutical care as "a covenantal relationship between a patient and a pharmacist in which the pharmacist performs drug use control functions (with appropriate knowledge and skill) governed by the awareness of and commitment to the patient's interest." Hepler and Strand, in 1990,[4] published a paper that provided a conceptualization of pharmaceutical care that stimulated widespread debate within the profession. A more detailed account of this history is provided by Posey.[21] It is the following definition that best characterizes Hepler and Strand's foundational conceptualization:

> Pharmaceutical care is that component of pharmacy practice which entails the direct interaction of the pharmacist with the patient for the purpose of caring for the patient's drug-related needs.[4]

Hepler and Strand emphasized that two activities must occur for pharmaceutical care to be delivered. First, the practitioner takes time to determine the patient's specific wishes, preferences, and needs concerning his or her health and illness. Second, the practitioner makes a commitment to continue care once it is initiated. From this fundamental premise it follows that "pharmaceutical care is the responsible provision of drug therapy for the purpose of achieving definite outcomes that improve a patient's quality of life."[4]

Hepler and Strand also placed considerable emphasis on the adoption of a strong patient focus, and the development of a therapeutic relationship in which both patient and practitioner work together to resolve complex issues. Moreover:

> Pharmaceutical care is a necessary element of health care, and should be integrated with other elements. Pharmaceutical care is, however, provided for the direct benefit of the patient, and the pharmacist is responsible directly to the patient for the quality of that care. The fundamental relationship in pharmaceutical care is a mutually beneficial exchange in which the patient grants the authority to the provider and the provider gives competence and commitment (accepts responsibility) to the patient.[4]

The concept of pharmaceutical care, as enunciated by Hepler and Strand, has received widespread acknowledgment as the foundational mandate for the profession of pharmacy. In this sense, *the profession has been redefined as a patient care practice profession* with a direct and manifest responsibility for patient care.

The Practice of Pharmaceutical Care Emerges

Although the concept of pharmaceutical care was widely accepted by the profession as early as 1990, the practice itself was not defined until 1998 by Cipolle, Strand, and Morley.[22] The definition of the practice resulted from a 5-year research project conducted from the University of Minnesota. The research involved 20 different community pharmacy practice sites and 54 practicing pharmacists. This project brought together the results of more than 20 years of research efforts that had been started by Strand in 1978.

Strand's work began with looking for a rational, systematic approach to decisions made in practice to treat with medications. Strand's research with physicians who were selecting treatment for essential hypertension failed to produce empirical evidence of a rational approach.[23] Therefore, Strand, with the assistance of Cipolle, beginning in 1978, and Morley in 1983, worked to develop a cognitive process in which the drug-related needs of patients could be approached systematically and comprehensively.

These efforts resulted in the creation of a problem-solving process applied to the use of drugs. It was presented initially as a means to document drug therapy decisions and was called the Pharmacists Workup of Drug Therapy.[24] This Workup, which has undergone continuous revision since its inception, has proven effective in structuring and framing drug use decisions. The Pharmacists Workup of Drug Therapy became the patient care process for the practice described in this volume and is now called the Pharmacotherapy Workup.[25]

This systematic problem-solving approach allowed Strand, Cipolle, and Morley to further focus their efforts to clearly define the responsibilities of a practitioner managing a patient's drug therapy. It became clear that such a practitioner had two primary responsibilities: (1) to assure that *all* of a patient's drug therapy was appropriate, the most effective possible, the safest available, and convenient enough to be taken as indicated, and (2) to identify, resolve, and most importantly, prevent any drug therapy problems that interfered with accomplishing the goals of therapy. These responsibilities were defined in 1990, and, became the foundation for pharmaceutical care practice.[26]

With the practice successfully defined in 1998, efforts could be directed toward changing the educational preparation of pharmacists to more closely meet the needs of practice. In addition, payment mechanisms for delivering these services would be necessary to continue to practice. Toward these ends, the American Medical Association approved reimbursement codes in 2004, the Federal Government passed the Drug Benefit of Medicare in 2006 and State Medicaid programs started to pay for the service in 2006. The practice of pharmaceutical care has now been shown to add value, improve care and has become a permanent fixture in the care of patients around the world.

SUMMARY

Medication management services require a professional practice as its ethical, clinical, and legal basis. Pharmaceutical care is this professional practice. A professional practice includes a philosophy, patient care process, and practice management system. In addition, a professional practice has standards, a specific vocabulary, and must "fit" with the other patient care professional practices. Pharmaceutical care meets these requirements and "fits" nicely into the primary care context that has emerged in the United States called the medical home. In other words, pharmaceutical care practice has finally found its home. Now it is necessary to understand each of the components of the professional practice in more detail, and we will start with the philosophy of practice in the next chapter.

REFERENCES

1. Rouse J. *Engaging Science: How to Understand Its Practices Philosophically.* Ithaca: Cornell University Press; 1996.
2. MacIntyre A. *Three Rival Versions of Moral Inquiry.* London: Duckworth; 1990.
3. MacIntyre A. *After Virtue.* 2nd ed. Notre Dame: University of Notre Dame Press; 1984.
4. Hepler CD, Strand LM. Opportunities and responsibilities in pharmaceutical care. *Am J Hosp Pharm.* 1990;47(3):533–543.
5. Strand LM. 1997 Remington lecture. Re-visioning the profession. *J Am Pharm Assoc.* 1997;NS37(4):474–478.
6. Cipolle RJ. Drugs don't have doses--people have doses! A clinical educator's philosophy. *Drug Intell Clin Pharm.* 1986;20(11):881–882.
7. Ricœur P. The conflict of interpretations. *Northwestern University Studies in Phenomenology and Existential Philosophy.* Evanston: Northwestern University Press; 1974.
8. Fleischman S. Language and medicine. In: Schiffrin D, Tannen D, and Hamilton HE, ed. *The Handbook of Discourse Analysis.* Oxford : Blackwell Publishing; 2003:470–502.
9. Bourdieu P. *Language and Symbolic Power.* 4th ed. Cambridge MA: Harvard University Press; 1995.
10. Glassman PA, Garcia D, Delafiel JP. *Outpatient Care Handbook.* 2nd ed. Philadelphia PA: Hanlelyl & Belfus; 1999.
11. EURACT. *The European Definitions of General Practice/Family Medicine.* European Academy of Teachers of General Practice; 2005.

12. Cassell EJ. *Doctoring: The Nature of Primary Care Medicine.* New York: Oxford University Press; 1997: p 3.
13. Starfield B. *Primary Care: Concept, Evaluation, and Policy.* New York: Oxford University Press; 1992.
14. WHO. Division of strengthening health services. In: *Cited in Starfield;* 1978.
15. Woodward K. '76 Primary health care model. In: Miller RS, ed. *Primary Health Care: More Than Medicine.* Englewood Cliffs NJ: Prentice Hall; 1983.
16. Lloyd W. *'76 Neighborhood Health Center.* New York: New York Academy of Medicine; 1977.
17. Hibbard H, Nutting P. *Research in Primary Care: A National Priority.* US Department of Health and Human Services; 1991.
18. PCPCC. In: McInnis T, Strand LM, Webb CE, eds. *The Patient Centered Medical Home: Integrating Comprehensive Medication Management to Optimize Patient Outcomes.*Patient Centered Primary Care Collaborative; 2010.
19. Brodie DC, Harvey AK. Whitney lecture. Need for a theoretical base for pharmacy practice. *Am J Hosp Pharm.* 1981;38(1):49–54.
20. Hepler CD. Unresolved issues in the future of pharmacy. *Am J Hosp Pharm.* 1988;45(5):1071–1081.
21. Posey LM. Pharmaceutical care: will pharmacy incorporate its philosophy of practice? *J Am Pharm Assoc.* 1997;NS37(2):145–148.
22. Cipolle RJ, Strand LM, Morley PC. *Pharmaceutical Care Practice.* New York, NY: McGraw-Hill; 1998.
23. Strand LM. Decision analysis of physician prescribing in the treatment of essential hypertension. In: *Department of Social and Administrative Pharmacy.* Minneapolis: University of Minnesota; 1978.
24. Strand LM, Cipolle RJ, Morley PC. Documenting the clinical pharmacist's activities: back to basics. *Drug Intell Clin Pharm.* 1988;22(1):63–67.
25. Cipolle RJ, Strand LM, Morley PC. *Pharmaceutical Care Practice: The Clinician's Guide.* 2nd ed. New York, NY: McGraw-Hill; 2004.
26. Strand LM, Morley PC, Cipolle RJ, Ramsey R, Lamsam G D. Drug-related problems: their structure and function. *DICP: Ann Pharmacother.* 1990;24(11):1093–1097.

chapter three

Toward a Philosophy of Pharmaceutical Care Practice

🔑 KEY CONCEPTS

1 The philosophy of practice is the most important concept of a professional practice, but the most difficult to grasp because it is the only component that is not tangible.

2 A philosophy of practice is the set of values that guides a practitioner's behavior to be ethically appropriate, clinically accurate, and legal. It defines the rules, roles, relationships, and responsibilities of the practitioner.

3 A philosophy of practice is specific to a practice, not the practitioner. A practitioner's philosophy of life is different and separate from the practice philosophy.

4 The philosophy of pharmaceutical care establishes the purpose for the practice that is to meet the social need to control drug-related morbidity and mortality by managing medications well.

5 The professional responsibilities defined by the philosophy of pharmaceutical care are to identify drug therapy problems, resolve them, and most importantly, prevent them from occurring in patients.

6 The philosophy of pharmaceutical care states that these responsibilities will be carried out in a patient-centered manner using the caring paradigm that has been defined by the professions of medicine and nursing. This paradigm requires that the practitioner comprehensively assess a patient's drug-related needs, that he develops a care plan that can address these needs, and that he follows up to determine that the desired outcomes are achieved and no harm has been done.

7 There are standards of professional behavior that determine if a practitioner is applying the philosophy of practice in practice. These standards should be met each time a patient is cared for by the practitioner.

All professional patient care practices (e.g., medicine, nursing, dentistry) have a philosophy of practice that serves as the basis for all that occurs in practice. This philosophy of practice guides the patient care process and the practice management components of the professional practice. The philosophy is the most challenging of the three components to grasp because it is the only one that is not tangible, it can only be seen in the behavior, attitude, and work of the practitioner. The philosophy of practice reflects the professional values that the practitioner holds—the values that guide his every day behavior and decision making in practice. As the philosophy of pharmaceutical care practice is new to pharmacists, we will spend time describing the meaning and importance of it in practice.

A PHILOSOPHY OF PRACTICE DEFINED

Definition   A philosophy of practice is the set of values that guides behaviors associated with certain acts—in this case, those of pharmaceutical care.

A philosophy defines the rules, roles, relationships, and responsibilities of the practitioner. Any philosophy of practice, which is to be taken seriously, must reflect the functions and activities of the practitioner and also critically provide direction toward the formation of a consistent practice. How a practitioner practices from day-to-day should reflect a philosophy of practice.

KEY CLINICAL CONCEPTS

A philosophy of practice helps a practitioner make decisions, determine what is important, and sets priorities over the course of the day by establishing which responsibilities need to be met, which ethical parameters apply, and which moral obligations exist.

Ethical dilemmas, management issues, and clinical judgments are all resolved with the assistance of a practitioner's philosophy of practice. This is why the philosophy of practice must be well understood and clearly articulated, so it is explicit and relied on when facing difficult problems.

A philosophy of practice is specific to a practice, not to the practitioner, and it is different from an individual's philosophy of life. A philosophy of life includes an individual's beliefs about politics, religion, child-rearing, and the work ethic, among many other things. And, in a democratic society individuals are allowed to have whichever philosophy of life he chooses, provided it does not lead to illegal behaviors. However, when an individual chooses to care for another individual's health, that person is obligated to make decisions and take actions according to a specific philosophy of professional practice. This philosophy will protect the patient from unprofessional or unethical behavior from the practitioner, and it will help to guide the practitioner to know his responsibilities and ethical obligations.

When a practitioner takes an oath to practice a profession, it is the philosophy of that practice the practitioner is promising to uphold. Therefore, all practitioners who purport to be engaged in a specific professional practice will hold the same philosophy of practice. This uniformity of philosophy, and therefore standardization of behaviors, can then result in consistently high-quality services and expectations from patients, which then leads to a new demand for the service. Additionally, the philosophy must be applied to all patients in that practice, and not applied selectively depending on convenience, time availability, or personal preferences. The philosophy of practice is the "prescriptive" component of a practice as it defines *what should be done.* A practice philosophy is "timeless" in that it does not change on a daily basis, nor is it different among and between practitioners. This is not to say that the philosophy is dogmatic and unchanging, but rather it is to be seen as a set of ideals, principles, concepts, and values held in common by "all practitioners" who draw upon this framework to define the nature of their practice.

KEY CLINICAL CONCEPTS

The philosophy of practice specific to pharmaceutical care describes a purpose for the practice that is to meet the social need to manage drug-related morbidity and mortality, with an explicit objective to care for a patient's drug-related needs by making it the practitioner's responsibility to ensure that all of a patient's drug therapy is appropriate, the most effective available, the safest possible, and is taken as indicated.

This is accomplished by identifying, resolving, and preventing drug therapy problems, which could interfere with successfully meeting a patient's drug therapy goals and producing positive patient outcomes. All of this needs to be done in a patient-centered manner using the caring paradigm that is at the center of all patient care professions.

This philosophy of practice remains only "wishful thinking," or abstract, until a therapeutic relationship is built with the patient, and the pharmacist engages in the patient care process to provide a service. There is always a tendency to want to "get on with the practice" when learning about pharmaceutical care. However, because everything about the practice emanates from the philosophy and reflexively returns to "push against" it, we need to understand the philosophy of pharmaceutical care in some detail.

THE PHILOSOPHY OF PHARMACEUTICAL CARE PRACTICE

The philosophy of pharmaceutical care practice was outlined in Chapter 2 but will be discussed in more detail here.

KEY CLINICAL CONCEPTS

The philosophy consists of four discrete elements, expressed as a commitment to (1) meet a social need with the practice, (2) fulfill specific responsibilities to achieve the goals of practice, (3) utilize a patient-centered approach to meeting this need, and (4) "care" for another through the development and maintenance of a therapeutic relationship.

This philosophy of practice allows patients and practitioners to know what to expect and through the philosophy of practice can the practitioner be held accountable for what he should do as well as what he actually does. This is why the philosophy of practice is so important in practice. We will now discuss each of the commitments involved in the philosophy of pharmaceutical care practice.

Meeting a Social Need

All professions must meet a unique social need to justify their elevated position and privileges in society. This need is at the heart of the philosophy of practice. In the case of pharmaceutical care practice the practitioner optimizes the use of medications and minimizes drug-related morbidity and mortality for society. The practitioner meets this social need by attending to the needs of patients, *one at a time*. This can be achieved only if the philosophy of practice is patient-centered, which means that all decisions made by the practitioner are made for the benefit of the patient first, and what is done by the practitioner is done in response to the patient's needs, and is not driven by self-interest or economic advantage.

Professional activities are rewarded when they meet a unique social need. This is accomplished when the practitioner applies specialized knowledge and skills to provide a service that addresses "client" problems. In the case of health care professionals, these unique needs are health-related. And, although all health care professionals are first and foremost in the business of keeping patients healthy, they usually do so by preventing, identifying, and resolving a unique set of health-related problems.

Meeting a unique social need balances the benefits realized by professionals. For example, society supports an extensive education for the professional student through public taxes. Society provides the professional with an exclusive right to earn a relatively high income, grants her an elevated status in the community, and generally accepts the autonomy with which professions govern themselves. Such privileges come with certain social responsibilities and accountability.

Fulfilling Specific Responsibilities

Traditionally, we have assumed that physicians optimize the use of medications and minimize drug-related morbidity, and sometimes nurses take on a portion of this responsibility, and less frequently pharmacists contribute to this goal. However, it is this fragmentation of responsibility, along with an ever-expanding range of new, more complex drug products that has created the need for a specific professional to be designated to correct this openly and comprehensively because only then can a specific individual be held accountable for its management. When such a person is "in place" can the level of drug-related morbidity and mortality experienced in society be minimized, and the cost of drug-related illness to society managed.[1] Therefore, we emphasize that the first premise of the philosophy of pharmaceutical care is that it is the pharmacist's essential responsibility to meet society's need to assure that patients are taking appropriate, effective, safe, and convenient drug therapy.

Pharmaceutical care prescribes the responsibilities that must be met through standards of practice (see Appendix 1 for these standards). These standards are non-negotiable and they must be met each time care is provided in order to contribute the value expected from this professional practice. All patients deserve to be taking medications that achieve their goals and optimize their experience, and it is the responsibility of the pharmaceutical care practitioner to ensure this is the case. The responsibility for drug therapy has to be accepted completely without caveats and conditions to be considered a professional mandate. Therefore, the philosophy of pharmaceutical care states that wherever there is drug therapy, there needs to be a practitioner ensuring the patient receives the appropriate product, dose, duration, and monitoring. This responsibility can be no more clearly stated than this. When a practitioner accepts this philosophy of practice, he accepts this professional role in society.

The Patient-centered Approach

To effectively meet the social need described above and the responsibilities outlined, it is necessary for the practitioner of pharmaceutical care to use a patient-centered approach to practice. This approach considers the patient as a "whole" individual whose health care needs generally, and drug therapy needs specifically, are the primary concern of the practitioner. The patient is seen as an individual with rights, knowledge, and experience, all of which are necessary for the practitioner to fulfill his responsibilities. Using this approach prevents the patient from being seen as a repository for drugs to be studied and also precludes the patient from being defined as a conglomerate of organ systems and drug reactions. Such objectification is not acceptable to the pharmaceutical care practitioner. This approach requires that the practitioner treat the patient as a partner in care planning, and always as the ultimate decision maker because the patient experiences the ultimate consequences of drug therapy.

A patient-centered approach means that *all* of the patient's drug-related needs are seen as the responsibility of the practitioner, not just those associated with a specific drug category or a specific disease state. All of the patient's concerns and expectations about his drug therapy become the practitioner's responsibilities.

> **KEY CLINICAL CONCEPTS**
>
> The patient-centered approach insists that the patient's needs, and not the practitioner's preferences, "drive" the practice of pharmaceutical care. In a pragmatic sense, this means that the practitioner will start with the patient's needs and provide care until they are all met.

The practitioner will make all of the decisions and take all of the actions necessary to meet the drug-related needs of the patient.

The term patient-centered has taken on an even greater significance, as the patient-centered medical home concept has become reality in the United States. Pharmaceutical care will integrate easily with the other services provided by members of the "medical home team" because the philosophy of practice for all members now is consistent and complimentary with the others. This magnifies the importance of understanding and applying the philosophy in practice. For these reasons, the next chapter will focus on the patient-centered concept and describe in detail the elements of pharmaceutical care that make it a patient-centered practice.

Caring as a Practice Paradigm

The term "caring" means many different things. However, when caring is used in the context of a philosophy of practice, its meaning is very specific. It indicates that the practitioner should accomplish three objectives for the patient. First, the practitioner comprehensively assesses the patient's needs, then brings all the resources he has available to meet those needs, and finally, determines whether the needs have been met or if any negative outcomes have occurred.

However, within the context of a philosophy of practice, the idea of care generally derives from two different, but complementary concerns:

1. the technical dimensions of taking care of patients
2. caring for or about a particular patient thereby demonstrating a concern for the well-being of another person.[2]

The first of these is reasonably well understood. Indeed, some may very well argue that it is too well "understood" and is reflected in our national preoccupation with "high-tech" solutions to all manner of health problems. Certainly, pharmacy has general agreement on such matters as they manifest themselves in the empirically driven use of pharmaceutical agents—the usual emphasis being on the actual therapeutic agent in question at any given time.

It is the second concern that provides pharmaceutical care with the focus on the "softer" side of practitioner purpose. To use a somewhat well-worn distinction, the first exemplifies the *science* of pharmacy-at-work, the second plumbs the depths of the *art* of practice.

Within the context of pharmaceutical care the emphasis/focus moves from product to person—from pharmaceutical agent to patient. We emphasize that this does not diminish the importance of pharmaceutical knowledge! In fact, we would argue that the responsibility to apply pharmaceutical knowledge to the benefit of another dramatically elevates the requirement to possess a comprehensive understanding of the pharmacological basis of therapeutics. But, it does refocus attention on the recipient of such technical knowledge. This change in focus is very clearly established in Cipolle's understanding that "drugs don't have doses—people have doses."[3]

Thus, the *patient* becomes the central focus for our interventions. Such a change of focus involves very serious cognitive, conceptual, and some would add emotional, shifts on the part of those committed to giving and receiving pharmaceutical care. Conventional boundaries, tracing their legitimacy to disciplines and professionally arrogated authority, must be critically examined and practitioners intending to practice pharmaceutical care should be prepared to ground technical knowledge within a broader philosophical and sociocultural context. Facts and values must both be examined as these affect persons who are more than biological, or organ systems.

In essence, the practitioner of pharmaceutical care will welcome the opportunity to participate in the development of a scientific humanism that emancipates both practitioner and patient from the often debilitating excesses of a "technical fix."

Rollo May, for example, defines caring as a state in which something matters. Care is seen as the antithesis of apathy and distance, and is the necessary source of eros. It is "the source of human tenderness."[4]

For May, and other humanists, care is not to be confused with sentimentality, for this emotion is reflecting on sentiment itself, rather than experiencing who is the subject of the caring attention. Care is essentially equated with compassion. But, it is important to note that within the humanistic tradition, the concept of care conveys a compassionate state of being and not merely an attitude.[4]

Within the humanistic psychology of Rogers and Maslow is found the essence of "otherness" in the caring relationship. To care for another person, in a meaningful sense, is to help with growth and "self-actualization." It is a process, a relationship wherein the cared for individual is deeply involved in his healing journey. Self-actualization, as a process, engages all those concerned in the healing process. Thus, "client-centered" therapy does, in a secular sense, what theological intervention achieves as it integrates mind, body, and spirit. Disjunctions between "care giver" and the "cared for" become blurred as the relationship brings two, or more, individuals together in a partnership intent on the resolution of a particular problem.[5,6]

Caring, then, involves a profound respect for the otherness of the other. It differs considerably from any paternalistic, authoritarian imposition of will or direction upon the other. Thus, with this in mind, therapeutic compliance is not to be seen as enforcement based on the authority of the practitioner, but is to be seen as a consequence of an alliance between *all* those concerned with the resolution of a particular problem. Perhaps the better term for this is adherence. Caring, as situated within the context of pharmaceutical care, finds its expression in helping the other come to care for herself. It requires a relationship where there is a sense of participation in the other, an awareness of that individual's particular need for growth and control over the therapeutic process. This is frequently minimized or dismissed completely as practitioners assume the more paternalistic posture of the "expert knows best."

Any effective and appropriate therapeutic alliance requires that the "voice" of the patient be heard and heeded. On matters that require empirical knowledge practitioners have a duty to inform, educate, and engage in listening to the patient's needs and preferences. Dialogue is essential, practitioner monologue is not. Mayerhoff, for example, emphasizes the importance of self-actualization:

> Caring, as helping another grow and actualize himself(sic) is a process, a way of relating to someone that involves development in the same way that friendship can only emerge in time through mutual trust and a deepening and qualitative transformation of the relationship.[7]

Gaylin offers a somewhat different viewpoint. His understanding of caring attempts to demonstrate that caring is biologically programmed and caring must be seen as a fundamental fact of human growth and development. His thesis weds biology to culture, and reaches out to humanistic philosophy in an attempt to argue a case for innate goodness.[8]

Perhaps the most substantive discourse on the subject of caring and relationships is to be found in nursing. Indeed, the literature is rich with intellectual argument and passion. Benner's work is of particular importance and goes directly to the heart of the matter:

> Caring is a relational word, and it shows up in relational contexts. Caring, if it means anything, always means something in a particular context, a particular relationship. Caring is incompatible with radically free individualism and autonomy. Caring means that others can lay claim on your time, your interests, your resources. It means that you cannot remain atomistic, unrelated, outside a community, or outside of relationships.[9]

Surely this captures the essence of any caring relationship. She continues:

> Caring unravels the control paradigm and forms one of the few cultural resistances against the anomie, dominance, and oppression of a technological self-understanding. Caring requires both listening and a form of knowing that goes beyond curiosity and dissection, beyond laying bare the facts. Caring requires a truth theory that is true to the knower and the known. Caring is embodied and embedded in a community or social network. Caring unleashes pleasure in the midst of work; a sense that some things are worth doing and some things are good in themselves—a uniting of means and ends.[9]

Moreover:

> Care sets up what matters, what counts as stressful, what can count as coping, what being related and situated means, and finally, what counts as giving and receiving help.[9]

Benner, in our view, provides us with one of the clearest, most comprehensive treatments of the caring concept particularly as it relates to the therapeutic relationship as we envisage it within pharmaceutical care.

Nurse theorists have now turned their attention to such important issues as the meanings attached to care, transcultural themes in caring, values, beliefs concerning care and practice (theory and practice relationships), the aesthetics of care, the economics and politics of care, the ethics of care, spiritual and religious dimensions of care, and the educational requirements for a "caring profession." These are but a few of the issues central to any caring practice.[10] Pharmacists will have to deal with these issues as they begin to practice pharmaceutical care.

Caring as Covenant

Hepler and Strand have asserted that pharmaceutical care is "provided for the direct benefit of the patient and the pharmacist accepts direct responsibility for the quality of that care."[11] Recall, they emphasize that pharmaceutical care "is based on a covenant between the patient, who promises to grant authority to the provider, and the provider, who promises competence and commitment to the patient."[11] To this we would add that the pharmacist is to be held *accountable* for her decisions and interventions.

The key term in the original Hepler and Strand position is "covenant." They use the term to signify a *bond* between the pharmacist and patient. This is the bond that "cements" the therapeutic relationship. It is to be seen as a common understanding of roles and responsibilities for both parties actively engaged in such a relationship. Essentially, it is an agreement, for all concerned, to work toward the resolution of all experienced and potential drug-related problems.

Within pharmaceutical care practice, and the reciprocity of the covenant, certain responsibilities are recognized, assumed, and accounted for, on the part of both practitioner and patient. The practitioner of pharmaceutical care agrees to assess the patient's needs, bring whatever resources are required to successfully address these needs, and follow-up to ensure that effective, good interventions have taken place. The patient agrees to at least two important things. First, he agrees to provide accurate and complete information (data) to the practitioner so that both individuals can make effective decisions. Also, the patient agrees to play an active role in the care provided. This means that the patient agrees to set goals, carry out agreed upon behaviors, and provide information required for beneficial care.

Cooper believes that "a covenant relationship brings the moral and personal aspects of nursing care together."[12] She notes that:

> a responsiveness to the presence of the patient and his or her needs, an acknowledgment of the indebtedness by the caregiver to the patient for the benefit of practice and engagement, and a recognition of the mutuality and reciprocity that distinguishes the relationship indicate a willingness by nurses to enter a covenantal relationship.[12]

Although the concept of a covenant does have a certain appeal, particularly as it fits well into accepted Judeo-Christian understandings of commitment, it does have some limitation. Bishop and Scudder, for example, contend that:

> A covenant is an agreement that both includes and excludes. For example, in the Judeo-Christian tradition, the people of the Covenant saw themselves as connected to each other through covenant but separate from those who were not of the Covenant.[13]

The central issue, they continue, is that the covenantal relationship is too restrictive in that it emphasizes the practitioner's responsibilities, but does not adequately address the patient's involvement. Thus, although we recognize the essential element of good faith implied in covenantal relationships and accept the positive implication for professional responsibility, and ultimately accountability, we also recognize the importance of the dialogue that frames the formation of covenantal relationships, or for that matter, those of a more contractual intent. Cooper expresses this well:

> Unlike a covenant relationship, a dialogical relationship does not assume a common purpose between both parties. Each person meets the other as they are present to each other as persons. They mutually respond to each other's presence in a relationship which recognizes the legitimate right of the other to be. This relationship has been described by Buber (1923) as an I-Thou relationship, in contrast to a I-It relationship in which the person is treated as a thing to be categorized and used. I-Thou relationships are cultivated and developed through dialogue.[12]

Covenant and dialogue clearly have a place in pharmaceutical care. Once the dialogical preconditions are satisfied, both practitioner and patient can enter into a covenantal relationship that is committed to open, not exclusive, conditions. Moreover, such a relationship must very seriously incorporate the desires, wishes, and needs of the patient. Such an alliance must move from the patient to the practitioner. However, we also recognize the essential dialogical preconditions that must frame the "agenda" and shape the nature of the relationship. We do not see covenantal and dialogical relationships as necessarily mutually exclusive. Rather, we see both as dimensions of the therapeutic relationship and central to effective pharmaceutical care.

Caring, then, initiated and sustained through dialogue, is fundamental to pharmaceutical care philosophy and practice. The covenantal ethic establishes commitment to, and respect for, persons. Certainly, close inspection of the dynamics of a covenantal relationship reveals that it is essentially dialogue that makes such a relationship possible and maximizes its inclusive probabilities. Hence, the relationship is not simply a mutual understanding, however arrived at. It is first and foremost, the process of how such a relationship is formed and sustained. Dialogue shapes expectations, desires, methods, and therapeutic commitment. It identifies needs, fosters well-being, and brings to the relationship on-going reflection on meaning and purpose. Dialogue explores the sense of trust, respect, truth-telling, and authenticity. For some, talk may be "cheap," but in a viable therapeutic relationship, not talking can be costly.

The Values Involved in Caring

Pharmaceutical care practice is inherently value-laden and the philosophy of practice defines those values that need to be applied in practice. Values, or that which we consider worthy, are central to all interventions in the lives of others. As Guttman observes: Values are embedded in all facets of the intervention process and both influence and serve as justification for the choice of the intervention goals and objectives.[14]

For the pharmaceutical care practitioner, this fact is of vital importance. Clinical intervention is much more than the accurate, competent application of technical knowledge to the resolution of health problems. It is also the value-laden context in which the clinician struggles with the process of decision making, judgment, and justification for choices made.

The first step to dealing with these situations successfully on a daily, patient-specific basis is to separate your personal values from the professional values that are required to provide care to others. This is difficult for new, young practitioners because in order to separate one set of values from another, one must be conscious of what one's personal values are. To become conscious of these values, it is necessary to engage in critical thinking in an area usually referred to as *values clarification.*

Values clarification is an essential step in the development of a pharmaceutical care practitioner as it leads to greater self-awareness. Practitioners who engage in a reflective process to become more conscious of what they value or consider worthy, do the following:

- Understand one's beliefs and behaviors, which include knowing what one does and does not support, and communicating this to others.
- Choose one's beliefs and behaviors by evaluating values received from others, which includes examining alternatives and their consequences, then deciding which are one's own.
- Act on these beliefs with a consistent pattern that reinforces actions supportive of the values.[14–16]

A personal set of values will include political views, religious beliefs, social norms, personal preferences, and influence from personal experiences. Practitioners must become consciously aware of these personal values so that they know when they create conflict in the practice setting. Problems can develop in practice when practitioners confuse personal values with professional values and when they impose personal values onto the patient. Personal values must be kept separate from professional values because personal values are private, whereas professional values are public and ascribed by the practicing community. This is the distinction between a personal philosophy of life and a professional practice philosophy.

From Values to Ethics

The leap from values to ethics is in reality a short one. Values help to shape what is individually conceived as right and wrong, and this drives the decisions and interventions made in practice. Ethics is a system of understanding what motivates and determines our behavior, based upon individual conceptions of right and wrong.[17] Moreover, ethics helps us to address the question "What should I do in this situation?" Ethics offers a formal process for applying moral dimensions to our actions when we are making decisions for and with another individual as we do in practice.[17]

A strong case can be made for including ethical reflection within the context of pharmaceutical care practice. Indeed, we argue that such a focus is essential to practice and is closely tied to care. Accepting responsibility for the outcomes of another person's drug therapies is not a complex commitment, but it is a serious commitment that requires frequent reflection and critique against a set of ethics.

Husted and Husted[18] put forward the following decision-making principles as *natural* in all interactions. These are especially relevant to health care providers to help guide behavior in practice:

- Every patient has a right to be treated according to her unique character.
- Every patient has a right to decide and act on her own values to fulfill individual life plans.
- Every patient has a right to expect complete objective information and the emotional support necessary to act effectively on that information.
- Every patient has the right, alone or through a health care professional, to the control of her time and effort.
- Every patient has a right to expect whatever benefit is possible in the health care setting and to expect no avoidable harm.
- Every patient has a right to expect that agreements established with the health care professionals will be kept.[18]

Such principles as these provide ethical justification for a certain standard of care. Hence, they are useful for practitioners to *push against* while exploring their personal values and ethical positions. Can you readily and unreservedly accept these principles? How do they affect your professional obligations, responsibilities, and duties to patients? What will you do when you cannot accept any one of these? These questions, and others, are important to ask at all stages of values/ethics exploration.

ETHICS IN PRACTICE

The practice of pharmaceutical care will create situations that have the potential to involve ethical dilemmas. Two individuals (patient and practitioner) perhaps from different cultures, with different values and levels of knowledge are meeting to address life-changing issues of disease and treatment. This is occurring in a society that is increasingly dependent on technology and that has limited financial resources coupled with an increased demand for services. Any one of these situations can lead to an ethical dilemma.

Every practitioner must be prepared to recognize situations with moral and ethical implications. This requires the practitioner be prepared with (1) insight of his or her own values, cultural norms, moral development, and ethical principles; (2) time, focused attention, and sensitivity to recognize subtle clues that may indicate a situation is laden with ethical components; and (3) the knowledge and aptitude for making logical, fair, and consistent decisions. Basic professional behavior can go a long way in helping to avoid ethical dilemmas. Each of these important behaviors is based on an ethical principle and is described in Table 3-1. Pharmaceutical care practitioners will learn these behaviors and make them a consistent part of everyday practice. It is useful to briefly discuss each of these and place them in the context of pharmaceutical care.

Beneficence   The ethical practitioner will want to do what is best for the patient. Although perhaps exceptionally well-informed on pharmacological matters, we have seen that in itself, this does not mean that the practitioner knows best. Clearly, when the centrality of the patient and her preferences are considered, deciding what is best under any circumstance involves more than professional opinion and alternatives. For example, deciding the burdens and benefits of therapeutic protocols cannot be carried out without the involvement of the patient.

Patients will decide what risks to take, what benefits they desire, and what burdens they are willing and able to endure.

Table 3-1 Basic professional behaviors expected in practice

Professional behavior	Ethical principle
Do the very best you can for every patient	Beneficence
In all cases, do no harm	Nonmaleficence
Tell the patient the truth	Veracity
Be fair	Justice
Be loyal	Fidelity
Allow the patient to be the ultimate decision maker	Autonomy/paternalism
Always protect your patient's privacy	Confidentiality

Although the *expert* may be capable of calculating the technical dimensions of risk and uncertainty based on empirical evidence, once this is communicated to the patient, she must decide the course of action. Beneficence—doing what is best for the patient—is therefore negotiated between two parties rather than imposed even if what is best for the patient seems to be *clinically obvious.*

A simple rule of thumb is to consider all available information, engage in free noncoercive discussion with the patient, facilitate decisions that derive from this individual, and serve his or her best interests.

Nonmaleficence All health care practitioners are familiar with the Hippocratic principle of *primum non nocere, or above all, do no harm.* This can be seen as linked to the principle of beneficence. However, while we may all agree that any principles opposed to inflicting harm must be accepted, it is reasonable to suggest that wherever there is risk, there is the potential to harm.[19]

At no time should the pharmaceutical care practitioner aggressively force a treatment on a patient. No matter what justification is offered, whether in the name of pharmaceutical science, clinical evidence, or practitioner preference, the clinician who performs without due regard for the patient's considerations acts with malfeasance. In this sense, the end does not justify the means.

Veracity It sounds simple to insist that practitioners tell the truth at all times. Keep in mind that there are many questions that must be explored. Should we tell the truth at all times? Is it ever ethical not to tell the patient the truth? Can telling the truth harm people? If so, under what circumstances can people be harmed? Can we lie when we consider it in the best interest of our patients? Does lying sometimes protect people? Why not deceive a patient if it promotes her health and recovery? Does this particular patient want bad news? Will a bleak prognosis harm the patient? Why not withhold certain information? Is nondisclosure a form of lying? Do we need to tell the patient everything? Don't we confuse patients with all this information?

These are but a few of the questions that emerge in any discussion related to truth-telling. There are no formulaic answers unless one adopts the position that the truth will be told at all costs regardless of the consequences.

Although we endorse the ethical principle of veracity, and believe honesty to be a highly regarded part of character, we also recognize that in practical terms, grounded in the realities of human suffering, individual practitioners are fallible creatures, and often lack the emotional strength necessary to tell the complete truth if they are convinced that it will harm the patient. Emotional strength, conscience, and often, clinical judgment can present barriers to truth-telling.

Those providing care devote considerable time reflecting upon the nature and practice of truth-telling and its place in the therapeutic relationship. Can there be trust based on deception and lies? Does it matter how small the lie, how insignificant the deception? What if it worked and the patient recovered? Those who provide care, respect patients, and recognize the importance of trust in the therapeutic relationship must ask themselves how they can transmit peace of mind to those who willingly place themselves in the hands of strangers.

Does it really come down to a personal choice? Not exactly. Truth-telling may be a skill that can be learned with practice. Providing patients with bad news is difficult and sometimes heartbreaking. It may seem easier to equivocate, be vague, or even mumble. Rest assured, in the end, *the truth will win out*. Individuals in trouble, often weak, vulnerable, and impoverished in spirit, seem to find the truth.

In the end, the principle of veracity can only serve the best interests of the patient. Sensitivity and thoughtful communication skills on the part of the pharmaceutical care practitioner can be learned and *polished* with experience.[20–22]

Once initial formative trust is established and a therapeutic relationship is developed, honesty should be unconditional and reciprocal. In order to accomplish this it is useful to make honesty a part of therapeutic discourse. Outline the expectation of truth, emphasize its importance, and nurture its development. Only when truth is a central piece of a relationship can a care plan be created with any hope of success.

Justice Justice is an ethical principle "that relates to fair, equitable, and appropriate treatment in the light of what is due or owed to persons. The principle of justice recognizes that giving to some may deny receipt to others."[15]

Frequently, patient circumstances raise serious considerations of fairness and justice. Not all patients can afford essential drugs. Is it appropriate to accept what are generally described as *the morals of the marketplace?* Clearly, practitioners, who are predominantly employees, cannot *give away the store.* What are their responsibilities to the poor who need assistance?

What of the uninformed patient who does not understand insurance options and limitations? Is it ethical to refuse to serve uninsured patients? This has become a serious issue when practitioners claim that insurance does not *pay enough* to cover expenses. Once again there is no easy fix for issues arising from questions of justice.

At the outset the problem is systemic in that the distribution of goods and services in a market-driven economy is always going to be inequitable, uneven, and—for many, of questionable fairness. Presently in the United States, we do not have a national health system, and there is no common acceptance of the idea that health care is a fundamental right. Given the prevailing realities of our social norms and values, pharmaceutical care practitioners must resolve problems within the context of what *is*, not what *ought to be.* Most practitioners are aware of such matters and will endorse a pragmatic approach to each case as it presents itself.

In effect, it is reasonable to expect the ethical pharmaceutical care practitioner to make every effort to treat all patients equally and assist those who are legitimately disadvantaged by locating information and programs that will meet their needs. This is not to suggest that all pharmaceutical care practitioners should become social workers, but rather to know the health care system in general and policies in particular and use this information to solve a patient's problems of access to care and pharmaceuticals.

Practitioners will be expected to adhere to the principle of equality in so much as they care for patients as equals regardless of ethnicity, class, gender, or sexual preference. Discrimination of any kind is unacceptable, unethical, and intolerable.

Fidelity   This is an ethical principle that relates "to the concept of faithfulness and the practice of keeping promises."[15] Pharmaceutical care practitioners are granted authority to practice by a society that regulates competition through licensure and thereby protects the self-interests of the profession. In a real sense, such a social contract provides privileges to an elite group, and in doing so demands accountability. Bukhardt and Nathaniel, while specifically referring to nurses, put the case well:

> The process of licensure is one that ensures no other group can practice within the domain of (pharmaceutical care) as defined by society and the profession. Thus, to accept licensure and become legitimate members of the profession mandates that (pharmaceutical care practitioners) uphold the responsibilities inherent in the contract with society.[15]

Although we have inserted *pharmaceutical care practitioner* where they had written *nurse*, the same conditions apply. Pharmaceutical care practitioners are expected to "be faithful to the society that grants the right to practice."[15]

Moreover, they are expected to:

- Keep the promise of upholding the professional code of ethics,
- to practice within the established scope of practice and definition of (pharmaceutical care),
- to remain competent in practice,
- to abide by the policies of employing institutions, and
- to keep promises to individual patients.[15]

To be a pharmaceutical care practitioner is to make and keep promises to patients. Of course, it can readily be seen that fidelity is related to trust as an essential part of any meaningful therapeutic relationship.

Promises can be hard to keep in patient care, particularly when they are based on hope or reassurance. The often heard *I promise—you will be all right*, meant to reassure, and perhaps motivate the patient all too often cannot deliver the promised outcome. In short, there can be no absolute promises, or immutable duty to keep them.[15] The ethical pharmaceutical care practitioner should keep in mind "that in every case, harmful consequences of the promised action should be weighed against the benefits of keeping the promise."[15]

Autonomy　No one is entirely self-governing. For the purpose of ethics discourse, however, the concept of autonomy refers to a patient having the freedom to make choices for him or herself. In this sense, it implies that an individual is free from coercion or threat and can make informed decisions as a free agent. This does not mean that other individuals play no role in influencing the choices people make. Rather, it means that individual choices are respected and subsequent interventions are predicated on respect. This is particularly true when the patient's choices conflict with those of the practitioner. Respect for patients is mandatory. Without it there can be no trust, no therapeutic relationship, and no care.

Of course everything has limits. In the case of autonomy, while respect should be ever present, there are serious considerations to be taken into account when formulating a care plan. Does the patient have a clear understanding of all important facts and values? How do I know if the patient is cognitively competent and can make informed, autonomous decisions? Is the confused patient acting autonomously? These questions may sound rhetorical, but they are frequently asked, and uncertainty is common. Some patients—children and the mentally incompetent, for example—are not thought capable of making autonomous decisions.

Respect for the patient's autonomy is essential in pharmaceutical care practice. Trust, and the necessary therapeutic relationship—the *covenant*[11]—cannot become a shared reality unless, and until, respect is established. Failure to take this foundational principle seriously makes a mockery of any claim to have provided care, and most certainly offers very little assistance that is meaningful to those seeking help.

Paternalism is not the answer   Setting aside the child or otherwise dependent patient, there are very few occasions when paternalism should be acted upon. Paternalism refers to "the practice of overriding or ignoring preferences of patients to benefit them or enhance their welfare."[23] Moreover, paternalism represents the judgment that beneficence takes priority over autonomy.[23]

Pharmaceutical care is committed to *informed* patient preference. As stated earlier, the pharmaceutical care practitioner and the patient form a therapeutic alliance where the patient is given to understand the pharmaceutical care practitioner's responsibilities and duties and, most importantly, understands her personal responsibilities in relation to those of the practitioner. In effect, both the practitioner and patient must have a clear understanding of the rules, roles, and responsibilities central to the therapeutic relationship. Without such an understanding there can be no meaningful relationship that produces positive outcomes.

The authoritative and univocal allocation of pharmaceutical fact and value does not result in productive communication.[24] It is equally doubtful that such an approach will result in too much informed consent or compliance.

Therefore, it can be argued that it is both ethically and therapeutically more appropriate to engage in dialogue and develop meaningful two-way communication that maximizes cooperation and meaningful understanding of all facets of the pharmaceutical care experience.

Respect for autonomy is not simply an ethical imperative, but it also receives a legal mandate in some instances. For example, the Patient Self-Determination Act of 1990[25] mandates that in all institutions receiving Medicare or Medicaid funding patients must receive written information explicitly stating

- their right to accept or refuse treatment;
- their rights under existing state laws regarding advance directives;
- any policies the institution has regarding the withholding of life-sustaining treatment.

The logical consequence of respect for autonomy and person can only be understood as respect for patient preference. Ethically, it should be the individual's desires, aspirations, and priorities that form the nucleus of pharmaceutical care. Such a view of patient-centered care sets an agenda where the pharmaceutical care practitioner acts as advocate for the patient's well-being.

Pharmaceutical care practice is not possible without due regard to the full implications of patient autonomy and informed consent. Indeed, upon reflection, it is noteworthy that pharmacotherapy is the most common form of treatment found on a daily basis, yet very little attention is focused on consent. Although surgery, a much less common invasion on mind and body, requires written consent based on substantive information, pharmacotherapy relies on a less rigorous process of an entirely verbal nature.

Patient-centered care requires an ethical and clinical commitment to a therapeutic relationship in which accurate, therapeutically optimal drug therapy and drug information is discussed. Options are examined, and the patient communicates a strong sense of understanding. The practitioner has acted ethically and in a clinically appropriate manner when both parties have reached a common understanding of purpose and goals, and a care plan has been jointly negotiated and agreed upon.

Confidentiality   The trust that is built between practitioner and patient is compromised without the assurance of confidentiality. The duty to protect patient confidentiality emerges from a relationship based upon trust.

As a clinician with clearly defined pharmaceutical care responsibilities, you have a duty to protect a patient's personal information from public view. This is a well-known fact of clinical life. The expectation of confidentiality is essential to further the free exchange of information between patient and practitioner and should not be taken lightly. Patients must feel that anything they say, the nature of their disease or illness, the medications they take, or any other matter they regard as *private* will be respected.

If the pharmaceutical care practitioner displays a respectful attitude and protects privacy at all times even a nondrug-related transaction can contribute to a relationship that embodies trust and eventually has some therapeutic value. It is simple—at all times, confidentiality is the rule.

These practice responsibilities, the patient-centered approach to pharmaceutical care, and the ethical principles involved in patient care all lead to a set of standards for professional performance. Although these standards are quite self-evident, their statement in an explicit and complete manner is necessary to finish the subject of practitioner responsibilities within the philosophy of practice.

Maintaining a patient's privacy is the greatest test of the respect a practitioner gives a patient. Practitioners can claim to be fair and loyal, they can argue they are patient-centered, they can attest to a positive therapeutic relationship, and yet if the patient's privacy is not protected, then they have failed on all of these accounts. Patient confidentiality has always been a concern in health care. However, since April 14, 2003, it is of even greater concern. New patient privacy standards were developed as a result of the Health Insurance Portability and Accountability Act (HIPAA).[26] The U.S. Federal Government intervened to establish a new standard for patient confidentiality with the HIPAA requirements. These guidelines require a higher expectation and a more diligent adherence to the precept of *always protect your patient's privacy.* HIPAA regulations are designed to protect the privacy and security of individual health information. Patients have the right to request a copy of their medication information. They also have the right to amend any information that is incorrect or incomplete. Patients also have the right to request that practitioners communicate about health matters in a specific way, for example, only by mail or e-mail, or at a certain location such as only at work or only at home. See summary of HIPAA rules at http://www.hhs.gov/ocr/privacy/hipaa/understanding/summary/privacysummary.pdf.

PROFESSIONAL RESPONSIBILITY EXPRESSED AS THE STANDARDS FOR PROFESSIONAL BEHAVIOR

KEY CLINICAL CONCEPTS

Caring for others is a privilege that is reserved for those individuals who are uniquely well prepared and who adhere to standards for professional behavior.

All health care professionals are expected to learn and execute a set of behaviors that set them apart because they are working with patients to make decisions that can have significant consequences. The behavior and the standards expected are described as the Standards for Professional Behavior. New practitioners need to internalize the meaning of each standard and become comfortable with the level of expectation associated with the successful application of each standard in practice. Table 3-2 summarizes the seven professional behaviors expected of all pharmaceutical care practitioners. These standards were adapted from nursing, medicine, dentistry, and veterinary models of standards for professional behavior.[25,27]

These standards refer to the behaviors expected of practitioners who belong to an identifiable group of professionals. Each practitioner is expected not

Table 3-2   Standards of professional performance for
pharmaceutical care practitioners

Category	Standard
Quality of care	The practitioner evaluates his or her own practice in relation to professional practice standards and relevant statutes and regulations.
Ethics	The practitioner's decisions and actions on behalf of patients are determined in an ethical manner.
Collegiality	The pharmaceutical care practitioner contributes to the professional development of peers, colleagues, students, and others.
Collaboration	The practitioner collaborates with the patient, family, and/or caregivers, and health care providers in providing patient care.
Education	The practitioner acquires and maintains current knowledge in pharmacology, pharmacotherapy, and pharmaceutical care practice.
Research	The practitioner routinely uses research findings in practice and contributes to research findings when appropriate.
Resource allocation	The practitioner considers factors related to effectiveness, safety, and cost in planning and delivering patient care.

only to adhere to the standards herself but to hold her colleagues accountable for similar behavior. Even though practitioners are seldom evaluated in any formal or consistent manner, all practitioners *know* whether a colleague is able to maintain these standards in practice on a daily basis.

One of the cornerstones of a profession is that it is self-regulating. Colleagues hold other colleagues accountable for the quality of the work that is performed. This starts with self-evaluation. It is important to be reflective in practice so that each practitioner comes to know the quality of her work. This helps each practitioner improve in practice and contributes to maintaining high standards of professional performance.

The standards of professional performance applied to the practice of pharmaceutical care are described below. The criteria to measure adherence to each standard are also described. These standards should be considered constantly, reflecting on each patient encounter and making adjustments as needed to provide quality pharmaceutical care.

Standard I: Quality of Care

> **STANDARD I:** THE PRACTITIONER EVALUATES HER OWN PRACTICE IN RELATION TO PROFESSIONAL PRACTICE STANDARDS AND RELEVANT STATUTES AND REGULATIONS.
>
> **Measurement criteria**
> 1. The pharmaceutical care practitioner uses evidence from the literature to evaluate performance in practice.
> 2. The pharmaceutical care practitioner seeks peer review on a continual and frequent basis.
> 3. The pharmaceutical care practitioner utilizes data generated from practice to critically evaluate performance.

A significant amount of discussion has already focused on ethical behavior in practice. Its presence here only helps to emphasize the relative importance of this behavior. Second to providing high-quality care is providing care in an ethical manner.

Standard II: Ethics

> **STANDARD II:** THE PRACTITIONER'S DECISIONS AND ACTIONS ON BEHALF OF PATIENTS ARE DETERMINED IN AN ETHICAL MANNER.
>
> **Measurement criteria**
> 1. The practitioner maintains patient confidentiality.
> 2. The practitioner acts as a patient advocate.
> 3. The practitioner delivers care in a nonjudgmental and nondiscriminatory manner that is sensitive to patient diversity.
> 4. The practitioner delivers care in a manner that preserves/protects patient autonomy, dignity, and rights.
> 5. The practitioner seeks available resources to help formulate ethical decisions.

It is common knowledge among experienced practitioners that it is impossible to become a great practitioner without the support and assistance of colleagues. This is especially true as a patient care provider. It is impossible to know everything, experience everything and make the *right* decision in all cases. Therefore, the need to be collegial becomes absolutely necessary. In the end it serves the patient's best interest, but it also serves the practitioner's purpose as well.

Standard III: Collegiality

> **STANDARD III:** THE PHARMACEUTICAL CARE PRACTITIONER CONTRIBUTES TO THE PROFESSIONAL DEVELOPMENT OF PEERS, COLLEAGUES, AND OTHERS.
>
> **Measurement criteria**
> 1. The practitioner offers professional assistance to other practitioners whenever asked.
> 2. The practitioner supports positive relationships with patients, physicians, nurses, and other health care providers.

Patient care, perhaps more than most other activity, is collaborative. The patient is complex. Patient care is complex. The health care system is complex. Collaboration makes all of this manageable, even enjoyable. The practice of pharmaceutical care has been developed to make collaboration relatively easy and productive. Take advantage of this and become comfortable with all patient care practitioners, for the patient's benefit.

Standard IV: Collaboration

> **STANDARD IV:** THE PRACTITIONER COLLABORATES WITH THE PATIENT, FAMILY, AND HEALTH CARE PROVIDERS IN PROVIDING PATIENT CARE.
>
> **Measurement criteria**
> 1. The patient is seen as the ultimate decision maker, and the practitioner collaborates accordingly.
> 2. The practitioner collaborates with the patient's health care providers whenever it is in the best interest of the patient.

The professional behavior described as education is closely associated with the first standard of providing care. It is virtually impossible today to remain competent without a rigorous schedule of continuing education and collegial interaction. You owe it to your patient, yourself, and your colleagues to invest both time and energy in remaining current with your knowledge and competent in your skills. The volume and rate of knowledge expansion makes this a necessity today.

Standard V: Education

STANDARD V: THE PRACTITIONER ACQUIRES AND MAINTAINS CURRENT KNOWLEDGE IN PHARMACOLOGY, PHARMACOTHERAPY, AND PHARMACEUTICAL CARE PRACTICE.

Measurement criteria

1. The practitioner uses the skills of reflecting on practice to identify areas where knowledge needs to be supplemented.
2. The practitioner continually updates knowledge with journal subscriptions, current texts, practitioner interactions, and continuing education programs.

The expectation that research will serve as the basis for decision making in practice is expressed as evidence-based practice. This is a requirement when a practitioner makes decisions that will impact another person.

Because our knowledge of drug therapy, human physiology, and pathology is incomplete, clinicians make decisions in areas of uncertainty on a daily basis. The appropriate method for dealing with this is to use our knowledge well, understand the limits of the knowledge, and be able to recognize when science is inconclusive on a topic.

Standard VI: Research

STANDARD VI: THE PRACTITIONER ROUTINELY USES RESEARCH FINDINGS IN PRACTICE AND CONTRIBUTES TO RESEARCH FINDINGS WHEN APPROPRIATE.

Measurement criteria

1. The practitioner uses research results as the basis for practice.
2. The pharmaceutical care practitioner systematically reviews the literature to identify knowledge, skills, techniques, and products that are helpful in practice and implements them in a timely manner.
3. The practitioner approaches practice with a perspective to conduct applied research in practice when appropriate.

All health care resources are limited whether it be time, personnel, knowledge, or access to the latest technology. Practitioners need to recognize this, but always put the patient's best interest first.

Standard VII: Resource Allocation

STANDARD VII: THE PRACTITIONER CONSIDERS FACTORS RELATED TO EFFECTIVENESS, SAFETY, AND COST IN PLANNING AND DELIVERING PATIENT CARE.

Measurement criteria

1. The pharmaceutical care practitioner is sensitive to the financial needs and resource limitations of the patient, the health care providers, and the institutions.
2. Decisions are made by the pharmaceutical care practitioner to conserve resources and maximize the value of those resources consumed in practice.

Becoming a patient care practitioner is about being prepared to meet, and exceed when necessary, professional practice standards on behalf of the patient. These activities become part of the clinician's personality, and executing them becomes a way of life. Pharmaceutical care practitioners will come to expect this behavior of themselves and colleagues. The following represent healthy practice behaviors for pharmaceutical care practitioners.

1. Insist on knowing or learning the facts before acting or speaking (*evidence-based practice*).
2. Always follow through—find the answer by looking for unknown information immediately—*never let unknowns last.*
3. Set an example both personally and professionally. People respect you, and they will emulate you—*act like it.*
4. Be a colleague who can be trusted.
5. Hold yourself and your colleagues to the standards of practice.
6. Attend to appearance and be conscious of the impact it has on others.
7. Practice ethically.

These seem to be "common sense" and therefore we take them for granted or assume they are in place and yet these standards need to be reflected upon constantly. Patients are able to detect even the smallest deviation during a patient encounter. The purpose of personal reflection is to detect it before they do!!!

SUMMARY

The philosophy of practice is what practitioners hold to be true and right as they provide care to patients. Having this philosophy, internalizing it and applying it each time a decision is made in practice is what gives practitioners the right to care for patients. The philosophy of a professional practice outlines the ethical obligations the practitioner has to the patient; it establishes evidence as the basis for decisions made in practice; and it provides the practitioner with the legal foundation he needs to make the very difficult decisions implicit in a patient care practice. Whenever confusion or uncertainly emerges, the philosophy can be used to guide the thought process through to a logical conclusion. This philosophy is applied in practice at each step of the patient care process. This becomes especially apparent when looking more closely at the patient-centered approach found in this philosophy of practice. The next chapter investigates what is involved in patient-centeredness with an emphasis on how to apply these concepts in practice.

REFERENCES

1. Manasse HR, Jr. Medication use in an imperfect world: drug misadventuring as an issue of public policy, Part 1. *Am J Hosp Pharm.* 1989;46(5):929–944.
2. Reich WT. Historical dimensions of an ethic of care in health care. In: Reich WT, ed. *Encyclopedia of Bioethics.* New York: Macmillan; 1995.
3. Cipolle RJ. Drugs don't have doses--people have doses! A clinical educator's philosophy. *Drug Intell Clin Pharm.* 1986;20(11):881–882.
4. May R. *Existential Psychology.* New York: Random House; 1960.
5. Rogers C. *On Becoming a Person.* Boston: Houghton Mifflin; 1961.
6. Maslow AH. *Toward a Psychology of Being.* Princeton NJ: D. Van Nostrand; 1962.
7. Mayerhoff M. *On Caring.* New York: Perennial Library; 1971.
8. Gaylin W. *Caring.* New York: Avon Books; 1976.
9. Benner P. The moral dimensions of caring. In: Stevenson J, Tripp-Reimer Y, eds. *Knowledge About Care and Caring.* American Academy of Nursing; 1990.
10. Leininger M. Historic and epistemologic dimensions of care and caring with future directions. In: Stevenson J, Tripp-Reimer Y, eds. *Knowledge About Care and Caring.* American Academy of Nursing; 1990.
11. Hepler CD, Strand LM. Opportunities and responsibilities in pharmaceutical care. *Am J Hosp Pharm.* 1990;47(3):533–543.
12. Cooper MC. Covenant relationships: grounding for the nursing ethic. *ANS Adv Nurs Sci.* 1988;10(4):48–59.
13. Bishop AH, Scudder JR. Dialogical care and nursing practice. In: Chinn P, ed. *Anthology of Caring.* National League of Nursing; 1988.
14. Guttman N. *Public Health Communication Interventions.* Thousands Oaks, CA: Sage Publications; 2000.
15. Bukhardt MA, Nathaniel AK. *Ethics and Issues in Contemporary Nursing.* New York: Delmar; 2002.

16. Simon SB, Howe L, Howard K. *Values Clarification: A Handbook of Practical Strategies for Teachers and Students.* New York: Hart; 1995.
17. Towsley-Cook DM, Young TA. *Ethical and Legal Issues for Imaging Professional.* St. Louis, MO: Mosby; 1999.
18. Husted GL, Husted JH. *Ethical Decision-Making in Nursing and Health Care.* 3rd ed. New York: Springer; 2001.
19. Hebert PC. *Doing Right: A Practical Guide to Ethics for Medical Trainees and Physicians.* Toronto: Oxford University Press; 1996.
20. Tindall WN, Beardsley RS, Kimberlin CL. *Communication Skills in Pharmacy Practice: A Practical Guide for Students and Practitioners.* 3rd ed. Malvern, PA: Lea & Febiger; 1994.
21. Lipkin MH, Putman SM, Lazare A, et al. *The Medical Interview: Clinical Care, Education, and Research.* New York: Springer; 1995.
22. Cole SA, Bird J. In: Schmitt W, ed. *The Medical Interview: The Three-Function Approach.* St. Louis, MO: Mosby; 2000.
23. Jonsen AR, Siegler M, Winslade WJ. *Clinical Ethics: A Practical Approach to Ethical Decisions in Clinical Medicine.* 5th ed. New York: McGraw-Hill; 2002.
24. Parrish II, RH. *Defining Drugs: How Government Became the Arbiter of Pharmaceutical Fact.* New Brunswick: Transaction; 2003.
25. ANA. *Standards of Clinical Nursing Practice.* Kansas City, MO: American Nurses Association; 1991.
26. HIPAA. In: USDHH Services, ed. *The Standards for Privacy of Individually Identifiable Health Information "Privacy Rule".* Washington, DC: OCP Privacy Rules; 1996.
27. Wilkinson JM. *Nursing Process: A Critical Thinking Approach.* 2nd ed. Menlo Park, CA: Addison-Wesley Nursing; 1992.

chapter four

Patient-Centeredness in Pharmaceutical Care

⚷ KEY CONCEPTS

1   Patient-centered behavior includes a number of constructs, but the most important one is that the patient comes first.

2   What the patient wants and needs is what drives the patient encounter.

3   Little can be accomplished until the practitioner understands the patient's concept of his illness and his medication experience, in the patient's words, so listen closely.

4   The therapeutic relationship is a partnership or alliance between the practitioner and the patient for the very specific purpose of optimizing the patient's medication experience.

5   The quality of the care provided will depend on the quality of the therapeutic relationship developed because the relationship will impact the information shared, the decisions made, and what you can learn from the patient.

6   The patient has both rights and responsibilities; practitioners must attend to both.

7   Adherence to a medication regimen is a test of the practitioner's ability to practice in a patient-centered manner.

8   Medication management services, when provided in a patient-centered manner, can achieve adherence rates of over 80%, consistently, because of the active participation of the patient.

9   Patient-centered adherence can be achieved when the practitioner takes into account the patient's individual needs, his rights, his responsibilities, and the practitioner's obligation to make decisions in a consistent, systematic, and comprehensive manner for each individual patient.

DEFINING PATIENT-CENTEREDNESS

The concept of patient-centeredness can be a difficult idea to "get your arms around," which makes it hard to operationalize it in practice. Because it is a concept that reflects so many general "feelings" among other things, it is important to ask, "Where do I begin to ensure I practice in a patient-centered manner"? Oliveira and Shoemaker provide a useful framework for thinking about this question.[1]

Fortunately, when you practice pharmaceutical care, you will always think in a specific, structured order. What you do for each patient has a clearly defined beginning, middle, and end.

> **KEY CLINICAL CONCEPTS**
>
> The order of thinking, making decisions and acting always is patient first, medical condition (diagnosis) second, and medications third.

This may seem a bit counterintuitive because this practice is mostly about medications; however, in order to get the medications right, you must understand that the patient-specific context in which you are going to make your decisions is most important. This translates in practice, to understanding what your patient wants and needs before you address their medical conditions and medications. This is why a physician starts a patient interview with, "What can I do for you today?" Only after the physician understands what is most important to the patient—why the patient came to see the physician—does he begin to understand the medical problem at hand. This is true in pharmaceutical care practice also. This is a service so what the patient wants is most important.

In order to understand what the patient wants and needs, it is necessary to understand how the patient thinks about his illness and his medications. What the patient thinks is usually different than what the physician or the pharmacist thinks; in fact, they tend to be so different that we call the patient's perspective, the illness, and the physician's perspective, the disease. We call the patient's perspective on medications, his medication experience, whereas we call the pharmacist's perspective on medications, pharmacotherapeutics. Remember how we argued in Chapter 2 that language matters? It makes all the difference. So, if we are going to practice in a truly patient-centered manner, then we will begin by understanding what our patient wants, what their concept of illness is, and perhaps most importantly in pharmaceutical care practice, what the patient's medication experience is. This is all explained below.

UNDERSTANDING THE PATIENT'S CONCEPT OF ILLNESS

To a physician or pharmacist, the collection of symptoms or laboratory values results in a diagnosis, which reflects a particular disease, ailment, or syndrome. To a patient, however, this is experienced as an "illness" as it is the patient's lived experience and has associated with it, many consequences, some negative and some positive. In fact, when the medical provider decides not to take the time to understand the meaning of the patient's illness, then a number of negative outcomes can result.

> The systematic inattention to illness is in part responsible for patient noncompliance, patient and family dissatisfaction with professional health care, and inadequate clinical care.[2]

Therefore, in order to understand how we might best utilize medications to treat a patient we must first understand how the patient thinks about his health and his illnesses. When we discuss health with patients, their attitude tends to be either positive or negative. In the cases it is positive, it is usually focused on the "ideal state." Such a notion is central to the old and well-worn definition offered in 1946 by the World Health Organization:

> Health is a state of complete physical, mental, and social well-being and not merely the absence of disease and infirmity.[3]

Until one becomes ill, this concept of health is frequently held by patients. And when asked about their health, patients often refer to their functional status and their ability to cope with life. This has significant meaning in different cultural contexts and is important to know when conducting interviews and assessments. In the second sense—the negative dimension—individuals see health as primarily the absence of disease, disability, and most certainly symptoms of pain and discomfort. The individual with this negative perspective on health will often focus entirely on symptoms, and the underlying causes of the problem can get lost in the search for specific treatment of generalized symptoms. So, an individual's conceptualization of a "healthy state" tells us something about his beliefs, values, attitudes, and expectations about illness. Moreover, this also serves as an introduction to what he will do to "fix" the problem he brings to the clinic.

Discussions on the general topic of health are valuable in that they allow the clinician to obtain important information about health behavior, ideas of wellness, and often reveal motives and past methods used to maintain what is considered to be a healthy state. Clearly this can be of considerable importance as you are developing a therapeutic relationship with the patient and working to involve the patient in his care plan. It will be very useful to understand what matters most in maintaining one's health to determine appropriate interventions to achieve the patient's goals of therapy when illness occurs.

Brown, Weston, and Steward[4] provide a particularly useful set of four dimensions that illuminate the relationship between illness experience and behavior. These dimensions can be directly related to the patient's medication experience and the drug therapy problems that are identified. They are as follows:

1. What are the patient's *ideas* about their illness? What meaning do they attach to the illness experience? Many persons endure illness as an irreparable loss; others may view it as an opportunity to gain valuable insight into their life experience. Is the illness seen as a form of punishment or, perhaps, as an opportunity for dependency? Whatever the illness, knowing it's meaning is paramount for understanding the patient.

2. What are the patient's *feelings*? Do the patients fear that the symptoms they present may be the precursor of a more serious problem such as cancer? Some patients may feel a sense of relief and view the illness as an opportunity for respite from demands or responsibilities. Patients often feel angry or guilty about being ill.

3. What are the *expectations* of the [clinician]? Does the presentation of a sore throat carry with it an expectation of penicillin? Do they want the [clinician] to do something or just listen?

4. What are the effects of the illness on *function*? Does it limit patients' daily activities? Does it impart their family relationships? Does it require a change in lifestyle?

At one level the meaning of an illness experience can be seen to be subjective and devoid of empirical considerations derived from the usual medical paradigms. A large part of the problem is to be found in the confusion between the concepts of "illness" and "disease." Disease is the physiological condition analyzed, interpreted, and diagnosed largely through the empirics of medicine. Illness, on the other hand, is the individual's experience of disease. In the case of medication experience we find both the empirical pharmacological agent imposed, and the subjective cognitive, emotional, sensate, experiences of the individual, who may or may not, take the medicine as prescribed. Either way, the individual in question experiences something and probably has a history of medication experience locked away inside of him or her.

KEY CLINICAL CONCEPTS

Patients have stories to tell and much to teach us. Their narratives open up a vast mine of usable information that can be used in formulating a care plan.

However, this only becomes meaningful, in a broad sense, when what the patient experiences and articulates is actually heard and used to benefit the patient. Listening to the patient reflect on sensations, emotions, anxieties, fears, and other manifestations of illness experience, and the therapeutic encounter, is essential if resolution is to occur. The narrative offered by the patient is an attempt to find meaning in illness and its treatment. It is a process directed toward understanding "what is going on." Thus, while it is often the case that meanings and experiences of illness are different for patient and clinician, there is a common purpose to understand what is actually "going on" from the patient's perspective.

Clinicians collect patient information. We take "histories" that with varying degrees of detail, depth, and comprehension we construct charts, which become the patient's "biography," a biography that often becomes the single foundation for all interventions. Now electronic devices have largely replaced paper records, but the quality of information gathered continues to depend on the quality of the interview, the nature of the questions asked and the answers given. Many times we record a few answers to what we consider vital, clinically relevant questions. The central problem here is that we ask and the patient answers. However, what we are looking for is more of an autobiography not a biography almost entirely constructed by a clinical "author."

We clinicians must avoid the situation where there is little dialogue and the patient is afforded little opportunity to "tell his story." By this we mean that the patient's story is usually much deeper than the typical clinical questions reveal. Kleinman's classic work *The Illness Narratives*[2] reveals the magnitude of this frequent tension between patient and clinician. Not all patients become in-depth *cases* with their input at center stage.

In any therapeutic encounter both patient and clinician attempt to impose order on what frequently appears to be "chaos." There is an attempt to make sense out of the multiplicity of signs, symptoms, and expressions of distress uttered by the patient. As Kleinman avers the "problem of illness as suffering raises two fundamental questions for the sick person and the social group: Why me? (the question of bafflement), and What can be done? (the question of order and control)." Patients have their own explanatory models of their illness. They have a story to tell about its causes, its duration, when it was first noticed, its possible outcomes, and how these will impact daily life.[2]

Also, it is not unusual to hear about treatment options from patients. This last theme has become noticeably more prevalent in the age of the Internet. Patients do their own "research" and arrive armed with beliefs, ideas, and specific information that they "found on the WEB" and which serve to enhance or elaborate their stories. The patient's explanatory model is an essential part of the therapeutic relationship. As we have repeatedly stated, it is imperative that the clinician understands the patient's explanatory model in order to meet on common ground and identify those parts of the story that will become clinically relevant to both parties and form the foundation for impending treatment. Sacks,[5] a physician, who became a patient, says it well:

> There were some difficulties about the "history" because they wanted to know the "salient facts" and I wanted to tell them everything, the entire story. Besides, I wasn't quite certain what might or might not be "salient" in the circumstances.

KEY CLINICAL CONCEPTS

Patient input, their personal stories, should become a central part of any medical and pharmacy history.

A collaborative partnership where the patients' story is heard and their conception of illness examined, leads to better treatment and more positive outcomes. Illness experience generally, and the medication experience in particular, both benefit from shared understanding. The underlying assumptions of both patient and clinician should be made explicit and critically examined by all concerned as they are incorporated into the treatment plan. Such mutual understanding can only improve treatment and adherence to any collaborative plan of action.

THE PATIENT'S MEDICATION EXPERIENCE

The medication experience is a relatively new concept in health care. Practitioners, as discussed a propos of the illness experience, have always completed medication histories and created medication records that list drug therapies taken in the past or are currently being taken. But, providers have not traditionally sought and utilized information from the patient about (1) how the patient *feels* about taking her medications, (2) how a patient makes her decisions about whether to take a medication or not, and, how she will actually take it. This level of inquiry requires time and attention to the details involved in the comprehensive management of a patient's medications. The work of Oliveira and Shoemaker has added important depth to our discussion of the medication experience.[6–8]

For quite some time physicians have recognized the need to understand the patient's interpretation, understanding, and feelings about her disease. Recall that this is illness experience and illness behavior, as discussed previously. So too must the pharmaceutical care practitioner understand the patient's perception of her medication and the impact these medications are having on her life. This is called the patient's medication experience.[6]

> **Definition** The *patient's medication experience* is the sum of all the events a patient has in his lifetime that involve drug therapy. This is the patient's personal experience with medications. This lived experience shapes his attitudes, beliefs, and preferences about drug therapy.

The patient's medication experience reveals how patients make personal decisions about medications. It includes the evidence of medications that were effective, and those that failed in the past, and it tells you what drug therapy is currently prescribed and how the patient is actually taking it, or, as the case may be, not taking it. There is no more important information about your patient than the medication experience. Because it describes his attitudes and beliefs about medications, it has a very powerful influence on the outcomes of drug therapy. In fact, a practitioner cannot make sound clinical decisions without a good understanding of the patient's medication experience.

> **KEY CLINICAL CONCEPTS**
>
> The patient's medication experience is the patient's personal approach to the use of medicines—why he believes or feels a certain way about drug therapy.

Some patients have little or no well-formed medication experience, others who have taken numerous medications may have developed distinct beliefs or preferences and habits. It is shaped by patients' traditions, religion, culture, and what they have heard and learned from others. All of these factors and others will influence whether patients take a medication or not, how they will use the medication, whether they believe it will be effective, and whether they believe the medication will be harmful. The patient's medication experience influences the confidence she has in your abilities to help, whether you are an experienced clinician or this is your first encounter.

Some patients will express a high level of frustration with past drug therapies that have failed to produce any benefit. This negative experience can influence that patient's expectations of your recommended drug therapy unless you recognize and directly address the individual's negative impressions. Also, patients may prefer not to use medications while at work or at school or during religious observances. Incorporating patient preferences into your pharmacotherapy decisions can greatly enhance adherence and outcomes.

The patient's medication experience can be strongly influenced by others including friends and family members. This is especially true of individuals who have little or no personal experience with medications. It is not only helpful to become familiar with your patient's understanding and beliefs concerning medications, but also learn how others influence those beliefs. Always consider these issues within the context of the particular individual's life experiences and world view.

> ### KEY CLINICAL CONCEPTS
>
> Your primary responsibility as a pharmaceutical care practitioner is to improve each patient's medication experience—to make it better than it was before you provided care.

The medication experience is the context in which you will do all of this work, and it is the portion of the patient's life you will influence most. Remember, each patient has a highly personal medication experience. Some patients will have a very short, concise medication experience because they are young, they have taken very few medications, or they have never been ill. Others, especially the elderly with multiple medical conditions, will have an extensive medication experience and require a significant amount of time to communicate it to you. Patience and empathy are of considerable value here.

Sometimes, these specific beliefs or preferences concern only a limited scope of pharmacotherapy, such as a patient with a chronic back ailment who has endured numerous therapeutic attempts with nonsteroidal anti-inflammatory drugs (NSAIDs) and now feels these medications will not be effective to manage her back pain. It will not be useful to make assumptions about your patient's medication experience or to generalize from one patient's experience to another. Taking the time to understand each patient's individual medication experience is a valuable investment in your time. Not putting forth the effort to understand a patient's medication experience will impede your decision-making ability and reduce the likelihood of your patient experiencing positive outcomes.

Some patients have strong religious beliefs that inhibit them from taking oral contraceptives to prevent pregnancy. Others may rely on traditional or folk medicines to maintain health and only seek conventional pharmacotherapy for acute illnesses. Practitioners learn to make decisions in all of these unique patient contexts. It is the reason each patient must be treated as an individual.

Understanding the Patient's Medication Experience in Practice

The first step to managing a patient's medications is to elicit the patient's medication experience. As we emphasized earlier, listen intently to the patient's story. Let us consider which pieces of the patient's story you will want to "target":

- What is the patient's general attitude toward taking medication?
- To what extent does the patient understand her medications?
- What does the patient want/expect from her drug therapy?
- What concerns does the patient have about her drug therapy?
- Are there cultural, religious, or ethical issues that influence the patient's willingness to take medications?
- What is the patient's medication taking behavior?

These are the some of the questions you will use to learn of your patient's medication experience. It is useful to take the time to understand the meaning behind each one.

Patient's general attitude toward taking medications   Keep in mind that the patient's medication experience represents the sum total of the impact of events in the patient's life that have formed the patient's impressions, beliefs, concerns, understanding, and preferences about the use of medications to manage specific health problems. Over time and with experience, patients develop attitudes toward and beliefs about drug therapy generally and the medications they are taking specifically. Negative attitudes and beliefs that patients may develop include "Drugs don't work, they only cause more problems," or "I don't take medications." Overly positive attitudes include "There must be a drug I can take to solve this problem." For example, individuals who use herbs may have a less positive perception of the safety of prescription therapies and a more favorable attitude regarding the impact of herbs on their health.[9-11] The word "natural" frequently is used to denote "safe"—a much misleading interpretation and a possibly dangerous one at that.

These beliefs and attitudes work to establish specific preferences that each patient has about taking medications. These preferences will directly impact whether or not a patient will take medication and how she will take the mediation. It is likely that you will need to influence the patient's attitudes and beliefs about drug therapy. It is also necessary to know what your patient believes before you attempt to change those beliefs or attitudes.

Patient's understanding of drug therapy The patient may present with a thorough and comprehensive understanding of all her drug therapies or may understand very little about the medications. Other patients will know more than you do about both their disease and their drug therapy. Your patient's level of understanding will determine the extent to which you will need to educate and explain effectiveness and safety instructions. Experienced practitioners are certain to elicit the patient's level of understanding before embarking on a time-consuming patient drug information and education campaign. Achieving the patient's goals of therapy depends on the patient having a clear understanding of why each medication is being taken, the name of each medication (in a way the patient understands), the dosage and dosing schedule for each medication, the clinical and laboratory measures that will be used to determine a successful outcome, and the clinical and laboratory measures that can be used to detect if any safety/risk issues occur. The pharmaceutical care practitioner must elicit enough information from the patient to determine how well she understands medications.

Patient's "wants" and expectations Establishing what your patient wants is the most productive place to begin an assessment. This is for two common-sense reasons. In order to provide a service that a patient feels is valuable, it must be perceived to be doing what she wants it to do. The best way to determine what another person wants is to ask. The other, and more pragmatic reason to begin an assessment by determining what your patient wants, is that virtually all patients already know, in varying measures, what this is. Every patient who walks into a clinic, an office, or a pharmacy is there for a purpose.

Some people may have difficulty describing what they want in terms that the practitioner can fully understand. Some may be hesitant to share their goals with someone with whom they have not yet established a strong therapeutic relationship. Some may feel as though what they want is not very important to the practitioner. Some patients may feel that the practitioner is too busy with other issues to deal with their personal concerns.

You may experience all of these situations in your practice, but it is important to reiterate that all patients you care for have a good idea of what they really want. The better you are at discovering what that is, the better you will serve your patients. If you provide services that people want, you will engender their loyalty. If you can determine what your patients want and reassure them that you intend to help them achieve a positive experience from their medications, then patients will have full confidence that you have their best interest in mind. This establishes the basis for the trust that is required to build a strong therapeutic relationship. It also assures your patient that you intend to be comprehensive in your care. A caveat: remember that sometimes what a patient wants is not necessarily what he needs. Needs and wants must be differentiated and resolved. Discuss these distinctly different issues with the patient.

For example, in the situation when the patient describes that she wants to "not have to take so many pills every day," the practitioner should make every effort to minimize the number or frequency of doses she is required to take every day. During the assessment, the practitioner may determine that other clinically important drug therapy problems need to be resolved; however, it is still important to address the patient's original stated request to reduce daily doses. There will be plenty of opportunity to interpret what the patient wants relative to your professional decision of what is needed, later in the assessment. However, if you fail to determine what your patient wants from her medications, you have no reference point, no starting place.

Patient concerns   Patients frequently express what they want in terms of concerns they have about the medication itself or how it must be taken.[12] Such concerns are frequently the reason they want to see a pharmaceutical care practitioner. Common concerns include risks of taking a certain medication, side effects experienced, and confusion over how to take a medication or why it is being taken. Concerns can be more expansive if the patient is afraid to take medications in general because of previous problems experienced. It is important to know all of a patient's concerns because they have a dramatic impact on the patient's medication taking behavior. Furthermore, patients who feel that their concerns are not being attended to by the practitioner often do not take medications as intended. Concerns related to medications are a major cause of nonadherence. Past experiences with medications have a significant impact on the patient's willingness to take them in the future, so take the time required to address this important issue.

For example, the patient may be afraid to take an antibiotic because a friend or another family member once had a bad experience with a drug that was also used to treat an infection. Even if the two antibiotics are completely different, such as amoxicillin and erythromycin, and even if the infections were different, such as pneumonia and urinary tract infection, you must recognize and address this patient concern to have a successful outcome. A concerned patient could raise highly controversial and ideological issues such as vaccines and autism. Be prepared to fully present the facts and listen to the patient's concerns.

Cultural, ethical, and religious issues   The impact that society has on shaping individual attitudes and beliefs has been widely documented and broadly accepted.[12-18] Therefore, it is important to understand the social context of each patient. Within that social context lie religious beliefs, traditions, and social expectations that can all impact a patient's attitudes and beliefs about the efficacy of the medication, its appropriateness, and the proper way to administer it. Again, this information is relevant because it shapes the patient's medication taking behavior or compliance. Practitioners frequently need to influence this behavior to optimize the patient's response to medications. Additionally, the practitioner must accommodate religious practices, traditional beliefs, and cultural norms that may be very different from her own. All of these belief systems may directly influence a patient's willingness to comply with the recommended drug therapy. Unfamiliarity with issues or differences in views commonly introduces ethical dilemmas into practice. For example, many Native Americans value a process of group decision making by the family that may need to be balanced with the concept of personal autonomy.[19]

Ethical dilemmas do not have to be negative experiences. They can serve as discussion topics between the practitioner and the patient. It is important to emphasize that the patient is always the final decision maker, and he must give consent to the practitioner's influence on whether and how to take a drug product.

Patient's medication taking behavior   All of the previous components of a patient's medication experience—a patient's expectations, values, concerns, understanding, beliefs, attitudes, preferences, culture, and religion—can influence what is described as the patient's medication taking behavior. A patient's medication taking behavior describes the decisions a patient makes and acts upon related to the use of drug products and dosage regimens. These behaviors include whether a patient chooses to obtain and take the medication, how the patient takes the medication, whether the patient chooses to refill a prescription, or if the patient chooses to adhere to the regimen. These behaviors frequently need to be positively reinforced to obtain the desired results from therapy. Some patients may not believe that the drug therapy the clinician recommended will work. Therefore, the patient may not even have the prescription filled or purchase the product. The practitioner needs this information to make good decisions. Some portions of your patient's description of her medication experience may be confusing or missing. Complicated brand and generic names, complex dosing schedules, and multiple instructions can all contribute to a patient having incomplete information or recall about the medication and how it was taken. It will require both time and patience to elicit this information.

Utilizing the Patient's Medication Experience to Optimize Therapeutic Outcomes

Pharmaceutical care, as a practice, cannot function without the practitioner having a firm grasp of the patient's medication experiences revealed by the patient himself. Without a clear detailed knowledge of the patient's past experiences, present wants and needs, and future aspirations and expectations, clinicians can, and do, make mistakes. One can readily see how adherence levels can sink so low when little of this information is sought and integrated into a care plan. Empowering the patient to proactively place himself "in charge" of his treatment, and assume the life-supporting responsibility of what is usually termed "self-care" is essential to positive outcomes. To think of this in a more mundane manner, consider the simple act of selecting paint for someone's house without asking or caring what his preferences are, what colors he likes or doesn't like. Although the consequences of drug preference and paint preference may differ in degree of risk, there is in both cases a required rational decision-making process, and we might add, a courtesy that should be followed.

Clearly, few clinicians will elicit or understand all (or sufficient) information concerning the medication experience in the beginning of their career. But, such information gathering is an ongoing enterprise, and each patient's biography will develop and become more illustrative as time passes and the clinician's skills improve. Remember, communication skills can and will improve as trust and an empathic caring self is revealed to the patient. Completing an assessment with any degree of meaning, acceptable to both patients and clinician, is very difficult with little shared frame of reference. Some say "talk is cheap," but it may be the most valuable asset a clinician has at his disposal. Chapter 6 will continue this discussion in reference to the specifics of conducting an assessment of a patient's medication needs.

THE PRACTITIONER AND THE PATIENT FORM A RELATIONSHIP

The ability of the practitioner to elicit the information described above depends on establishing a meaningful relationship with the patient where personal, intimate feelings and beliefs can be shared. This is, indeed, a special relationship that is developed only with a patient care provider. This relationship is one of the most important "tools" a practitioner can have when practicing pharmaceutical care. In fact, it is our experience that the quality of care you are able to provide will depend entirely on the nature of the therapeutic relationship you develop with each patient.

The Therapeutic Relationship Defined

The relationship that develops between the patient and the practitioner is termed *the therapeutic relationship*.

> **Definition**   The therapeutic relationship is a partnership or alliance between the practitioner and the patient formed for the purpose of optimizing the patient's medication experience.[20]

The therapeutic relationship requires recognition of certain responsibilities on the part of the patient and the practitioner. It is based on trust, respect, authenticity, empathy, and commitment. We use the term *therapeutic* because this distinguishes it from other relationships including familial, friendly, customer, or professional. The therapeutic relationship has the specific purpose of facilitating the exchange of information and expertise so that patients can achieve the best possible results from drug therapies. The first function of the face-to-face interaction with the patient is to build and maintain an effective therapeutic relationship. Although it may be more difficult, a therapeutic relationship is also necessary if the care is provided telephonically. This will take additional skill and practice.

An effective relationship takes the form of a partnership with the patient. This partnership serves as the foundation for the entire assessment process as well as future follow-up evaluations. There will always be a relationship between practitioner and patient, and it is your responsibility to maintain the quality of that relationship. A good therapeutic relationship means that you can provide good care to your patient, whereas an excellent therapeutic relationship allows you to provide excellent care. Therefore, it should come as no surprise that a badly maintained therapeutic relationship often results in unsatisfied patients and even litigation. The therapeutic relationship can make this much of a difference.

The nature of the information that is shared by your patient can be quite technical, often personal, occasionally embarrassing, and frequently difficult to describe. Therefore, the therapeutic relationship must be supported by trust, honesty, cooperation, sensitivity, empathy, and confidentiality. It will take time to develop a relationship with these qualities, but the continuous nature of pharmaceutical care practice facilitates the establishment and growth of a positive therapeutic relationship. Achieving a positive therapeutic relationship is an active rather than passive process. It is an act of caring for and about a person. It focuses on the whole person and not simply a biological specimen, organ system, disease state, or drug product in any reductionist sense.

Therapeutic relationships will vary because each patient is different, and each practitioner is different. However, there are certain characteristics and behaviors that facilitate building the therapeutic relationship with your patient. There are characteristics about yourself and behaviors toward your patient that make a noticeable difference in the quality of relationship that can be built. These are listed in Table 4-1.

This list includes characteristics and behaviors that are central to the philosophy and practice of pharmaceutical care. The therapeutic relationship links a practitioner's philosophy of practice to the real world of the patient.

Table 4-1 Characteristics and behaviors associated with the therapeutic relationship

Characteristics about yourself	Behaviors you manifest toward your patient
Honesty/authenticity/open communication	Putting the patient's needs first
Empathy/sensitivity	Offering reassurance Seeing the patient as a person
Patience and understanding	Mutual respect/trust
Competence	Cooperation/collaboration
Assuming responsibility for interventions	Caring
Being held accountable for the decisions and recommendation made	Building confidence Supporting the patient Offering advocacy Paying attention to the patient's physical and emotional comfort

In essence, the relationship with the patient is how a practitioner brings his philosophy of practice to the care that is provided.

The Importance of the Therapeutic Relationship

All practitioners should make every attempt to create a collaborative, patient-centered, therapeutic relationship with their patients. Foremost in this relationship is good communication and a thorough evaluation of patient feedback. For the clinician (physician, pharmacist, nurse, physician assistant, etc.), the centrality of the patient, her autonomy, and self-determination are critical to the care provided. Understanding what these concepts mean and their problems or possible limitations (e.g., cognitively impaired individuals) is essential to forming a therapeutic relationship. The ability to (a) note nonverbal cues, (b) listen attentively, (c) focus critically and reflexively on all information exchanged, (d) pay attention to all emotions displayed and see these as an important part of any communicative act, (e) provide feedback promptly, and (f) develop a level of trust that becomes an integral part of the therapeutic regimen are all indispensable components of a caring culture.

Dialogue is therapeutic! Patient preferences and clinician recommendations can conflict. Patient preferences must be heard and respected, and when appropriate, integrated into any treatment plan. When values, ideas, and recommendations conflict without finding a resolution for them, nonadherence is possible. The issues in question must be discussed and to the best of everyone's ability resolved. What is the patient's preference based on? What does the clinician prefer? If there is any conflict, can it be worked out to everyone's satisfaction? If not, why not? Are the patient's preferences rational, logical, or harmful? Can the clinician examine her preferences and recommendations addressing the same questions?

In any therapeutic relationship there is a "search for meaning," sometimes deeply philosophical, often at a more pragmatic level emphasizing what patients refer to as "commonsense," and frequently involving highly personal experiences even of a spiritual nature.[2] Everyone tries to make sense of their experiences. Patients bring to the therapeutic arena a considerable amount of experience, both good and bad, and seek answers to many troubling questions. Illness is transformative, as is medication taking. It changes worldviews, attitudes, expectations, values, conceptions of self, and many other attributes that define the afflicted and influence those whose purpose it is to offer assistance. Indeed, some illnesses define a significant part of identity as in: "I'm a diabetic" or, "I'm an epileptic." Such power of transformation and ascription found in the illness and medication experience cannot be ignored. Oliveira reveals this and more in her work with patients receiving pharmaceutical care services.[21]

> **KEY CLINICAL CONCEPTS**
>
> The time and effort invested in developing strong therapeutic rela-
> tionships will serve you well in practice. This relationship will make
> it easier to elicit necessary information from the patient, positively
> influence the patient's decisions, and learn from the patient.

The Patient as the Primary Source of Information

In all patient care practices the patient is the primary source of information.
The patient either knows everything the practitioner needs to learn about the
case or has primary access to the necessary information. Often we think of
the medical chart, laboratory values, or the physician as the primary source of
information, but all of these sources are secondary to the patient herself. The
medical chart is often a translation of patient information.

Laboratory values can be helpful, and whenever we need them, we can
obtain them from the patient or request that the patient obtain them from
the physician's office. Often we can generate the data firsthand in practice by
gathering it ourselves (i.e., blood pressure, glucose, cholesterol), or by ordering the test directly from the laboratory.

The stronger your therapeutic relationship is with the patient, the more
likely you can gather all of the personal medication use and history information necessary to make sound clinical decisions.

> **KEY CLINICAL CONCEPTS**
>
> One of the most important results of a positive therapeutic rela-
> tionship between a patient and a practitioner is the shared deci-
> sion making applied to goals of therapy.

Goals of therapy establish the direction, the intensity, the risks, and even
the duration of drug therapies to be employed. Negotiation and agreement
between patient and practitioner must be accomplished for positive outcomes
to be possible. Through the therapeutic relationship, patients must be willing
to participate in establishing achievable goals of therapy.

It would be a mistake to underestimate the value of the patient's input into
the assessment of drug-related needs and the identification and resolution of
drug therapy problems. Over 75% of all drug therapy problems identified and
resolved in pharmaceutical care practice are resolved directly with the patient.

This is similar to other primary care providers in which the vast majority of issues are resolved between patient and practitioner. The quality of the therapeutic relationship will greatly impact your ability to accomplish these objectives.

The Patient as Decision Maker

The patient is the ultimate decision maker in his or her health care. This is especially true for drug therapy decisions. Prescribers decide only what medication and dosage regimen to suggest, and the patient makes all the other decisions. Patients decide what medications—both prescription and nonprescription—they will actually take and what they will not. Patients also decide how much to take, how frequently to take it, and how long they will continue to take it. Because only the medication that the patient *decides to take* has an impact on the patient's condition, the patient's decision-making process is very important to understand.

The practitioner has to positively influence the patient's decisions to create a positive medication experience. This requires a good therapeutic relationship. If you ever have difficulty influencing your patient's decisions about drug therapy, reevaluate your relationship with the patient. It usually holds at least part of the explanation.

The relationship between a patient and a health care professional should always be therapeutic in its most literal sense. We are always striving to help the patient achieve the most positive therapeutic results possible. However, drug therapy can be dangerous or frightening. It can be confusing. It can be distressing to some patients. These emotions are implicit in the pharmaceutical care process, and therefore, a significant portion of what the practitioner contributes to the patient is made possible only through a close, respectful, mutually rewarding therapeutic relationship. In situations of uncertainty, it will help to recall direction provided by Cipolle: "Treat each patient as you would treat your own grandmother."[22]

The Patient as Teacher

Practitioners will learn more from their patients than they learn from most textbooks. Books, professors, and experts can teach you a significant amount, but only your patient can teach you what you need to know about himself and the impact drug therapy has. Never assume your patient has the same values and views about his drug therapy as you do. Learn what the patient's views are and use his information to develop better goals and assure positive outcomes. Patients have a wealth of information about their diseases and drug therapy. This is especially true for patients with chronic diseases. Not only have they lived the experience firsthand, but they can often describe how drug therapy actually impacts their daily lives.

Patients frequently have multiple medical problems and are using several medications. Each patient presents a new combination or mixture of diseases, illnesses, personal characteristics, and drug therapies. This is an experience we can retrieve only from the patient. You will benefit tremendously if you allow your patients to teach you about their diseases and their drug therapy. It is an efficient and effective way to learn. In contrast to material learned from a textbook, practitioners retain all that they learn from their patients. The asset that allows you to learn optimally from your patients is a strong therapeutic relationship.

Pharmaceutical care practice, like all other patient care practices, includes a qualified practitioner, a patient in need, and the work that occurs between them.

All of the work focuses on the patient. Although you will collaborate with the patient's other providers and caregivers to ensure that she receives coordinated care in an efficient manner, your responsibility is to the patient.

The Patient's Rights

In a patient-centered practice, the patient's rights and responsibilities will be foremost in our mind as we make decisions. They will be primary as we consider the actions to be taken, and will not be relegated to a piece of paper that is posted on the wall in the waiting room. A patient-centered practitioner is cognizant of what the patient has a right to expect and what their responsibilities include.

What the Patient Can Expect

Although your patient may not have previously experienced pharmaceutical care, he or she will have received care from other health care practitioners and will have learned to expect certain behaviors from a clinician. These expectations often remain unspoken; however, you can be certain that your patients will look for the following behaviors from you each time care is provided. These expectations and your ability to meet them will have a significant impact on the quality of the therapeutic relationship you will develop with your patient.

Patients expect you to care about what they want

Experienced practitioners acknowledge what the patient wants and address these wants directly. Patients may not be able to express what this is in the most sophisticated clinical terms, and they may not have the same understanding as you regarding what would be therapeutically best, but they know what they want. When patients feel they are getting what they want, they are usually satisfied. *Patients only care how much you know, when they know how much you care.* There will be times when what your patient wants conflicts with what you consider to be in the patient's best interest. Successful resolution of these dilemmas requires that you put the patient first. What you think your patient needs is applied in the context of what your patient wants, what your patient expects, and what your patient is willing to do.

Patients will expect you to put their needs first, before your own
Patients expect their drug-related needs to dictate what you do and when you do it. Patients' needs establish your priorities and direct your clinical activities. When you fully recognize that your patient's needs are the focus of what you do, you will understand what it means to have a patient-centered practice. This is the cornerstone of pharmaceutical care practice.

Patients expect compassion and understanding of them as individuals
All patients are different. Each has unique beliefs, experiences, emotions, and understandings of health and the use of medications. Patient care practitioners hold the patient's personal beliefs and customs in high regard. You will have to be informed about patients' beliefs and customs from many different cultural backgrounds because the decisions you will make must be sensitive to them and reflect your patient's wishes. Taking time to understand the individual patient's medication experience will demonstrate your interest in the patient.

The patient expects you to possess the technical knowledge and the clinical experience and confidence it takes to apply that knowledge to their individual case
Compassion is only part of what the patient expects. You must be competent in your work. The patient will expect a similar experience and level of service from all pharmaceutical care practitioners. Patients should be able to expect practitioners to have and to meet specific practice standards that are consistently and comprehensively applied to all patients. Patients will expect pharmaceutical care practitioners to be competent at what they do, to create a written record of the care that is provided, and to follow-up to verify that the desired goals of therapy have been achieved. When you see a patient for the second time, he or she will expect you to remember what was said and done the last time—or at least to have a written record of it.

Patients expect to receive the appropriate medication for their medical problems, and they expect the medication to work

Because you have the knowledge and skills to meet this expectation, patients have a right to expect you to do whatever is necessary to ensure that they achieve the results they want from their medication. They expect you to provide this without taking unnecessary risks in the process. This does not seem difficult, but the data suggest that in today's health care system, we are having a difficult time meeting this expectation.[23] If the drug therapy is not effective, the patient expects you to find one that will be. If the drug product needs to be changed, they expect you to change it. If the dose needs to be altered, they expect you to alter it so it is effective, yet safe. There are several medications that are efficacious for most medical conditions or illnesses. Find one that works for the patient.

Patients will expect you to be realistic and honest about what they can expect from their medications

All patients are unique, so some will want to know everything about their medications: how they work and what they do, both positively and negatively. Virtually all patients want to have some level of understanding about the goals of therapy so that they will know if their drug therapy is working. Some patients will want you to make all the decisions without explaining much at all about their drug therapy other than how to take it. You will have to determine the level at which your patient wants to understand details about drug therapy. When you put a drug product (a chemical entity) about which we know a great deal into a patient (a complex biological system), the outcome cannot be predicted with full certainty. The more experience you have, the better you will be at predicting the outcome. There is so much that is still under investigation concerning drug therapy. In most situations there is no *right* answer. We are always making our best clinical judgment at the time. The patient has a right to know how certain you are about the potential positive and negative outcomes of drug therapy. You selected the drug therapy based upon effectiveness and safety, so be certain to explain how often this product works. If the data indicate that the drug is effective in 75% of cases, then your patient can expect it to work in three out of four cases.

Patients will expect you to be their advocate for all their drug-related needs

This will require that a special relationship develop between you and your patient, similar to the relationship patients have with other patient care providers. This relationship will demand that you respect every patient and his or her values, views, preferences, and wishes when making decisions about medications. What the patient wants and needs become your major concerns in practice. Your patients should be able to expect that you will provide the very best drug therapy possible. They should expect that you will provide the most effective drug therapy available in every circumstance. They will also expect you to keep their safety as a high priority. As a clinician, your advocacy for effectiveness and safety takes precedence over other considerations such as convenience and cost.

Patients will expect you to be accountable for the decisions you make and the advice you give

Whatever happens to the patient as a result of pharmacotherapy, positive or negative, you must take responsibility. The outcomes of drug therapies are your responsibility. Encourage the patient to contact you when questions arise or problems develop. Although you will work closely with the patient and his or her prescribing practitioners, always take responsibility for the outcomes resulting from drug therapy. The patient needs to know that you will be there for him or her regardless of the outcome. The patients need to know that you will find solutions to his or her problems.

Patients will expect you to know when to refer them to someone with different expertise

Don't try to be a dietician, an exercise physiologist, or a psychiatrist. It is important that you know the scope and breadth of your responsibilities (pharmacotherapy) and that you know where the boundaries of your expertise lie. Modern pharmacotherapies can improve the lives and overall health of many people. Focus your attention on maximizing the benefits of all drug therapies. Consultation and referrals serve a vital role in today's health care system. When referring a patient to another health care practitioner, it is important to be clear about the purpose of the referral, provide all of the relevant drug therapy documentation you have describing your patient's needs, and help your patient understand what questions to ask or what service to seek.[24]

The Patient's Responsibilities

With rights come responsibilities. It is important to be cognizant of your patients' expectations and aware of their responsibilities. Meeting the patient's drug-related needs requires the patient's participation and cooperation. Simply stated, you can expect your patients to

1. provide you with accurate and complete information
2. participate in establishing the goals of therapy
3. contribute to the care plan as agreed upon (act on the education and instructions they received, collect important outcome parameters, keep appointments)

4. maintain a diary of medication use, signs, and symptoms, and test results if needed to evaluate effectiveness, safety, and compliance
5. notify you of changes and/or problems with their drug therapy so you can act on them before they become harmful
6. ask questions whenever they arise.

The therapeutic relationship will allow you to uphold your patients' rights and benefit from their responsibilities. Work to make it a good one.

ADHERENCE AS A TEST OF PATIENT-CENTEREDNESS

Nowhere in the practice of pharmaceutical care are the concepts of understanding the medication experience and establishing a quality therapeutic relationship more important than in affecting your patients' behavior toward adherence. Adherence has been talked about and researched to such a degree that it has almost become "an end in itself," without regard to the outcomes the medications are meant to achieve. However, having said that, it must be recognized that adherence can make all the difference in achieving these outcomes.

> While no single strategy will guarantee that patients will fill their prescriptions and take their medicines as prescribed, elevating adherence as a priority issue and promoting best practices, behaviors and technologies may significantly improve medication adherence in the U.S. Enhancing Prescription Medication Adherence: A National Action Plan (National Council of Patient Information and Education, 2007)

The problem of medication adherence has been the focus of numerous research projects and marketing campaigns initiated by the pharmaceutical industry, academics, health care administrators, economists, practitioners, and others and has produced a significant volume of results. However, in spite of this substantial effort to both elucidate the dynamics of nonadherence and develop methods of remedy, the level of adherence has not positively improved to any significant degree since the groundbreaking work of Sackett in the 1970s.[25]

Wertheimer and Santella[26] help to quantify the problem:

- Sixty percent of all patients cannot identify their own medications
- Thirty to 50% of all patients ignore or otherwise compromise instructions concerning their medications

- Twelve to 20% of patients take other people's medicines
- Hospital costs due to patient nonadherence are estimated at $8.5 billion annually

Additionally, as a Center for Health Transformation report[23] discusses:

- Approximately 125,000 Americans die annually (342 people every day) due to poor medication adherence
- Ten to 25% of hospital and nursing home admissions are caused by the inability of patients to take their medications as prescribed and directed[24]
- The rates of nonadherence to prescription medication therapy have remained stagnant over the past three decades, and recent reviews have shown that as many as 40% of patients still do not adhere to their treatment regimens[27] and up to 20% of all new prescriptions go unfilled.[28]

Not only are there clinically identifiable consequences to nonadherence, there are also economic costs. It has been estimated that the annual cost of nonadherence in the United States approximates $290 billion, and as the population ages is likely to significantly increase.

The work of Cramer,[29] Pittman,[30] Osterberg and Blaschke,[31] Fleming,[24] Atreja et al.,[27] McHorney,[32] Bushnell,[33] Mattke,[34] Fortney,[35] and Ho et al.[36] confirms that the problem of nonadherence is very much with us. Indeed, a broader reading of the data beyond our shores indicates that the problem has universal significance.

Defining Adherence

Adherence is essentially a behavioral issue that has communication at its core. Most health care providers would agree that effective, safe, therapeutic intervention depends on communicating clearly, accurately, and with patient affirmation and consent. Medication, because of its benefits and risks, must be consumed in specific dosages, at individualized times and for a clearly determined period of time. This can be quite interruptive, discouraging, frustrating, confusing, tiring, and can, and often does, lead to nonadherent behavior. Pharmaceutical care is able to positively impact nonadherence in a number of ways. But first, consider the meaning of these terms.

For purposes of this discussion we define adherence in the following manner:

> Adherence is defined as the patient's ability and willingness to take a therapeutic regimen that the practitioner has clinically judged to be appropriately indicated,

adequately efficacious, and, based on all available evidence, can produce the desired outcomes without any harmful effects.

A critical examination of "classical" adherence literature reveals that all too often, the focus becomes that of "blaming the victim." The "bad patient" did not comply with the doctor's orders. The emphasis is on the paternalistic role of the physician and the subservience of the patient. Although our rhetoric has changed and denials of this attitude are rampant, it does resonate with the real nature of what still remains of the "doctor–patient" relationship. The critique of this relationship, particularly from bioethicists, is well documented, and at present is experiencing a dramatic exposure throughout the health care system as we try to organize patients into "medical homes." We are quickly realizing that the U.S. health care system is anything but a home, where one can be safe and comfortable and find solutions from the problems of the world. But, while structural changes occur at a modest rate, patients continue to be somewhat passive actors reacting, for better or worse, to the pronouncements of clinicians.

This scenario of "bad patient" and "right prescriber" sets up an explosive situation for a couple of obvious reasons. First, Conrad discovered, as we do every day in practice, that patients have rational, well-thought-out reasons for not taking their medications.[37] Secondly, our data indicate that 70% of patients receiving medication management services have a drug therapy problem that needs resolving. These problems occur with the following distribution: inappropriate medications being used 27%, ineffective medications being used 29%, unsafe medications 27%, and finally nonadherence of 17%. Essentially these data, which have been reproduced all over the world, indicate that providers may be responsible, either directly or indirectly, for 83% of the drug therapy problems being identified and solved today, whereas patients participate, directly or indirectly, in 17% of them!! This is something to consider.

MEDICATION MANAGEMENT AS A SOLUTION TO NONADHERENCE

As described above, medication management services (provided as pharmaceutical care practice) have been shown to consistently decrease noncompliance levels to less than 20%, and in some cases to as low as 9%.[20] How can this be achieved in view of the literature, which demonstrates how difficult it is to achieve levels of less than 50%? There are four primary reasons why medication management services can accomplish this and each will be discussed below.

First, and perhaps most importantly, patients receiving medication management services are not encouraged to be compliant with their medications until an assessment has been completed. This assessment must determine first, if the medications being taken are appropriate for the medical conditions being treated; second, that the medications are the most effective available; and third, that the medications are the safest possible. Only after these decisions are validated, is the patient's behavior assessed to determine whether the patient is being adherent or not. If the drug therapy is found to be inappropriate, ineffective, or unsafe, then the patient should not be encouraged to be compliant until changes can be made to address these drug therapy problems. Too many times an assumption is made that all the medications prescribed and taken by the patient are correct; but too frequently, in one out of two patients, this is not the case. This will be explained in more detail below.

The second reason nonadherence levels can be decreased so dramatically is that the patient is put at the center of the care that is delivered. The patient is encouraged to play a very active role in the decisions that are made to treat the patient's medical conditions. The patient helps to establish goals, assists in determining the most appropriate interventions, and collects information to monitor outcomes. This active participation keeps the patient involved in what is happening and gives the patient some control over a situation that often makes the patient feel "out of control."

The third reason that medication management services can decrease nonadherence so significantly is that the pharmacist understands that a quality service starts by revealing the preferences, beliefs, expectations, and concerns of the patient about his medications. This practitioner comes to understand the patient's medication experience and uses this information to individualize the care that is delivered to each patient. When a patient's care is individualized to this extent, the outcomes improve considerably.

And, the final reason medication management services can result in adherence levels of 90% is that the pharmacist providing the service works to establish a meaningful, therapeutic relationship with the patient. Through this therapeutic relationship comes the trust and respect that is necessary for adherence to be achieved.

Adherence Is Assessed Last, Not First

Patients have rarely been taught much about medications and, for the most part, have never been taught how to think about their medications in an empirical, pharmacological manner. This may have been reinforced because physicians have not traditionally been taught to think about medications in a systematic, comprehensive way.[17] Therefore, it would be difficult for physicians to share well-organized information about medications with patients when they frequently do not have it themselves. And, medications have always been considered the domain of the physician and they have taken on a mysterious, secretive quality so much so that patients don't feel comfortable asking questions or sharing information about their medication experience.

It is not a trivial matter to mention the difficulty found in pronouncing and spelling the names of drugs. Anyone who has taught pharmacy students or other health care professions (who by any measure are a bright and resourceful lot) has found that the language of pharmaceuticals has mind-bending properties that are confounding enough to try the patience of any linguist. We know from experience that many clinicians often "stutter" pronunciations of some drugs and we certainly observe numerous patients "tongue-tied" and frustrated as they try to provide verbal identities to their medications. A glance at a number of antiepileptic medications, for example—ethosuximide, lamotrigine, or levetiracetam, gives the impression that struggling to pronounce their names could in itself produce seizures. Perhaps this is another example of iatrogenesis.

It is unethical, almost unthinkable to imagine that we would encourage our patients to take medications that are inappropriate, ineffective, or unsafe, and yet, that is exactly what is occurring repeatedly every day. As we mentioned earlier, one out of two ambulatory patients who enter a retail pharmacy to have a prescription prepared is taking a medication that is inappropriate, ineffective, or unsafe. However, we frequently assume that everything is fine and continue to encourage them to be "compliant" every day with these medications. This happens so frequently that we can no longer encourage patients to adhere to their regimen unless all of the patient's drug therapy has been assessed, comprehensively and systematically, an individualized care plan has been developed, and the patient is followed up to determine that the drug therapy is appropriate, effective, safe, and can be taken as intended. In other words, medication management services have to become the standard of care for patients in our health care systems.

This seems to be simple and basic. Yet, patients have many different prescribers, medications are becoming increasingly complex, patients are developing numerous comorbidities because of their age and longevity, and they are adding many nonprescription medications to the mix. This leaves patients confused, changing their dosage regimens, stopping their medications, and often refusing to participate in this whole exercise. It doesn't have to be this way.

A successful approach to fixing this dilemma may be to make it all simpler and more understandable to both the patient and prescriber. Pharmaceutical care practice is built on a logical way to think about medications. And, this can provide both the patient and the practitioner a common language for communicating medication information. We believe this can have a significant impact on decreasing medication nonadherence.

When medication management services are delivered, all of a patient's medications are evaluated, together, in a very logical order that ensures a patient is given medication and is taking medication that is appropriate for the medical conditions she is experiencing, effective for the condition it is treating and safe for those with comorbidities and many medications. The assessment is done in this systematic way. Only when a medication is deemed appropriate, is it evaluated for effectiveness. Then, only when the medication is determined to be the most effective available, does the practitioner determine the safety of the medication. Then, when all of these criteria have been met, the patient's adherence is evaluated to determine if the medication can be effective and safe in the dose and manner in which the patient is ACTUALLY TAKING THE MEDICATION. In practice, the patient's adherence behavior is never evaluated until the practitioner has determined that what the patient has been given (and is taking) is appropriate, can be effective, and will remain safe. This is the logical way to think about medications. This is the basis for building a different approach to achieving medication adherence.

Patient-centered Adherence

Behavioral change on the part of the patient is the sine qua non of improved adherence. We do not refer here to the questionable ethics of the Pavlovian approach to "behavior modification." Rather, a more cooperative collaborative approach is called for. Not surprisingly, such an approach requires change on the part of the patient and also the clinician! So, we do not direct our attention to a limiting, and oppressive, patient-only approach, where the "deviant" patient must master better ways to be compliant and dutiful to "doctors orders." On the contrary, we argue that altering the behavior of both clinicians and patients is a major step forward.

When patients visit a physician and leave with a prescription, which they take to a pharmacy and exchange for medication, they usually have every intention of using this to improve their health and quality of life. For many patients, however, this positive expectation is, for whatever reason, disrupted, altered, or rejected. The reasons for this are not too difficult to ascertain. The following list, by no means exhaustive, provides some insight into the reasons found in more than three decades of research:

- The patient does not understand the instructions
- The patient, for whatever reason, prefers not to take the medication
- The patient forgets to take the medication
- The medication costs too much for the patient to purchase

- The patient cannot appropriately swallow or self-administer the product
- The drug is not available for consumption
- Patients take the medication for the wrong reason
- Patients with comorbidities, on many medications, often become confused and indecisive, thus "put off" taking them
- Patients all too frequently have a poor understanding of the science involved in goals of therapy and the expectations of healthy outcomes
- Patients can be "pharmacologically" illiterate or do not understand the particular language used by clinician and others
- Mathematics and measurement involved in dosages and the patient does not always understand frequencies of administration; hence, dose and duration are often problematic as is safety and efficacy
- Patients frequently have a poor understanding of their health problems
- Patients frequently hold beliefs contrary to any empirically based allopathic paradigm
- Cultural beliefs and practices can, and do, impact the patient's decision to take or not take medicines
- Religious beliefs and practices can inhibit adherence
- Complex therapeutic regimens can be confusing and frightening
- Cognitive factors (especially in older patients) can lead to poor or nonadherence

Although all of these factors can play a role in decisions not to adhere to a medication regimen, much can be done by the practitioner to prevent this. Perhaps the goal of all practitioners should be patient-centered adherence.

The practice of pharmaceutical care not only provides us with the opportunity to improve adherence, but expects us to approach it from a different perspective than has been taken for the past three decades. This approach is so different, in fact that the traditional meaning of adherence does not really "fit" with the paradigm of the practice. Therefore, we will refer to this new concept as patient-centered adherence.

Definition Patient-centered adherence is achieved once the pharmaceutical care practitioner ensures that only those medications which are determined to be appropriate, effective and safe for the individual patient are being used and that the individualized care plan developed with the patient takes into account the unique medication experience of that patient. Then the patient is able to actively participate in the decisions made to treat medical conditions with medications, as well as participate in the development of the care plan to achieve the goals of therapy, and the patient is able and willing to take responsibility for the actions he/she needs to take to achieve optimal outcomes.

This definition reveals concepts, which are central to understanding patient-centered adherence. Moreover, these concepts involve more active and more explicit involvement by both patient and provider. Although these concepts may not seem new as they are implicit in current understandings of adherence, it is the explicit presence of them and the change in behavior that is required that creates the patient-centered adherence paradigm. A more detailed look at each of the concepts will help to reveal this paradigm.

This paradigm eliminates our assumption that everything the practitioner has done is right and good for the patient and all the patient has to do is to obey the directions of the practitioner. Conrad[37] has demonstrated that patients change the doses of their medications and stop medications for very intelligent, logical reasons. These reasons are that the medications that health care providers frequently suggest for patients, and the medications patients select for themselves, are frequently inappropriate, ineffective, and unsafe because of multiple prescribers, comorbidities, and the lack of a logical decision-making process that can make sense of it all. And, finally, the patient has to have input into the decisions and actions to assure that patient-centered adherence can be achieved.

Patient Participation in Achieving Adherence

It is important to reiterate that the patient is the ultimate decision maker in his health care. Prescribers decide only what medication and dosage regimen to recommend, and the patient makes all the other decisions. Patients decide what medications—both prescription and nonprescription—they will actually take and what they will not. Patients also decide how much to take, how frequently to take it, and how long they will continue to take it, and, they make these decisions every day.

KEY CLINICAL CONCEPTS

The practitioner has to positively influence the patient's decisions to create a positive medication experience. This requires a good therapeutic relationship.

If you ever have difficulty influencing your patient's decisions about drug therapy, reevaluate your relationship with the patient. The relationship between a patient and a health care professional should always be therapeutic in its most literal sense. We are always striving to help the patient achieve the most positive therapeutic results possible. However, drug therapy can be dangerous or frightening. It can be confusing. It can be distressing to some patients. These emotions are implicit in the pharmaceutical care process, and therefore, a significant portion of what the practitioner contributes to the patient is made possible only through a close, empathic, respectful, mutually rewarding therapeutic relationship, and all that this entails.

Achieving Patient-centered Adherence

Perhaps more than anything, pharmaceutical care practice brings the patient who has a certain set of beliefs, expectations, and concerns together with a practitioner who may have a completely different set of values and level of knowledge about drug therapy, and provides the two of them with a common way to think about medications and a common way to talk about medications.

This should lead to the best decisions possible, which will bring about a significantly higher level of patient-centered adherence. This happens best when the patient can share her medication experience, when she is able to express her drug-related needs that day, and when the practitioner translates this information into drug therapy problems that the pharmaceutical care practitioner is able to identify, resolve, and prevent with the active participation of the patient. In Table 4-2 we represent this translational process. If you begin on the left with the patient's medication experience that is translated into the patient's drug-related needs on any single day and are then assessed by the pharmaceutical care provider to determine if any of the drug therapy problems in the right hand column are occurring. This translational process, which actively involves the patient and the practitioner, is able to focus everyone's efforts on how to resolve the drug therapy problem to achieve the intended goals of therapy. More about drug therapy problems will be discussed in Chapter 5.

At this point we would like to introduce another caveat: patients very often do not confine their actions to taking only prescription medications. Drug substances obtained by prescription often mix with over-the-counter products such as food supplements, vitamins, dietary products, and topical ointments and creams to name a few possibilities. Also, there is growing interest in, and enthusiasm for, alternative/complementary remedies. This category, regardless of your personal beliefs and practices, does involve a great

Table 4-2 Translating the patient's medication experience into drug therapy problems

Patient's medication experience	Patient's medication-related needs	Patient's drug therapy problems
UNDERSTANDING of the medication and why it is being used and how to use it as intended	The medication is APPROPRIATE for the medical condition being treated	1. Additional drug therapy is needed 2. Unnecessary drug therapy needs to be discontinued
EXPECTATIONS of the positive and potential negative outcomes from the medication	The medication is likely to be the most EFFECTIVE available	3. The medication is the wrong drug 4. The dosage is too low
CONCERNS about taking the medications	The medication is SAFE for the patient, his medical conditions and other medications	5. Adverse drug reaction is experienced 6. The dosage is too high
BEHAVIOR of the patient in terms of adherence	The patient is able and willing to ADHERE to the regimen	7. Patient is nonadherent

many risks for the patient. Although specifically focusing on the prescribed medication, and all its possible complications, the practitioner will want to know what other treatment options the patient is actively pursuing. Of major concern is the role that herbal medicine plays in the patient's attempts to alleviate symptoms or produce a "cure."[38,39]

Along with a more scientifically based pharmaceutical regimen (with all its flaws) patients are increasingly taking such things as: aloe vera for herpes, artichoke for high cholesterol, billberry for phlebitis and menstrual pain, block cohosh for menopause and colds, cranberry for urinary tract infection, horse chestnut for varicose veins, grape seed for the prevention of cancer, passion flower for anxiety, St. John's Wort for depression, saw palmetto for benign prostate hyperplasia, willow for general pain and fever-fern to prevent migraine. These are but a few of the possible herbal remedies that dot the therapeutic landscape.[38] These herbal remedies, and more, cannot be ignored. Not only are many of these controversial in their claims, but they do offer potential risks when taken in conjunction with other pharmaceuticals. Monitoring potential risk, both involving the claims and action of herbal medicine, and their potential for herb–drug interaction is important. For example, although devil's claw is presently seen by researches as good for musculoskeletal pain, does it interact with NSAIDs? Does garlic, considered good for high cholesterol, interact with statins? Simple questions, but asking them about any herb the patient sees as an essential part of his personal pharmacopeia, can and will, identify numerous medication needs.

Gathering information from the patient and placing it in a coherent, well-organized framework is necessary to translate his presentation of what he considers his drug-related needs into a problem-solving format. During this important act of translation the practitioner must assess the patient's level of understanding of drug therapy generally and the specifics of her past and present regimen.

Does the patient understand why she needs a particular medication, and why she should take it? Does she understand, to the best of her ability, how it works and what it will do for her? Is she aware of the costs and benefits? Does she express any reservations, risks, or misunderstandings? In short, is she fully engaged in her therapy, or is she a mere bystander? If the drug is *indicated*, we assess her understanding of what this means.

Are the patient's expectations consistent with the stated *effectiveness* of the medication? Are the expressed concerns that the patient has about taking the medication consistent with the safety profile of it? How comfortable is she with safety issues? Is there any reason, found in her past medication experience, to suggest that there is doubt and possible nonadherence? If there is, can you do anything to ally such doubt, suspicion, or general resistance? This organized, structured translation of patient-specific information into a framework that facilitates the practitioner's problem-solving responsibilities is the essence of a rational structured approach to drug therapy that is central to pharmaceutical care practice.

In sum, the practitioner depends, in large part, on the patient's provision of information required to make a comprehensive assessment of drug therapy needs, and to formulate a plan of action to do something about any should they arise. The process whereby the practitioner elicits this information is the patient care process that forms the interactive dynamic that is the therapeutic relationship. The specifics of this process are discussed in detail in Chapters 5 through 8.

This translation from the patient's medication experience to understanding her medication-related needs to identifying drug therapy problems is the essence of medication management services. Having this framework allows the patient and the practitioner to think about medications in a similar manner and to communicate with each other using a similar vocabulary. Most importantly, it allows for the patient and the practitioner to develop together a personal treatment plan for the patient that is based on the rational treatment plan of the practitioner. This is a tremendously important step in

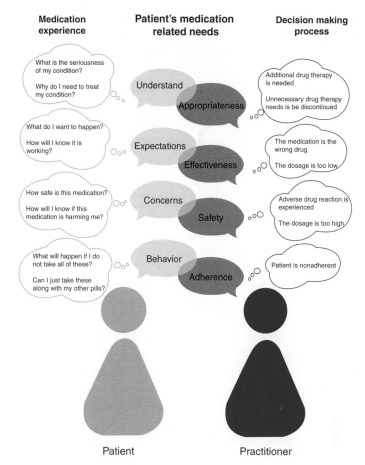

Figure 4-1 Communication and problem solving between patient and practitioner.

achieving patient-centered adherence. Figure 4-1 describes the thoughts and communication approaches used simultaneously by the patient and the practitioner. The patient comes to the encounter with her own, personal medication experience and a set of questions for the practitioner (understanding, expectations, concerns, behavior). These personal questions are in the patient's order of priority. On the other hand, the practitioner is skilled at clinical problem solving and comes to the encounter with a set of areas of clinical inquiry (appropriateness, effectiveness, safety, and adherence). It is the skill of the practitioner plus the strength of the therapeutic relationship that allows these two different languages and approaches to drug therapy to result in an understanding of the patient's drug-related needs and the identification of drug therapy problems.

With this framework for thinking about medications, patients can learn to discuss their understanding, expectations, concerns, and behavior as it relates to medications with anyone. The questions that are listed apply to all patients, all medical conditions, and all medications. If we expect patients to participate in their care, and if we seriously intend to make our practices patient-centered, then we have to provide patients with the tools to gain knowledge, learn a foreign vocabulary, construct questions, and change their own behavior. This tool is just the beginning of what needs to occur.

SUMMARY

All practitioners in the health care system are facing the fact that patient-centeredness has received a lot of "lip-service" but very little behavior has actually changed. This can no longer continue. The structure of the health care system is finally putting the patient at the center in the primary care context (called the medical home in the United States). Coordinated care focused on meeting the patient's needs is finally becoming a reality across the United States. All of these structural changes make it quite explicit that there is much work to be done on the practitioner's part. There is a need to better understand the meaning of patient-centeredness and to practice in a manner that treats the patient as the raison d'être for care being provided. Now the challenge is to apply these concepts in practice. The following four chapters will provide you the opportunity to do just that.

REFERENCES

1. Ramalho de Oliveira DR, Shoemaker SJ. Achieving patient centeredness in pharmacy practice: openness and the pharmacist's natural attitude. *J Am Pharm Assoc.* 2006;46(1):56–64; quiz 64–66.
2. Kleinman A. *The Illness Narratives.* New York: Basic Books; 1988.
3. WHO. *Constitution.* Geneva, Switzerland: World Health Organization; 1946.
4. Brown JB, Weston WW, Stewart M. Exploring both disease and the illness experience. In: Stewart M, ed. *Patient-Centered Medicine.* Thousand Oaks, CA: Sage Publications; 1995:31–43.
5. Sacks O. *A Leg to Stand On.* London: Picador; 1991.
6. Shoemaker SJ, Ramalho de Oliveira D. Understanding the meaning of medications for patients: the medication experience. *Pharm World Sci.* 2008;30(1):86–91.
7. Shoemaker SJ, Ramalho de Oliveira D, Alves M, Ekstrand M. The medication experience: Preliminary evidence of its value for patient education and counseling on chronic medications. *Patient Educ Couns.* 2011;83(3):443–450.

8. Ramalho de Oliveira D, Shoemaker SJ, Ekstrand M. Getting to the root of drug therapy problems: looking to your patient's medication experience. *J Am Pharm Assoc.* 2012 (in press).

9. Whyte SR, Van der Geest S. *Social Lives of Medicines.* Cambridge: Cambridge University Press; 2002.

10. Moerman D. *Meaning, Medicine and the 'Placebo effect'.* Cambridge: Cambridge University Press; 2002.

11. Nichter M, Vuckovic, N. Agenda for an anthropology of pharmaceutical practice. *Soc Sci Med.* 1994;39(11):1509–1525.

12. Smith RC. *The Patient's Story: Integrated Patient-doctor Interviewing.* Boston MA: Little Brown and Company; 1996.

13. Brown P. *Perspectives in Medical Sociology.* 2nd ed. Prospect Heights, IL: Waveland Press; 1989.

14. Conrad P, Kern R. *The Sociology of Health and Illness: Critical Perspectives.* 2nd ed. New York: St. Martin's Press; 1986.

15. Morley PC, Wallis R. *Culture and Curing: Anthropological Perspectives on Traditional Medical Beliefs and Practices.* London: Peter Own; 1979.

16. Radley A. *Making Sense of Illness.* London: Sage Publications; 1998.

17. Henderson GE. *The Social Medicine Reader.* 2nd ed. Vol. 2. Durham: Duke University Press; 2005.

18. Farmer P. *Partner to the Poor.* Berkeley CA: Berkeley University of California Press; 2010.

19. Coulehan JL, Block MR. *The Medical Interview: Mastering Skills for Clinical Practice.* 4th ed. Philadelphia PA: F.A. Davis Company; 2001:155–169.

20. Cipolle RJ, Strand LM, Morley PC. *Pharmaceutical Care Practice: The Clinician's Guide.* 2nd ed. New York, NY: McGraw-Hill; 2004.

21. Oliveira D. Pharmaceutical care uncovered: an ethnographic study of pharmaceutical care practice. In: *Department of Social and Administrative Pharmacy.* Minneapolis MN: University of Minnesota; 2003.

22. Cipolle RJ. Drugs don't have doses—people have doses! A clinical educator's philosophy. *Drug Intell Clin Pharm.* 1986;20(11):881–882.

23. *The 21st Century Intelligent Pharmacy Project: The Importance of Medication Adherence.* Center for Health Transformation; 2010.

24. Fleming WK. Pharmacy management strategies for improving drug adherence. *J Manag Care Pharm.* 2008;14(6 suppl B):16–20.

25. Sackett DL, Haynes RB, Gibson ES, et al. Randomized clinical trial of strategies for improving medication compliance in primary hypertension. *Lancet.* 1975;1:1205–1207.

26. Wertheimer AI, Santella TM. Medication compliance research: still so far to go. *J Appl Res Clin Exp Ther.* 2003;3(3):254–261.

27. Atreja A, Bellam N, Levy SR. Strategies to enhance patient adherence: making it simple. *MedGenMed: Medscape Gen Med.* 2005;7(1):4.

28. Anderson S. C. *Sebok Pharmacy Lecture.* 2010.

29. Cramer JA. A systematic review of adherence with medications for diabetes. *Diabetes Care.* 2004;27(5):1218–1224.

30. Pittman DG, Tao Z, Chen W, Stettin GD. Antihypertensive medication adherence and subsequent healthcare utilization and costs. *Am J Manag Care.* 2010;16(8):568–576.

31. Osterberg L, Blaschke T. Adherence to medication. *N Engl J Med.* 2005;353(5):487–497.

32. McHorney CA. The Adherence Estimator: a brief, proximal screener for patient propensity to adhere to prescription medications for chronic disease. *Curr Med Res Opin.* 2009;25(1):215–238.

33. Bushnell CD, Zimmer LO, Pan W, et al. Persistence with stroke prevention medications 3 months after hospitalization. *Arch Neurol.* 2010;67(12):1456–1463.

34. Mattke S, Martorell F, Hong SY, Sharma P, Cuellar A, Lurie N. Anti-inflammatory medication adherence and cost and utilization of asthma care in a commercially insured population. *J Asthma.* 2010;47(3):323–329.

35. Fortney JC, Pyne JM, Edlund MJ, Mittal D. Relationship between antidepressant medication possession and treatment response. *Gen Hosp Psychiatry.* 2010;32(4):377–379.

36. Ho PM, Magrid DJ, Shetterly SM, et al. Medication nonadherence is associated with a broad range of adverse outcomes in patients with coronary artery disease. *Am Heart J.* 2008;155(4):772–779.

37. Conrad P. The meaning of medications: another look at compliance. *Soc Sci Med.* 1985;20(1):29–37.

38. Singh D, Edzard E. *Trick of Treatment: The Undesirable Facts About Alternative Medicine.* New York: W.W. Norton and Company; 2008.

39. Bausell RB. *Snake Oil Science: The Truth About Complementary and Alternative Medicine.* New York: Oxford University Press; 2007.

Drug Therapy Problems

⚷ KEY CONCEPTS

1 Identifying, resolving, and preventing drug therapy problems are the unique contributions of the pharmaceutical care practitioner.

2 Identifying a drug therapy problem is a clinical judgment that requires the practitioner to identify an association between the patient's medical condition and the patient's pharmacotherapy.

3 Medication management services add value to the care of individual patients by identifying, resolving, and preventing drug therapy problems.

4 There are seven distinct categories of drug therapy problems.

5 How the practitioner describes the drug therapy problem influences the selection of interventions to resolve the problem.

6 A correctly stated drug therapy problem includes (a) a description of the patient's condition or problem, (b) the drug therapy involved, and (c) the specific association between the drug therapy and the patient's condition.

7 Drug therapy problems should be assessed for their severity, acuteness, and significance to the patient to determine how quickly the resolution of the problem must occur.

8 When multiple drug therapy problems exist, prioritize them and begin with the problem that is most important to the patient and/or is critical to the health of the patient.

9 Patients who have no drug therapy problems still require a care plan and follow-up evaluation to ensure that the goals of therapy continue to be met and no new drug therapy problems develop.

Drug therapy problems are the clinical domain of the pharmaceutical care practitioner. The purpose of identifying drug therapy problems is to help patients achieve their goals of therapy and realize the best possible outcomes from drug therapy. In the following sections, we will discuss the terminology, components, and categories of drug therapy problems and their central importance to the practice of pharmaceutical care and medication management services.

DRUG THERAPY PROBLEMS: TERMINOLOGY

The identification of drug therapy problems is the focus of the assessment and represents the key decisions made in that step of the patient care process. Although drug therapy problem identification is technically part of the assessment process, it represents the truly unique contribution made by pharmaceutical care practitioners. Therefore, a separate discussion has been devoted to describing drug therapy problems so that you can learn to identify, resolve, and most importantly, prevent drug therapy problems in your practice.

Drug therapy problems are a consequence of a patient's drug-related needs that have gone unmet. They are central to pharmaceutical care practice.

Definition   A drug therapy problem is any undesirable event experienced by a patient that involves, or is suspected to involve, drug therapy, and that interferes with achieving the desired goals of therapy and requires professional judgment to resolve.[1,2]

If not resolved, drug therapy problems have clinical consequences. As clinical patient problems, drug therapy problems require professional (clinical) judgment to resolve. The characteristics of requiring professional judgment place drug therapy problems at par with other clinical problems in medicine, dentistry, and nursing.

Every health care practitioner is responsible for helping patients with problems that require a certain level of professional sophistication to identify, prevent, or resolve. Societies have made dentists the primary health care practitioner responsible for identifying and resolving dental problems. Not all dental problems require the sophistication of a licensed dentist to resolve, but those dental problems that an individual patient cannot identify (diagnose) or resolve on his or her own require the knowledge and skills of a dentist.

KEY CLINICAL CONCEPTS

Identifying drug therapy problems is to pharmaceutical care, what making a medical diagnosis is to medical care. It is the most important contribution you can make. Drug therapy problems represent the major responsibility of the pharmaceutical care practitioner.

It must be emphasized here that the most important role for the pharmaceutical care practitioner is to *prevent* drug therapy problems from occurring. This is surely the most valuable service a practitioner can provide to his or her patient.

Pharmaceutical care practitioners use the term *problem* to denote an event associated with or caused by drug therapy that is amenable to detection, treatment, or prevention. A drug therapy problem is a clinical problem, and it must be identified and resolved in a manner similar to other clinical problems. *Patients have drug therapy problems—drug products do not have drug therapy problems.*

COMPONENTS OF A DRUG THERAPY PROBLEM

To identify, resolve, and prevent drug therapy problems, the practitioner must understand how patients with drug therapy problems present in the clinical setting. The patient's drug therapy problem always has three primary components:

1. An undesirable event or risk of an event experienced by the patient. The *problem* can take the form of a medical complaint, sign, symptom, diagnosis, disease, illness, impairment, disability, abnormal laboratory value, or syndrome. The event can be the result of physiological, psychological, sociocultural, or economic conditions.[1,2]
2. The *drug therapy* (products and/or dosage regimen) associated with the problem.
3. The *relationship* that exists (or is suspected to exist) between the undesirable patient event and drug therapy. This relationship can be
   a. the consequence of drug therapy, suggesting a direct association or even a cause and effect relationship
   b. the need to add or modify drug therapy for its resolution or prevention.[1]

KEY CLINICAL CONCEPTS

Stating the problem and identifying the cause require that all three components be known. This step involves clinical judgment by the practitioner.

There is no "right answer" as to whether or not a drug therapy problem exists. There is only the practitioner's clinical judgment and rationale for the decision. This is the reason pharmaceutical care can contribute uniquely to patient care. No other practitioner can identify and resolve drug therapy problems as routinely and comprehensively as the pharmaceutical care practitioner.

Example   "Mr. M.'s elbow pain is not being effectively controlled because the dosage of ketoprofen he has been taking for the past three days is too low to provide relief."

"My patient is experiencing orthostatic hypotension with mild to light headaches each morning because the 2 mg dose of risperidone she takes in the morning is too high."

"My patient has lost her ability to taste secondary to her captopril therapy."

"Mrs. W. requires additional calcium supplements in order to prevent osteoporosis."

Having one set of standard definitions and one set of distinct categories for all drug therapy problems help to define a fixed and manageable set of professional responsibilities for the pharmaceutical care practitioner.

All patient problems involving medications can be categorized into one of seven types of drug therapy problems. These include any and all side effects, toxic reactions, treatment failures, or the need for additive, synergistic, or preventive medications, as well as adherence problems and noncompliance. The seven categories of drug therapy problems are described in Table 5-1.

Practitioners frequently perceive that an infinite number of drug therapy problems exist given the rapidly expanding array of drug products available, the growing number of diseases being recognized and diagnosed, and the growing numbers of patients entering our health care system. The existence of an endless list of possible drug therapy problems might seem logical due to the fact that, during 2008, there were 4 billion prescriptions dispensed from community pharmacies throughout the United States and over 44,000 hospitalized patients

Table 5-1   Description of drug therapy problems categories

1.	The drug therapy is unnecessary because the patient does not have a clinical indication at this time.
2.	Additional drug therapy is required to treat or prevent a medical condition in the patient.
3.	The drug product is not being effective at producing the desired response in the patient.
4.	The dosage is too low to produce the desired response in the patient.
5.	The drug is causing an adverse reaction in the patient.
6.	The dosage is too high, resulting in undesirable effects experienced by the patient.
7.	The patient is not able or willing to take the drug therapy as intended.

die each year resulting from medical errors.[3] Although there are many thousands of drug products available, billions of prescriptions dispensed each year, and numerous acute and chronic diseases managed with drug products, there are only seven different categories of drug therapy problems.

Several drug therapy problem classifications have been proposed and described in the literature. With minor exceptions, all of these support the assessment of **indication, effectiveness, safety,** and **adherence** first described by Strand and colleagues.[2] Some authors have suggested adding a miscellaneous category in order to include prescription processing (system) errors. However, when there are no clinical problems identified in a specific patient, professional judgment usually is not required and therefore adds confusion rather than clarity to the core patient-centered responsibility of the practitioner providing medication management services.[4–11]

These seven categories should not be confused with the traditional criteria for categorizing medication errors, which describe the correct drug, correct dose, correct route, correct frequency, and correct duration according to a prescription. This prescription-focused approach establishes the prescribing and delivery of the drug product and not the patient's clinical condition as the focus of the problem. Drug products do not cause toxicity until they are taken by a patient. Drug products cannot prevent diseases unless they are taken at the appropriate time and at the appropriate dosage by patients. Drug products cannot cure a disease unless and until a sufficient dosage is provided to and taken by the patient. Drug therapy cannot be considered to have failed to manage a disease unless it was actually taken by the patient. Therefore, drug therapy problems always involve the patient, the medical condition, and the drug therapy that connects them.

This categorization of drug therapy problems was first defined, described, and developed in 1990 by the research group at the Peters Institute of Pharmaceutical Care at the University of Minnesota.[2] The seven categories of drug therapy problems have been examined, critiqued, and applied to practices in a variety of settings, cultures, and languages.[12–15]

KEY CLINICAL CONCEPTS

Knowing that there are only seven basic categories of drug therapy problems is a powerful concept for students and practitioners. These categories define the set of problems that might be caused by drugs and/or that can be resolved by drug therapy, and therefore describe the scope of responsibilities of the pharmaceutical care practitioner.

Table 5-2   Unmet drug-related needs as drug therapy problems

Drug-related needs	Categories of drug therapy problems
INDICATION	1. Unnecessary drug therapy 2. Needs additional drug therapy
EFFECTIVENESS	3. Ineffective drug 4. Dosage too low
SAFETY	5. Adverse drug reaction 6. Dosage too high
ADHERENCE	7. Nonadherence or noncompliance

The first two categories of drug therapy problems are associated with the INDICATION. The third and fourth categories of drug therapy problems are associated with EFFECTIVENESS. The fifth and sixth categories of drug therapy problems are associated with SAFETY. The seventh category deals with patient ADHERENCE. This order of problem assessment (indication, effectiveness, safety, and adherence) is significant in that it describes the rational decision-making process of the Pharmacotherapy Workup (Table 5-2).

You will note that the first six categories of drug therapy problems describe clinical problems that the patient experiences resulting from the *actions of drug therapy* on his or her health. These six categories are differentiated from the seventh in a unique and important way. The seventh category, adherence or noncompliance, results from the *actions the patient* makes concerning his or her willingness or ability to use the medication as instructed.

These categories of drug therapy problems are not specific to pharmacological class, area of practice specialty, medical service, or level of practitioner education or training. Drug therapy problem categories are also not specific to a unique patient group based on age, disease state, or health care plan. Hospitalized patients do not have different categories of drug therapy problems than ambulatory patients. Hospitalized patients might have more critical, unmet drug-related needs and they might require urgent resolution of their drug therapy problems, but all of the drug therapy problems identified in hospitalized patients fall into the same seven categories. The categories apply across all patient, practitioner, and institutional variables.

All practitioners who provide pharmaceutical care must be able to identify, prevent, and resolve any and all of the seven types of drug therapy problems for a given patient. When the practitioner concludes that a patient has a drug therapy problem, he or she is obligated to work with the patient and other health care practitioners, if necessary, to resolve that problem.

Categorizing drug therapy problems into seven categories can be an empowering process for a number of reasons. First, categorizing drug therapy problems serves as the focus for developing a systematic process of problem solving whereby the practitioner contributes significantly to the overall positive health outcomes of patients. A systematic process will not only aid the practitioner in achieving successful outcomes on an individual patient basis but could also aid pharmacoepidemiologists in the development of a national or even international database concerning drug therapy problems.[16] Second, these categories help to clarify and demarcate the professional responsibilities and accountability of the pharmaceutical care practitioner. This is most helpful in a team-oriented health care delivery system. Few practicing physicians, nurses, health care administrators, or payers need to be convinced that drug therapy problems are important, their prevention is necessary, and their resolution is in need of an expert.[13] In today's health care system, drug therapy problems are recognized as important patient problems to be solved. Within the national guidelines for patient-centered medical home services, drug therapy problem identification and resolution are recognized as the primary function of comprehensive medication management services. Third, this process illustrates how adverse drug reactions are but one category of drug therapy problem, and it also puts adherence and noncompliance into an appropriate clinical perspective. It becomes clear that practitioners must proactively identify, resolve, and prevent drug therapy problems of all types in order to ensure that each patient experiences effective and safe pharmacotherapy.

The fourth function of this categorization is to provide the clinical work of the pharmaceutical care practitioner with a vocabulary consistent with that used by other healthcare professionals. By defining the practitioner's function in terms of identification, resolution, and prevention of a patient's drug therapy problems, her function is placed in a patient care context consistent with the responsibilities of other health care practitioners. Recall, in pharmaceutical care practice, the patient—and not the drug product—is the major focus of the practitioner's energies, skills, knowledge, decisions, and actions.

Evidence-based medicine is facilitated by these logical drug therapy problem categories. The logical and comprehensive categorization of drug therapy problems facilitate the application of population-based evidence to an individual patient's problems. The development of new drug products and the generation of new pharmacological knowledge are based on the same set of fundamental pharmacological principles as drug therapy problems: clinical indication, effectiveness, safety, and compliance. When a new drug product is developed for commercial use, numerous rigorous research studies must be conducted in order to demonstrate the *safety* and *efficacy* when used to treat a specific *indication*. Therefore, the wealth of information and evidence generated in populations of patients during the drug development process

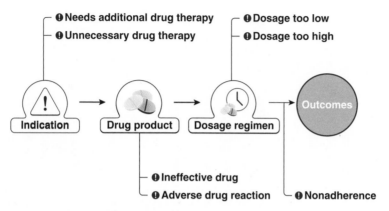

Figure 5-1 Drug therapy problem identification.

can be applied directly in the provision of pharmaceutical care to individual patients.

Drug therapy problems can and do occur at any stage of the patient's medication use process (Figure 5-1). Therefore, the practitioner must anticipate drug therapy problems in order to prevent them.

The sequence of how drug therapy problems are identified is important. The order in which you make decisions is of the utmost importance to ensure that your assessment is comprehensive and your clinical decisions are rational. Remember, in pharmaceutical care practice, decisions concerning an INDICATION are addressed first, then decisions concerning EFFECTIVENESS can be established, followed by SAFETY considerations. These categories of drug therapy problems describe the action (or result or outcome) that the drug therapy is having on the patient. Finally, ADHERENCE problems represent the willingness and ability of the patient to use the medication as intended.

CATEGORIES AND COMMON CAUSES OF DRUG THERAPY PROBLEMS

As with most clinical problems, drug therapy problems cannot be resolved or prevented unless the cause of the problem is clearly understood. It is necessary to identify and categorize not only the drug therapy problem but also its most likely cause. Only then can the practitioner apply clinical judgment and proceed with confidence to its resolution or prevention. The common causes of drug therapy problems are listed in order of frequency and summarized in Table 5-3.

Table 5-3 Common causes of drug therapy problems

Drug therapy problem category	Drug therapy problem cause
Unnecessary drug therapy	Duplicate therapy: multiple drug products are being used for a condition that requires only single drug therapy.
	No medical indication at this time: there is no valid medical indication requiring drug therapy at this time.
	Nondrug therapy more appropriate: the medical indication is more appropriately treated with nondrug therapy.
	Addiction/recreational drug use: drug abuse, alcohol use, or smoking is causing the problem.
	Treating avoidable adverse reaction: drug therapy is being taken to treat an avoidable adverse drug reaction associated with another medication.
Needs additional therapy	Preventive therapy: preventive drug therapy is required to reduce the risk of developing a new condition.
	Untreated condition: a medical condition requires the initiation of drug therapy.
	Synergistic therapy: a medical condition requires additional pharmacotherapy to attain synergistic or additive effects.
Ineffective drug	More effective drug available: the drug is not the most effective for the medical condition and a different drug is needed.
	Condition refractory to drug: the medical condition is refractory to the drug product and a different drug is needed.
	Dosage form inappropriate: the dosage form of the drug product is inappropriate.
	Contraindication present: the drug product is contraindicated in this patient.
	Drug not indicated for condition: the drug product is not an effective product for the indication being treated.
Dosage too low	Ineffective dose: the dose is too low to produce the desired response.
	Needs additional monitoring: clinical or laboratory parameters are required to determine if the dosage is too low for the patient.
	Frequency inappropriate: the dosage interval is too infrequent to produce the desired response.
	Incorrect administration: the drug product was not administered by the appropriate route or method.
	Drug interaction: a drug interaction reduces the amount of active drug available resulting in lack of effectiveness in this patient.
	Incorrect storage: the drug product was stored incorrectly and lost potency.
	Duration inappropriate: the duration of the drug therapy is too short to produce the desired response.

Adverse drug reaction	Undesirable effect: the drug product causes an undesirable reaction that is not dose-related.
	Unsafe drug for the patient: a safer drug product is required due to patient risk factors.
	Drug interaction: a drug interaction causes an undesirable reaction that is not dose-related.
	Incorrect administration: the drug product was administered by the incorrect route or method resulting in an adverse reaction.
	Allergic reaction: the drug product caused an allergic reaction.
	Dosage increase/decrease too fast: the drug dosage was administered or escalated too rapidly resulting in an adverse reaction.
Dosage too high	Dose too high: the dose of the drug is too high for the patient, resulting in toxicity.
	Needs additional monitoring: clinical or laboratory parameters are required to determine if the dosage is too high for the patient.
	Frequency too short: the dosing frequency is too short for the patient.
	Duration too long: the duration of drug therapy is too long for this patient.
	Drug interaction: a drug interaction increases the amount of active drug available resulting in toxicity in this patient.
Adherence	Does not understand instructions: the patient does not understand how to properly take or use the drug product and dosage regimen.
	Cannot afford drug product: the patient cannot afford the drug therapy recommended or prescribed.
	Patient prefers not to take: the patient prefers not to take the drug therapy as instructed.
	Patient forgets to take: the patient does not remember to take sufficient doses of the medication.
	Drug product not available: sufficient supply of the drug product is not available to the patient.
	Cannot swallow/administer drug: the patient is not able to swallow or administer the drug therapy as intended.

A pharmaceutical care practitioner should have a tacit understanding of the common causes of drug therapy problems because their identification is the essence of pharmaceutical care practice. By identifying the cause of the drug therapy problem, the practitioner, other health care providers, and the patient can rationally construct a care plan to resolve that drug therapy problem, thereby making it possible for the patient to achieve his goals of therapy.

Patient Data

Throughout this volume we will use examples of practice-based data generated within pharmaceutical care practices. All of these data are new since the first and second editions of our book. These new data were made available from Medication Management Systems, Inc (MMS) (www.medsmanagement.com). (Note that the authors of the book are all founders of Medication Management Systems, Inc and Robert Cipolle and Linda Strand also serve on the Board of Directors of MMS.)

The examples of practice data all come from a database created by aggregating results from 19 different medication management services. These patients received medication management services by qualified practitioners who were providing services in community pharmacies, hospital-based clinics, free-standing medical clinics, health systems, or pharmacy benefit management company call centers. All of these practices used the Assurance System to document the drug-related needs of their patients, the care provided those patients, the drug therapy problems identified and resolved, and the clinical and economic outcomes. This Assurance Database contains 22,694 patients with 50,142 documented encounters. All patients received services between April 2006 and September 2010.

In the 22,694 patients receiving medication management services, there were 88,556 drug therapy problems identified and resolved. Documentation within the Assurance System allows practitioners to track drug therapy problems by category, cause, and interventions required to resolve the drug therapy problems, and by resolution date. In addition, the Assurance System facilitates the documentation of health care savings realized by the provision of medication management services. Table 5-4 lists the drug therapy problems by category and frequency.

These 88,556 drug therapy problems represent an average of four drug therapy problems per patient over the course of their care. The range of drug therapy problems ranged from 0 to 94 drugs therapy problems over the 54 months of care. A full 85% of these patients had ≥1 drug therapy problems at some time while receiving medication management services. Five or more drug therapy problems were identified and resolved in 27% of patients (n = 6027 patients) and 10% of these patients had ≥10 drug

Table 5-4 Drug therapy problems identified in 22,694 ambulatory patients

Drug therapy problems category	Number of drug therapy problems	Percentage
Unnecessary drug therapy	4544	5
Needs additional drug therapy	29,794	34
Ineffective drug	6834	8
Dosage too low	20,602	23
Adverse drug reaction	9528	11
Dosage too high	4854	5
Adherence	12,400	14
Total	88,556	100

therapy problems. This large number of drug therapy problems demonstrates the vital need that pharmaceutical care practice fills in the overall health of patients. Note that the most frequent unmet drug-related need (drug therapy problem) identified in these patients was the need for additional (new) drug therapy to be initiated in order to prevent or treat a medical condition. The most common of these were patients needing vaccinations to prevent the development of influenza or pneumococcal pneumonia.

It is noteworthy that the second most frequent drug therapy problem identified and resolved in patients receiving medication management services was that the dosage of the medication they were taking was too low to achieve the goal of therapy and produce the desired outcomes. Inadequate dosing of prescription as well as nonprescription medications is a large and costly problem throughout our health care systems. Excluding drug therapy problems in which the patient presented with a new indication requiring new drug therapy or a need to add preventive drug therapy to the patient's regimen dosage too low constitute 35% of problems with patients' existing drug therapies. Underdosing of patients is so common that we now expect it in virtually every patient receiving medication management services. In these patients, the number of instances in which the drug dosing was assessed to be inadequate was almost equal to the total number of patients. That means, on average, every patient in pharmaceutical care practices has at least one medication that is being taken at a dosage that will not achieve the desired goals of therapy, and therefore will never achieve the intended positive outcome unless and until the dosage is adjusted to meet the patient's individual requirements.

Let us consider the "costs" associated with dosages that are too low. Imagine a patient who is feeling ill and decides to enter the health care system to receive treatment for a new condition. Once the decision is made, she must arrange for an appointment at her clinic. This may require taking time off of work or taking personal (leisure) time away from scheduled activities. At the appointed time, she goes to the clinic and sees her physician. The physician must go through the medical workup and history including the differential diagnostic assessment, physical examination, and required laboratory tests to determine the most likely cause for her illness. Once a diagnosis is selected, a specific drug treatment is initiated. The physician describes the condition, the risk of not treating it, and how he expects to manage the condition over the next several months. The patient then visits a pharmacy and gets her prescription filled. The pharmacist explains the instructions and makes certain the patient understands what the medication is for and how to use it. The pharmacist also reviews the patient's other medications to ensure that the new therapy does not interact with her other medications.

If the dosage regimen of this latest (new) prescription medication is inadequate (drug therapy problem = dosage too low) to achieve the goals of therapy, then the patient is likely to continue to suffer the ill feelings that brought her to her primary physician in the first place. After feeling no better after several days, what can she do other than return to the clinic and be seen again by her physician? This time the physician is obligated to revisit the differential diagnostic list and either repeat previous lab values or obtain new laboratory studies to determine the most likely cause of the patient's continued illness. Much if not all of the efforts of the original clinic visit are repeated or expanded in an attempt to identify the cause of the continued illness. All of these health care expenses are caused by the fact that the patient's "real" problem was a drug therapy problem caused by the dosage of the drug selected to treat the patient's medical condition was given at a dosage (dose or dosing interval) too low to achieve the goals of therapy. Our data and the experience of virtually all of those in pharmaceutical care practices show that patients are receiving inadequate dosage of medication far too often. The selection of a "first-line" medication must also be accompanied by the determination of the optimal (individualized) dosage for each patient. Remember: "Drugs do not have doses, people have doses."[17]

Examined another way, many of the drugs we use in today's practice are being used in a manner in which patients endure the cost of the medication and are at risk to experience the side effects of the product, but because their dosage is too low, they do not benefit from the improvement of their medical condition or illness. Individualizing a patient's dosage regimen requires understanding not only "recommended doses," but practitioners must have command of appropriate initial dosing regimens based on patient demographic parameters, comorbidities, and other risk factors. Practitioners must also have a full understanding of how to adjust medication dosages in attempts to achieve the desired goals of therapy for every patient. Should the dose be increased by 10% or doubled if the patient's initial response is not adequate? How long should we wait in order to assess if or to what extent the dosage change has been effective? Lastly, practitioners must also be aware of what the maximum dosage of a medication is that can or should be used for this patient. In summary, not only do drugs not have doses, but patients can each have three dosage regimens: (1) appropriate initial dosage, (2) dosage adjustments to ensure goals are achieved, and (3) maximum dosage.

These data also reveal the impact that pharmaceutical care practices can have on patients' willingness and ability to adhere to their medication regimens. There is a very different picture of nonadherence among patients receiving medication management services compared to those who do not receive the service. In the patients receiving medication management services, only 14% of their drug therapy problems were considered to be due to nonadherence with their drug regimens (Table 5-4). This differs considerably from the published literature on patient adherence, compliance, and/or concordance with their medications. In many studies, nonadherence or noncompliance is reported to be 40% up to 60% depending on the patient population and/or the complexity of the drug regimens.

Table 5-5 lists the number of patients who experienced each of the seven categories of drug therapy problems. There were 22,694 patients evaluated at a total of 50,142 documented visits and who experienced a total of 88,556 drug therapy problems. The average number of drug therapy problems per patient was four, whereas 10% of patients (n = 2257) had 10 or more drug therapy problems over the course of their care.

Table 5-5 Number of patients with drug therapy problems by category in 22,694 ambulatory patients

Drug therapy problem	Number of patients	Percentage of total (n = 22,694)
Unnecessary drug therapy	3069	13.5
Needs additional drug therapy	13,325	58.3
Different drug needed	4330	19.1
Dosage too low	8296	36.6
Adverse drug reaction	6003	26.5
Dosage too high	3309	14.6
Adherence	6354	28.0

Our data from many different practices, in many different practice settings, over many thousands of patient encounters indicate that patients who receive comprehensive medication management services have substantially higher adherence rates and therefore are much more likely to experience the full benefit of all of the medications they are taking. The 12,400 encounters in which a drug therapy problem of nonadherence was identified occurred in 6354 of the 22,694 patients over the 4-year time frame of these pharmaceutical care practices. This means that there were no adherence problems in 72% of these patients receiving medication management services at any time during their therapy. Keep in mind that these patients were taking an average of nine medications to treat or prevent an average of six different medical conditions, and adherence was individually assessed by qualified practitioners during personal visits with each patient and supported by that patient's medication possession ratio (based on refill history) when available. This improved level of adherence to medication instructions in patients in pharmaceutical care practices has the potential to dramatically improve the outcomes of medications across all patients, all drug products, and all disease states. These higher adherence rates are a direct result of the application of the logical drug therapy decision-making process that is the underlying principle of pharmaceutical care practice.

The Assurance System allows practitioners to document the specific cause of each drug therapy problem as well as the medication(s) involved in each problem. Table 5-6 lists the common causes of drug therapy problems within each of the seven categories of drug therapy problems. [listed by frequency within category]

Drug Therapy Problem 1: Unnecessary Drug Therapy

The drug therapy is unnecessary because the patient does not have a clinical indication at this time.

The following is a list of common causes of drug therapy problems involving patients who are taking unnecessary drug therapies. These common causes of drug therapy problems are listed in order of frequency of occurrence in practice:

- Multiple-drug products are being used for a condition that requires single-drug therapy.
- There is no valid medical indication for the drug therapy at this time.
- The medical condition is more appropriately treated with nondrug therapy.
- Drug abuse, alcohol use, or smoking is causing the problem.

Table 5-6   Drug therapy problems by cause in 22,694 ambulatory patients

Drug therapy problem category	Drug therapy problem cause	Number of drug therapy problems	Percentage of drug therapy problems
Unnecessary drug therapy	Duplicate therapy	2031	2.3
	No medical indication at this time	1711	1.9
	Nondrug therapy more appropriate	603	0.7
	Addiction/recreational drug use	109	0.1
	Treating avoidable adverse reaction	90	0.1
Needs additional therapy	Preventive therapy	14,081	16.0
	Untreated condition	7943	9.0
	Synergistic therapy	7770	8.8
Ineffective drug	More effective drug available	4111	4.6
	Condition refractory to drug	1321	1.5
	Dosage form inappropriate	1107	1.3
	Contraindication present	188	0.2
	Drug not effective for condition	107	0.1
Dosage too low	Ineffective dose	9266	10.5
	Needs additional monitoring	6660	7.5
	Frequency inappropriate	2476	2.8
	Incorrect administration	1616	1.8
	Drug interaction	334	0.4
	Incorrect storage	146	0.2
	Duration inappropriate	94	0.1
Adverse drug reaction	Undesirable effect	4813	5.4
	Unsafe drug for the patient	2236	2.5
	Drug interaction	1665	1.9
	Incorrect administration	706	0.8
	Allergic reaction	62	0.1
	Dosage increase/decrease too fast	46	0.1
Dosage too high	Dose too high	2952	3.3
	Needs additional monitoring	1128	1.3
	Frequency too short	374	0.4
	Duration too long	304	0.3
	Drug interaction	96	0.1
Adherence	Does not understand instructions	3384	3.8
	Cannot afford drug product	3267	3.7
	Patient prefers not to take	2334	2.6
	Patient forgets to take	1736	2.0
	Drug product not available	1326	1.5
	Cannot swallow/administer drug	353	0.4
	Total =	88,556	

Table 5-7 Drugs most frequently assessed to be unnecessary

Rank order	Unnecessary drug therapy
1.	Vitamin E
2.	Ascorbic acid (vitamin C)
3.	Omeprazole
4.	Aspirin
5.	Multiple vitamins with minerals
6.	Folic acid
7.	Omega-3 fatty acids
8.	Cholecalciferol (vitamin D)
9.	Ibuprofen
10.	Metformin

- Drug therapy is being taken to treat an avoidable adverse reaction associated with another medication.

The Pharmacotherapy Workup guides the practitioner to be thorough and to consider if the patient is taking unnecessary drug therapies.

The average number of medications taken by these patients was nine, but many patients take even more on a daily basis. In these patients, 10% of the encounters were with patients taking ≥15 medications on a continuous basis. Table 5-7 displays the drugs most frequently assessed to be unnecessary by the pharmaceutical care practitioner.

Note that nine of the 10 drug products assessed to be unnecessary do not require a prescription and are seldom recorded in the patient's medical record. Personal contact with the patient is required to assess if the patient is taking medications that are not necessary.

Drug Therapy Problem 2: Needs Additional Drug Therapy

Additional drug therapy is required to treat or prevent a medical condition or illness from developing.

The following is a list of common causes of drug therapy problems involving patients who require additional drug therapies to meet their needs:

- Preventive drug therapy is required to reduce the risk of developing a new condition.

- A medical condition requires the initiation of drug therapy.
- A medical condition requires additional pharmacotherapy to attain synergistic or additive effects.

KEY CLINICAL CONCEPTS

Patients taking no medications can have drug therapy problems. Prevention chronic medical conditions is a major objective of pharmaceutical care practice.

As new and innovative drug regimens are designed and demonstrated to be efficacious at preventing many diseases, it is important that patients receive appropriate preventive medications. We now have confirmed evidence that daily, low-dose aspirin use can prevent secondary heart attacks (myocardial infarction) and/or strokes in patients with certain risk factors. There are numerous trials demonstrating that fractures and other injuries can be minimized by the use of daily calcium and Vitamin D supplements to slow or prevent bone loss (osteoporosis) in women. Safer and more efficacious immunizations are constantly being developed to prevent serious infectious diseases including measles, mumps, rubella, influenza, and hepatitis. Table 5-8 lists several examples of drug therapies commonly used to prevent disease or illness.

The delivery of comprehensive medication management services requires the practitioner to provide proactive care rather than simply react to prescriptions, changes in drug orders, or questions from patients or other care providers. Not only does this patient-centered, drug therapy problem identification method facilitate providing preventive care, but the patient remains the focus of all inquiries and investigations. This exemplifies a major difference between pharmaceutical care practice as a rational approach to identifying and resolving drug therapy problems and most traditional methods that are based on a review of a list of prescription medications, often referred to as a drug review or even medication reconciliation.

A patient-centered focus must be established and maintained if the practitioner is to adequately identify potential risk factors or problems, especially those for which no drug has yet been prescribed or recommended. If the practitioner's efforts are limited simply to reviewing a list of medications that has already been prescribed for, or consumed by, the patient, then there is little chance that all the potential problems that the patient might be at a high risk to develop will be identified, and certainly not prevented.

Table 5-8 Pharmacotherapy as prevention

Preventive drug therapy	Clinical indication
Aspirin	Secondary prevention of heart attack and/or stroke
Calcium and vitamin D supplements	Prevention of osteoporosis
Folic acid supplements during pregnancy	Prevention of neural tube defects
Influenza vaccine	Prevention of the flu
Pneumococcal vaccine	Prevention of pneumococcal pneumonia
Filgrastim (Neupogen)	Prevention of infection in patients receiving some chemotherapy regimens
Sun screens	Prevention of sun-induced skin disorders and burns
Dimenhydranate	Prevention of motion sickness
Amoxicillin	Endocarditis prophylaxis in dental patients with cardiac lesions or prosthetic heart valves
Colchicine	Prophylactic therapy for patients with frequent attacks of gouty arthritis
Propranolol	Prophylactic treatment for recurring migraine headaches
Atorvastatin	Primary prevention of cardiovascular disease in patients with multiple cardiovascular disease risk factors or diabetes

Example The patient is at high risk to contract pneumonia and therefore requires a pneumococcal vaccine.

The drug products most frequently associated with the seven categories and the specific causes of drug therapy problems vary considerably. Within the category of additional drug therapy needed, the three primary causes are preventive medication indicated, untreated indication, and synergistic therapy indicated. The 10 most frequent drug products associated with these common drug therapy problems are listed in Tables 5-9 to 5-11:

Table 5-9 Medications most often added as preventive therapies

Rank order	Needs additional: indicated as preventive therapy
1.	Influenza vaccine
2.	Pneumococcal vaccine
3.	Insulin
4.	Aspirin
5.	Tetanus toxoid vaccine
6.	Metformin
7.	Calcium with vitamin D
8.	Zoster vaccine
9.	Sunscreens
10.	Glucagon

Drug Therapy Problem 3: Ineffective Drug

The drug product is not being effective at producing the desired response or outcome.

The following is a list of common causes of drug therapy problems involving patients who are taking drugs that are not effective:

- The drug product is not the most effective for the indication being treated.
- The medical condition is refractory to the drug product.

Table 5-10 Medications most often added to treat a new condition

Rank order	Needs additional: indicated for untreated condition
1.	Acetaminophen
2.	Simvastatin (Zocor)
3.	Varenicline tartrate (Chantix)
4.	Aspirin
5.	Nicotine
6.	Calcium carbonate with vitamin D
7.	Lisinopril
8.	Gabapentin
9.	Loratadine
10.	Metformin

Table 5-11 Medications most often added for additive or synergistic effects

Rank order	Needs additional: indicated as additive/synergistic therapy
1.	Metformin
2.	Albuterol sulfate (inhaler)
3.	Omega-3 fatty acids
4.	Insulin
5.	Exenatide (Byetta)
6.	Lisinopril
7.	Acetaminophen
8.	Fluticasone and salmeterol (Advair)
9.	Pioglitazone
10.	Glipizide

- The dosage form of the drug product is inappropriate.
- Contraindication is present.
- The drug is not effective for the medical problem.

Choosing the drug regimen that will be the most effective for an individual patient involves an important set of clinical decisions.

KEY CLINICAL CONCEPTS

Effectiveness can only be realized if an appropriate drug product is selected and the dosage used is sufficient to produce the desired outcome in a particular patient.

It is important to keep in mind that if a drug product has been demonstrated to be efficacious in 75% of patients with a certain medical condition, then it is likely that 25% of your patients with that same condition will not respond positively. Therefore, even if a drug product is thought to be the first-line therapy or the "drug of choice," it will not be effective for all patients. In our patient group, 4330 patients (19%) were taking a drug product assessed to be ineffective for them. Most frequently, these medications were being used unsuccessfully to manage diabetes, osteoporosis, hypertension, hyperlipidemia, or insomnia.

> **KEY CLINICAL CONCEPTS**
>
> Selecting a drug product for a patient that is likely to be effective requires a thorough understanding of the pathophysiology of the patient's disorder and the pharmacology of the drug product being considered.

The pharmaceutical care practitioner must keep up to date with new products and the primary literature to ensure that the best choices are being made for a particular patient.

The concept of the drug of choice is an overly simplistic view of clinical pharmacology and pharmacotherapeutic principles. New agents are developed constantly and some are shown to be more efficacious than previously existing drug products. Entire approaches to therapy can change over time. As an example, in the 1970s, the drug therapy of choice for peptic ulcer disease was antacids. This changed to H_2-inhibitors, such as cimetidine and ranitidine, during the next decade. In the 1990s, many ulcer patients were found to respond to combination antibiotic therapy due to *Helicobacter pylori* involvement. By 2002, the third and fourth leading prescription drug sales in the United States were Prevacid (lansoprazole) and Prilosec (omeprazole), both proton pump inhibitors used to treat and prevent peptic ulcer disorders. In 2009, over 13 million prescriptions for Prevacid and 38 million prescriptions for omeprazole were written in the United States. Table 5-12 lists the 10 drugs most frequently assessed to be ineffective and not achieving the goals of therapy in individualised patients.

Drug Therapy Problem 4: Dosage Too Low

The dosage is too low to produce the desired response or outcome.

The following is a list of common causes of drug therapy problems involving patients whose dosage regimens are insufficient to produce the desired effects:

- The dose is too low to produce the desired response.
- Needs additional monitoring to determine that the dosage is too low.
- The dosage interval is too infrequent to produce the desired response.
- Incorrect administration of the drug.
- A drug interaction reduces the amount of active drug available.
- Incorrect storage of the drug.
- The duration of drug therapy is too short to produce the desired response.

Table 5-12 Medications most frequently assessed to be ineffective for the patient

Rank order	Ineffective drug
1.	Calcium with Vitamin D
2.	Acetaminophen
3.	Omeprazole
4.	Insulin
5.	Zolpidem (Ambien)
6.	Metformin
7.	Simvastatin
8.	Loratadine
9.	Cetirizine
10.	Ibuprofen

Example The patient's 10-mg daily dose of glipizipe (Glucotrol) is too low to provide adequate control of her blood glucose.

The most frequent drug therapy problem associated with lack of effectiveness is seen in patients who receive a dosage regimen that is not sufficient to produce the desired pharmacological result. A dosage regimen has multiple parts and includes the drug product, the dose, the dosing interval, and the duration of therapy. All of these components must be appropriate for your patient in order to produce the desired outcome. Too often patients are given a drug product that is considered to be efficacious in a population, but the dosage regimen is not sufficient to benefit the individual patient.

Making certain that patients are taking an adequate dosage of their medications to produce the desired effects is a responsibility of the practitioner. One size does not fit all, and one dose does not work for all patients. Student practitioners need to understand that published dosing guidelines are usually generated through highly controlled research studies, and therefore can only be used as initial guidelines for drug dosing. Patients will require varying amounts of medications in order to produce the desired pharmacological effects.

People like to use safe drug therapies. *It is easy to make drug therapies safe, simply underdose everyone.* If the patient takes too little of the right drug, there is only a small likelihood of experiencing any undesirable effects. On the other hand, there is virtually no chance that the patient will benefit from an insufficient dosage regimen.

Allopathic practitioners do not intentionally provide insufficient doses for a patient. However, published dosing guidelines are often so conservative that patients suffer through ineffective drug therapy because they are instructed to take the "recommended" dose. The tools, knowledge, and successful approaches to the dosing of drugs based on patient-specific parameters play an important role in the provision of pharmaceutical care.

There are also many instances in which patients are started on drug therapies using a very low or conservative dosage regimen in order to "see what happens." This logical and often safe approach requires that the practitioner is fully committed to follow-up at scheduled intervals to evaluate the patient's status and make any necessary dosage adjustments. Without this critical follow-up evaluation step, the patient is destined to suffer unnecessary periods of inadequate treatment and continued illness if the dosage received is too low to produce the desired outcomes.

Similarly, patients may not be taking the dose of a drug product often enough to fully realize the benefit. If the dosing interval is too prolonged, the beneficial effects of the drug may disappear before the effects of the next dose appear. Adjusting the dosing interval is a common intervention to resolve some drug therapy problems.

Drug therapy problems caused by dosage regimens that are too low are the second most frequently encountered problems in pharmaceutical care practice. The 10 drugs most frequently prescribed for patients with doses that were too low to achieve the desired goals of therapy and therefore did not achieve the intended positive outcomes are listed in Table 5-13:

Table 5-13   Medications most frequently underdosed in ambulatory patients

Rank order	Dosage too low: dose too low
1.	Insulin
2.	Metformin
3.	Gabapentin
4.	Lisinopril
5.	Exenatide (Byetta)
6.	Simvastatin
7.	Furosemide
8.	Fluticasone and salmeterol (Advair)
9.	Hydrochlorothiazide
10.	Sertraline

Note that these are all drug products that are used very commonly in practice and for which there is considerable evidence of their efficacy and considerable dosing information available. Nevertheless, patients continue to be treated with inadequate dosages resulting in continued morbidity and mortality. What seems to be missing from our health care systems is the application of a rational, comprehensive, and effective method to ensure that each patient receives drug therapy at a dosage likely to produce the intended desired outcomes.

Drug Therapy Problem 5: Adverse Drug Reaction

The drug is causing an adverse reaction.

The following is a list of common causes of drug therapy problems involving patients who are taking drug products that are not safe for them:

- The drug product causes an undesirable reaction that is not dose-related.
- A safer drug product is required due to risk factors.
- A drug interaction causes an undesirable reaction that is not dose-related.
- Incorrect administration of the drug product.
- The drug product causes an allergic reaction.
- The dosage regimen was administered or changed too rapidly.
- The drug product is contraindicated due to risk factors.

Example The patient has developed a rash covering his upper torso and arm caused by the co-trimoxazole (sulfamethoxazole and trimethoprim) he was taking to treat a wound infection.

If the patient has a negative reaction to a drug product it is considered an adverse drug reaction. The resolution calls for discontinuing that product and identifying one that would likely be effective and would also be safer for the patient. Compare this type of drug therapy problem with those undesirable events that are caused by the patient receiving too high a dose. In these cases, the remedy is most often to reduce the dosage regimen. It is important for pharmaceutical care practitioners to distinguish between undesirable events that are dose-related and those that are not. The 10 drug products most frequently involved in adverse drug reactions are listed in Table 5-14.

The lack of a uniform definition and the collective inability of the health care system to create and support an effective infrastructure to identify, document, resolve, and report adverse drug reactions has resulted in an amazingly

Table 5-14   Medications most frequently involved in adverse drug reactions

Rank order	Adverse drug reaction
1.	Quetiapine fumarate (Seroquel)
2.	Doneprzil hydrochloride (Aricept)
3.	Memantine (Namenda)
4.	Metformin (Glucophage)
5.	Simvastatin (Zocor)
6.	Clopidogrel bisulfate (Plavix)
7.	Lisinopril (Prinivil))
8.	Tramadol HCl (Ultram)
9.	Levothyroxine sodium (Synthroid)
10.	Amlodipine besylate (Norvasc)

sparse amount of practical information that practitioners can apply to protect patients from serious and life-threatening experiences. The need for a uniform definition is clearly illustrated in the list of terms used to describe various types of undesired reactions to medications. Table 5-15 lists terms commonly used to describe adverse drug reactions. The category of "safety" in the taxonomy of drug therapy problems finally provides a standard vocabulary for and approach to adverse drug reactions in patients.

Table 5-15   Terms used to describe adverse drug reactions

Adverse events	Excessive therapeutic effects
Adverse drug reactions	Erroneous use and accidents
Adverse reaction	Iatrogenic disease
Complications	Iatrogenic illness
Drug-induced illness	Negative therapeutic effects
Drug-induced disease	Pathological reaction
Drug-induce injury	Prescribing errors
Drug intolerance	Side effects
Drug interaction	Super infection
Drug misadventure	Unwanted pharmacological effects

Drug Therapy Problem 6: Dosage Too High

The dosage is too high, resulting in undesirable toxic effects.

The following is a list of common causes of drug therapy problems involving the patient whose dosage regimen of a drug is too high and is therefore resulting in unacceptable risk or harm:

- Dose is too high.
- Need additional monitoring to determine if dosage is too high.
- The dosing frequency is too short.
- The duration of drug therapy is too long.
- A drug interaction occurs resulting in a toxic reaction to the drug product.

> **Example** The patient developed bradycardia and second-degree heart block resulting from a 0.5-mg daily dose of digoxin used for congestive heart failure. This dose was too high due to his advanced age and declining renal function.

Drugs often exert their pharmacological activities at many different sites in the body or within several organ systems or enzymatic pathways at the same time. Some of these known pharmacological activities will be considered beneficial for the specific indication of the patient. The other predictable, but undesirable pharmacological actions are considered side effects. However, *drugs do not know why we sell them, or why we use them.* Drugs merely exert their pharmacology on the patient; sometimes the results are intended and beneficial, sometimes they are not. Therefore, it is important for the pharmaceutical care practitioner to have an extensive and in-depth understanding of the pharmacology of the drugs his or her patient is taking. Most side effects are predictable, and therefore often preventable extensions of the known pharmacology of the drug.

A drug therapy problem resulting from patients receiving a dosage that is too high for them is also a serious health care problem. For patients in pharmaceutical care practices, 5% of the problems were from dosages that were too high. Table 5-16 lists the prescription medications frequently associated with drug therapy problems of the category dosage too high.

Drug therapy problems resulting from dosage that are too high are common and are associated with considerable patient discomfort, suffering, and expense. These drug therapy problems are distinguished from adverse drug reactions because the cause and therefore their resolutions differ. Drug therapy problems resulting from dosages that are too high for the patient are most commonly resolved by reducing the dose or by administering the drug less frequently. On the other hand, adverse drug reaction types of drug therapy

Table 5-16   Drugs most frequently given at too high of a dose for the patient

Rank order	Dosage too high
1.	Insulin
2.	Metformin (Glucophage)
3.	Lisinopril (Prinivil)
4.	Glipizide (Glucotrol)
5.	Furosemide
6.	Simvastatin (Zocor)
7.	Atenolol
8.	Levothyroxine sodium (Synthroid)
9.	Hydrochlorothiazide
10.	Darbepoetin alfa (Aranesp)

problems are not related to the dosage of the medication, and therefore their resolution most often requires the discontinuation of the offending drug product and replacement with an agent from a different pharmacological class.

For approximately 5% of drug therapy problems, the practitioner determined that the unwanted effects were dose-related and could be resolved by adjusting the dosage regimen downward. Distinguishing dose-related effects from adverse drug reactions that cannot be resolved by reducing the dosage is important. Over the course of their care, 15% of patients experienced a drug therapy problem caused by a dosage regimen that was too high for that particular patient. This is contrasted with the 37% of patients who had a drug therapy problem due to a dosage too low. These data also demonstrate the great need to evaluate patients for the negative outcomes of drug therapies as well as the intended positive outcomes.

Drug Therapy Problem 7: Adherence (Noncompliance)

The patient is not able or willing to take the drug therapy as intended.

The following is a list of common causes for patients not to adequately comply with the drug therapy instructions. The causes are listed from most frequently to least frequently encountered in practice:

- The patient does not understand the instructions.
- The patient cannot afford the drug product.
- The patient prefers not to take the medication.

- The patient forgets to take the medication.
- The drug product is not available for the patient.
- The patient cannot swallow or self-administer the drug product appropriately.

Example   The patient is not able to remember to instill her timolol eye drops twice daily for her glaucoma.

When a practitioner decides that the patient's drug therapy problem is an adherence problem, he or she must be certain that the patient's medication regimen has been judged to be therapeutically indicated, effective, and safe. Recall, the term *compliance* is used to mean compliance with a dosage regimen, not with the orders of a paternalistic or authoritarian figure. When pharmaceutical care practitioners conclude that a patient is being nonadherent they mean the following:

Definition   Nonadherence (noncompliance) is defined as the patient's inability or unwillingness to take a drug regimen that the practitioner has clinically judged to be appropriately indicated, adequately efficacious, and able to produce the desired outcomes without any serious harmful effects.

There is a reason for all nonadherence, and it is the practitioner's responsibility to discover that reason. The cause, or reason, for noncompliance determines the interventions and care that are necessary to alter or improve the patient's outcome. Keep in mind if the patient stops taking a drug because it was not being effective, it is an effectiveness problem—not a compliance problem. Similarly, if your patient stopped taking her medication because it was making her too dizzy to stand up, it is likely a safety problem and not a compliance problem. Less than 15% of all drug therapy problems are compliance problems. Our research and clinical experience indicates that the majority (>85%) of drug therapy problems involve problems with indication, effectiveness, and/or safety.

Noncompliance among patients receiving prescription medications has been studied quite extensively. This common drug therapy problem has most often been examined from the point of view of the practitioner rather than from the more influential attitude of the patient. Considerable efforts have been expended to identify the social characteristics of patients that might be indicators of who will and who will not comply with a given medication regimen. Most social factors, including age, sex, race, social class, marital status, and religion, have proven to be of low value in identifying compliant and noncompliant patients.[18]

In order to successfully follow any set of instructions, patients must first understand them. Practitioners often use language and terminology that is unclear to, or not understood by, the patient. Sometimes, patients have different definitions of terms, and these differences can result in misunderstandings, confusion, and noncompliance.

Patients can have very different interpretations of common phraseology used in prescription directions, such as "two times a day." What message are you trying to send to your patient with instructions such as "take this medicine twice a day?" Most often the intended message is two doses, taken about 12 hours apart. However, without being explicit about these instructions, patients may interpret "two times a day" quite differently. Consider what time frame is intended when common activities such as telephoning a friend or checking your e-mail twice a day are described.

KEY CLINICAL CONCEPTS

Not only are patients capable of making rational decisions, they actually make numerous decisions concerning their own health and well-being throughout the various stages of the diagnostic and therapeutic processes.

Each patient decides whether to be concerned about signs, symptoms, or the discomfort present and decides to agree, or not to agree, with the diagnosis that is presented. Furthermore, patients decide whether they believe that the proposed therapy is likely to achieve their desired outcome.

Patients decide how they will comply with medications. Patients tend not to take medications that they do not understand. They usually do not take drug therapies that they believe will not benefit them. Patients also do not take drugs if they have safety concerns about the product. Similarly, people do not begin taking a medication without their own preconceived ideas, nor do they enter a health care system without such preferences. They have their own health care beliefs, ideas about medications, and most importantly, they have ideas about what they want and when they want it. Patients weigh the advantages and disadvantages of drug therapy, the risks and benefits, and the possible discomfort of changing their own behavior against the likelihood of a positive outcome.

As with any person who is asked or expected to follow a set of directions, the patient must determine for herself whether doing what the practitioner has recommended is really going to be in his or her best interest. If patients believe that it will be, then they are likely to do their best to comply with the instructions. On the other hand, patient package inserts and coaching by clinicians will be of little value if patients do not perceive that a condition can cause harm or discomfort, or if they do not believe that the recommended therapy will reduce the threat or discomfort caused by the ailment.

When patients choose not to take a medication as intended, they have what they consider to be a good reason for not accepting advice and complying with their prescription instructions. Practitioners must internalize the fact that patients' perceptions and health care belief systems discovered during the assessment process are major driving forces that ultimately influence the decision to seek care or not, and to follow instructions and advice or not.

Patient behavior associated with taking medications has a significant impact on pharmacotherapy outcomes. The last category of drug therapy problems describes patient actions when they do not or cannot adhere to the instructions.

The rate of nonadherence among patients receiving comprehensive medication management services care is low. This category of drug therapy problem is resolved through interventions such as explaining how the medication works (pharmacology) and how the patient will know if it is being effective (goals of therapy), and making the instructions clearly understandable to the patient, providing the patient with a daily medication diary, medication administration reminders, calendars, pill boxes, and access to free medication programs or price reduction programs offered by some manufactures or governmental agencies. The medications most frequently involved in problems of nonadherence are presented in Table 5-17.

Table 5-17 Medications most frequently involved in problems of nonadherence

Rank order	Adherence (overall)
1.	Simvastatin (Zocor)
2.	Metformin HCl (Glucophage)
3.	Atorvastatin calcium (Lipitor)
4.	Insulin-various
5.	Fluticasone and salmeterol (Advair)
6.	Lisinopril (Prinivil, Zestril)
7.	Albuterol—inhalers (Proventil, Ventolin, ProAir)
8.	Exenatide (Byetta)
9.	Levothyroxine sodium (Synthroid)
10.	Rosuvastatin calcium (Crestor)

Table 5-18   Medications with instructions that patients often did not understand

Rank order	Adherence—patient does not understand instructions
1.	Albuterol—inhalers (Proventil, Ventolin, ProAir)
2.	Fluticasone and salmeterol (Advair)
3.	Metformin HCl (Glucophage)
4.	Insulin—various
5.	Mycophenolate mofetil (CellCept, Myfortic)
6.	Simvastatin (Zocor)
7.	Omeprazole
8.	Levothyroxine sodium (Synthroid)
9.	Aspirin
10.	Lisinopril (Prinivil, Zestril)

Of the patients who had problems complying with the instructions for their medications, four causes of noncompliance were among the most frequently encountered. Eleven percent (2551 patients) reported that they did not understand the instructions that they were given as to how to properly take or administer their medications. This was the cause identified in 27% of the cases of noncompliance. Both prescription and nonprescription products were involved (Table 5-18).

One thousand seven hundred twenty-seven patients (8%) explained that they understood the rationale for the treatment but preferred not to take the medication. In these situations, the practitioners intervened with some alternate form of drug therapy that the patient agreed to use (Table 5-19).

In our sample of 22,694 patients, 2120 patients (9%) found that their drug therapies were too costly, and therefore did not follow the instructions. Less expensive products were identified and substituted in these cases (Table 5-20).

The fourth most common cause of noncompliance was that the patient forgot to take the medication. Five percent of patients did not remember to take their drug therapies as intended (Table 5-21).

Many patients receiving pharmaceutical care have to manage multiple drug therapies. More than 30% of patients require 10 or more different drug regimens, several of which require multiple doses each day. Simplifying a patient's drug regimens can have a dramatic impact on the patient's ability to follow all of the instructions properly.

Table 5-19 Medications patient often preferred not to take

Rank order	Adherence—patient prefers not to take the drug product
1.	Metformin HCl (Glucophage)
2.	Simvastatin (Zocor)
3.	Fluticasone and salmeterol (Advair)
4.	Lisinopril (Prinivil, Zestril)
5.	Insulin—various
6.	Atorvastatin calcium (Lipitor)
7.	Furosemide
8.	Hydrochlorothiazide
9.	Gabapentin (Neurontin)
10.	Exenatide (Byetta)

In Australia, pharmacists providing medication management services in patients living in residential care facilities and also for patients living in their own home found a large number of drug therapy problems (mean = 5 per patient) involving a wide range of medications. Patients at home had more drug therapy problems (mean = 5) than patients living in a residential care facility (mean = 4).[16]

These practice-based results create an interesting picture of how medications are presently being used within the health care system. Far more people

Table 5-20 Medications patient often could not afford to purchase

Rank order	Adherence—patient cannot afford the drug product
1.	Simvastatin (Zocor)
2.	Atorvastatin calcium (Lipitor)
3.	Lisinopril (Prinivil, Zestril)
4.	Rosuvastatin calcium (Crestor)
5.	Insulin—various
6.	Esomeprazole magnesium (Nexium)
7.	Fenofibrate (TriCor)
8.	Losartan potassium (Cozaar)
9.	Fluticasone and salmeterol (Advair)
10.	Ezetimibe and simvastatin (Vytorin)

Table 5-21 Medications patient often forget to take as instructed

Rank order	Adherence—patient forgets to take the drug product
1.	Metformin HCl (Glucophage)
2.	Simvastatin (Zocor)
3.	Fluticasone and salmeterol (Advair)
4.	Exenatide (Byetta)
5.	Mycophenolate mofetil (CellCept, Myfortic)
6.	Lisinopril (Prinivil, Zestril)
7.	Prednisone
8.	Insulin—various
9.	Tacrolimus (Prograf)
10.	Metoprolol tartrate (Lopressor, Toprol-XL)

can benefit from additional drug therapies to prevent or treat illnesses than are presently recognized. Drug therapies are frequently used at dosages not sufficient to provide effective therapy. Patients often have not been adequately instructed on the optimal way to use their medications. These problems occur at a frequency sufficient to keep many pharmaceutical care practitioners busy helping patients achieve the results they want from their medications.

Drug Interactions

It is also interesting to examine the medications most frequently associated with drug therapy problems that are caused by drug–drug interactions. Note that drug interactions can cause drug therapy problems in several categories. Drug interactions can result in reducing the effectiveness of a medication, increasing the toxicity of a medication and/or resulting in an adverse drug reaction. Table 5-22 lists the 10 drug products most frequently causing drug–drug interactions that required the practitioner to intervene and change or adjust the patient's drug regimen(s):

STATING DRUG THERAPY PROBLEMS

When you identify and describe a patient's drug therapy problem, you are adding new and unique information about the patient's case. How the practitioner describes the drug therapy problem is of paramount importance.

Table 5-22 Medications involved in drug interactions requiring interventions

Rank order	Drug interactions
1.	Clopidogrel bisulfate (Plavix)
2.	Omeprazole
3.	Aspirin
4.	Calcium carbonate or calcium citrate
5.	Levothyroxine
6.	Warfarin
7.	Ibuprofen
8.	Pantoprazole sodium (Protonix)
9.	Simvastatin (Zocor)
10.	Tramadol

Therefore, it is important to describe the patient's drug therapy problem in a concise, accurate, and informative manner.

A statement describing the patient's drug therapy problem(s) consists of three components:

1. A description of the patient's medical *condition* or clinical state.
2. The *drug therapy* involved (causing or solving the problem).
3. The specific *association* between the drug therapy and the patient's condition.

In the context of an individual patient, the identification of a drug therapy problem establishes the practitioner's responsibilities to that patient. This will not only determine the solution to be employed but often dictates other components of the care plan, including clinical and laboratory parameters to be evaluated and the schedule for follow-up visits.

The way in which a drug therapy problem is stated, described, and documented can greatly influence the care of a patient. Simply stating that a patient is experiencing "toxicity" from drug therapy is not very useful. The type of toxicity (i.e., nephrotoxicity, leucopenia, thrombocytopenia, pseudomembranous colitis, diarrhea, bleeding) and the specific drug associated with this undesirable event are essential to know. Also, describing if the patient is experiencing a dose-related or nondose-related reaction should be identified as part of the description of the patient's drug therapy problem.

Experienced practitioners are mindful of the benefit of stating drug therapy problems in a format that is most useful and with an appropriate level of specificity for the patient's condition at the time of intervention. It is not very useful to describe the patient's drug therapy problem as "the drug she is taking for her high cholesterol is not working." Describing all of the components of your patient's drug therapy problems is more useful. "The Lipitor (atorvastatin) therapy that she has been taking for the past 3 months for hyperlipidemia has only resulted in a 5% reduction of her total cholesterol using an aggressive dosage of 80 mg daily."

The terminology used to describe a drug therapy problem can also greatly influence how a patient or other health care practitioners perceive and resolve the problem.

KEY CLINICAL CONCEPTS

The description of the patient's drug therapy problem directly influences the changes that will be made in the patient's pharmacotherapy regimens.

Terminology that implies cause and effect must be differentiated from terminology that implies a weaker association. Consider the different interventions that might be initiated to resolve drug therapy problems stated through the following pairs of examples:

- The 29-year-old patient is having continued breakthrough seizures due to subtherapeutic phenytoin concentrations.
  This drug therapy problem requires an increase in the patient's phenytoin dosage.
- This 29-year-old patient is noncompliant with phenytoin therapy, as she forgets to take her medication, and she is experiencing continued seizure activity.
  This drug therapy problem would be resolved by providing the patient with a daily medication reminder device or a medication diary to help keep track of her medication use.
- This 61-year-old male business executive is experiencing gastrointestinal bleeding caused by aspirin therapy.
  Determining the clinical indication for his aspirin therapy and substituting another medication that is less likely to cause gastrointestinal bleeding would resolve this drug therapy problem.

- This 61-year-old male patient, who is presently taking low-dose aspirin as prophylaxis to prevent a second myocardial infarction, has a history of several episodes of gastrointestinal bleeding from peptic ulcers.
  Using an enteric-coated aspirin product and frequently evaluating him for any gastrointestinal symptoms would prevent this drug therapy problem.
- This 43-year-old female patient, who is being treated for pneumonia with gentamicin therapy, has poor renal function.
  This drug therapy problem would be prevented by adjusting her dose and interval to provide desired peak and trough gentamicin serum concentrations and by determining her individual pharmacokinetic parameters for gentamicin.
- This 43-year-old female patient with pneumonia has acute renal failure secondary to gentamicin therapy.
  This drug therapy problem can be resolved by discontinuing the gentamicin therapy treating the pneumonia with a different antibiotic that is not harmful to the kidneys.

These examples illustrate the importance of clarity when stating or describing drug therapy problems.

PRIORITIZING DRUG THERAPY PROBLEMS

Once identified, each drug therapy problem can be prioritized as to the urgency with which it needs to be addressed. This prioritization depends upon the extent of the potential harm each problem might inflict on the patient, the patient's perception of the potential harm, and the rate at which this harm is likely to occur. If multiple drug therapy problems are to be dealt with sequentially, the patient should be involved in the decision as to the priority given to each drug therapy problem.

The logic applied to identify, prioritize, and resolve drug therapy problems in complex patients is based on organizational intelligence and is the best approach to problem solving.[19] In patients with multiple drug therapy problems, some problems are identified but are considered to be of a lower priority, and the effort to resolve them is delayed until drug therapy problems with a higher priority are first addressed. However, it remains essential to document those drug therapy problems assigned a lower priority, so they eventually receive the attention required and are not forgotten.

Prioritizing drug therapy problems is an essential skill because of the high frequency with which you will encounter patients who have more than one drug therapy problem at the same time. Our research shows that approximately 21% of patients have multiple drug therapy problems when initially assessed by the pharmaceutical care practitioner.

Once the list of drug therapy problems is prioritized according to risk to the patient, the list is reviewed and the following issues addressed:

1. Which problems must be resolved (or prevented) immediately and which can wait?
2. Which problems can be resolved by the practitioner and patient directly?
3. Which require the interventions by someone else (perhaps a family member, physician, nurse, care giver, or some other specialist).

Obviously, pharmaceutical care practitioners hold a great deal of the responsibility for identifying drug therapy problems. Much of this responsibility stems from their special knowledge and experience in the fields of pharmacology, pharmacotherapy, pathophysiology, and toxicology. However, patients often identify their own drug therapy problems. This occurs through self-diagnosis, self-examination, and introspective comparisons with previous states of health, or the condition of friends, colleagues, acquaintances, and family members.

Patients will help to prioritize drug therapy problems and they can also help you identify them initially. When a patient has, or at least feels he or she has identified a drug therapy problem, it must receive the full attention of the clinician. Many elderly patients reveal that they will discontinue taking prescribed medications, without seeking the advice of a health care professional, if they perceive they are not experiencing the beneficial effects of the drug. This may be considered to be "rational noncompliance."[20] When a patient self-identifies a drug therapy problem, the practitioner must make it a priority. One might ask in a patient-centered practice: "Who better to recognize drug therapy problems than the patient?"

PATIENTS WITH NO DRUG THERAPY PROBLEMS

It is the practitioner's responsibility to identify any and all drug therapy problems that the patient has. Or, the practitioner may conclude, with substantive evidence, that the patient does not have any drug therapy problems at the present time. A conclusion that no drug therapy problems exist means that all the patient's drug therapies are clinically indicated, the dosage regimens are producing the desired results, and they are not causing any intolerable side effects. A finding that there are no drug therapy problems present will also be interpreted as the patient understands, agrees with, and is compliant with all of his or her drug regimens and instructions. Finally, the decision that the patient has no drug therapy problems at this time indicates that all of the patient's drug-related needs are being met, and no adjustments in drug products or drug dosage regimens are required.

In cases when the patient does not have a drug therapy problem, the pharmaceutical care practitioner focuses on assuring that the goals of therapy are being met and that the patient is not at high risk of developing any new problems. Providing continuous care requires the assurance of progress toward achieving and maintaining the desired goals of therapy. Patients who have no drug therapy problems at this time still require a care plan and follow-up evaluation to ensure that goals of therapy continue to be met and no new drug therapy problems develop. Therefore, care plans and follow-up evaluation activities continue even when no drug therapy problems are found, similar to a yearly check-up with the dentist to identify any new dental problems (cavities, gingivitis, or excessive build-up of plaque) that may occur.

DOCUMENTING DRUG THERAPY PROBLEMS

The standard for documenting the patient's drug therapy problems is that each problem identified is added to the patient's record and includes the medical condition, illness, or complaint involved, the drug therapy or therapies involved, and the likely cause of the drug therapy problem. Drug therapy problems are most efficiently documented within the care plan for each medical condition involved. The interventions required to resolve the drug therapy problem will also be associated with that care plan. The action that is taken (increase dosage, discontinue drug therapy, add preventive drug to regimen) also needs to be recorded. Sometimes it is helpful to record the individuals involved in resolving the drug therapy problem (patient, family, physician, nurse).

Documenting the economic impact of identifying and resolving a drug therapy problem at the time the service is provided is helpful to provide evidence of the economic impact of new medication management services. Recording instances in which clinic, specialist, or hospitalization visits were avoided because the drug therapy has been improved, can help to justify the cost of a new or expanding medication management service. These additional service management records can be maintained separately from the patient's personal care records and summarized quarterly or annually. The Assurance Pharmaceutical Care system maintains records that facilitate information retrieval and data consolidation, as well as providing the summary reports needed to evaluate the practitioner's services and support improvements and expansion in that service. These are described in Chapter 9.

SUMMARY

The identification, resolution, and prevention of drug therapy problems are the responsibility of the pharmaceutical care practitioner and are the central value of all medication management services. Drug therapy problems are clinical problems because they affect individual patients and require professional judgment to resolve. The rational assessment of a patient's drug-related needs follows the logic of *indication, effectiveness, safety,* and *adherence.* The centrality of drug therapy problems to the practice of pharmaceutical care cannot be overemphasized. It is essential that practitioners who intend to provide medication management services understand each type of drug therapy problem as well as their common causes. The disciplined thought required in pharmaceutical care practice guides the practitioner to first make certain that all of the patient's indications for drug therapy are being appropriately treated and that no unnecessary drug therapy is being taken. Then, the practitioner can logically consider product selection and/or dosage adjustment to maximize the effectiveness of the medication. The practitioner must then make certain that all drug therapies will be as safe as possible for the patient. It is important to re-emphasize that only after these first three primary pharmacotherapy principles have been fully addressed, are adherence and cost issues considered.

The data generated from patients seen in practice present interesting observations. It is instructive to note that adherence problems are not those most frequently associated with drug therapies seen in clinical practice. Patients requiring the practitioner to provide appropriate drug therapies for preventive and treatment purposes occur most frequently. Also, it is important to note that in today's health care system, patients are underdosed and not achieving desired goals of therapy three to four times more frequently than they are overdosed. Providing patients with drug therapies at doses that are not sufficient to produce a clinical benefit is a major problem in the care of many.

The responsibility to identify, resolve, and prevent drug therapy problems is a "compass" to focus the practitioner's clinical activities in cases that involve patients with numerous, complex, and difficult therapeutic dilemmas. Constant referral to the seven categories of drug therapy problems ensures that consistent and rational, comprehensive medication management services are being provided, and effective care plans can be established for even the most complicated patient.

REFERENCES

1. Cipolle RJ, Strand LM, Morley PC. *Pharmaceutical Care Practice.* New York, NY: McGraw-Hill; 1998.
2. Strand LM, Morley PC, Cipolle RJ, Ramsey R, Lamsam GD. Drug-related problems: their structure and function. *DICP.* 1990;24(11):1093–1097.
3. Kohn LT, Janet C, Donaldson MS. *To Err is Human: Building a Safer Health System.* Washington, DC: National Academy Press; 2000.
4. Smith CP, Christensen DB. Identification and clarification of drug therapy problems by Indian health service pharmacists. *Ann Pharmacother.* 1996;30(2):119–124.
5. Nickerson A, MacKinnon NJ, Roberts N, et al. *Drug-therapy problems, inconsistencies and omissions identified during a medication reconciliation and seamless care service. Healthc Q.* 2005;8(Spec No):65–72.
6. Manley HJ, McClaran ML, Overbay DK, et al. Factors associated with medication-related problems in ambulatory hemodialysis patients. *Am J Kidney Dis.* 2003;41(2):386–393.
7. Simonson W, Feinberg JL. Medication-related problems in the elderly: defining the issues and identifying solutions. *Drugs Aging.* 2005;22(7):559–569.
8. Roughead EE, Barratt JD , Gilbert AL. Medication-related problems commonly occurring in an Australian community setting. *Pharmacoepidemiol Drug Saf.* 2004;13(2):83–87.
9. Gordon K, Smith F, Dhillon S. Effective chronic disease management: patients' perspectives on medication-related problems. *Patient Educ Couns.* 2007;65(3):407–415.
10. van Mil JW, Westerlund LO, Hersberger KE, et al. Drug-related problem classification systems. *Ann Pharmacother.* 2004;38(5):859–867.
11. Westerlund T. *Drug-Related Problems: Identification, Characteristics and Pharmacy Interventions.* Goteborg: Gotebrorgs University; 2002.
12. Tuneu Valls L. Drug-related problems in patients who visit an emergency room. *Pharm Care Espana.* 2000;2(3):177–192.
13. Mant A. *Thinking About Prescribing: A Handbook for Quality Use of Medicines.* Sydney, Australia: McGraw-Hill; 1999.
14. Rovers JP. *A Practical Guide to Pharmaceutical Care.* 2nd ed. Washington, DC: American Pharmaceutical Association; 2003.
15. Hepler CD, Segal R. *Preventing Medication Errors and Improving Drug Therapy Outcomes: A Management Systems Approach.* Boca Raton, FL: CRC Press; 2003.
16. Rao D, Gilbert A, Strand LM, et al. Drug therapy problems found in ambulatory patient populations in Minnesota and South Australia. *Pharm World Sci.* 2007;29(6):647–654.
17. Cipolle RJ. Drugs don't have doses—people have doses! A clinical educator's philosophy. *Drug Intell Clin Pharm.* 1986;20(11):881–882.
18. Sackett DL, Haynes RB. *Compliance With Therapeutic Regimens.* Baltimore, MD: The Johns Hopkisn University Press; 1976.
19. Descartes R. *The Formulation of a Rational Scheme of Knowledge in Discourse on Method and the Meditations.* Hanrmondsworth, UK: Penguin Classics; 1968.
20. Conrad P. The meaning of medications: another look at compliance. *Soc Sci Med.* 1985; 20(1):29–37.

The Assessment

⚷ KEY CONCEPTS

1 The purpose of the assessment is to determine if the patient's drug-related needs are being met and if any drug therapy problems are present.

2 Know your patient by understanding his or her medication experience before making any decisions about his or her drug therapy.

3 Elicit only relevant information necessary to make drug therapy decisions.

4 Always assess the patient's drug-related needs in the same systematic order. First determine if the **indication** is appropriate for the drug therapy. Second, evaluate the **effectiveness** of the drug regimen for the indication. Third, determine the level of **safety** of the drug regimen. Only after determining that the drug therapy selected or being used by the patient is appropriately indicated, effective, and safe do you logically evaluate the patient's **adherence** to the medication regimen.

5 Documentation includes the practitioner's assessment of how well the patient's drug-related needs are being met and a description of the drug therapy problems present.

PURPOSE, ACTIVITIES, AND RESPONSIBILITIES

The primary purpose of the assessment is to determine to what extent the patient's drug-related needs are being met. In order to accomplish this, the practitioner gathers, analyzes, researches, and interprets information about the patient, the patient's medical conditions, and the patient's drug therapies. Individuals can have drug-related needs whether they are taking medications or not.

This chapter describes how all of these activities combine to create an assessment of the patient's drug-related needs. A consistent format will be used to describe the standards of care and the corresponding measurement criteria that apply to the assessment step of the patient care process.

The assessment step in the patient care process is the most important of the three: (1) the assessment, (2) the care plan, and (3) the follow-up evaluation. It requires work on the part of the clinician and cooperation on the part of the patient. There are standard sets of issues and questions the practitioner must constantly think about and analyze throughout the assessment. The assessment interview is the means through which the practitioner encourages the patient's participation in the patient care process. The assessment interview influences all other components of the patient care process. It influences communication, data accuracy, clinical decision making, ethical judgments, patient adherence, patient satisfaction, practitioner satisfaction, and clinical outcomes.

KEY CLINICAL CONCEPTS

The personal, one-to-one nature of the assessment process creates the context to demonstrate caring and patient-centeredness.

There are essential clinical skills that each practitioner must develop in order to conduct a productive assessment. These include inquiry, listening, and observational skills. You must be committed to learning and teaching yourself the skills needed to assess the drug-related needs of your patients.

To be successful, you must understand and master the basic skills as well as the pharmacotherapy knowledge required to conduct a comprehensive assessment of your patient's drug-related needs because over a 40-year career, a clinician will conduct over 160,000 patient assessments.[1]

The thoroughness and organization of the assessment play a major role in determining how effective you will be as a practitioner and whether your patients will receive the maximum benefit from your work. All of your subsequent activities, clinical decisions, care planning, interventions, and evaluations are dependent upon your ability to fully assess your patient's drug-related needs and identify drug therapy problems.

There is structure to the assessment so the practitioner can be logical, systematic, and comprehensive in the work that must be accomplished.

The activities and responsibilities of the assessment are shown in Table 6-1.

KEY CLINICAL CONCEPTS

During each assessment interview the three responsibilities of developing the therapeutic relationship, assessing drug-related needs, and identifying drug therapy problems are simultaneously at work, and each function influences the other two.

Table 6-1 Activities and responsibilities during the assessment

Activities	Responsibilities
Meet the patient	Establish a therapeutic relationship
Elicit relevant information from the patient and other health records	Determine who your patient is by learning about the reason for the encounter, the patient's medication experience, patient demographic information, and other clinical data
Make rational drug therapy decisions using the Pharmacotherapy Workup	Determine whether drug-related needs are being met (indication, effectiveness, safety, adherence) Identify drug therapy problems

Practitioners in training need to expend considerable effort to develop the knowledge and skills required for each of these essential tasks; however, you can work on developing one skill at a time so as not to become overwhelmed with the task at hand.

During every assessment, the pharmaceutical care practitioner must collect information and make clinical decisions concerning the relevance of the patient's demographics, medication experience, immunization history, allergies and history of adverse drug reactions, medication history, and current medical conditions and drug therapies. This is accomplished through clinical assessment and inquiry skills and the use of the Pharmacotherapy Workup.[2,3]

The Pharmacotherapy Workup directs you through a logical decision-making process that allows you to evaluate the appropriateness, effectiveness, and safety of each of the patient's medications, and determine the ability and willingness of the patient to be compliant with the drug therapy.

The assessment and inquiry functions are accomplished by the use of two sets of questions. One is a structured set of questions the practitioner must learn to ask him or herself about the patient, diseases, and drug therapies and their interrelatedness. The other set is the questions the practitioner can address directly to the patient to elicit the information necessary to properly assess all of the patient's drug-related needs. It is important to learn how to effectively collect information directly from your patient. A few basic skills can help in this most important clinical endeavor. The mark of an effective practitioner is one who can combine the skills of asking appropriate assessment questions and analyzing the patient, disease, and drug data in a logical, structured manner.

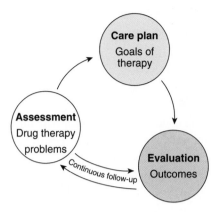

Figure 6-1 Unique contributions of the patient care process in pharmaceutical care practice.

This is a good time to consider the unique contributions that pharmaceutical care practice brings to our existing patient care processes (Figure 6-1). Patients who receive pharmaceutical care have their drug therapy problems identified and clearly described so that the entire team can work together to resolve them. Goals of therapy are individualized, made explicit and agreed upon so that each member of the care team can contribute to achieving these goals. The outcomes of drug therapy are documented so that everyone can learn what is most effective and safe.

Now we can begin to understand the process involved in assessing a patient's medications.

Standard of Care 1: Collection of Patient-specific Information

Standards of care have been developed for the major activities in pharmaceutical care practice: the assessment, care plan, and follow-up evaluation. These standards apply to the care that the practitioner provides for individual patients. These standards are applicable to all practice sites, diseases, patients, and drug therapy categories because they represent the generalist practitioner's responsibilities to provide pharmaceutical care.

The standards of care and measurement criteria are presented throughout this chapter as well as the two that follow so the practitioner knows the performance level expected at each step when providing pharmaceutical care. The complete set of standards for the practice of pharmaceutical care can be found in Appendix 1. The first standard of care for the assessment (there are three in all for the assessment) is given below.

STANDARD 1: THE PRACTITIONER COLLECTS RELEVANT PATIENT-SPECIFIC INFORMATION TO USE IN DECISION MAKING CONCERNING ALL DRUG THERAPIES.

Measurement criteria

1. Pertinent data are collected using appropriate interview techniques.
2. Data collection involves the patient, family and caregivers, and other health care providers when appropriate.
3. The medication experience is elicited by the practitioner and incorporated as the context for decision making.
4. The data are used to develop a pharmacologically relevant description of the patient, the patient's health status, and the patient's drug-related needs.
5. The relevance and significance of the data collected are determined by the patient's present conditions, illnesses, wants, needs, and preferences.
6. The medication history is complete and accurate.
7. The current medication record is complete, accurate, and includes indication, drug product, dosage regimen, and result to date.
8. The data collection process is systematic, comprehensive, and ongoing.
9. Only data that are required and used by the practitioner are elicited from the patient.
10. Relevant data are documented in a retrievable form.
11. All data collection and documentation is conducted in a manner that ensures patient confidentiality.

MEETING THE PATIENT

The first responsibility involved in the patient–practitioner interaction is to establish an effective therapeutic relationship so the practitioner can collect, analyze, and use relevant patient-specific information to understand who the patient is and what he or she wants and needs. Meeting and greeting your patient is a very important step in establishing this relationship.

You must meet and greet a person you may have never met before, describe all of his or her drug-related needs, identify drug therapy problems, design a plan to resolve those problems as well as to achieve therapeutic goals, and make certain that your patient experiences the maximum effectiveness from every medication. To accomplish all of this, it is important to create a positive experience for each patient. The therapeutic relationship begins the moment you first meet your patient. Patients must feel that you are free to identify with the patient before the patient will feel free to identify with you as their pharmaceutical care practitioner. As patients and practitioners begin to develop a shared identity, that is the essence of a therapeutic relationship.[4] Make greeting him or her a positive experience for both of you.

Introducing Yourself

How you introduce yourself sends a very distinct message. If you are a student, make certain your patient understands that you have a preceptor, mentor, or staff member who is fully responsible for the care being provided and is available if needed.

Decide how you want to be addressed. Your patients most often address you in the same manner in which you introduce yourself. Consider whether you want your patients to use your given name, surname, and/or applicable prefixes. Your patients will usually follow your lead. As an example, you might introduce yourself as *Sally, Sally Brown, Ms. Sally Brown, Dr. Sally Brown,* or *Dr. Brown.* Keep in mind that written materials you provide to your patients might also have your name on them, and it will be helpful if you are consistent. Furthermore, your colleagues and other staff in the patient care areas will also address you in the presence of your patients, and it will be less confusing if everyone calls you by the same name and/or title.

Addressing your patient in a proper manner is essential to begin a positive, respectful relationship. Addressing adult patients as Mr., Ms., or Mrs. is most often appropriate. Children usually prefer to be addressed by their first names. Correct pronunciation of your patient's name is important to him or her. If you are unsure of how to correctly say or pronounce it, ask how he or she would like to be addressed and how he or she pronounces his or her name.

During the assessment interview the patient's perception of your professional expertise is based on many factors, including your dress and demeanor, quality and relevance of your comments, your ability to elicit relevant information, your willingness to listen, your ability to provide meaningful information, feedback, and explanations, as well as your attitude and confidence. If you are well prepared to meet and help your patient, you will find your patients are forthcoming, open, and appreciative of your work.

The Physical Environment

The assessment interview can be personal and involve the exchange of sensitive information. The physical environment you choose to practice in reflects you and the choices that you make as a practitioner. A semiprivate or private space must be provided for you to conduct an assessment of your patient's drug-related needs. Unlike a physical examination, the assessment of a patient's drug-related needs rarely requires a fully private area. An environment in which the patient feels comfortable and assured that others cannot hear the conversation is often sufficient. However, some patients will need to speak with you in private about some drug-related issues, and therefore it is advisable to have a fully private space available for those occasions. The private or semiprivate area must be separate from any commercial business that also occurs in the setting (Minnesota Statute 256B.0625 Subd. 13h;2005).

Keep the area where you meet with patients clean and organized. It is their space, not yours. Only have materials available that you intend to use to help patients such as informational brochures, patient records, and access to the Internet, or samples of products or drug administration devices for demonstration. If you have large supplies of these items, only keep a minimal supply in the patient care area. Keep in mind that most of these items are new to your patients and can be distracting during the assessment interview.

A comprehensive assessment requires focused work on the part of the practitioner. First, you will need to focus on your patient and his needs. This means that how you feel personally, how your day is going, what is on your mind, what you were just doing, and what you will be doing later must all be set aside. Your patient has come to see you. You need to give each patient your full and undivided attention. This person trusts that you will do your very best to help. The patient believes you can and do care about his well-being. He will believe that you have the skills and knowledge to help. He needs to feel comfortable and know that at this moment you are committed to helping with whatever drug-related issue he may have.

Taking Notes

You will often need to take notes during the assessment. At times you may want to record the patient's words verbatim as he or she describes the medication experience. Documentation is an essential standard of practice that you must meet. It is important that your patient feels comfortable with this. Take the time to explain how essential it is for your records to reflect what is truly happening with the patient and his or her medications.

Assure your patient that all records you make are considered confidential. You can only make good decisions and provide good advice with good data. Well-meaning decisions based upon bad or missing information can become bad decisions. When you use a computer to document care, be careful not to focus your attention on the machine at the expense of your patient. Once you have computerized your pharmaceutical care records, you will find that only very minimal note taking is required.

ELICITING INFORMATION FROM THE PATIENT

During the assessment, a significant amount of information is needed from the patient. It is important to be clear about what information is relevant to the patient's case so that only the information you will use is gathered, otherwise time and resources are wasted. The information that is necessary for the assessment is represented in Table 6-2.

All of this information is necessary in all patient encounters; however, each patient is different and will require a different level of detail in each of these data categories.

Table 6-2   Patient information required for the assessment

Demographic information	Patient's medication experience	Clinical information
Age	Patient's attitude toward taking medications	Reason for the encounter
Weight and height	Description of what the patient wants, understands, believes, and any concerns about medications	Relevant medical history
Gender		Relevant medication history
Pregnancy status		past treatment failures
Living arrangements		past treatment successes
Occupation	The patient's medication taking behaviors	Review of systems
Contact information	Allergies to medication	to assess drug side effects
Address	History of adverse reactions to medications	to identify other problems
Telephone number	Other special needs	Relevant laboratory values
E-mail	Social drug use (caffeine, tobacco, alcohol)	to assess effectiveness
	Current medication record for all medical conditions	to assess safety
	Indication	
	Drug product	
	Dosage	
	Outcome	

Getting Started

The first two challenges for the student practitioner are to learn what information is necessary to help each patient and how to effectively gather the necessary patient-specific information. The *what* includes information that describes the personal characteristics of the patient that influence the use and outcomes of drug therapies. The *how* involves becoming skilled in eliciting patient-specific information by employing open-ended questions that help the patient to tell his or her story and then delving into relevant areas in search of sufficient detail to make the necessary clinical decisions.

Elicitation techniques that encourage the patient to state his or her full range of concerns and questions and that help the patient stay actively involved in the assessment process lead to a more valid assessment of needs and problems, more comprehensive data, greater patient satisfaction, better patient compliance, and more positive clinical outcomes.

Introductions such as the following can be useful to inform your patient of what to expect:

- I would like to talk with you today in order to gather some information about your health in general and medications specifically, so we can determine how best to meet your needs.
- Today we will review all of your drug therapies, so we can make certain that you get the results you want from all of your medications.

Keep in mind that your primary goal is to determine what your patient wants and needs from you. You will find it helpful to present open-ended questions during most of the assessment interview. Open-ended questions ask what, when, why, where, who, and how. They allow the patient to fully respond and facilitate complete descriptions of needs, wants, concerns, and experiences.[1,5,6]

The first information you will need from your patient is the reason for the present encounter. The following questions may help to initiate this discussion:

- What can I do for you today?
- How can I help you today?

If you have provided care for this patient in the past, you can open today's assessment with:

- I am glad you came to see me today. Tell me how you have been feeling since the last time we talked.
- Tell me how well your new medications have been working for you.

Reason for the Encounter

> **KEY CLINICAL CONCEPTS**
>
> The patient's primary reason(s) for the encounter anchors and directs the practitioner's assessment process. The primary reason for the encounter can be variable and may be an illness that must be managed with drug therapy, a disease, a complaint, a question, a concern, or a new condition that has developed.

The patient's view of the primary reason for the encounter is vital information in the assessment of drug-related needs and is often documented directly in the patient's words.

The patient's primary concern is the focus of a patient-centered assessment. The portion of your patient's medication experience that is the primary reason for the present encounter is what your patient is most concerned about today, and you must give it your first and full attention. This is the most current information that you have available. Other past information may also be valuable, but the truly current information is found in the patient's description of the primary reason for seeking your help today.

The history of the present problem can yield the most essential data you will need in your identification of the patient's drug therapy problems. Again, it is important to emphasize that the patient and the patient's view of his or her situation frequently serve to guide the assessment and identification of drug therapy problems. This is similar to the physician's assessment of a patient to determine the medical problem or diagnosis. The wealth of information that can be contained in your patient's *story* of the present problem includes its severity, context, location, quality, timing, modifying factors, and associated signs and symptoms.[7]

It is important to understand that during an assessment interview, all of the relevant information should be obtained, but the clinician rarely conducts an assessment in a strict section-by-section order. Patients provide information in the order and depth that makes the most sense to them. The clinician must be flexible enough to pursue a topic with the patient and later in the interview, return to obtain any additional information that might be required. This is why it is necessary for every pharmaceutical care practitioner to be completely familiar with all the components of the Pharmacotherapy Workup.

The most efficient way to do this is to allow patients to tell you their story in their own words. This uncovers the information you will use to provide pharmaceutical care within the patient's understanding and relevance. The practitioner must help to guide the storytelling to include the necessary clarity, completeness, and detail to make drug therapy decisions. Practitioners are often tempted to take total control of the assessment interview, but this invariably leads to practitioners not analyzing factors that are important to the patient.

If you are talking, your patient is not talking. If your patient is not talking, you are not gaining new information. As a student practitioner you are learning a new way of thinking and of making decisions in the best interest of patients regarding their diseases and their medications. Learning new methods of thinking and acting can be demanding at times and require practice. As you gain more knowledge and experience, you will become more confident and more efficient. Experience requires learning at every opportunity and integrating what you have learned with what you already know. Take every opportunity with a patient to learn the most you can from his or her unique medication experience: what was effective, what failed, what they liked, what they did not like, and why. Adding the information from their stories to your clinical experience is difficult at first, but it begins with the assessment interview.

Early in your assessment as you explore the primary reason for the encounter, you will want to understand how important resolving this problem or condition is for your patient. You will need to determine when it began, previous attempts to treat it, and the results or outcomes of any previous therapeutic approaches. You will always need to explore fully what self-care steps your patient has taken in an attempt to control or resolve his or her problem. If your patient has had limited success in the past, you will want to discover how much faith your patient has in drug therapy, so you can determine if you can confidently recommend continuation. On the other hand, if your patient has attempted to treat his or her condition with little or no positive results, you must recognize that repeating this same drug therapy or recommending continuation of that same medication will have a negative influence on the therapeutic relationship and probably result in poor compliance.

The information describing your patient's presenting signs and symptoms, illness, condition, or problem will focus much of the remaining assessment. Your patient's primary complaint, question, or illness serves as the *beginning* and the *ending* of the assessment. It will focus your inquiry and initiates connections with other patient-specific data you might need to gather later in the assessment. Furthermore, to conclude the assessment you must provide your patient with your clinical judgments about his or her primary presenting problem or question.

Patient Demographics

The individual characteristics of each patient create the context for all of your clinical activities. Patient demographic information is needed to see each patient as a unique individual. The purpose of the patient demographic portion of your assessment is to determine who your patient is and to provide a description of him at the time of the assessment. Your goal is to observe and elicit information describing the personal characteristics of the patient that are relevant to making drug therapy decisions. As you are initiating a therapeutic relationship and beginning to understand the patient's medication experience, you can begin to understand how your patient makes decisions as to if and when to take medications.

> **KEY CLINICAL CONCEPTS**
>
> The individuality of your patient and understanding his or her personal medication experience is an essential component in any patient-centered practice.

Your patient's demographic data consists of the information that allows you to treat him or her as a unique individual. Who is this patient? What makes this person unique and therefore have different drug-related needs than the last patient you met? Relevant information includes all of the data that will be useful to select and individualize drug therapies, doses, and instructions, establish goals of therapy, construct care plans, and suggest lifestyle changes. This information will also be used to determine the optimal timing, methods, and intensity of follow-up visits to evaluate actual positive and negative outcomes of drug therapies.

The patient demographics portion of your assessment can vary from requiring a few pieces of vital statistics to in-depth collection and analysis of information to personalize your clinical decisions concerning the patient's drug-related needs. The initial patient demographic information most often includes age, gender (to assess risk factors including pregnancy), height, weight, and ethnicity/cultural/language origin to ensure effective communication and understanding.

Age of the patient Age is a vital statistic when providing pharmaceutical care as it is often applied to both the discovery of the indication for drug therapy and the appropriate choice of pharmacotherapy to manage the disease

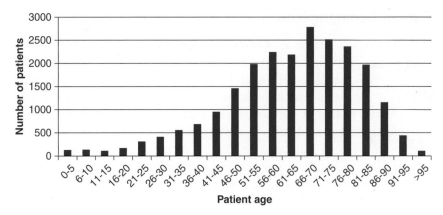

Figure 6-2 Number of patients by age (n = 22,694 patients, median = 66 years old).

or illness. The patient's age is also required for selecting appropriate products and dosage forms suitable for his or her age group, and for dosing guidelines (pediatric, geriatric). The appropriate approach to drug therapy for pneumonia is different in a 7-week-old patient, a 7-year-old patient, and a 70-year-old patient. Age is best identified and documented as birth date, so that age can be continuously updated as you provide care year after year.

In our patient data, females constituted 63% of these patients and 37% were males. Their ages ranged from 1 to 101 years old, with a mean age of 63 years (median = 66 years). The above chart shows the distribution of these patients by age (in groupings of 5 years) (Figure 6-2).

Height and weight Each patient's height and weight should be documented so that it can be used for dosage individualization. In many situations observational estimates of body weight are sufficient, but for extremely obese patients, or infants and children, and when using medications that require precise dose to body weight determinations, the exact weight of your patient must be known.

Much of the drug dosing literature considers a normal or average adult body weight to be 70 kg and a body surface area of 1.73 m². Lean or ideal body weight is often a better determinant for drug dosage than total or actual body weight, especially in obese patients. A patient is considered to be overweight if his or her body mass index (BMI) is 25 to 29.9 kg/m² and obese if the BMI is ≥30 kg/m².[8] Lean body weight can be estimated for dosage individualization of specific medications. There are simple methods to estimate lean body weight, BMI, or body surface area using equations based on height and weight measurements (Table 6-3).[8,9]

Table 6-3 Estimates for body weight, mass, and surface area in adults

Ideal body weight males (kg) = 50 + [2.3 × inches > 5'0"]

Ideal body weight males (kg) = 50 + 0.91 (height in cm −152)

Ideal body weight females (kg) = 45.5 + [2.3 × inches > 5'0"]

Ideal body weight females (kg) = 45 + 0.91 (height in cm −152)

Body mass index (kg/m^2) = (weight in kg)/(height in meters)^2

Body surface area (m^2) = ((height in cm) × (weight in kg/3600))$^{1/2}$

Living situation The patient's living situation is often a key factor in determining drug-related needs. Who lives with the patient and who cares for the patient? Does your patient have children who live at home, and are their ages important to consider for safety purposes (childproof tops, storage of medications)? Does the patient live with his or her parents, spouse, or significant other? Does he or she live alone? Who is responsible for administering medications and making health care decisions? Do other family members have a history of certain diseases, illnesses, or other risk factors (smoking, alcohol use, eating disorder) that may negatively affect your patient's drug therapy outcomes (coronary artery disease, depression, allergies)?

Family background, health insurance, and other special needs that might require specific accommodations are also helpful to gather during the assessment.

Questions to help you understand more about your patient might include the following:

- How would describe your family situation?
- What type of work do you do?
- Is anyone else at home also ill?
- How much assistance with taking your medications do you receive from other family members?
- What arrangements for transportation do you have to make to come to these appointments?
- What issues or problems do you have with insurance coverage for the medications that you need?

Your patient's occupation and socioeconomic status can have a dramatic influence on drug-related needs and subsequent outcomes. Does your patient's occupation put him or her at risk for certain diseases, injuries, or drug therapy problems? Drowsiness from antihistamines often found in cough and cold products might have a different impact on your patient if he or she is a commercial airline pilot or over-the-road truck driver, as opposed to your next patient who is a studio musician or a librarian.

Pregnancy and breast-feeding   Practitioners are often confronted with inquires concerning the safety of medication use in pregnant or breast-feeding patients. The decisions in these situations involve weighing the therapeutic benefits of the drug to the mother against its risk to the developing fetus or infant.

When conducting an assessment of a pregnant patient, the practitioner should record the due date. Most pregnant women know their due date, and this allows the practitioner to determine which trimester the patient is in during any subsequent evaluations. Risk to the fetus is difficult to predict; however, exposure to harmful drugs during the first trimester is most dangerous.

We often lack sufficient data and clear answers about the use of most medications during pregnancy or breast-feeding because the outcomes of such use are rarely studied and are difficult to collect. The amount of new information on drug effects on the fetus continues to grow. The risks that a drug poses to the fetus have been assigned to a risk factor level of A, B, C, D, or X. In this system, which is used by the U.S. Food and Drug Administration (FDA), the lowest level of risk is noted as risk factor A that is felt to be safely used during pregnancy, whereas the risk factor designated as X indicates that there is strong evidence of fetal abnormalities caused by the drug.[8,10] Each category is described in Table 6-4.

The vast majority of substances used for therapeutic purposes can pass from the mother to the fetus. In general, substances of low molecular weight diffuse freely across the placenta due primarily to the concentration gradient. The safety of medications used by mothers who are breast-feeding infants must also be assessed for the potential risk to the infant. In patients who are breast-feeding, the risks from a specific medication are usually much clearer, although we often must infer risk and benefit from data generated on related drug products. If the drug is generally safe to give directly to the infant, then it is generally thought to be safe to give to the mother during lactation.[10] Table 6-5 lists the pregnancy risk factor levels for commonly used medications.

Understanding the Patient's Medication Experience

Understanding the patient's medication experience is necessary in order to provide patient-centered care. The patient's medication experience is the personal context for all of your patient-specific clinical decisions. The better you understand it, the better your decisions will be and the more effective

Table 6-4   Risk factors: drug use during pregnancy*

Category A: Controlled studies in women fail to demonstrate a risk to the fetus in the first trimester (and there is not evidence of a risk in later trimesters), and the possibility of fetal harm appears remote.

Category B: Either animal-reproduction studies have not demonstrated a fetal risk, but there are not controlled studies in pregnant women, or animal reproduction studies have shown an adverse effect (other than a decrease in fertility) that was not confirmed in controlled studies in women in the first trimester (and there is no evidence of a risk in later trimesters).

Category C: Either studies in animals have revealed adverse effects on the fetus (teratogenic, embryocidal, or other) and there are no controlled studies in women, or studies in women and animals are not available. Drugs should be given only if the potential benefit justifies the potential risk to the fetus.

Category D: There is positive evidence of human fetal risk, but the benefits from use in pregnant women may be acceptable despite the risk (e.g., if the drug is needed in a life- threatening situation or for a serious disease for which safer drugs cannot be used or are ineffective).

Category X: Studies in animals or human beings have demonstrated fetal abnormalities, or there is evidence of fetal risk based on human experience or both, and the risk of the use of the drug in pregnant women clearly outweighs any possible benefit. The drug is contraindicated in women who are or may become pregnant.

* http://www.safefetus.com/fda_category.asp.

you can be in managing your patient's medications. A detailed description of the medication experience can be found in Chapter 4. You will be expected to know more about the patient's medication experience than any other member of the health care team.

The patient's description   No two patients have exactly the same medication experience. Even patients who have never taken any medications have some attitudes or beliefs concerning drug therapy that they acquired from friends, family, or the media.

KEY CLINICAL CONCEPTS

The patient's medication experience is the most specific information you have available to make an assessment of your patient's drug-related needs.

Table 6-5 Pregnancy risk factor ratings for commonly used medications*

Rank	Drug	Risk factor
1.	Hydrocodone/APAP	C
2.	Lisinopril†	C
3.	Simvastatin	X
4.	Levothyroxine	A
5.	Amoxicillin	B
6.	Azithromycin	B
7.	Hydrochlorothiazide	B
8.	Amlodipine besylate	C
9.	Alprazolam	D
10.	Metformin	B
11.	Omeprazole	C
12.	Atenolol	D
13.	Furosemide oral	C
14.	Metoprolol tartrate	C
15.	Sertraline	C
16.	Zolpidem tartrate	C
17.	Metoprolol succinate	C
18.	Oxycodone w/APAP	C
19.	Prednisone oral	C
20.	Citalopram HBR	C
21.	Ibuprofen	C
22.	Fluoxetine	C
23.	Gabapentin	C
24.	Warfarin	X
25.	Tramadol	C
26.	Clonazepam	D
27.	Lisinopril/HCTZ†	D
28.	Lorazepam	D
29.	Cephalexin	B
30.	Cyclobenzaprine	B
31.	Amoxicillin/Clavulanate potassium	B

(Continued)

Table 6-5 (*Continued*) Pregnancy risk factor ratings for commonly used medications*

Rank	Drug	Risk factor
32.	Trimethoprim/sulfamethoxazole	C
33.	Ciprofloxacin HCl	C
34.	Fluticasone nasal	C
35.	Triamterene w/HCTZ	C
36.	Pravastatin	X
37.	Trazodone HCl	C
38.	Propoxyphene-N/APAP	C
39.	Alendronate	C
40.	Fexofenadine	C
41.	Lovastatin	X
42.	Carvedilol	C
43.	Paroxetine	D
44.	Meloxicam†	C
45.	Diazepam	D
46.	Ranitidine HCl	B
47.	Fluconazole	C
48.	Naproxen	C
49.	Doxycycline	D
50.	Amitriptyline	C

* Source: SDI/Versipan, VONA, full year 2009, Drug Topics Resource Guide.
† Manufacturer considers lisinopril category C during first trimester and category D if used during second or third trimester.
‡ Manufacturer considers meloxicam category C early in pregnancy, but category D ≥ 30 weeks gestation.

The medication experience includes the patient's preferences, attitudes, general understanding of his or her drug therapy, concerns about it, expressed expectations of desired outcomes, and the patient's medication taking behavior. An initial objective of the assessment is to understand your patient's preferences and attitudes concerning medications and to what extent they influence the decision-making process. Your patient will ultimately decide if and how to use medications.

Your understanding of your patient's preferences, needs, expectations, and concerns will form the basis for the majority of what will follow in the assessment, care plan, and evaluation. It is important to remind yourself that these early patient impressions are most important because they reflect how the patient sees the situation. You may discover that some other issue is more important or more critical, but you must always return to your patient's initial impressions because that is the basis for his or her decision-making process. Your clinical decisions, impression, advice, and knowledge must be related to the patient's view of his or her medication experience. Remember, the more you understand the patient's medication experience, the more likely it is that you can positively influence it. A primary goal of medication management services is to improve your patient's medication experience.

The information you discover while inquiring about your patient's medication experience will direct virtually all your subsequent thinking and questioning. In order to have this positive influence, you will need to assess your patient's overall understanding of his or her medical conditions or illnesses and how they are or can best be managed by drug therapies. Discovering the patient's understanding will help you determine what additional information and education you must provide.

During the assessment, you will need to inquire and make judgments about the following questions:

- What is your patient's level of understanding of his or her disease or illness, drug therapies, and therapeutic instructions?
- What concerns does your patient have about his or her health in general or medical conditions and drug therapies in particular?
- What concerns does your patient have about side effects, toxicities, adverse events, or allergies?
- What does your patient dislike about his or her drug therapies?
- What unique preferences about drug therapies does your patient have?
- Are your patient's expectations and goals realistic and achievable?
- To what extent does your patient want to be an active participant in his or her care?
- To what degree is the cost of drug therapy, clinic visits, hospitalizations, or treatment failures, a concern for your patient?

You will want to inquire as to what the patient expects to gain or accomplish from his or her drug therapies. What are the patient's goals of therapy? You will also need to determine if the patient's expectations are realistic. Your clinical judgment concerning these important areas of inquiry will establish the scope of patient information you will need to fully understand your patient's medication experience and to begin to establish a strong and positive therapeutic relationship. The three components of your patient's medication experience are (1) the patient's description of his or her wants, needs, concerns, understanding, and beliefs about health in general and drug therapies specifically, (2) the patient's medication history, and (3) the patient's current medication record.

Medication history Your comprehensive assessment of the patient's medication history will include immunization status, social drug use, allergies, adverse reactions and other special needs, and a history of relevant medication use.

Immunization record Even to this day, most patient care documentation systems, and in fact many electronic health care record systems in general, do not adequately address individual immunization records. In the United States, tracking vulnerable children to ascertain their immunization status is largely left to the school systems. However, because one of your primary responsibilities as a pharmaceutical care practitioner is prevention, an assessment of your patient's immunization history is an essential part of the assessment.

With the exceptions of clean water, sanitation, and nutrition, the most effective mechanism that modern health care has developed to prevent disease and human suffering is immunization. Diseases such as polio, mumps, diphtheria, tetanus, pertussis, rubella, and many forms of hepatitis and influenza can be effectively prevented if patients are properly immunized. Immunization standards vary throughout the world, but they are commonly designed to ensure adequate protection against diseases that can reach epidemic proportions. Ensuring that your patient is adequately immunized is certainly a health care priority and a primary patient care responsibility in pharmaceutical care practice. Immunization recommendations differ with age, risk factors, and geography (http://www.cdc.gov/vaccines/). There are versions designed for families and parents, so the entire family can understand the recommended vaccination schedule. (http://www.cdc.gov/vaccines/who/teens/for-parents.html).

Social drug use The definition of drug use in the context of pharmaceutical care is quite extensive but implies a therapeutic use. Knowing your patient's exposure to caffeine, nicotine, alcohol, and drugs of abuse will avoid detrimental drug interactions, dosage errors, and even toxic reactions. When providing pharmaceutical care, you will need to assess your patient's use or exposure to these compounds and determine the impact this exposure may be having on the health and well-being of this individual.

Use of these drugs may be a habit that the patient would like to discontinue, and, if so, you can be an invaluable resource in meeting the patient's drug-related needs.

When inquiring about tobacco use, you can ask:

- Are you now, or have you ever been, a smoker?
- Is this something you would find difficult to give up?
- How would you describe your attempts to cut down or quit in the past?

Effective smoking cessation programs and products are widely available and can have a positive influence on a patient's quality of life and outcomes. Comprehensive smoke-free legislation in Scotland in 2006 has not only reduced the rate of respiratory symptoms among workers in bars, but has also significantly lowered the hospital admission rates for asthma among both pre-school and school-age children.[11] The pharmaceutical care practitioner can provide this service. Moreover, poor outcomes from comorbidities, especially respiratory and cardiovascular disorders, can often be prevented through a comprehensive assessment and management of the patient's smoking and/or alcohol use. Similarly, constant exposure to drugs of abuse and the associated addictive behaviors of tolerance, withdrawal symptoms, self-deception, loss of will power, and distortion of attention can place your patient at risk to experience serious medical, financial, compliance, or other drug therapy problems. It is essential to maintain patient confidentiality when assessing social drug use. Only collect and document information that is relevant to the drug-related decisions you will be making.

Allergies and adverse reactions "First do no harm" is the tenet of all health care practitioners. An essential part of any assessment of a patient's drug-related needs is your patient's drug allergies and a history of adverse drug reactions. This information will help to manage your patient's risk and thus prevent future drug therapy problems. The reason to distinguish between a drug allergy and an adverse reaction is that how you define the risk will dictate how you make drug therapy decisions to resolve or prevent it.

For example, if your patient has a history of an allergic reaction to penicillin, this usually implies that it is not safe to expose him or her to penicillin (or related products) ever in the future. Reexposing the patient who is allergic to penicillin, to a penicillin-containing product can be life threatening. Doing so would likely place your patient at immediate risk for a known, severe, and possibly life-threatening allergic reaction. This might include an anaphylactoid or anaphylactic reaction.

A history of an adverse drug reaction most commonly involved a negative or undesirable effect that your patient experienced with a specific drug product in the past. These types of reactions are important to document, so you and others who provide care for the patient can consider the risks and benefits of using that particular agent again. In most cases, an allergic reaction to a drug product requires that the patient not receive that drug or related agents in the future. However, if your patient has experienced an undesirable adverse effect caused by a drug product that was not deemed to be allergic in nature, in future decisions that product may be considered appropriate despite the past adverse reaction.

For example, if your patient experienced nausea and gastric discomfort when taking erythromycin to treat a skin infection, then you need to consider that adverse reaction when selecting antibiotics for that patient in the future. However, this adverse reaction does not necessarily preclude you from using erythromycin or related macrolide antimicrobials to treat future infections in that patient. Erythromycin might certainly be considered a viable treatment in your patient who experienced nausea from erythromycin as long as the first episode was appropriately assessed and documented as an adverse effect, and not as an allergic response.

To make these important clinical distinctions between allergic reactions and other predictable adverse drug reactions, you will need to be familiar with the presentation, timing, and common drugs involved in allergic reactions. Similarly, you will need to be familiar with commonly encountered negative reactions to drugs, especially those that can be successfully managed by dosage adjustments or other means without necessitating withholding that medication from your patient in the future.

In the case of adverse reactions to drug products, you must assess whether your patient could not tolerate the medication, or a particular dosage form, and what reservations your patient might have about being reexposed to this particular medication.

Questions that might help to elicit this important information include:

- What happened when you took that drug?
- What happened when you stopped taking the drug?
- Have you ever taken that same medicine again?

Health alerts, health aids, and special needs   Many patients have some special or unique needs that must be identified and incorporated into the assessment of specific drug therapy requirements. These often include physical limitations such as sight and/or hearing impairment. This might require larger than usual print for instructions or face-to-face follow-up rather than telephone communications. Patients requiring contact lenses or eyeglasses for vision correction may appreciate larger or bolder print for instructions, and may be very interested in new products or advances in contact lens technologies or lens care products as they become available.

Although the general description of the patient often includes observable physical characteristics such as age, gender, race, ethnicity, height, and weight, it may also be helpful to note any other noticeable, presenting characteristics such as nervousness and difficulties with speech, hearing, or sight. Being aware of language or communication difficulties can be helpful when trying to explain complicated instructions to patients or other family members.

Such language differences and cultural contexts can become barriers to your ability to optimize your patient's medication experience and achieve positive therapeutic outcomes. Your patient may benefit from a translator who can help you to assess the patient's drug-related needs. The use of a trained translator may be preferred to a family member because familial relationships may interfere with the communication of necessary information.

Physical limitations, including requiring a cane, walker, or wheelchair, must be noted and might require home visits, delivery of services, or mail services for medications and supplies to ensure that the patient receives all of the support and care required.

History of relevant medication use   The drug therapies that patients have taken in the past (usually during the last 6 months) can provide useful information. The assessment of past drug treatments is conducted for two primary reasons. First, to determine if the present problem has been treated before with medications and if so, what was the outcome or result. The best information a practitioner can have is that a certain drug regimen has already been used by the patient and was effective for a similar episode. If it was effective before, it is likely to be effective again.

The other usefulness of past drug treatment information is to determine if the patient has experienced any treatment failures and unwanted side effects to medications used in the past. If so, then it is important to not reexpose the patient to those drug therapies that have already failed or caused harm. Gathering a comprehensive medication history will help the practitioner avoid repeating mistakes, treatment failures, and side effects of the past. If it caused the patient harm in the past, it is likely to cause harm if used again.

To be most useful, past drug treatment information should include the indication for the drug, the drug regimen actually taken, the response to that therapy, and why the therapy was discontinued if relevant. For drug therapies taken in the distant past, it is often difficult to ascertain the exact dose and dosing intervals, and sometimes exact dates are not known.

Questions that can help to elicit this information are given below:

- How well did that medication work for you in the past?
- What happened when you took that drug in the past?
- How would you feel about using the same medication again?
- How would you feel about using the same medication but changing the amount we use in order to get a better result this time?

Current medication record In order to make sound, rational decisions about drug therapy, you must have assessed your patient's current medical conditions and all current drug therapies. Your patient's medication record includes (1) the indication for drug therapy, (2) all of the drug products your patient is taking for that indication, (3) specifically how the patient is actually taking them, and (4) the patient's response to the drug therapy. All four of these pieces of patient-specific information are required to make a rational, clinical assessment of the effectiveness and safety of your patient's drug therapies.

Medications: prescription, nonprescription, herbals A complete medication record is most useful if it includes all prescription medications, all nonprescription products, professional samples, medications obtained from friends or family members, vitamins, nutritional supplements, home remedies, traditional medicines, and natural and homeopathic remedies. Indeed, it includes all substances being taken by the patient for therapeutic purposes. A comprehensive assessment will involve inquiries into conditions that your patient might be treating or preventing with vitamins or minerals, nonprescription cough and cold preparations, laxatives, antacids, topical ointments, creams, or lotions, oral contraceptives, aspirin, acetaminophen, ibuprofen, and dietary or herbal supplements. As some of these products are used on such a routine basis, many patients do not consider them treatments and will need to be asked directly to have them considered in the comprehensive assessment.

KEY CLINICAL CONCEPTS

Establishing the appropriate indication or *connection* between each drug product that your patient uses and the corresponding medical condition, disease, or illness is a necessity in the provision of pharmaceutical care.

You cannot assess the effectiveness of a drug if you do not know why it is being used (indication). For many patients this will be the first time that any practitioner has put forth the effort to collect, organize, assess, and document *indications* and associated *drug therapies.* These data are invaluable, not only for you as a pharmaceutical care practitioner, but also to medical, nursing, emergency, and dental practitioners, as well as other health care providers.

The comprehensive medication record will become the information centerpiece for you to make clinical decisions concerning your patient's drug-related needs. To be most useful, the medication record should clarify the associations between the patient's indications for drug therapy, the drug product and dosage regimens, and the patient's response to each medication regimen. This is accomplished by establishing the fundamental connections between the three important categories of information; that of patient, disease, and drug. All three types of information are necessary in order to make rational decisions and successfully manage a patient's drug therapies.

Recall the essential elements current medical conditions are as follows:

- *Indication:* The active medical condition, illness, disease, signs, and/or symptoms being treated or being prevented by the use of medications.
- The drug *Product* your patient is taking.
- The *Dosage* regimen your patient is actually using.
- *Outcome:* How your patient is responding to the medication—what progress toward desired goals of therapy has been achieved to date.

Example   "My patient's hypertension has been adequately controlled for the past 4 months with chlorthalidone 25 mg taken each morning."

Example   In order to prevent stage fright, he takes 20 mg of oral propranolol 1 hour before his public-speaking engagements, and it has been effective for him.

Indication   *A drug without an indication is just a bottle of pills.* Assessing all of a patient's medications requires adequate data and an organized, yet comprehensive, thought process. It is essential to establish and document the clinical indication for every medication your patient is taking. The concept of *indication* for drug therapy is intended to encompass all of the clinical reasons that a patient might require drug therapy. The concept of indication is broader than simply a diagnosis or a disease.

A diagnosis is a medicolegal term used primarily by physicians to describe his or her best medical judgment describing the patient's pathology or illness. A diagnosis is established after the medical practitioner meets with the patient, conducts an interview, history and physical examination, collects and interprets all relevant laboratory test results, and sometimes confers with colleagues. We use drugs in a much broader scope within the health care system.

The clinical indication combines patient-specific information and disease (or illness) information. Therefore, indications are unique to patients. Your patient may be taking a common drug like lisinopril for hypertension (indication), however if she is pregnant, the lisinopril may be contraindicated. You can only assess the effectiveness and safety of your patient's medications by understanding your patient's indications.

Medications are used for many purposes throughout the health care system. We use medications to prevent diseases (influenza), to treat diseases (breast cancer), slow the progress of a disease (diabetes), to correct laboratory abnormalities (low serum potassium), to provide comfort (nausea) and relieve pain (analgesia), and we use medications to assist in the diagnostic process (antianxiety for magnetic resonance imaging). All of these situations are considered clinical indications for drug therapy. In pharmaceutical care practice, the term indication refers to the clinical reason the patient is taking or needs to take a medication. This is often different from the FDA use of the term indication. The FDA and therefore the pharmaceutical industry restricts the use of the term indication to refer only to the approved labeling and marketing of a product based on data submitted by the industry and reviewed by the FDA. In fact, when a product is used for a clinical condition that the FDA has not approved, it is termed "off-label" use. This should not be confused with the clinical use of the term indication. In practice, the term indication is used for the clinical condition for which the practitioner, prescriber, and/or patient have decided to use the product. (Note: This use may or may not be FDA approved and therefore may or may not be "off label.")

We often initiate drug therapy before a firm diagnosis is established. We may use medications to assist in establishing the diagnosis. Drug therapy is also used to provide comfort during other treatments. Many preventive medications are used before the signs and symptoms or any evidence of the disease are present.

Therefore, indication reaches well beyond disease or medical diagnosis, and includes the following uses for drug therapy.[12]

- Cure a disease or illness
- Prevent a disease or illness
- Slow the progression of a disease or illness
- Supplement nutritional, electrolyte, hormonal, or other deficiencies
- Correct abnormal laboratory test results
- Provide comfort or temporary relief from signs and symptoms of a disorder
- Assist in the diagnostic process

During the assessment, it is vital that the intended indication for each medication is identified, verified, if necessary, and associated with the appropriate medication(s). This connection is required for all drugs in all patients. It is neither efficient nor safe to assume an indication. Propranolol, a commonly used beta-blocker, can be used to treat hypertension, essential tremors, hypertropic subaortic stenosis, pheochromocytoma, stable angina, and tach-yarrhthmias. It is also used to prevent migraine headaches.

The effectiveness of a drug product can only be assessed if you know the intended indication. Most pharmacy claims data do not include the indication for the drug; therefore, it becomes the practitioner's responsibility to establish what the indication is and to assess the clinical appropriateness of the indication.

The clinical indication is necessary to establish goals of therapy, and goals of therapy are necessary to evaluate outcomes. Establishing and assessing the appropriateness of the indication directs the rest of the pharmaceutical care process. The care plan is dependent on the indication, as are all subsequent evaluations. Identifying and deciding whether the indication is clinically appropriate for the patient is the first clinical judgment you will make within the pharmaceutical care assessment.

Your patient's, sources of drug products can vary and include purchasing nonprescription (over-the-counter or OTC) products, using physician samples, and obtaining medication directly from friends or family members. Samples and drug products provided by friends and family members represent approximately 5% of the products patients use to manage their health.

You will need to assess the appropriateness of the entire drug therapy including the drug product, dosage form, the dosage regimen your patient is expected to take, the dosage the patient is actually taking, the method of administration, and the duration of therapy. You will assess when the patient started the particular drug regimen, and, if applicable, when it was or should be discontinued is also important to consider and document in the medication record.

The medication record also contains a brief description of the clinician's impression of any evidence as to the effectiveness of each drug regimen, as well as any associated side effects. For every indication and medication combination you must assess the status of both positive and negative outcomes. In most situations the single most influential determinant a practitioner will use in clinical decision making is direct, patient-specific evidence as to the actual effectiveness, or toxicity, of a particular drug regimen(s). Therefore, each assessment you conduct of a patient's drug-related needs must consider and document any evidence of drug therapy outcomes, be they successes or failures.

KEY CLINICAL CONCEPTS

A comprehensive medication record is organized by therapeutic indications and includes clinical evidence of outcomes.

This type of comprehensive and organized personal medication summary rarely exists in any other place in the health care system. It is a valuable instrument, not only for you as a pharmaceutical care practitioner, but also for other health care practitioners who care for your patient. Also, patients express thanks and voice appreciation when you provide them with a copy of this type of clear, organized information about all of their medications. Our experience is that patients respond very positively when this record is made available to them as part of their personalized pharmaceutical care plan.

Patient Data

MEDICAL CONDITIONS: In our group of patients receiving medication management services (n = 22,694) 51% of patients had five or more medical conditions being managed with drug therapies. One in five (20%) of patients had ≥10 medical conditions requiring drug therapy. There was an average of six medical conditions evaluated per encounter over these 50,142 patient encounters.

Other Clinical Information

Medical history The primary purpose of the past medical history portion of the assessment is to describe and make appropriate connections between what your patient needs today and the influence of relevant past health events. The past medical history contains information about past serious illnesses, hospitalizations, surgical procedures, pregnancies, deliveries, accidents, or injuries. Data about important past medical conditions can lend useful information to the comprehensive assessment. Any information in the patient's history or background that suggests a high risk or predisposition to develop a serious condition, or that would represent a contraindication to future drug therapies, should be described as part of the patient's past medical history. It is important to note that past successful or failed drug therapies are often the best predictors of future drug therapy outcomes for individual patients.

> **Example** Patients who have a history of peptic ulcer disease are at higher risk for gastrointestinal erosion from nonsteroidal anti-inflammatory agents than are patients with no past history of peptic ulcer disease.

In order to make an appropriate transition from inquiring about your patient's current needs to questions about past medical history, you will find it helpful to guide your patient with the following:

- Ok, I think I understand what has been happening over the last few weeks; now, tell me about your health in the past.

- Tell me about any serious illnesses or medical problems you have had in the past.
- How has your health been in the past?

Gathering information about your patient's past medical history is often one of the most challenging for new practitioners. These data are usually well understood by the patient due to the fact that they have already occurred, and your patient has developed a full understanding of these past events. Your patient feels comfortable with this section of the *story*. This portion of the patient's explanations can become quite lengthy and may not add new relevant information to the assessment of current needs. Another challenge to keep in mind is that your patient is here for today's drug-related needs and today's drug therapy problem(s). There is a tendency, especially on the part of practitioners in their early stages of skill development, to overcollect and sometimes even overinterpret the importance of some historical data.

Before you finish the assessment and determine if drug therapy problems exist, you need to be certain that you have been comprehensive in your fact finding. A brief, but systematic, oral review of systems will serve that purpose.

KEY CLINICAL CONCEPTS

An oral review of systems has two main purposes: (1) to uncover significant symptoms or problems that have not already been revealed during the assessment interview, and (2) to screen for any side effects, toxicities, or other undesirable/adverse reactions your patient may be experiencing, but does not necessarily associate with a medication.

Review of systems   An efficient review of systems is organized around body systems. Some practitioners begin with the head and work anatomically through the body. Beginning practitioners will find it useful to consult a list of relevant questions or illnesses so as to not miss an important finding. Positive responses by your patient need to be explored by more focused questions.

The review of systems also allows you to explore in more depth any positive findings from earlier portions of the assessment. The length of the review of systems depends on what information you have gathered up to this point. It should require no more than a few minutes for most patients.

The review of systems is designed to function as a screen for a large number of potential drug therapy problems that the patient may have or be at risk to develop. You will want to explain to the patient that this is a separate part of the assessment and helps you make certain that nothing important is omitted.

You will want to direct the patient to report common, recurrent, or particularly troubling symptoms.

- I need to ask you a series of short questions to help make sure we do not miss any important information about how well your medications are working for you or any trouble they may be causing.

You will be examining and establishing connections between actions of the medications the patient is taking and signs and symptoms reported. The review of systems is therefore an excellent opportunity to check with the patient for any common side effects he or she may have, but did not associate with any drug therapies.

Example   By asking your patient if she has experienced any stomach discomfort, diarrhea, constipation, or vomiting during the past 2 weeks, you can make a clinical judgment as to whether she has experienced any bothersome gastrointestinal side effects from her antibiotic therapy or from any other medication.

The review of systems is used to organize new findings, and your interpretation of any abnormal or unexpected results ensures that a comprehensive review has been conducted. For each new finding in your review of systems, you will constantly be asking yourself "Is this something that is being caused by a drug, or is this something that I can treat with a drug?" As described earlier, patients will not always have the ability to identify or describe all of their drug-related needs, and you will need to systematically investigate and assess the patient's medical conditions, complaints, and concerns. The review of systems may include physical findings, descriptions and experiences offered by your patient, and laboratory values, in addition to baseline information required for later comparison to evaluate effectiveness and safety. When recording your findings in the review of systems, include the objective, empirical data as well as your interpretation of the clinical significance of the result.

For example, is the headache your patient has had for the past 3 days being caused by the ketoprofen she is taking for her tendonitis? Are your patient's myalgias being caused by atorvastatin (Lipitor) he is taking to manage his hyperlipidemia? Is the cough the patient has asked for help to treat being caused by the captopril he is taking to manage his hypertension?

For each portion in the review of systems we have developed key questions, or areas of inquiry, that are useful. All positive findings should be documented to permit efficient retrieval at a later date, either by you when initially providing care for your patient or by colleagues who subsequently participate in the patient's care. These questions are by no means exhaustive, but are designed to serve as examples of important probes focused on identifying additional drug-related needs at the patient-specific level. The list of questions that you will find helpful to establish your review of systems techniques is shown in Table 6-6.

Vital Signs: Every patient has a temperature, a pulse, a systolic and diastolic blood pressure, and a respiratory rate. These data are always available, can be collected at very little or no cost, and are often important in drug therapy decision making. Your interpretation transforms these data into information that can be useful in the provision of pharmaceutical care. Remember, many of the most commonly used medications can cause undesirable increases or decreases in your patient's vital signs. Additionally, these most important monitoring parameters are used to evaluate the outcome of drug therapies in almost all patients.

The discipline that is required of you, as a pharmaceutical care practitioner, demands that each section of the review of systems be considered in order to avoid errors of omission. Only with this type of professional discipline and serious attention to detail can patients be confident that all of their drug-related needs are being addressed.

At this point in your assessment you will be establishing your clinical impressions of your patient's drug-related needs and how you can best meet them. However, up to now, you have been gathering information from your patient, primarily in response to information he or she has offered to tell you. You have been listening intently and creating a comprehensive list or mental picture of your patient's drug-related needs, wants, expectations, concerns, and understanding. It is now time to make the clinical decision, are all your patient's drug-related needs being met or does your patient have a drug therapy problem.

THE PHARMACOTHERAPY WORKUP

Now that you have a pharmacologically relevant understanding of your patient, you have the context in which to make patient-specific clinical decisions. Individualized, logical, and systematic drug therapy decisions represent your professional contribution to patient care. It is drug therapy problem identification, resolution, and prevention that will serve as your unique contribution to your patient. Because drug therapy problems interfere with your patients' ability to reach their goals of therapy, it is of the utmost importance that you acquire the hypothetical-deductive reasoning skills and knowledge necessary to identify, resolve, and prevent drug therapy problems in order to have a positive impact on their health and welfare.

Table 6-6 Pharmacotherapy Workup: review of systems

Assessment questions:

Are there deviations from normal that could be due to drug therapy (side effects)?

Are there deviations from normal that should be incorporated into the care plan or follow-up evaluation?

Vital Signs: Temperature: Heart Rate: Blood Pressure: Respiratory Rate:

Eyes, Ears, Nose, & Throat
- Do you have any problems with your eyes or eyesight?
- Do you need to wear glasses or contacts?
- Any troubles with your contacts?
- Are you being treated for glaucoma, eye infections, ear infections, cold sores, or dental pain?
- Are you experiencing coughs, colds, sore throats, sinus infections, or seasonal allergies?

Cardiovascular
- Have you had any trouble with your heart; any abnormal rhythms (dysrhythmias), chest pain, dizziness, blood pressure problems?
- What was your blood pressure the last time it was measured?
- Have you ever had your cholesterol checked? What are your cholesterol levels?

Pulmonary
- Are you having any problems with your lungs?
- Do you experience shortness of breath that bothers you?
- Are you now or have you ever been treated for pneumonia, bronchitis, influenza, chronic obstructive pulmonary disease (COPD), pulmonary emboli, or chest pain?

Digestive
- Are you experiencing trouble with your stomach, heartburn, gastritis, or ulcers?
- Any stomach pain, trouble with your bowels, nausea, diarrhea, or vomiting?

Endocrine
- Do you have any thyroid problems?
- Have you ever had your blood glucose checked?
- Have you ever been told you have high blood glucose or diabetes?

Genitourinary
- Are you having any problems urinating?
- Any pain or urine discoloration?

(Continued)

Table 6-6 (*Continued*) Pharmacotherapy Workup: review of systems

- Are you experiencing yeast infections, dysmenorrhea, or urinary tract infections?
- What are you doing to prevent osteoporosis?
- Have you had a prostate test recently?
- Some people who use this medication experience some change in their sexual function; have you noticed any changes?

Kidney
- Have you had any problems with your kidneys?
- Have you ever been told you have kidney disease?

Liver
- Have you noticed any signs of jaundice such as yellowing of the eyes or skin?

Hematological
- Do you bruise easily?
- Have you ever been told you have anemia?
- Do you take a multivitamin with iron?
- Do you take a folic acid supplement?

Musculoskeletal
- Do you have any problems with your joints or muscles?
- Do you exercise regularly?
- Any pain, swelling, or tenderness?
- Do you have any arthritis or arthritis-like pain?
- What medications do you use for relief of minor pain or discomfort?

Neurological
- Any problems with weakness, numbness, tingling, balance, or walking?
- Have you had trouble with seizures?
- Any difficulty with memory?

Psychiatric
- Any problems with anxiety, mood, depression, panic disorder, or attention deficit disorder?
- What do you do to relieve stress in your life?

Skin
- Are you having any problems with your skin?
- Are you bothered by itching, rashes, acne, eczema, or sores?
- Do you use any topical medications like ointments, creams, or salves?

Standard of Care 2: Assessment of Drug-related Needs

STANDARD 2: THE PRACTITIONER ANALYZES THE ASSESSMENT DATA TO DETERMINE IF THE PATIENT'S DRUG-RELATED NEEDS ARE BEING MET, THAT ALL THE PATIENT'S MEDICATIONS ARE APPROPRIATELY INDICATED, THE MOST EFFECTIVE AVAILABLE, THE SAFEST POSSIBLE, AND THE PATIENT IS ABLE AND WILLING TO TAKE THE MEDICATION AS INTENDED.

Measurement criteria

1. The patient-specific data collected in the assessment are used to decide if all of the patient's medications are appropriately indicated.
2. The data collected are used to decide if the patient needs additional medications that are not presently being taken.
3. The data collected are used to decide if all of the patient's medications are the most effective products available for the conditions.
4. The data collected are used to decide if all of the patient's medications are dosed appropriately to achieve the goals of therapy.
5. The data collected are used to decide if any of the patient's medications are causing adverse effects.
6. The data collected are used to decide if any of the patient's medications are dosed excessively and causing toxicities.
7. The patient's behavior is assessed to determine if all medications are being taken appropriately in order to achieve the established goals of therapy.

If your patient's drug-related needs are not being met, then a drug therapy problem exists. Identifying drug therapy problems requires professional judgment, discipline, a thorough understanding of your patient as a whole person, drug and disease knowledge, communication skills, and a systematic approach to the patient care process. It is unique to pharmaceutical care practice that both the empirical problem and your patient's perception of the problem become the focus of your deductive energies.

The Pharmacotherapy Workup   There is considerable information to be learned about patients, pathophysiology, and pharmacotherapy, but in order to understand how to apply this information to help an individual patient, you need an organizing framework. You need a framework in which to think about your patient-specific information, your knowledge of patients, diseases, and drug therapy, and the decisions you have to make. This is called the Pharmacotherapy Workup, and you will use it for making drug therapy decisions each time you care for a patient.

The Pharmacotherapy Workup represents the cognitive work involved in pharmaceutical care. During the Pharmacotherapy Workup you will systematically and repeatedly consider the questions dealing with indication, effectiveness, safety, and adherence. This disciplined way of examining patient–disease–drug findings is central to making sound decisions as to the optimal pharmacotherapy for any clinical situation. All health care professionals who accept the responsibility to work with patients to help manage their medications need to have mastery of the Pharmacotherapy Workup. The complete Workup can be found in Appendix 3.

Managing Medications: Assessing the Appropriateness of the Indication for the Patient's Drug Therapy

In pharmaceutical care practice, every indication for a drug is assessed to determine if it is clinically appropriate or not for this patient with this condition at this time. The following table presents the 25 most common clinical indications for drug therapies that were assessed in pharmaceutical care practices in ambulatory care clinics. These 25 common indications represent approximately 78% of all of the various clinical indications in these patients receiving medication management services (Table 6-7).

Note that on average, these patients had six clinical indications (medical conditions, Figure 6-3) for drug therapies at the same time (comorbidities).

Figure 6-4 introduces the most basic structure of the Pharmacotherapy Workup and the first step of the decision making that must occur. This basic structure illustrates the connections that must be established to determine if each drug product the patient is taking has an indication that is appropriate for the patient's medical problem and if each indication that requires drug therapy is being managed appropriately. The associations that must be established between these variables are illustrated in Figure 6-4 through 6-9.

The intended use of the medication is the starting point in drug therapy problem identification. You must first make the connections between the indication (medical condition), the drug product, the dosage regimen, and the outcome. These represent the minimum data set needed to successfully manage a patient's medications. For each medication being taken by the patient, consider: Is there is a medical condition or illness present requiring drug therapy. What drug product is being used to manage the condition? What dosage is actually being taken? What has the patient's response been?

Table 6-7 Twenty-five most common indications for drug therapy

Rank	Indication
1.	Hypertension
2.	Diabetes
3.	Hypercholesterolemia
4.	Vitamin supplements/nutritional deficiencies
5.	Esophagitis (gastroesophageal reflux disease)
6.	Osteoporosis treatment/prevention
7.	Depression
8.	Secondary prevention of myocardial infarction/stroke (aspirin)
9.	Pain-generalized
10.	Allergic rhinitis
11.	Insomnia
12.	Arthritis pain
13.	Vaccination
14.	Constipation
15.	Asthma
16.	Hypothyroidism
17.	Anxiety
18.	Edema
19.	COPD (chronic obstructive pulmonary disease)
20.	Heart failure
21.	Backache
22.	Tobacco use disorder
23.	Psychosis
24.	Diarrhea
25.	Atrial fibrillation

If there is not a clinical indication requiring the drug therapy, then the drug therapy is *unnecessary*. If there are any therapeutic indications that are not presently being treated, the patient may *need additional drug therapy*. During this step of the Pharmacotherapy Workup, you are constantly asking yourself if the patient's problem is caused by drug therapy or if the problem is something that can be treated (or prevented) with drug therapy.

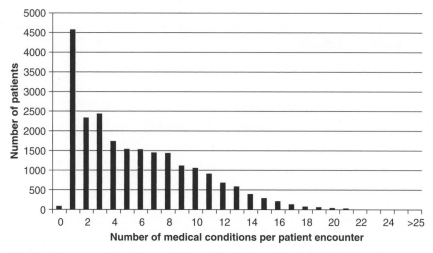

Figure 6-3 Number of patients by the number of medical conditions per patient.

Establishing that the patient has a clinically appropriate indication for the medication is of prime importance. It is virtually impossible to provide rational, personalized, valuable recommendations concerning a patient's drug therapy if you cannot identify the indication. Assuming what the indication might be from knowing only the drug product is dangerous and often leads to misleading and confusing decisions. You cannot optimize drug therapy if you do not know what is to be accomplished (goals of therapy). In the case of nonprescription drug product use, the patient (or the patient's family member or caregiver) has an indication in mind. The best method to gather this information is to ask the patient directly for what purpose he or she is using the product and what he or she is trying to achieve.

In the case of drug therapies that require a prescriber to initiate therapy, it is most helpful if you can educate the patient to ask why the prescriber is initiating this drug therapy. If your patient is not certain of the clinical intent of the medication, it is your responsibility to determine the intent

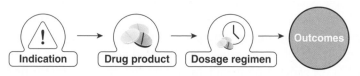

Figure 6-4 Associations within the Pharmacotherapy Workup.

of the prescriber. This can be accomplished through direct communication between you and the prescriber or by instructing the patient to ask the prescriber at the next office visit.

It is helpful for prescribers to write the indication within their dosing instructions. For example, "Take one tablet every morning to control blood pressure." Or, "Take one capsule every eight hours for lower back pain." Asking a prescriber to incorporate the intended use within the instructions can be extremely valuable. There is always an intended use (indication) for a drug prescribed by a practitioner who is licensed to prescribe drugs. The intended use is best known at the time the decision is made to prescribe a drug. Similarly, the patient always has an intended use in mind when he or she decides to self-initiate drug therapy that does not require a prescription. In any case, the indication is a vital piece of information in the identification and resolution of drug therapy problems.

If the patient has an indication that is appropriate for each medication and if each of the patient's medical problems is being treated or prevented with drug therapy, then you are ready to evaluate the patient's medications for effectiveness.

> **Note**   If the patient does not have a clinically appropriate indication or needs additional drug therapy to treat or prevent a medical condition, then you have identified a drug therapy problem.

Managing Medications: Determining the Effectiveness of the Drug Regimen

Figure 6-5 introduces the two main determinants of drug therapy outcomes: effectiveness and safety. Whenever a medication is used, its results can be described by determining the effectiveness and the safety experienced by the patient. To be responsible to: (1) manage a patient's medications and

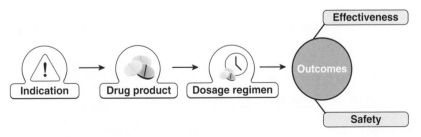

Figure 6-5   Drug outcomes: effectiveness and safety.

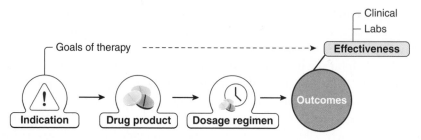

Figure 6-6 Achieving goals of therapy determines effectiveness within the Pharmacotherapy Workup.

(2) achieve the desired outcomes from drug therapies, means that you accept the responsibility to evaluate and make clinical judgments about both the effectiveness and safety of all of your patient's drug therapies.

Drug therapy is effective if it is achieving the intended goals of therapy. Effectiveness is determined by evaluating the patient's response compared to the desired goals of therapy for each indication. In today's health care system these goals of therapy are not often explicitly stated. To evaluate effectiveness you must establish *goals of therapy*. Goals of therapy are based on: (1) the *signs and symptoms* experienced by patients, or (2) the abnormal *laboratory values* associated with the underlying disorder or (3) a combination of signs, symptoms, and laboratory test results. Figures 6-6 and 6-7 introduce the information needed to evaluate the effectiveness of your patient's medications.

By comparing the desired goals with actual patient status at this time you can judge whether the drug therapy is being effective or not.

> **Note**   If the patient's drug therapy is not being effective (not achieving the goals of therapy), then the patient has a drug therapy problem.

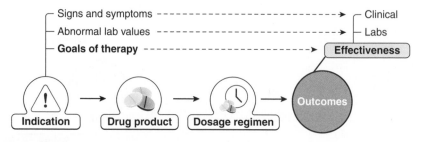

Figure 6-7   Effectiveness parameters within the Pharmacotherapy Workup.

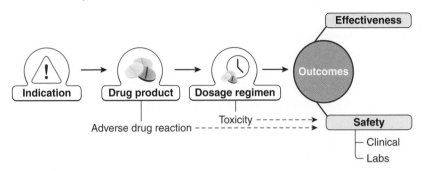

Figure 6-8   How safety decisions are made within the Pharmacotherapy Workup.

When the drug therapy is not effective for the patient, the practitioner will consider two of the most frequent reasons: "Is this the wrong product for this patient's condition?" or "is the dosage regimen too low to produce the desired effects?" Once again ask yourself "Is this problem caused by a [ineffective] drug or is this a problem I will resolve with [more] drug therapy?"

The next objective is to determine if your patient is experiencing any safety issues secondary to drug therapy.

Managing Medications: Establishing the Safety of the Drug Regimen

Drug products and dosage regimens can cause adverse drug reactions and/ or toxicities in patients. *Adverse drug reactions* are either (1) undesirable or unintended responses to the known pharmacology of the drug product or (2) idiopathic effects experienced by the patient. *Toxicities* are the result of dosages that are too high for your patient. (Figure 6-8)

The first safety consideration is reflected in the following question: "Is this undesirable effect the patient is experiencing caused by a drug he/she is taking?" The next safety consideration is whether the undesirable effect is related to (or proportional to) the dosage of the drug the patient is taking. Within the Pharmacotherapy Workup, practitioners must make clinical judgments as to whether an unwanted effect is dose related or not. If the patient's drug therapy problem is related to the dosage of the product, then the resolution is to continue to use the same product, but to reduce the dosage regimen. The dosage regimen can be reduced by giving the patient a smaller dose or by instructing the patient to take the dose less frequently. Most drug therapy problems caused by taking too much of the correct drug product are predictable because they are extensions of the known pharmacology of the drug product. In general, dose-related problems are resolved by lowering the dose, whereas those reactions not dependent on the amount of a drug the patient takes are resolved by switching to another drug product.

The safety of your patient's drug therapy is assessed by evaluating clinical parameters (signs and symptoms) or laboratory values to determine if any are associated with the unwanted effects of the drug therapy. Practitioners constantly ask: "Is this safety problem caused by too much of a drug?" Or, "Am I going to resolve this safety problem by using a different drug?"

Note If you have identified a medication or dosage of the medication that is unsafe, a drug therapy problem exists.

If the patient's drug therapy is effective and safe in your clinical judgment, then you are ready to assess the patient's adherence with the medication regimen (Figure 6-9).

Understanding Patient Adherence (Compliance)

The disciplined thought process that is described in the Pharmacotherapy Workup requires practitioners to make clinical decisions about indication, effectiveness, and safety issues before they evaluate the patient's compliance.

Note Although we are aware of the controversy surrounding the term "compliance," we have chosen to continue its use in some cases. There

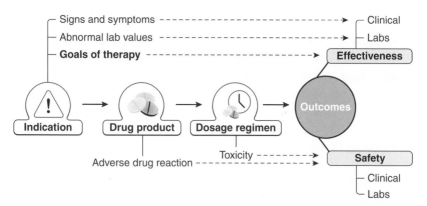

Figure 6-9 Effectiveness and safety parameters of the Pharmacotherapy Workup.

is no consensus on alternative wording (adherence, concordance), and the term is used here specifically to mean compliance with a dosage regimen, not compliance with the orders of a paternalistic or authoritarian figure.

Therefore, noncompliance is considered a problem only after the drug therapy is deemed to be clinically indicated, judged likely to be effective in achieving the goals of therapy, and safe in that it is not causing or likely to cause any harm to the patient. *In the practice of pharmaceutical care, a noncompliant patient refers to someone who is not able or willing to take an appropriate, effective, and safe medication as intended.* Patients have personal reasons for the decisions they make about whether or not to take the medication. Your responsibility is to discover that reason, so you can help to optimize the patient's medication experience.

Noncompliance represents a distinct category in that it describes the behavior of the patient, not the actions or effects of the drug therapy. Effective pharmacotherapy requires the medication be consumed in a particular dosage, at specified times, and for a specific period of time. Therefore, patients who are exhibiting a drug therapy problem of noncompliance need to be cared for in the context of altering their behavior. Identifying and resolving compliance problems are important responsibilities of every practitioner.

Patient Data

MEDICATIONS: Our patients were taking numerous medications to treat or prevent multiple medical conditions. The average was nine medications evaluated per patient. These medications were being used to treat or prevent an average of six medical conditions per patients. The number of medications per patient encounter varied from 0 to 49. In practice, not every medication is evaluated at every medication management encounter. In these patients an average of seven medications were evaluated at each encounter, with 30% of encounters requiring 10 or more medications be evaluated to ensure their effectiveness and safety. The following chart displays the number of medications evaluated in these patients by the number of documented encounters (total = 50,142 encounters) (Figure 6-10).

The pharmacological classes of these medications included virtually every type of product used to treat or prevent diseases. Based on generic product indicator (GPI) codes, the most frequently encountered medications were antidiabetic, antihyperlipidemic, antihypertensive, and analgesic medications. These four classes represented approximately 25% of all medications (total medications = 317,965). The following table lists the 25 most frequent

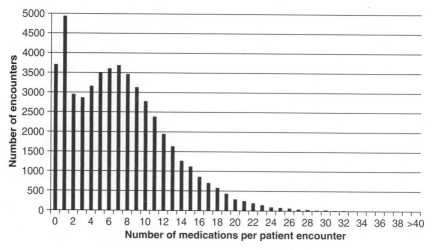

Figure 6-10 Number of medications evaluated by the number of documented encounters.

pharmacological classes of the medications taken by patients requiring pharmaceutical care. Medications from these 25 most frequently encountered classes represent 75% of all medications taken by patients receiving medication management services (Table 6-8).

The most frequent medications used by patients receiving medication management services were aspirin, metformin, simvastatin, lisinopril, and insulin (glargine). The following table presents the 25 medications most frequently encountered in patients receiving medication management services (based on GPI codes, 10 digits). These 25 medications accounted for 37% of all of the medications used by these patients. It is essential for practitioners who are responsible to work directly with patients to manage their medications to have a thorough understanding of the appropriate use, initial dosing, dosage adjustments, maximum dosages, monitoring parameters for effectiveness and for safety for all of these commonly used medications (Table 6-9).

The Assurance System allows practitioners to document and assess all medications the patient is taking regardless of the source of the product (prescription, nonprescription, dietary supplement, professional samples, or herbal products). In addition to the numerous prescription medications required by patients seen in these pharmaceutical care practices, they also take many nonprescription (or OTC) medications. It is essential that practitioners recognize the ever-growing use of nonprescription medications and the extensive practice of self-medication by patients in order to address their illnesses and prevent the worsening of medical conditions. This group of 22,694 patients receiving medication management services was taking

Table 6-8   Most frequent medications used by patients receiving
medication management services (by pharmacological class)

Rank	Pharmacological class
1.	Antidiabetic agents
2.	Antihyperlipidemic agents
3.	Antihypertensive agents
4.	Analgesics-non-narcotic
5.	Minerals and Electrolytes
6.	β Blockers
7.	Antidepressants
8.	Ulcer drugs
9.	Diuretics
10.	Vitamins
11.	Antiasthmatic and bronchodilator agents
12.	Vaccines
13.	Calcium channel blockers
14.	Analgesics-anti-inflammatory
15.	Analgesics-opioids
16.	Anticonvulsants
17.	Antihistamines
18.	Nutrients
19.	Dermatologicals
20.	Hematopoietic agents
21.	Laxatives
22.	Thyroid agents
23.	Psychotherapeutic agents
24.	Alternative medicines
25.	Nasal agents (systemic and topical)

78,782 nonprescription medications (mean = 3.5 OTC med per patient). In
addition, the practitioners documented the use of 1977 dietary supplements
being used by 502 different patients. In those patients who use dietary supplements on a regular basis, that represented an average of four supplements
per patient. The dosing, effectiveness, and potential for harm must be fully
assessed in all patients using dietary supplements as therapies or as general

Table 6-9 Most frequently used medications by patients receiving medication management services

Rank	Medication
1.	Aspirin
2.	Metformin
3.	Simvastatin
4.	Insulin
5.	Lisinopril
6.	Acetaminophen
7.	Omeprazole
8.	Metoprolol
9.	Calcium with vitamin D
10.	Furosemide
11.	Multiple vitamins
12.	Omega-3 fatty acids
13.	Amlodipine besylate
14.	Albuterol sulfate
15.	Atorvastatin
16.	Levothyroxine
17.	Influenza vaccine
18.	Hydrochlorothiazide
19.	Pneumococcal vaccine
20.	Glipizide
21.	Gabapentin
22.	Fluticasone-salmeterol
23.	Ibuprofen
24.	Atenolol
25.	Pioglitazone

support of their health. Similarly, 300 different patients were attempting to manage their medical conditions using physician samples given out in their medical clinics. These prescription medications are not recorded in any pharmacy claims systems and seldom appear in any medical records. This can be very problematic for patients who require multiple other medications to treat comorbid conditions. Practitioners, who are responsible to manage all

Table 6-10 Most frequently used nonprescription (OTC) medications in patients receiving medication management services

Rank	Nonprescription medications
1.	Aspirin
2.	Multiple vitamins
3.	Glucosamine-chondroitin
4.	Acetaminophen
5.	Omega-3 fatty acid (fish oil)
6.	Calcium with vitamin D
7.	Ibuprofen
8.	Ferrous sulfate
9.	Docusate sodium
10.	Loratadine

of a patient's medications, must inquire about the use of profession samples in order to assess their potential impact on the patient.

Most common nonprescription medications taken by patients receiving medication management services are listed in Table 6-10.

In addition to prescription medications and nonprescription products, many patients use dietary supplements on a daily basis to help manage their health. These products can often interact with or enhance the effects of other medications the patient is taking and therefore must be included in any comprehensive assessment of a patient's drug-related needs. In our sample over 243 encounters patients involved using dietary supplements on a chronic basis. The most common dietary supplements taken by patients receiving medication management services are listed in Table 6-11.

Table 6-11 Most frequently used dietary supplements in patients receiving medication management services

Rank	Dietary supplements	Rank	Dietary supplements
1.	Zinc	6.	Cinnamon
2.	Coenzyme Q_{10}	7.	Echinacea
3.	Ginger root	8.	Acidophilus
4.	Flaxseed	9.	Lysine
5.	Cayenne pepper	10.	Chromium

Table 6-12 Most frequently used physician samples in patients receiving medication management services

Rank	Physician sample medications
1.	Insulin pens (FlexPen, SoloSTAR)
2.	Byetta (exenatide)
3.	Actos (pioglitazone)
4.	Albuterol inhalers (ProAir, Ventolin, Proventil)
5.	Diovan (valsartan)
6.	Crestor (rosuvastatin)
7.	Advair (fluticasone and salmeterol)
8.	Lyrica (pregabalin)
9.	Spiriva (tiotropium)
10.	Vytorin (ezetimibe and simvastatin)

In addition to prescription and nonprescription medications and dietary supplements purchased and used by these patients, we also found that in 702 encounter patients were managing their medical conditions with physician samples. Their physician at no charge provides these prescription medications to the patient. The products are supplied to the physician or clinic by the pharmaceutical manufacturer and usually contain a limited number of tablets, capsules, or inhalers. Due to the limited supply, patients with chronic conditions are often required to return to the clinic frequently to obtain an additional supply or eventually a prescription for the product in order to purchase the medication through the normal drug delivery system. Physician samples can be problematic in that their use is not captured in any prescription claim systems, and therefore are not recognized by other health care providers as being part of the patient's drug regimen. Pharmaceutical care practice calls for the assessment of all medications taken by the patient (regardless of source), and therefore physician samples used by patients receiving medication management services are important to assess and document. The following are the most frequent medications provided as physician samples to patients receiving medication management services (Table 6-12).

DRUG THERAPY PROBLEM IDENTIFICATION

In the process of assessing your patient's drug-related needs, it is possible that you will identify a situation where things are not as they should be. Perhaps your patient may be taking a medication, but there is no valid clinical indication for it. Perhaps your patient is not benefiting from the medication he or she is taking. Your patient may be experiencing an adverse effect from one or more medications. Or, perhaps your patient cannot afford the medication that was prescribed, so he or she is not taking it. When you discover that your patient's medications are not appropriately indicated, as effective as they need to be, safe, or taken as intended, you have identified a drug therapy problem.

The last standard of care that prescribes appropriate practitioner behavior refers to the identification of drug therapy problems.

Standard of Care 3: Identification of Drug Therapy Problems

STANDARD 3: THE PRACTITIONER ANALYZES THE ASSESSMENT DATA TO DETERMINE IF ANY DRUG THERAPY PROBLEMS ARE PRESENT.

Measurement criteria
1. Drug therapy problems are identified from the assessment findings.
2. Drug therapy problems are validated with the patient, family, caregivers, and/or health care providers, when necessary.
3. Drug therapy problems are expressed so that the medical condition and the drug therapy involved are explicitly stated and the relationship or cause of the problem is described.
4. Drug therapy problems are prioritized, and those that will be resolved first are addressed.
5. Drug therapy problems are documented in a manner that suggest the goals of therapy and desired outcomes within the care plan.

Figure 6-11 illustrates where drug therapy problems can exist throughout the decision-making framework. This figure makes it clear that drug therapy problems can occur at each step of the patient's medication use process.

Each time a drug therapy problem occurs, the goals of therapy are compromised and cannot be met. Therefore, successful medication management requires the resolution of these drug therapy problems before positive outcomes can be expected. This is the reason why the identification, resolution, and prevention of drug therapy problems is the most important responsibility of the pharmaceutical care practitioner.

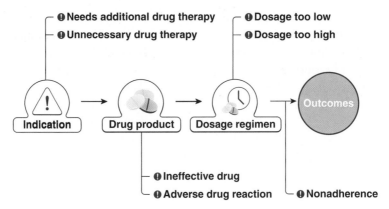

Figure 6-11   Drug therapy problem identification.

DOCUMENTING THE ASSESSMENT

It is essential that you document each visit and each encounter with every patient. In health care "if you did not document it, you did not do it." Your actions, interventions, advice, warnings, and drug therapies are all designed to impact another person. You are professionally obligated to keep a record of the care you provide for patients. At first, this task can seem labor intensive and monotonous, but all of the time and effort spent documenting your initial assessment will yield great dividends at all follow-up evaluation visits.

Recording the findings from your assessment is best done at the time you see the patient or shortly thereafter. Waiting for a more convenient time to record essential patient information, clinical findings, and decisions will only lead to errors of omission or confusion in your documentation. The expectation of most health care providers is that your documentation will be complete the same day you see the patient or provide the care. When first learning this skill, it is often useful to create a written paper record (see Appendix 3). This allows you to learn what information you use to make your clinical decisions and how to make the appropriate connections between patient, disease, and drug information. When caring for many patients it is very difficult to maintain accurate and up-to-date records using a paper system. Computerized documentation systems have been developed to support busy practitioners. All of the patient data in this book originated from the clinical documentation by practitioners using the Assurance System.

The information you will find useful to record includes name, address, and contact information for the most common forms of communication including telephone, cell phone, and e-mail. Correct spelling of your patient's name is important and demonstrates respect. Some patients may change their names when married or divorced. Obviously, your patient's name is a personal characteristic that you must value whenever you speak with your patient, communicate in writing, or for record keeping purposes.

Contact information is used to mail, telephone, or e-mail information to your patient. These are not clinical data and can be collected by support personnel, gathered through an electronic interface, or simply supplied by the patient or a family member. You may need the patient's address to mail health information to the patient or for billing purposes. The patient's preferred telephone numbers, or parent(s)' in the case of pediatric patients, may be useful in order to conduct convenient follow-up evaluations in the future or to contact the patient with new or additional information. Many of your patients might prefer to be contacted using e-mail, and if that is their preferred method of routine communication, then you will want to accommodate them by recording an e-mail address.

Patient demographic information usually does not change too much and need only be recorded at the first encounter. Age is best recorded using birth date, so all care providers can determine the patient's correct age at any future visit. Weight changes can be noted as some drug dosing guidelines are based on body weight, usually in kilograms. Pregnancy status is essential to note as drug safety becomes an overriding issue in pregnant and breast-feeding patients. Health insurance information changes frequently in the United States and constant efforts are required to keep current plan and policy numbers as well as eligibility.

The patient's primary reason for the encounter should hold a prominent place in your assessment record. Each visit may be for a different reason and therefore new or additional information may be required.

Your record of the patient's description of her medication experience is often best described in the patient's own words. This reduces your chances of over- or under-interpreting patient comments or descriptions of concerns or beliefs about using medications to manage health. This is helpful to note if you need to attend to any specific or unique patient needs that are revealed in your patient's description of her medication experience. The immunization status can simply be noted as to any vaccinations your patient needs to receive if that is the case. Drug allergies warrant thorough description as to the offending agent, the time frame of the reaction, the sequelae, and any treatment that was required. Some record systems place the drug allergy documentation in the very front in a bright color to notify all health care practitioners of this important risk factor.

Your record of your patient's current medical conditions and associated drug therapies can be considered the centerpiece of your assessment documentation. This will often be the first and only place in which all of your patient's medical conditions or illnesses, the drug products, and dosages actually being used are gathered and organized in the same place. This record has five components for every medical condition: indication, drug product, dosage regimen, length of therapy, and response. The dosage regimen to be recorded is that actually taken by your patient. If it is different from that prescribed, note the difference. It is important for all health care decisions to be made based on what dosage the patient is actually taking. The responses to be documented include both positive results and any side effects experienced by the patient. Drug therapies are organized and grouped by medical condition. Tobacco, alcohol, and other social drug use are documented in terms of amounts or frequency of use.

Your pharmaceutical care record should also document relevant past medical events including surgeries, illnesses, accidents, and special dietary needs/restrictions if they contribute to your drug therapy decision making.

You will need to record all pertinent findings from the review of systems. Positive findings as well as relevant negative findings are briefly noted. The absence of side effects or expected drug actions should be noted here.

KEY CLINICAL CONCEPTS

Documenting your drug therapy problem decisions requires a clear record of the patient's problems or medical conditions, the drug therapy that is involved, and the relationship (cause and effect) between the two. Noting the cause of the drug therapy problem in the assessment is most valuable, as it will guide future changes in your patient's drug therapies whether you or other clinicians implement them.

It is often useful to write a brief, two to three sentence summary of the assessment in the record to summarize the most important information and findings.

A comprehensive record that includes the description of your patient, his or her medication experience, the medical condition(s), associated drug therapies, actual dosages, and the results as of the present visit, as well as any drug therapy problems you identify, is required to contribute in a consistently positive path to the patient's good health.

SUMMARY

Patient care requires time, commitment, knowledge, skills, and compassion. When managing a patient's medications, the assessment step will require most of your time and energy. The assessment is the most important step in the care process because it establishes a relationship and the direction, urgency, and resources that will be committed to a patient's drug-related needs.

Understanding a patient's medication experience depends on the quality of the therapeutic relationship established between you and your patient. The patient's medication experience is the personal basis on which your patient makes drug therapy decisions. You will use the Pharmacotherapy Workup to make your clinical drug therapy decisions, but the more you understand and pay attention to your patient's past experience, preferences, and concerns about medications, the more likely you will have a positive impact on the long-term outcomes of drug therapies.

As a pharmaceutical care practitioner you bring new knowledge and skills to patient care. You will contribute in many ways, but essentially you are adding and verifying the clinical appropriateness of the indication for every medication, the medication's effectiveness and safety, and the patient's compliance. You are also contributing uniquely by the identification of the patient's drug therapy problems. This straightforward approach to managing medications places all of your patients' drug therapies into a rational context and greatly increases the probability of positive outcomes.

REFERENCES

1. Lipkin ML, Putnam S, Lazare A. *The Medical Interview: Clinical Care, Educaiton, and Research.* New York: Springer; 1995.
2. Strand LM, Cipolle RJ, Morley PC. Documenting the clinical pharmacist's activities: back to basics. *Drug Intell Clin Pharm.* 1988;22(1):63–67.
3. Cipolle RJ, Strand LM, Morley PC. *Pharmaceutical Care Practice: The Clinician's Guide.* 2nd ed. New York, NY: McGraw-Hill; 2004.
4. Prochaska JO, Norcross JC. *Systems of Psychotherapy: A Transtheoetical Analysis.* 7th ed. Belmont, CA: Books/Cole, Cengage Learning; 2009.
5. Coulehan JL, Block MR, Biblis MM. *The Medical Interview: Mastering Skills for Clinical Practice.* Philadelphia, PA: F.A. Davis Company; 2001.
6. Billings JA, Stoeckle JD. *The Clinical Encounter: A Guide to the Medical Interview and Case Presentation.* Chicago: Year Book Medical Publishers; 1989.

7. Cole SA, Bird J. In: Schmitt. W., ed. *The Medical Interview: The Three-Function Approach.* St. Louis, MO: Mosby; 2000.

8. Lacy CF, Armstrong LL, Goldman MP, Lance LL. *Lexi-Comp's: Drug Information Handbook.* 17th ed. New York: McGraw-Hill; 2010–2011.

9. Rowland M, Thomas TN. *Clinical Pharmacokinetics Concepts and Applications.* 3rd ed. Philadelphia: Lippincott Williams & Wilkins; 1995.

10. Hale TW. *Medications and Mothers' Milk.* 11th ed. Amarillo, TX: Pharmasoft; 2004.

11. Mackay D, Haw S, Ayres JG, Fischbacher C, Pell JP. Smoke-free legislation and hospitalizations for childhood asthma. *N Engl J Med.* 2010;363(12):1139–1145.

12. Cipolle RJ, Strand LM, Morley PC. *Pharmaceutical Care Practice.* New York, NY: McGraw-Hill; 1998.

The Care Plan

⚷ KEY CONCEPTS

1 A care plan is developed for each of the patient's medical conditions being managed with pharmacotherapy.

2 Care plans include goals of therapy, interventions, and a schedule for the next follow-up evaluation.

3 A goal of therapy is the desired response or endpoint that you and your patient want to achieve from pharmacotherapy.

4 The care plan includes interventions to resolve the drug therapy problems, interventions to achieve goals of therapy, and any necessary interventions to prevent drug therapy problems.

5 Pharmacotherapy interventions include; initiating new drug therapy, discontinuing drug therapy, or increasing the dosage, decreasing the dosage regimen, or changing the product.

6 Additional interventions to achieve the goals of therapy can include; patient education, medication adherence reminders/devices, referrals to other health care practitioners, or initiating a monitoring plan including how to use the equipment to measure outcome parameters.

7 The last activity in the care plan is scheduling a follow-up evaluation with the patient to determine the progress toward achieving the goals of therapy and desired outcomes.

8 Documentation of the care plan shows the relationship between the goals of therapy and the interventions made to achieve the goals.

PURPOSE, ACTIVITIES, AND RESPONSIBILITIES

The purpose of the care plan is to determine, with the patient, how to manage his or her medical conditions or illnesses successfully with pharmacotherapy and includes all the work that is necessary to accomplish this. The activities and responsibilities involved in care planning are described in Table 7-1.

Table 7-1 Care planning activities and responsibilities

Activities	Responsibilities
Establish goals of therapy	Practitioner and patient negotiate and agree upon desired endpoints and time frame for pharmacotherapies.

Determine appropriate interventions to:
    resolve drug therapy problems
    achieve goals of therapy
    prevent new problems
	Consider therapeutic alternatives and select patient-specific pharmacotherapy, patient education, and other nondrug interventions.

Schedule follow-up evaluations	Establish a schedule for follow-up evaluation that is clinically appropriate and convenient for the patient.

Standard of Care 4: Development of Goals of Therapy

There is a standard for each of the activities in the care plan. The first of these follows:

STANDARD 4: THE PRACTITIONER IDENTIFIES GOALS OF THERAPY THAT ARE PATIENT-CENTERED

Measurement criteria

1. Goals of therapy are established for each indication managed with drug therapy.
2. Desired goals of therapy are described in terms of the observable or measurable clinical and/or laboratory parameters to be used to evaluate effectiveness and safety of drug therapy.
3. Goals of therapy are mutually negotiated with the patient and other health care practitioners when appropriate.
4. Goals of therapy are realistic in relation to the patient's present and potential capabilities.
5. Goals of therapy include a time frame for achievement.

The structure of a care plan functions as a framework for the cooperative efforts of all those involved in the management of a patient's medications especially regarding the goals of therapy. The care plan allows you to work with the patient, who may have different expectations or understanding of his or her medication. Most often the care plan serves as a negotiated agreement or a *joint venture* between the practitioner and the patient. In the case wherein care is provided using a team approach, the team functions as a single entity when negotiating a care plan. When family members, guardians, friends, or other caregivers act on the patient's behalf or in conjunction with the patient, it is helpful if this patient is represented by a single voice when negotiating the details of a care plan with a practitioner.

Organizing care plans and clearly stating goals of therapy can benefit all patients in all settings. In the ambulatory setting, care plans and goals of therapy must be communicated and understood by several individuals including patients, family members, physicians, pharmacists, nurses, and other caregivers. Evidence in intensive care units (ICU) revealed that the daily use of "goals" reduced the length of stay in the ICU by 50%.[1] In the ICU, the team included physicians, nurses, respiratory therapists, and pharmacists. To manage the work required to care for patients in an ICU, the entire care team must agree upon the goals of therapy, the tasks to be performed, and the communications plan.

KEY CLINICAL CONCEPTS

In most clinical practices, care plans are organized by *medical condition*. In pharmaceutical care, care plans are organized by *indications* for drug therapy (i.e., pain management, sinusitis, prevention of osteoporosis). This structure allows the practitioner to constantly be aware of the indications the patient has for drug therapies and how best to manage each of them.

It is important to note that patients often have multiple medical conditions requiring drug therapy. Some conditions are acute and can be resolved with effective drug therapy, whereas many are chronic disorders requiring long-term medication management plans. Therefore, the practitioner constructs a separate care plan for each indication. This allows for more organized decision making and facilitates follow-up evaluations. Establishing separate care plans for separate indications facilitates record keeping in that changes in one or two drug therapies can be noted in the appropriate care plan, while not affecting or confusing the information in the plans treating the patient's other disorders. This organization of care plans by indication becomes more important as patient complexity increases. Being responsible for the outcomes of drug therapies in a patient with six medical conditions and nine separate drug therapies requires strict organization to avoid confusion, mistakes, and errors of omission.

Multiple drug therapies for the same indication are grouped together within the same care plan. This allows you to evaluate the impact of the entire pharmacotherapeutic approach for each condition, and thus make rational decisions about changes that might be required. Our data indicate that it is very common for patients to require multiple drug therapies at the same time. Pharmaceutical care practitioners in the ambulatory setting provide care for patients taking from one to as many as 20 or more medications. The median is more than 11 medications per encounter when prescription, nonprescription, herbal, and vitamin supplements are all taken into account.

The major questions you must consider to construct a successful care plan are as follows:

1. What goals of therapy are you and your patient trying to achieve with pharmacotherapy?
2. What are you going to do, or how are you going to intervene, to resolve any drug therapy problems identified during the assessment?
3. What interventions (drug therapies, devices, patient education) are you going to provide to ensure that your patient achieves the desired goals of therapy?
4. When are you going to follow-up with your patient to determine the actual outcomes of drug therapies and other interventions?

Common things are common. As a new practitioner, it is helpful to become familiar with the most common drug-related needs your patients will have. In ambulatory practices, several indications for drug therapy occur frequently. Table 7-2 lists the most frequent indications for drug therapy in patients receiving medication management services in ambulatory practice settings (same as Table 6-7). This list can serve as an excellent study guide because patients with combinations of these conditions will be encountered numerous times throughout your practice career. These 25 indications represent 78% of all the indications treated in this patient sample.

ESTABLISHING GOALS OF THERAPY

Goals of therapy allow all those involved in a patient's drug therapy to participate constructively. Goals of therapy are necessary in order to produce and document positive outcomes. For each medical condition, you and the patient must agree upon clear and concise goals of therapy. Establishing goals of therapy is an essential step toward ensuring a patient will maximally benefit from drug therapies.

When goals of therapy are agreed upon and described explicitly, not only can the patient work toward achieving them, but so can supportive family members, caregivers, and other health care practitioners.

Table 7-2 Most common indications for drug therapy in patients receiving medication management services

Rank	Indication
1.	Hypertension
2.	Diabetes
3.	Hypercholesterolemia
4.	Vitamin supplements/nutritional deficiencies
5.	Esophagitis (gastroesophageal reflux disease [GERD])
6.	Osteoporosis treatment/prevention
7.	Depression
8.	Secondary prevention of myocardial infarction/stroke (aspirin)
9.	Pain-generalized
10.	Allergic rhinitis
11.	Insomnia
12.	Arthritis pain
13.	Vaccination
14.	Constipation
15.	Asthma
16.	Hypothyroidism
17.	Anxiety
18.	Edema
19.	Chronic obstructive pulmonary disease
20.	Heart failure
21.	Backache
22.	Tobacco use disorder
23.	Psychosis
24.	Diarrhea
25.	Atrial fibrillation

The goals of drug therapy can be to:

1. Cure a disease
2. Reduce or eliminate signs and/or symptoms
3. Slow or halt the progression of a disease

4. Prevent a disease
5. Normalize laboratory values
6. Assist in the diagnostic process

Most drug therapies are used to manage chronic diseases that are not curable with our existing drug products. Examples include; diabetes, arthritis, hypertension, hyperlipidemia, and hypothyroidism. The goals of therapy for these disorders will include reducing or eliminating the patient's signs and symptoms, the normalization of laboratory values, and slowing the progression of the disease. Table 7-3 contains examples of common disorders and the goals of therapy that most frequently apply.

KEY CLINICAL CONCEPTS

Goals of therapy have a specific structure and always include the following components:

1. clinical *parameters* (signs and symptoms) and/or laboratory values that are observable, measurable, and realistic;
2. a desired *value* or observable change in the parameter;
3. a specific *time frame* in which the goal is to be met.

Goals of therapy have the qualities of being realistic, observable, measurable, and describable by the patient and/or the practitioner. Patient-centered goals of therapy must be also associated with a time frame describing when each goal should be achieved. This time frame is important to your patients as it lets them know *what* to expect and *when* to expect it. The time course for achieving patient-specific goals of therapy also serves as a guide to establishing an appropriate schedule for you and your patient to evaluate the impact or outcomes of drug therapy. It is not very useful to say your goal is for the patient to feel better soon. What is meant by *feel better*? When is *soon*? A goal of therapy might be stated as "The patient's elbow pain will be eliminated within 24 hours," or "The patient's diastolic blood pressure will be reduced to between 75 and 85 mmHg within 30 days," or "The patient will have no more than two episodes of seizures within the next month," or "The patient's serum potassium will increase to between 3.5 and 4.5 meq/L within 48 hours."

The patient's presenting signs and symptoms often form the foundation for the patient-centered goals of therapy within the care plan.

For example, a patient who suffers from allergic rhinitis and presents with nasal congestion, runny nose, and eye itching, but no cough or loss

Table 7-3 Examples of the goals of therapy for common medical conditions

Goals of therapy	Medical condition
Cure a disease	Urinary tract infection
	Diarrhea
	Streptococcal pneumonia
Reduce of eliminate signs and/or symptoms	Allergic rhinitis
	Major depression
	Low back pain
Slow or halt the progression of disease	Diabetes
	Ischemic heart disease
	Alopecia
Prevent a disease	Osteoporosis
	Stroke
	Measles
Normalize laboratory values	Hypokalemia
	Anemia
Assist in the diagnostic process	Anxiety with magnetic resonance imaging procedures
	Intraocular pressure tests for glaucoma

of taste; the patient-specific goals of therapy might include the relief of the patient's complaints of nasal congestion, runny nose, and eye itching in a time frame of 48 hours.

Given this type of patient-centered goal, a rational approach to pharmacotherapy is possible. Goals of therapy should be realistic and observable or measurable. Eliciting goals of therapy and obtaining agreement with the patient can be facilitated with the following discussion questions.

- What would you like to achieve with your medications?
- What are your goals for this therapy?
- How do you feel about trying to achieve…with a new drug therapy?

There are generalized goals of therapy that have been established for many medical conditions by groups of practitioners and researchers who specialize in the treatment of a particular disorder. These general guidelines (Table 7-4) have been established in the literature and verified in practice and can be used as initial goals until patient-specific goals of therapy can be negotiated and agreed

Table 7-4 Goals of therapy for common medical conditions

Medical condition and general guidelines for goals of therapy	Comments and time frame
HYPERTENSION	

Systolic <140 mmHg[5]
  115–140 mmHg
Diastolic <90 mmHg
  75–90 mmHg
<130/80 mmHg for patients with diabetes or chronic kidney disease
<140/90 mmHg with cardiovascular disease[10]
	The aim of reducing blood pressure is to minimize end-organ damage including heart disease (angina, myocardial infarction, heart failure), stroke, renal impairment, and/or retinopathy.
	Evaluate effectiveness of drug therapy monthly for the first 3–6 months following initiation or change in antihypertensive therapy.

HYPERLIPIDEMIA	

Total cholesterol <200 mg/dL
  (SI <5.17 mmol/L)
Low-density lipoproteins (LDLs)
  <160 mg/dL (SI < 4.14 mmol/L) in patients without risk factors
<130 mg/dL (SI < 3.36 mmol/L) in patients with two risk factors[7]
<100 mg/dL (SI < 2.59 mmol/L) optimal and considered the goal in patients with diabetes and in patients with coronary heart disease and two additional risk factors
High-density lipoproteins (HDL)
  >40 mg/dL (SI > 1.03 mmol/L)
Triglycerides
  <150 mg/dL (SI <1.69 mmol/L)
	Goal of therapy varies depending on other patient risk factors including hypertension, smoking, family history of coronary heart disease, males >40 or female >45, and HDL <40 mg/dL.
	Peak effects on lowering lipids can be evaluated 4–6 weeks after starting or changing drug therapy.
	Statins can be expected to lower LDL 18–55% and triglycerides 7%–30%.
	Niacin therapy can be expected to lower LDL 5%–25% and triglycerides 20%–50%.
	Once goals are achieved, continuous follow-up evaluation every 6 months to 1 year is recommended.

DIABETES	
Glycosolated hemoglobin (A1c) A1c < 7% Blood glucose Fasting or preprandial 80–120 mg/dL (4.0–7.0 mmol/L) 2 hours postprandial 100–140 mg/dL (5.0–10.0 mmol/L or 5.0–8.0 mmol/L if A1c not at goal)[8,9]	The aim of glycemic control is to reduce risk of microvascular complications including poor wound healing, retinopathy possibly leading to blindness, polyuria, polydipsia, polyphagia, and diabetic ketoacidosis. A1c is used to evaluate glucose control over the past 2–3 months.

(Continued)

Table 7-4 (*Continued*) Goals of therapy for common medical conditions

Medical condition and general guidelines for goals of therapy	Comments and time frame

Blood pressure
  Systolic < 130 mmHg
  Diastolic < 80 mmHg
  110–129/65–79 mmHg in pregnant patients with diabetes
LDL
  LDL ≤ 100 mg/dL
  LDL < 70 mg/dL for patients with overt cardiovascular disease (CVD)
  LDL ≤ 2.0 mmol/L
Total cholesterol (TC)/high-density lipoprotein cholesterol (HDL) ratio
TC/HDL ratio < 4.0
HDL
  HDL > 50 mg/dL in women
  HDL > 40 mg/dL in men
Triglycerides
  < 150 mg/dL
Plasma Apo B (apolipoprotein)
  Apo B < 0.9 g/L[8]
	Timely adjustments to and/or additions of antihyperglycemic agents should be made to attain target A1c within 6 to 12 months.
	A1c should be measured every 3 months when glycemic targets are not being met and when diabetes therapy is being adjusted.
	Once A1c is at goal, testing every 6 months is recommended

HYPOTHROIDISM Achieve normal thyroid function, reverse any biochemical abnormalities, and provide relief of symptoms that may include lethargy, weakness, loss of ambition and energy, dry skin, cold intolerance, weight gain, constipation, coarse hair, periorbital puffiness, muscle cramps, myalgias, abnormal menses, decreased libido. Thyroid-stimulating hormone (TSH) TSH generally elevated in primary hypothyroidism. Goal is to reduce TSH to reference range of 0.4–4.5 mU/L	Usual replacement dose of levothyroxine is 1.6–1.8 µg/kg/day (lean body mass) In patients <50 years old and without cardiac disease, may start with 50–100 µg/day of levothyroxine or with full replacement dose. In older adults, initial starting dose of 25–50 µg/day. In patients with cardiovascular risk factors or history of coronary artery disease begin dosing with 12.5–25 µg/day. Increase 12.5–25 µg/day every 4–6 weeks Resolution of symptoms usually begins in 2–3 weeks after beginning levothyroxine.

(*Continued*)

Table 7-4   (*Continued*) Goals of therapy for common medical conditions

Medical condition and general guidelines for goals of therapy	Comments and time frame
Low TSH levels (0.1–0.4 mU/L) in patients >60 years old may increase risk of osteoporosis or atrial fibrillation[11]	Optimal TSH levels (0.4–4.5 mU/L) may not be achieved for 6–8 weeks. If dosage changes are required, allow 4–6 weeks to determine effectiveness of new therapy. Full effects may require 4–6 months.
ASTHMA Maintain normal activity levels. Prevent symptoms of wheezing, cough, dyspnea, and/or chest tightness. Maintain normal, or improve spirometry. Spirometry goals vary with severity of asthma levels 1 through 4. Level 1: FEV1 or PEF >80%–85% of patient's personal best or predicted value Level 2: FEV1 or PEF >80% of patient's personal best or predicted value Level 3: FEV1 or PEF >60%–80% of patient's personal best or predicted value Level 4: FEV1 or PEF <60% of patient's personal best or predicted value FEV1, Forced expiratory volume in one second; and PEF, Peak expiratory flow.	Early evaluation based on FEV1 at 30 minutes after use of inhaled β_2-agonists is a useful predictor of outcome. Patient usage of inhaled β_2-agonists on a daily or weekly basis is used to evaluate effectiveness of pharmacotherapeutic plan. Use of short-term β_2-agonists on a daily basis indicates addition of inhaled corticosteroids therapy is needed. When inhaled corticosteroids are added for long-term control, improvements observed in 1–2 weeks with maximum effectiveness evaluated in 4–8 weeks. Following a severe exacerbation requiring hospitalization, return to normal lung function may require 3–7 days. Once stable, patient's drug therapy should be evaluated every 3–6 months.
GERD Alleviate or eliminate patient's symptoms which often include esophagitis (heart burn), hypersalivation, belching, regurgitation after eating	Symptom relief generally observed within 2 weeks. However, prolonged treatment (8–16 weeks) required to achieve healing and minimize recurrence.

(*Continued*)

Table 7-4 (*Continued*) Goals of therapy for common medical conditions

Medical condition and general guidelines for goals of therapy	Comments and time frame
Decrease frequency and duration of GERD Heal the injured mucosa prevent recurrence	
ALLERGIC RHINNITIS Reduction or elimination of signs and symptoms that may include rhinorrhea, sneezing, nasal congestion, postnasal drip, and/ or conjunctivitis	Therapeutic benefits of nasal steroids can be seen within a few days, but may require 2–3 weeks to see maximum response. Antihistamines generally produce maximum benefit when administered a few hours before exposure to allergen.
DEPRESSION Improvement of patient's target signs and symptoms identified before starting drug therapy including depressed mood, loss of interest and enjoyment, fatigue, reduced energy, reduction in self-confidence, appetite, disturbed sleep, reduced concentration, and attention. Aim is to reduce symptoms and help patient return level of functioning present before the onset of illness.	Adverse effects of antidepressant drugs may occur immediately, while symptoms of depression may not improve for several weeks. Antidepressants typically require 1–4 weeks to begin to be effective. Full effect may take 6 weeks, and in some cases improvement may continue for several months. Some symptoms can improve quickly, with energy and interest improving within 10–14 days. Mood improvement often requires 2–4 weeks. Continuous follow-up evaluations every 6–8 weeks to ensure continued control.

upon by those involved in the care of the patient.[2–4] These include such published parameters as goals for blood pressure in patients with hypertension,[5,6] goals for serum lipids in patients with hyperlipidemia,[7] and recommended goals for glycemic control in patients with diabetes.[8,9] To optimize each patient's medication experience, patient-specific goals must be established, agreed upon, and documented in the patient's individualized care plan(s).

As a blueprint to achieve positive outcomes, the care plan includes your decisions as to how specific goals of therapy will be achieved and when this should be accomplished. All of the activities that you perform are called interventions. These interventions may directly involve drug regimens, or they may utilize education, technology, exercise, or dietary instructions.

INTERVENTIONS

In order to resolve or prevent a drug therapy problem, practitioners intervene with, or on behalf of, the patient to make changes in the patient's drug regimen. In general, these resolution actions (interventions) involve starting new drug therapies, increasing dosages, decreasing dosages, discontinuing drug therapies, providing patient-specific drug information/explanations, or referring the patient to another health care practitioner who has the expertise to resolve a complex problem.

Patient Data

In our sample of 50,142 documented patient encounters, 80% of the interventions to resolve drug therapy problems occurred directly between the patient and the pharmaceutical care practitioner. The other 20% of inventions to resolve drug therapy problems required direct contact with the patient's prescriber (usually the primary physician). Many pharmaceutical care practitioners have collaborative practice agreements with physicians or medical practice groups allowing the modification of a patient's drug regimen within published guidelines without the direct approval of the physician. In those practices without collaborative practice agreements, the physician must be contacted whenever the resolution of the patient's drug therapy problem needed the modification of any product that requires a prescription.

In those cases requiring the patient's physician to get directly involved in resolving the patient's drug therapy problem, the most frequent action needed was the initiation of new medication for the patient that required a new prescription. Table 7-5 lists the interventions requiring the direct involvement of the patient's physician.

KEY CLINICAL CONCEPTS

The majority of drug therapy problems identified by pharmaceutical care practitioners are resolved by actions taken directly between the pharmacist and the patient.

Table 7-5 Interventions requiring direct communication with the patient's physician

Physician action required to resolve the drug therapy problem	Percentage of total physician actions
Initiate new drug therapy	43
Change the dosage regimen	18
Change the drug product	15
Discontinue the drug regimen	12
Institute a monitoring plan (labs)	12

Most frequently, the pharmaceutical care practitioner instructs the patient on how to best use the product to achieve the desired goals of therapy. Patients often need assistance in eliminating barriers to obtaining needed medications due to cost or administrative barriers put in place by payers. Table 7-6 describes the actions taken by the practitioner and the patient to resolve drug therapy problems.

Resolving some drug therapy problems require the pharmaceutical care practitioner to refer the patient to a specialist or some other health care provider with specialized expertise. If the patient's problem is acute or critical, the patient may be referred to an emergency department or to a hospital. In

Table 7-6 Interventions implemented directly by patient and/or practitioner

Patient–pharmacist actions required to resolve the drug therapy problem	Percentage of total patient interventions
Patient-specific instructions on proper use of medication	33
Removal of barriers to obtain medication	21
Initiation of new drug regimen	15
Change in dosage regimen	11
Initiation of a monitoring plan	8
Change in drug product	4
Discontinue drug therapy	4
Drug administration device provided	1
Other	3

Table 7-7   Medication management referrals

Referrals to	Number of referrals
Physician office	1415
Specialist office	497
Emergency department/hospital	93

the short tem, these referrals add health care costs. In the longer term, these early referrals reduce overall health care expenses. Table 7-7 lists the most frequent referrals made by pharmaceutical care practitioners.

Health Care Savings and Return-on-Investment

When pharmaceutical care, practitioners document the interventions required to resolve the patient's drug therapy problem, the Assurance System tracts the health care savings and costs associated with each action. These savings and cost data are conservative and only take into account expenses and savings that would have occurred over the next 90 days following the visit. Based on national data from 2008,[12] there was $11,437,130 saved through the provision of pharmaceutical care to these 22,694 patients. The average health care savings was $504 in medical expenditures per patient. Medical savings were the net of dollars saved and dollars spent for referrals. These savings resulted from avoided medical office and specialist office visits, emergency department visits, and hospitalizations due to drug therapy problems.

The medical savings were partially offset by the net use of more medications in these patients. Although there was $1,356,618 saved by eliminating unnecessary, ineffective, or unsafe medications, these practitioners also added medications to prevent illnesses, increased dosages to achieve desired goals of therapy, and improved adherence. These added medication costs totaled $2,928,679. The net for medications was an increase in drug expenditures of $1,570,061.

KEY CLINICAL CONCEPTS

Overall, the average health care savings associated with these pharmaceutical care practices was $435 per patient. There was an average savings of $197 per patient encounter.

Table 7-8 Medical and drug savings and costs documented in pharmaceutical care practices

	Savings ($)	Costs ($)	Net ($)
Medical services	14,157,270	2,720,149	11,437,120
Drugs	1,358,618	2,928,679	–1,570,061
Totals	15,515,890	5,648,828	9,867,062
Per encounter	309	113	197
Per patient	684	249	435

The average charge for medication management was $82.62 over the 50,142 document encounters. The overall return-on-investment (ROI) was 2.4:1. An ROI of 2.4:1 means that for every dollar paid for pharmaceutical care services, $2.40 of health care expenses can be avoided.

The net health care savings for patients >65 years of age was $3,995,449. The ROI for the patients >65years of age was slightly higher at 2.6:1. Patient-centered services dedicated to the identification and resolution of drug therapy problems has a positive ROI and makes medication management services one of the most cost effective new services in our health care system.

Table 7-8 is a summary of the medical and drug savings and costs documented in pharmaceutical care practices.

Health care savings can be achieved by the identification and resolution of drug therapy problems. Savings are not realized in every case, but improving the overall outcomes associated with drug therapies has a positive impact on the economics of health care delivery. Using the Assurance System, practitioners can document health care savings realized by the resolution of drug therapy problems. Also, when a referral is made to another health care provider (physician, emergency department, or hospital), the added health care costs of those referrals are recorded. The conservative standard of only counting savings and costs that would occur over the following 90 days is used. This validated method[13] yielded over $9.8 million in health care savings in these 22,694 patients. This average of $434.79 in savings per patient, makes medication management services one of the best investments we can make in our health care system. Table 7-9 describes the savings and costs associated with the provision of pharmaceutical care.

The next standard of care for developing a care plan refers to the interventions required to optimize the patient's medication experience.

Table 7-9 Healthcare savings and costs outcomes from interventions to resolve drug therapy problems

Health care savings[12,14]	Number of events	Savings ($)	Health care costs	Number of events	Costs ($)	Net ($)
Office visit avoided ($182)	33,895	6,168,890	Office visit referral	2,044	372,008	5,796,882
Specialist visit avoided ($564)	1,791	1,010,124	Specialist visit referral	497	280,308	729,816
Employee work day saved ($320)	616	197,120	Employee work day lost	10	3,200	193,920
Laboratory services avoided ($50)	817	40,850	Laboratory monitoring added	5,408	270,400	−229,550
Urgent care avoided ($182)	1,232	224,224	Urgent care referral	18	3,276	220,948
Long-term care avoided ($17,438/90 day stay)	9	156,852	Long-term care referral	14	243,992	−87,140
Emergency department visit avoided ($821)	2,610	2,142,810	Emergency department referral	41	33,661	2,109,149
Hospital admission avoided ($29,046)	145	4,211,670	Hospital referral	52	1,510,392	2,701,278
Home care visit avoided ($182)	26	4,732	Home care referral	16	2,912	1,820
Drug savings (varied)	13,845	1,358,618	Drug costs added	32,224	2,928,679	−1,570,061
Totals		15,515,890			5,648,828	9,867,062

Standard of Care 5: Statement of Interventions

> **STANDARD 5:** THE PRACTITIONER DEVELOPS A CARE
> PLAN THAT INCLUDES INTERVENTIONS TO RESOLVE
> DRUG THERAPY PROBLEMS, ACHIEVE GOALS OF
> THERAPY, AND PREVENT DRUG THERAPY PROBLEMS.
>
> **Measurement criteria**
> 1. Each intervention is individualized to the patient's conditions,
>   drug-related needs, and drug therapy problems.
> 2. All appropriate therapeutic alternatives to resolve drug therapy
>   problems are considered, and the best are selected.
> 3. The plan is developed in collaboration with the patient, his family
>   and/or caregivers, and health care practitioner.
> 4. All interventions are documented.
> 5. The plan provides for continuity of care by including a schedule for
>   continuous follow-up evaluation.

Patient-centered care plans designed to manage a patient's medications can contain interventions to:

- start drug therapy
- stop drug therapy
- increase doses
- decrease doses
- provide personalized patient instructions or education
- refer patients to another practitioner or specialist

The patient's care plan is constructed by selecting the interventions that will help the patient to achieve the desired goals of therapy. These interventions will resolve any drug therapy problems identified during the assessment, optimize the patient's medication experience, and prevent drug therapy problems. Finally, all care plans must contain a scheduled plan for the follow-up evaluation.

The interventions portion of the care plan represents the creative portion of the clinical problem-solving process. Based on the patient's value system and his sense of what is important, you and your patient collaborate to establish a prioritized list of activities designed to effectively and efficiently address all drug-related needs. The interventions you select are grounded in patient preferences, selected according to patient needs, and limited by patient tolerance. Therefore, the higher the level of patient participation and the more creative you can become at individualizing the care plan to meet your patient's unique needs, the higher the success rate will be. This success is not only evaluated as compliant behavior but also in terms of patient outcomes that are positive when measured at follow-up visits.

Interventions to Resolve Drug Therapy Problems

KEY CLINICAL CONCEPTS

The resolution of drug therapy problems is given highest priority within a pharmaceutical care plan. Drug therapy problems need to be resolved because they interfere with patients realizing their goals of therapy and meeting their drug-related needs.

For example, if your patient is not realizing the full effectiveness from her prescribed antihistamine to manage seasonal allergic rhinitis because the dose is too low, the dosage regimen must be increased before there is any realistic hope of achieving a positive outcome.

Similarly, if your patient is experiencing dose-related side effects from her antihistamine, the dosage regimen must be modified in order for her to receive appropriately indicated drug therapy that is both effective and safe.

The patient's drug therapy problems must be dealt with early in the care planning process. With the goals of therapy firmly in mind, you can decide how you will intervene on the patient's behalf in order to resolve the drug therapy problem.

Interventions designed to resolve drug therapy problems include the full spectrum of modifications in drug dosage regimens. These might include initiating new drug therapy, changing the drug product, altering the dose and/or the dosing interval, or discontinuing drug therapy. Each of these decisions is a balance between potential benefit to the patient (achieving goals of therapy) and potential harm to the patient through the selection of a specific drug product and/or dosage regimen. The drug product and/or dosage regimen determines the safety parameters you will evaluate at follow-up visits.

In clinical practice, drug therapy problems are considered resolved when the practitioner initiates or executes an intervention. Therefore, drug therapy problems are documented as being resolved at the time the intervention is initiated. After appropriate interventions have been chosen to resolve the patient's drug therapy problem, additional interventions and individualized drug therapies to achieve the goals of therapy can be implemented to optimize the patient's medication experience.

It is important to include the patient at each step in the decision-making process. The following questions can facilitate this discussion:

- How do you feel about making these adjustments in your medications?
- Is this a change that you think you can manage in your daily use of this medication?
- What do you think would be the best way to improve your therapy?

In patient-centered practices, 75% to 80% of interventions to resolve drug therapy problems are negotiated and agreed upon directly between the patient and the practitioner. The original prescriber is involved in the remaining 20% to 25% either through direct contact or via preapproved protocols or collaborative practice agreements.

Interventions to Achieve Goals of Therapy

Once the drug therapy problem is fully addressed in the patient's care plan, the goals of therapy for the primary indication can again be considered. The intent of the goals of therapy is to provide direction to a variety of activities for the patient and the practitioner. The goals of therapy become the agreed upon target of the prescriber's drug therapy, the patient's non-prescription drug therapy, other interventions, and the patient's adherence behavior.

Interventions to achieve the goals of therapy can include new drug regimen(s) the patient should receive, changes in drug therapy that are required, patient-specific education or information, referrals to specialists, instructions on how to properly use prescription drug products, nonprescription drug products, and how to use other remedies, products, and devices.

The patient's ability and willingness to obtain the drug products is an important consideration in a patient's care plan. A care plan is of little value if the patient is unable to acquire the medication, unable to afford the medication, unable to take the medication, or simply refuses to fill a prescription. All of these issues can cause additional drug therapy problems.

Interventions to Prevent Problems

Each patient's care plan must also address the need to prevent the development of new drug therapy problems. This is an area that can be confusing to some when first beginning to practice. Actions required to prevent a problem are in direct response to risk factors identified during the assessment of the patient's drug-related needs. These interventions are unique to each patient's situation.

In the course of clinical practice, practitioners always design drug therapies and patient education to avoid preventable side effects or risks known to be associated with certain drug therapies or diseases. If these are routine and standard practice, then they do not necessarily become part of the patient's individualized care plan. Examples include initiating antihypertensive therapy with a minimal dosage to prevent orthostatic hypotension or warning patients about drowsiness associated with some antihistamine products. Practitioners also routinely recommend that patients take certain medications with food to avoid stomach upset. These types of product-associated activities are due to the pharmacological or chemical properties of the drug and/or the disease but are not unique to the patient. These would be considered standard or routine instructions and would be provided for all patients taking those medications.

The types of preventive actions to be considered in this step are interventions that are necessary due to unique risk factors that your patient has. What do you need to do because of your patient's specific circumstances to make certain that nothing harmful occurs while taking medications?

For example, if your 29-year-old female patient is pregnant, you may decide to make certain that she is getting enough folic acid and other vitamins during her pregnancy. Additionally, you may also need to suggest that she reduce consumption of caffeinated and alcoholic beverages during her pregnancy and not take prescription or nonprescription drug products without checking with you first.

These interventions are preventive because she is pregnant. Neither would likely be considered if she was not pregnant. Only a comprehensive, disciplined assessment can identify patient risk factors that indicate the need for preventive interventions.

Prevention interventions are too often avoided by patients because of the delay in observable positive patient outcomes and the cost of the preventive intervention itself. This is unfortunate because the cost of the disease itself can be much greater. Interventions designed to prevent the development of a drug therapy problem can take the form of the initiating drug therapies, vitamins, diets, immunizations, educational programs (either directly to the patient or the patient's caregiver), or recommendations made on behalf of the patient to the prescriber (see Tables 7-5, 7-6, and 7-7).

Therapeutic Alternatives

> ### KEY CLINICAL CONCEPTS
>
> There is seldom, if ever, only one best intervention. The best drug, the best dose, the best approach is always patient-specific.

Clinicians train themselves to consider several options that might be useful for each patient. They will weigh these options in their minds or discuss them with colleagues and decide which are best for this patient at this time. Here, practitioners apply the rational process of the Pharmacotherapy Workup. For a given indication, the clinician considers effectiveness as the first criterion when selecting among therapeutic alternatives. The next consideration of therapeutic alternatives involves safety issues. This is when your pharmacotherapy knowledge and evidence-based information are applied to the care of individual patients. Which drug product in combination with what dosage regimen is most likely to achieve the goals of therapy? This is an important clinical decision-making process.

During the learning phase, it is useful to always identify at least three different therapeutic alternatives for every drug therapy decision you make with your patients. This helps you to learn about drugs that you may not otherwise encounter, and it helps you to learn to investigate, compare, and contrast the evidence supporting efficacy and safety of drug products used for similar indications. When you make recommendations to prescribers for changes in your patient's drug therapy, you will want to provide alternatives that you consider acceptable. Always indicate which is preferred and why.

Drug therapy alternatives constitute a unique knowledge base that the pharmaceutical care practitioner brings to the patient's case, whether practicing independently or as part of a team. In general, drug therapies are considered as viable therapeutic alternatives if there is evidence (in the literature and/or your own clinical experience) of efficacy in managing the patient's medical condition. The list of therapeutic alternatives is then assessed according to the safety risk to the patient. Practitioners must make these benefit-to-risk decisions continuously for their patients.

Practitioners who accept the responsibility for the outcomes of a patient's drug therapy (the definition of pharmaceutical care practice) must constantly consider all of the potential therapeutic alternatives that might benefit each individual patient. Keep in mind that the evidence we have concerning the efficacy of many drug products we use for even the most common conditions (hypertension, depression, allergic rhinitis, chronic pain, diabetes) is that they will be effective in 60% to 85% of patients. So, even the most popular, first-line, drug-of-choice will fail in a substantive number of your patients. There really is no "drug-of-choice" anymore than there is a car-of-choice or purse-of-choice or fruit-of-choice.

In medication management services, it is the responsibility of the practitioner to consider all of the viable therapeutic alternatives, not only to be able to select the best initial therapy, but also to be prepared with an alternative if and when the first therapy does not produce the desired outcome.

Cost Considerations

> **KEY CLINICAL CONCEPTS**
>
> Cost is an important management issue, but effectiveness and safety always take precedence in the decision-making process of a patient-centered practitioner.

After you have considered the evidence of efficacy and safety, then cost and convenience considerations can be applied. The least expensive drug therapy is the one that is most effective and does not cause the patient harm.

The cheapest drug is the one that works. Cost considerations should become important only after you have generated therapeutic alternatives based on effectiveness and safety. Any drug therapy that is ineffective for a patient or results in toxicity is too expensive.

Considering drug product costs before efficacy and safety considerations is not rational and can often be harmful and wasteful. Too often, if the differences between the clinical efficacies and/or safety of various drug therapy alternatives have not been well documented, they are considered to be the same. Not knowing the evidence as to whether one therapy is more efficacious than another, and assuming they are the same, is not clinically appropriate. This results in choosing the less expensive of the alternatives. Drug costs are easy to determine and require no clinical judgment. The rational decision-making process within the Pharmacotherapy Workup requires the practitioner discover and incorporate comparative efficacy data and safety data in order to make the optimal clinical decisions about drug therapies.

SCHEDULE AND PLAN FOR FOLLOW-UP EVALUATIONS

The last standard of care for care plan development refers to the follow-up evaluation that must be scheduled with each patient.

Standard of Care 6: Establishing a Schedule for Follow-up Evaluations

STANDARD 6: THE PRACTITIONER DEVELOPS A SCHEDULE TO FOLLOW-UP AND EVALUATES THE EFFECTIVENESS OF DRUG THERAPIES AND ASSESSES ANY ADVERSE EVENTS EXPERIENCED BY THE PATIENT.

Measurement criteria

1. The clinical and laboratory parameters to evaluate *effectiveness* are established, and a time frame for collecting the relevant information is selected.
2. The clinical and laboratory parameters to evaluate the *safety* of the patient's medications are selected, and a time frame for collecting the relevant information is determined.
3. A schedule for the follow-up evaluation visit is established with the patient.
4. The schedule and plan for follow-up evaluation is documented.

"If you don't follow-up, you don't care." The final component that practitioners negotiate during the care planning process is the schedule and plan for follow-up evaluation. Every intervention in a care plan may have a positive impact on the patient, a negative impact, or no demonstrable impact at all. Only through a well-constructed comprehensive follow-up evaluation can the practitioner and the patient learn whether the pharmacotherapies, drug information, and other interventions have met the patient's drug-related needs and resulted in the intended positive patient outcomes.

KEY CLINICAL CONCEPTS

Practitioners providing medication management services are responsible to follow-up and evaluate the impact and outcomes of the drug therapies provided.

The appropriate time for the patient and the practitioner or team to meet again must be established. At this time, the progress of the intervention, drug therapy regimens, changes in products and dosage regimens, devices, information, and referrals provided for the patient will be evaluated. It is important to be explicit. The more precise you are about when to have the next clinical encounter, the better. Being precise about the follow-up evaluation helps the patient understand your commitment to achieving the goals of therapy that have been established.

The plan for the follow-up evaluation addresses three basic questions:

1. When should the follow-up evaluation occur?
2. How will you determine if positive outcomes have occurred? (effectiveness)
3. How will you determine if negative outcomes have occurred? (safety)

Timing of Follow-up Evaluations

Deciding *when* to see your patient again to determine the effectiveness and safety of the therapy is a clinical decision. The optimal timing for the next follow-up evaluation is often difficult for new practitioners to determine. Most textbooks and guidelines cannot provide precise timetables for scheduling the follow-up visit, as each patient's situation involves different combinations of drug therapies, comorbidities, and risk factors. The clinical decision as to the optimal time to schedule follow-up visits should be based on the most likely period for the desired benefits to manifest themselves, balanced with the most likely time for harm or side effects to appear.

Evaluating effectiveness requires an understanding and appreciation for the onset of action and the time to maximum effect of each of your patient's medications.

Evaluating safety requires an understanding and appreciation for what the side effects are and when they are likely to occur. Therefore, the clinical decision as to when to schedule the next follow-up evaluation becomes the balance between: "When am I likely to see the beneficial effects?" versus "When am I likely to see the adverse effects or toxicity?" A rule of thumb for new practitioners is "Use whichever of these two occur sooner to schedule the next follow-up."

There are primary factors used by experienced practitioners to determine the appropriate time to follow up with any given patient. There are also the "red flags" that require more aggressive (earlier and more frequent) follow-up schedules. In general, the patient's medical condition list, the current medications, the patient overall health status, and the patient's ability and reliability to manage their own health are used to decide when it is necessary to follow-up with the patient. If the patient's case has some unique situations, often referred to as "red flags," then earlier and more often follow-up schedules are indicated. Examples include a patient who has had a very negative medication experience (past treatment failures or adverse outcomes), or if the patient's clinical status has been worsening over the past few visits, then a more aggressive follow-up schedule is indicated. Also, patients who struggle to understand or lack the full capability required to execute the care plan or fully utilize the health care system, also deserve a more aggressive follow-up schedule. Finally, there are several medications that for many years have been associated with a high risk of hospitalization including digoxin, warfarin, oral corticosteroids, antiplatelet, hypoglycemics and insulin.[15] Patients taking these medications and who are not at goal also deserve to be seen more often than guidelines might suggest.

During the learning phase, it is helpful to remember the adage: *Follow-up early and follow-up often.* In general, the more evidence, experience, and confidence you have that the care plan will result in positive outcomes and not result in undesired toxicity, the longer the time interval between follow-up evaluations. On the other hand, the less supportive evidence, data, information, clinical experience, and confidence that you and/or your patient have in the care plan, the sooner and more frequent the follow-up evaluations should be scheduled. Using the standard of "treat every patient as you would treat your own grandmother" to select your follow-up schedule. Early learners can ask themselves: *"If I had my grandmother on this care plan, when would I check on her (follow-up) to determine how she is doing (effectiveness and safety)?"*

DOCUMENTING THE CARE PLAN

Documentation of the care plan is required. Recording the care plan(s) allow(s) you to organize even the most complex pharmacotherapeutic approaches into a format that patients and other practitioners can easily understand and follow. Care plans are documented separately by medical condition or illness. A patient who is managing two chronic conditions and one acute illness with five total medications will have three care plans.

The care plan document lists the indication and includes a brief summary of the patient's signs and symptoms. Goals of therapy must be a prominent part of every care plan. One of the most valued additions that medication management services make to the patient's health records is explicitly stated goals of therapy (see Appendix 3).

Students may want to record two or three therapeutic alternatives that are considered for each indication to ensure that the most rational options have been considered. Experienced practitioners do not often record alternatives considered but not selected.

The care plan needs to be complete and should follow the structure of drug product(s) and dosage instructions including dose, route, frequency, and duration. Any special dosing instructions that will help the patient maximally benefit from the drug therapy should be included in the care plan. If the drug therapy is a change from earlier regimens, it should be noted and dated in the care plan. Multiple drug therapies for the same condition are contained in the same care plan. Any changes in drug products, dosage regimens, or instructions should be recorded so that the patient's care plan is continuously current and includes all forms of pharmacotherapy the patient is receiving (prescription, nonprescription, food supplements, vitamins, herbals).

Other interventions to support the specific pharmacotherapy should also be recorded. These often include health advice, exercise, dietary changes, or instructions on the proper use of medication administration devices or drug monitoring devices.

The care plan should include the schedule for the next follow-up evaluation including effectiveness and safety parameters to be evaluated.

SUMMARY

In summary, the care plan is used to organize all of the patient's pharmacotherapies and other interventions to optimize the drug therapy. The foundation of each care plan is the goal of therapy. Drug, device, and educational interventions and all future follow-up evaluations are coordinated within the care plan to achieve the patient's goals of therapy. Goals of therapy are necessary and guide multiple practitioners (team) to provide collaborative care. The patient and practitioner need to negotiate and agree upon goals of therapy, selected interventions including drug products, dosage regimens, instructions, as well as schedule future follow-up evaluations. The patient must clearly understand which interventions the practitioner will be responsible for and which will be the patient's responsibility. Finally, the patient needs to understand what improvements in signs and symptoms and what changes in laboratory tests can be expected from the drug therapies and how they will be used to evaluate effectiveness and safety at the next follow-up evaluation visit.

REFERENCES

1. Pronovost P, Berenholtz S, Dorman T, Lipsett PA, Simmonds T, Haraden C. Improving communication in the ICU using daily goals. *J Crit Care*. 2003;18(2):71–75.
2. Dipiro JT, Talbert RL, Yee GC, Matzke GR, Wells BG, Posey LM. *Pharmacotherapy a Pathophysiologic Approach*. 7th ed. New York: McGraw-Hill; 2008.
3. Gray J. *Therapeutic Choices*. 4th ed. Ottawa Ontario: Canadian Pharmacists Association; 2003.

4. Youngkin EQ, Sawin KJ, Kissinger JF, Israel DS. *Pharmacotherapeutics A Primary Care Guide.* 2nd ed. Upper Saddle River, NJ: Pearson Prentice hall; 2005.

5. NIH. *Prevention, Detection, Evaluation, and Treatment of High Blood Pressure.* U.S. Department of Health and Human Services, National Institutes of Health, National Heart, Lung, and blood Institute, National High Blood Pressure Education Program; 2003.

6. Chobanian AV, Bakris GL, Black HR, et al. Seventh report of the Joint National Committee on Prevention, Detection, Evaluation, and Treatment of High Blood Pressure. *Hypertension.* 2003;42(6):1206–1252.

7. NIH. *Detection, Evaluation, and Treatment of High Blood Cholesterol in Adults (Adult Treatment Panel III).* U.S. Department of Health and Human Services, Public Health Service, National Institutes of Health, National Heart, Lung, and Blood Institute. NIH Publication No. 01–3305, May 2001, 2001.

8. Blumer I. *Canadian Diabetes Association 2008 Clinical Practice Guidelines for the Prevention and Management of Diabetes in Canada: Executive Summary.* Canadian Diabetes Association; 2009:1–15.

9. Ali I, Ross SA. Targets for glycemic control. *Can J Diabetes.* 2008;32(S1):29–31.

10. Tobe S, Lebel, M.. *CHEP Recommendation for the Management of Hypertension.* Canadian Hypertension Education Program; 2010:1–39.

11. Vaidya B, Pearce SH. Management of hypothyroidism in adults. *BMJ.* 2008;337:a801.

12. Chowdhury SR. *Expenses per Visit for Ambulatory Visits and Inpatient Stay for 2008.* Rockville, MD: Agency for Healthcare Research & Quality-Center for Financing, Access, and Cost Trends; 2010.

13. Isetts BJ, Brown LM, Schondelmeyer SW, Lenarz LA. Quality assessment of a collaborative approach for decreasing drug-related morbidity and achieving therapeutic goals. *Arch Intern Med.* 2003;163:1813–1820.

14. Genworth. *Genworth 2011 Cost of Care Survey.* New York: Genworth Financial; 2011.

15. Budnitz DS, Lovegrove MC, Shehab N, Richards CL. Emergency hospitalizations for adverse drug events in older Americans. *N Engl J Med.* 2011;365:2002–2012.

Follow-up Evaluation

🔑 KEY CONCEPTS

1   The purpose of the follow-up evaluation is to determine the patient's outcomes in relation to the desired goals of therapy.

2   Parameters that reflect both effectiveness and drug safety are evaluated at each follow-up visit.

3   The evaluation of effectiveness of pharmacotherapy includes measurable improvement in clinical signs and symptoms and/or laboratory values.

4   The evaluation of the safety of pharmacotherapy includes evidence of adverse drug reactions and/or toxicity.

5   Patient adherence and its influence on outcomes are determined during the follow-up evaluation.

6   The outcome status of the patient's medical condition being treated or prevented with drug therapy is determined and described.

7   The patient is reassessed to determine if any new drug therapy problems have developed since the last follow-up visit.

8   The follow-up evaluation is the step in which actual results and outcomes from drug therapies are documented.

INTRODUCTION

The follow-up evaluation is an essential step in the care process. It is the step in which actual results and outcomes from drug therapies are observed, evaluated, and documented. This is the important step where you see the results of your previous work. The time and energy invested in your assessment of the patient's drug-related needs benefits you at the follow-up evaluation. Although most follow-up visits require a brief amount of time compared to some initial assessments, the follow-up evaluation is the step in which you gain new clinical experience and knowledge.

The follow-up evaluation solidifies your commitment to your patient, strengthens the therapeutic relationship, and demonstrates your willingness to work with your patient to achieve the desired goals of therapy. The primary purpose of every follow-up evaluation is to determine the patient's outcomes that have resulted from the drug therapies and care plans you have provided. Be sure to evaluate both effectiveness and safety parameters each time. The follow-up evaluation is such an important step that you need to "follow-up early and follow-up often."

Table 8-1 Follow-up evaluation activities and responsibilities

Activities	Responsibilities
Elicit clinical and/or laboratory evidence of actual outcomes and compare them to the desired goals of therapy.	Evaluate the effectiveness of the patient's drug therapies.
Gather clinical and/or laboratory evidence of adverse effects or toxicity to determine safety of drug therapy.	Evaluate the safety of the patient's drug therapies.
Document clinical status and any changes in pharmacotherapy that are required.	Make clinical judgment as to the clinical status of the condition being managed with drug therapy.
Assess the patient for any new problems.	Evaluate patient adherence and identify if any new drug therapy problems have occurred.
Schedule the next follow-up evaluation.	Provide continuous care.

PURPOSE, ACTIVITIES, AND RESPONSIBILITIES

The purpose of the follow-up evaluation is to determine the patient's outcomes from drug therapy and compare these results with the patient's goals of therapy. The follow-up evaluation activities and responsibilities are described in Table 8-1.

Standard of Care 7: Follow-up Evaluation

STANDARD 7: THE PRACTITIONER EVALUATES THE PATIENT'S OUTCOMES AND DETERMINES THE PATIENT'S PROGRESS TOWARD THE ACHIEVEMENT OF THE GOALS OF THERAPY, DETERMINES WHETHER ANY SAFETY OR ADHERENCE ISSUES ARE PRESENT, AND ASSESSES WHETHER ANY NEW DRUG THERAPY PROBLEMS HAVE DEVELOPED

Measurement criteria

1. The patient's outcomes from drug therapies and other interventions are documented.
2. The effectiveness of drug therapies is evaluated, and the patient's status is determined by comparing the outcomes within the expected time frame to achieve the goals of therapy.
3. The safety of the drug therapy is evaluated.

4. Patient adherence is evaluated.
5. The care plan is revised, as needed.
6. Revisions in the care plan are documented.
7. Evaluation is systematic and ongoing until all goals of therapy are achieved.
8. The patient, family, and/or caregivers, and health care practitioners are involved in the evaluation process, when appropriate.

The only way to know whether the drug therapy of your patient is effective and/or safe and the care plan is achieving the desired goals of therapy is to conduct a follow-up evaluation.

KEY CLINICAL CONCEPTS

You have not provided pharmaceutical care unless and until you have followed up with your patient to determine what has happened as a result of your clinical decisions, drug therapy advice, and care planning.

Caring is demonstrated through the activities of the follow-up evaluation. It adds new information to the patient's medication experience and potentially to the practitioner's pharmacotherapeutic knowledge base.

Although all practitioners provide drug therapy advice and instructions with the best of intentions, these well-meaning activities do not always have positive outcomes. Follow-up evaluation activities represent a new step in the health care system that does not routinely occur within the dispensing process and frequently does not occur even in the medical care process.

It is difficult to overemphasize the importance of the evaluation step in the patient care process.

KEY CLINICAL CONCEPTS

The follow-up evaluation is where and when practitioners gain *clinical experience*. Follow-up evaluations provide the evidence of effectiveness and safety. Follow-up evaluations strengthen the therapeutic relationship, have a positive influence on your patient's medication experience, and demonstrate the caring process. *"No one cares how much you know, until they know how much you care."*

Observing what resulted from your clinical decisions constitutes clinical experience. Throughout the assessment and care planning steps of the Pharmacotherapy Workup, you have been assessing your patient's drug-related needs. You have been acting on what you think your patient's drug therapy problems are, and you have been intervening by doing what you think has the best probability of achieving your patient's goals of therapy. All of this rational clinical thinking produces actual (real) results (outcomes). Learning from real results, good or bad (effectiveness or safety), is the working definition of clinical experience. New knowledge is gained during each follow-up evaluation. The follow-up evaluations are the most productive times for clinicians to learn which medications and which dosage regimens are most effective, and which cause harm.

The outcomes of drug therapies, drug therapy decisions, drug information, referrals, and other interventions are unknown until the practitioner conducts a follow-up evaluation with the patient. Your clinical decisions, drug therapies, and advice can produce any one of the following three outcomes:

- The intended positive clinical result
- A negative clinical result
- No demonstrable change

If the result is positive, you have learned that a certain drug regimen was effective in a specific clinical situation, and you will never forget it. If the result is negative, you have learned that a certain drug regimen failed to produce the desired outcome. Either result provides the greatest learning that a student practitioner can experience. The same holds true for learning about the adverse effects of drug therapies. If the patient experiences an adverse effect and describes that to you, or if you observe it at the follow-up evaluation, then that information is added to your long-term clinical database.

KEY CLINICAL CONCEPTS

During the follow-up evaluation, the practitioner is looking for evidence of effectiveness, safety, and any new problems that may have occurred since the last visit.

At each follow-up, the practitioner is looking for *good, bad,* and *new.* In general, the good (effectiveness) comes in the form of the improvement of the signs, symptoms, or laboratory tests associated with the disease or illness. The bad (safety) comes in the form of adverse and harmful toxic effects from drug therapies. The new comes from new medical conditions or new drug therapy problems that have developed since the last follow-up evaluation.

EVALUATING EFFECTIVENESS OF DRUG THERAPIES

During the follow-up evaluation, the practitioner and the patient compare the goals of therapy with patient outcomes. The most frequent parameters used to evaluate the clinical outcomes that result from a patient's drug therapy are clinical and/or laboratory parameters (Figure 8-1).

Clinical Parameters: Improvement in Patient Signs and Symptoms

Changes in clinical parameters are frequently used to determine the effectiveness of drug therapy. Positive clinical outcomes are most often associated with the disappearance or diminution of the patient's presenting signs and symptoms. Clinical parameters of the disease or illness often include clinical manifestations such as levels of pain, anxiety, mood changes, inflammation, or frequency and severity of cough, seizures, bleeding, sleep disturbances, tremors, and shortness of breath. Changes in these parameters are determined by asking the patient to describe them at the follow-up evaluation, then comparing the patient's response to what was observed and documented during the initial assessment or the most recent patient encounter.

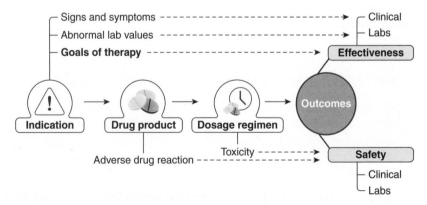

Figure 8-1 Pharmacotherapy Workup.

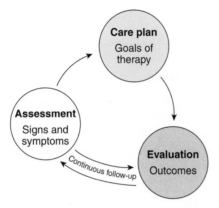

Figure 8-2 The relationships in the patient care process.

The practitioner's observational and clinical inquiry skills are applied during the follow-up evaluation in a similar manner to that during the assessment interview. The practitioner must have the clinical knowledge and ability to gather relevant information from the patient so that an evaluation of the clinical effectiveness of the patient's drug therapies can be made. The process of outcomes evaluation is straightforward. What clinical parameters were used to establish the goals of therapy? What is the status of those same parameters today? The practitioner establishes the relationships between (1) the original presenting signs and symptoms of the disease or illness, (2) the clinical parameters used to establish the goals of therapy, and (3) the improvement in those same clinical parameters (outcomes) at the time of follow-up (Figure 8-2).

Table 8-2 presents examples of common disorders in which effectiveness of pharmacotherapy is evaluated based on changes in clinical signs and symptoms.

Laboratory Parameters: Improvement in Laboratory Test Results

Outcome evaluations often rely on changes in laboratory values. In some diseases or conditions there are few or no clinical manifestations and outcome judgments are based primarily on improvements in laboratory test results. Hyperlipidemia is a common example where measurements of the patient's serum lipids (cholesterol, low-density lipoproteins—LDL, high-density lipoproteins—HDL, and triglycerides) serve as the parameters to determine the effectiveness of drug therapy. Patients seldom exhibit clinical symptoms

Table 8-2 Clinical signs and symptoms used to evaluate effectiveness of pharmacotherapy

Therapeutic indication	Clinical parameter
Depression	Mood changes, feelings of sadness, energy level, interest or enjoyment in usual or favorite activities, insomnia, agitation, fatigue, ability to concentrate, thoughts of death
Anxiety	Level of restlessness, irritability, muscle tension, sleep disturbance, ability to concentrate
Cough	Severity and frequency of cough, interruption of daily activities or sleep
Rash	Changes in color, size, inflammation, and itching
Osteoarthritis	Changes in pain in weight-baring joints including hip, knee, spine, and hands. Changes in stiffness in other joints
Back pain	Changes in level, quality and intensity of pain, weekly episodes of pain, worse pain over the past week, ability to ambulate, sleep, work, and changes in ability to function including activities of daily living at work and in social settings

associated with hyperlipidemia. Therefore, *effectiveness* evaluations are often based on laboratory measurements (Table 8-3).

Practitioners must understand the impact that drug therapies have on specific laboratory tests in order to determine if they are effective. The timing of when to collect the sample for the laboratory test is an important clinical decision. Often the practitioner must decide if the question to be answered at the follow-up evaluation is: "Will this drug regimen have any beneficial effect for my patient?" In this case, the practitioner would want to know how soon any positive effect could be measured. The more common question is: "How much of an impact will this drug regimen have on my patient?" In this case, the practitioner would want to know when the maximum effect can be measured.

For example, most HMG CoA reductase inhibitors (statins) begin to improve serum lipid determinations within a few days (5–14 days), but generally several weeks (3–6 weeks) are required to see the full extent of the changes in serum lipids. Waiting only 1 to 2 weeks after initiating lipid-lowering pharmacotherapy to measure changes in serum lipids might provide information as to whether the selected therapy is likely to have any effect at all on the patient's lipid profile. However, waiting 6 weeks or longer is more likely to provide evidence as to the extent of the benefit the patient is likely

Table 8-3 Laboratory test results used to evaluate effectiveness of pharmacotherapy

Therapeutic indication	Laboratory parameters
Hyperlipidemia	Total cholesterol, LDLs, HDLs, triglycerides
Hypertension	Systolic and diastolic pressure, mean arterial pressure, pulse rate
Anemia	Complete blood cell count, hemoglobin, hematocrit, red blood cell count, mean corpuscular volume, reticulocyte count, serum iron, serum B_{12}
Cardiac dysrhythmias	Electrocardiogram (ECG, EKG)
Diabetes	Blood or plasma glucose, hemoglobin A1c, lipids, blood pressure, renal function tests including serum creatinine and blood urea nitrogen

to experience from the drug regimen. In the first case, the laboratory test is used to evaluate whether *any* effectiveness is likely and in the second case, the laboratory test result is used to determine the *extent or degree* of benefit the patient has received from the drug therapy.

Follow-up evaluations of patients with acute disorders can serve to evaluate the final patient outcomes. Follow-up evaluations for patients with chronic conditions serve to establish the present status of the patient's condition being managed with drug therapy. Patients with chronic conditions require longitudinal, continuous follow-up that is initially designed to ensure that the drug therapy has, in fact, produced the desired effects (effectiveness), followed by less frequently scheduled evaluations designed to ensure that the patient remains stable and the drug therapy continues to benefit the patient. Typically, follow-up evaluation schedules are more frequent at first, until the goals of therapy are achieved (desired blood pressure, cholesterol, or level of pain), and then are scheduled less frequently in order to determine that the maintenance drug therapy continues to effectively manage the patient's condition.

EVALUATING THE SAFETY OF DRUG THERAPIES

The follow-up evaluation requires proactive practitioner involvement. That is to say, it is here that practitioners assertively assume the responsibility to reach out to patients and demonstrate caring behavior. Experienced pharmaceutical care practitioners understand that it is their responsibility to determine if drug therapies are, in fact, safe for their patients, and the best way to ensure safety is to determine whether the patient is experiencing any negative effects.

It is unacceptable only to wait for the patient to contact you if he or she has any side effects from the drug therapies that you provided. This type of passive approach is inconsistent with the values of pharmaceutical care practice and results in over $175 billion in drug-related morbidity and mortality each year.[1-3] To conduct a comprehensive, adequate follow-up evaluation requires active communication with each patient and feedback concerning any problems. Such feedback either validates the care plan or questions its appropriateness, thereby leading to improvements in the patient's medication experience.

Drug products are produced and made available for patient use because they possess a set of pharmacological actions. Most drugs exhibit several related pharmacological activities ("allopathic"), some beneficial, some undesirable. Which are considered beneficial and which are considered undesirable depend upon the therapeutic indication (why we are using the drug). However, when you use a drug at doses high enough to exhibit its pharmacological activities, any and all of those pharmacological actions can and will occur. Those actions that are desirable help to achieve the goals of therapy. The undesired actions are most often called adverse effects or side effects.

For example, aspirin is known to have analgesic, antipyretic, and anti-inflammatory properties. It impairs prostaglandin biosynthesis. Aspirin inhibits cyclooxygenase-1 (COX-1) associated with gastrointestinal irritation, renal effects, and irreversible inhibition of platelet aggregation, and also inhibits cyclooxygenase-2 (COX-2) that provides aspirin anti-inflammatory properties. When a patient is treated with aspirin, all of these effects occur to varying degrees. If the intended therapeutic indication is to manage pain (analgesia), then the platelet inhibitory activities, which can aggravate bleeding, are undesirable and would be considered a side effect. On the other hand, if the patient is using aspirin as secondary prevention of a heart attack (myocardial infraction) or stroke (cerebrovascular accident), then the platelet pharmacology is the desired action, and renal and gastrointestinal activities would be considered negative consequences. *The aspirin does not know why you are using it. It just exerts all of its pharmacological activities in every patient who takes it.*

That is why students need to learn all of the pharmacological action of the drug products they recommend to patients. Understanding the pharmacology, at a mechanism of action level, is required to determine what beneficial effects as well as what undesirable (safety) effects need evaluation at each follow-up visit. The practitioner and the patient need to know the intended therapeutic indication and evaluate it for effectiveness. At the same time the practitioner must expect drug therapies to exert *all* of their known pharmacological actions. This is why we keep repeating: "*Learn your pharmacology, learn your pharmacology, and learn your pharmacology.*"

Clinical Parameters: Patient Signs and Symptoms as Evidence of Drug Safety Problems

KEY CLINICAL CONCEPTS

Patients manifest undesirable actions of drugs in many ways. The practitioner's follow-up evaluation must include determining if any of the patient's clinical manifestations are due to adverse drug effects or toxic reactions related to excessive dosage of the medication.

The vast majority of medications used in modern medicine are taken orally. Therefore, it is not surprising that gastrointestinal irritation is a common problem with medications. The direct effects of the drug on the gastrointestinal lining often cause nausea, vomiting, and diarrhea. Similarly, many undesirable drug effects manifest as skin eruptions or rashes. Drugs that exhibit some of their pharmacological activities within the central nervous system can cause patients to become drowsy, somnolent, dizzy, agitated, or confused.

The two major categories of undesirable effects are unpredictable adverse reactions associated with the *product* itself and those reactions related to the *dosage* of the drug. The unpredictable effects include allergic reactions, hypersensitivity reactions, or idiosyncratic adverse events. The substantially more frequent category of undesirable drug effects results from the predictable, pharmacological action of the drug regimen and is related to the dosage of the drug.

In general, adverse effects of drug therapies manifest as clinical signs or symptoms and/or as alterations in laboratory test results. The practitioner evaluates clinical parameters and/or laboratory parameters during each follow-up evaluation in order to determine the safety of the patient's drug therapy (Figure 8-3).

Laboratory Parameters: Abnormalities in Laboratory Test Results as Evidence of Drug Safety Problems

It is common to require the measurement of specific laboratory tests as part of a follow-up evaluation to determine the safety of the patient's drug therapies. Drug toxicities can often be identified before severe or permanent harm is caused by evaluating laboratory tests parameters on a scheduled basis.

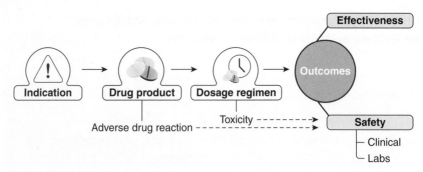

Figure 8-3   Evaluating the safety of drug therapy.

Several of the drug products commonly used to manage hyperlipidemia can cause liver damage, including atorvastatin, simvastatin, pravastatin, and lovastatin. Tests to determine the presence and extent of hepatic damage (ALT: alanine aminotransferase, AST: aspartate aminotransferase) are recommended at baseline and every 12 weeks as part of the follow-up evaluation of patients using these agents to lower cholesterol and other lipids. If the results of these hepatic injury tests become elevated to greater than two to three times normal, the drug therapy may need to be discontinued and different therapeutic alternatives need to be used to manage the patient's hyperlipidemia.

Another example of using laboratory test results to evaluate the risk of drug therapy would be measuring serum potassium in patients receiving digoxin therapy. The cardiac toxicity of digoxin is more pronounced in the presence of hypokalemia, hypomagnesemia, and hypercalcemia. The risk of digoxin toxicity is reduced if serum electrolyte concentrations are evaluated at follow-up and maintained within the desired normal ranges.

It is important for practitioners to understand the laboratory test parameters that are most useful in detecting drug toxicity and to make certain that these tests are appropriately scheduled as part of the patient's follow-up evaluation. Key activities in the follow-up evaluation step of the care process include the collection, interpretation, and evaluation of clinical and laboratory parameters to judge effectiveness and safety of the patient's drug therapy.

The positive clinical impact of pharmaceutical care practice has been well documented. The elimination of drug therapy problems from a patient's medication regimen can have a dramatically positive impact on the patient's health and well-being. Not all drug therapy problem resolutions result in cost savings that can be measured within even 1 to 2 years. However, clinical improvement in general and the achievement of specific goals of therapy can be documented and analyzed. Some goals of therapy are used as surrogates for improved health and positive outcomes. For example, the achievement of a desired cholesterol of <200 mg/dL (<5.2 mmol/L) is used to evaluate a patient's risk of developing coronary heart disease or a stroke. Therefore, logic would suggest that for patients with elevated cholesterol (total cholesterol and low density lipoproteins-LDL) lowering the patient's cholesterol would lower risk. This relationship can be complicated as we now have data suggesting that patients with peripheral arterial disease can benefit from treatment with a statin regardless of their baseline lipid levels.[4] So, evaluating the impact that statins have on your patients by how much their cholesterol levels or their LDL levels are lowered may not tell the whole story. It often requires years of therapy to realize the full measurable benefit from some drug therapies. Similarly, it can take years of exposure to a medication in many thousands of patients to be able to fully evaluate the toxicity of the product.

In pharmaceutical care practices, we can track the changes in patient risk factors due to medication use. Patients with hypertension can be evaluated at each visit to determine if the antihypertensive medication regimen is appropriately controlling the patient's systolic and diastolic pressures. Most guidelines call for blood pressures to be maintained at or slightly below 140/90 mmHg in patients with uncomplicated hypertension. However, for patients with diabetes, renal disease, and heart failure the lowering of the blood pressure to a value of 130/80 mmHg is recommended. These same guidelines call for the selection of specific drugs to be used to lower blood pressure in patients with "compelling indications" such as heart failure or diabetes. Blood pressure control is an example in which the desired goal of therapy and even the medications used to achieve the goal can be different for patients with different medical conditions or combinations of diseases. Therefore, each patient's situation must be evaluated individually to ensure that the appropriate medications are being used to achieve the appropriate goals of therapy.

Patient Data: Outcomes

Evaluating the outcomes of drug therapy requires comprehensive documentation of related medications, laboratory values, and changes in clinical signs and symptoms over time. In the Assurance System practitioners can record changes in parameters used to evaluate the impact of drug therapy for each medical condition the patient has. As an example, to evaluate the outcomes that drug therapies are having on a patient with diabetes, you need to be able to evaluate glycemic control (blood glucose and hemoglobin A1c), blood pressure control (<130/80 mmHg), and lipid lowering (LDL <100 mg/dL, 2.6 mmol/L). In order to fully evaluate the outcomes associated with drug therapies in patients with diabetes, all of these values (and more if the patient also has other comorbidities) must be monitored, evaluated, and documented over time. Using the Assurance System practitioners providing care for patients with diabetes can track improvements or lack of improvement in all of these laboratory measurements over time. This allows the practitioners to easily evaluate the impact that the patient's drug regimens are having on the various surrogate endpoints and make necessary adjustment in drug selection or dosing to achieve the desired goals.

In 4700 patients with diabetes, blood pressures were measured over time and documented in the patients' electronic therapeutic record. At their most recent visit, 95% of their values for diastolic blood pressure were at goal (<80 mmHg). Systolic pressures were at goal in 71% of the most recent measurements (<130 mmHg). In these same patients glycemic control was evaluated by measuring their A1c values. Their most recent A1c values were at goal (<8%) in 85% of patients with diabetes. Their most recent A1c values were at a more aggressive goal of <7% in 58% of cases. As described earlier, lipid control is also an important factor in reducing risk for patients with diabetes. Their most recent cholesterol (total) was at goal (<200 mg/ dL, 5.2 mmol/L) in 88% of these patients with diabetes. In 77% their LDL was at goal (either <100 mg/dL, 2.6 mmol/L or <70 mg/dL, 1.8 mmol/L if indicated). Triglycerides were at goal in only 57% of these patients with diabetes indicating that many patients require individualized drug regimens, often combinations, in order to adequately control cholesterols and triglycerides.

Patients with hyperlipidemia most often are treated with a statin or a combination of lipid-lowering agents. Practitioners followed over 3300 patients with hyperlipidemia to evaluate the clinical outcomes of their drug therapies. In this group, their most recent cholesterol (total) was at goal in 86% of patients. The most recent LDL was at goal in 80% of patients with hyperlipidemia, whereas triglycerides were at goal in 58% of these patients with hyperlipidemia. Similarly, the HDL most recently documented was at goal (>40 mg/dL, 1.1 mmol/L) in 61% of these patients. Table 8-4 summarizes these clinical outcomes data in patients with diabetes and in patients with hyperlipidemia.

In order to evaluate the clinical impact that pharmaceutical care practices can have on patients, practitioners document several laboratory-monitoring parameters serially over time. Blood pressures, lipids, and hemoglobin A1c are the most common values followed in these patients. Across all 19 of these pharmaceutical care practices, the A1c was reduced by an average of 0.4% ($P < 0.01$). Statistically significant reductions in systolic blood pressure, total

Table 8-4 Outcome data in patients with diabetes and patients with hyperlipidemia

DIABETES most recent value at GOAL					
Systolic	Diastolic	A1c < 8%	A1c < 7%	Cholesterol	LDL
71%	95%	85%	58%	88%	77%
HYPERLIPIDEMIA most recent value at GOAL					
Cholesterol	LDL	HDL	Triglycerides		
86%	80%	61%	58%		

cholesterol, LDL, and triglycerides were also documented. Table 8-5 describes these outcome data across all 19 pharmaceutical care practices. The average difference in values by practice are measured from baseline (the earliest measured value) to the most recent value (the latest measured value) in patients with multiple measurements.

Table 8-5 Outcomes of key laboratory values in patients receiving medication management services

Number of Patients	Average earliest value	Average latest value	Average difference by practice	P value
A1c n = 2109	7.7 %	7.2 %	0.4 %	<0.01
SYSTOLIC n = 3852	132 mmHg	129 mmHg	4 mmHg	<0.05
DIASTOLIC n = 3765	76 mmHg	75 mmHg	1 mmHg	ns
CHOLESTEROL n = 1804	172 mg/dL	168 mg/dL	10 mg/dL	<0.05
LDL n = 1665	98 mg/dL	92 mg/dL	7 mg/dL	<0.01
HDL n = 1694	49 mg/dL	48 mg/dL	1 mg/dL	ns
TRIGLYCERIDES n = 1673	169 mg/dL	145 mg/dL	21 mg/dL	<0.05

DETERMINING THE CLINICAL OUTCOME STATUS

In pharmaceutical care practice, the practitioner is responsible for the outcomes of drug therapies. To determine if this fundamental professional responsibility is being met, practitioners must make a clinical judgment about patient outcomes. Each follow-up evaluation contains the practitioner's clinical judgment as to how effective the care plan and the associated drug therapies have been in achieving the goals of therapy for each of the patient's medical conditions. From the information gathered at the follow-up evaluation, the practitioner and the patient can evaluate the outcomes to that point in time.

KEY CLINICAL CONCEPTS

The practitioner is responsible to document the progress (or lack of progress) in achieving the goals of therapy.

In a comprehensive medication management service, the status of each medical condition being managed by medications is evaluated at each follow-up encounter. This provides a longitudinal picture of the effectiveness of the patient's drug therapy over time. For patients with acute disorders, the follow-up evaluation often serves as the determination of the final outcome. More commonly, for patients with chronic conditions, continual or serial follow-up evaluations over time serve to establish the improvement or decline in the status of the patient's condition being managed with drug therapy during that same time frame.

In practice, many patients have multiple conditions and require drug therapy to manage both acute and chronic conditions simultaneously. Therefore, practitioners require a working vocabulary of terms that can be used to effectively describe and document the outcome and status of patients' conditions being managed with medications. A standard set of definitions for pharmacotherapy outcomes has been established and is discussed below in detail.[5,6]

Outcome Status Terminology

The standard terminology used to describe clinical outcome status resulting from drug therapies is precise and represents both the decisions and actions on the part of the practitioner and the patient.

The standard outcome terms describe two characteristics of the patient's drug therapy:

1. the progress, or lack of progress, in achieving the desired goals of therapy at the time of the follow-up evaluation;
2. the action, if any, taken to adjust the patient's drug therapies.

A summary of the outcome status terminology with standard definitions is given in Table 8-6.

Table 8-6 Summary of outcomes status terminology and definitions[5,6]

Pharmacotherapy outcome status	Definition
RESOLVED	Goals of therapy have been achieved. Drug therapy has been completed and can now be discontinued. Usually associated with therapy for acute disorders.
STABLE	Goals of therapy have been achieved. The same drug therapy will be continued with no changes. Usually associated with therapy for chronic disorders.
IMPROVED	Adequate progress is being made toward achieving the goals of therapy at this point in time. The same drug therapy will be continued with no changes.
PARTIALLY IMPROVED	Some measurable progress is being made toward achieving the desired goals of therapy, but adjustments in drug therapy are required to better achieve the goals. Usually dosage changes or the addition of additive or synergistic therapies are required.
UNIMPROVED	No or only minimal progress in achieving goals of therapy can be demonstrated at this time. It is judged that more time is needed to evaluate the full response of this drug regimen. Therefore, the same drug therapy will be continued at this time.
WORSENED	There has been a decline in the health status while receiving the current drug therapy. Some adjustments in drug regimen (product and/or dosage) are required.
FAILURE	The goals of therapy have not been achieved despite adequate dosages and adequate duration of therapy. Discontinuation of the present medication and initiation of new drug therapy are required.
EXPIRED	The patient died while receiving drug therapy.

Before we describe each outcome term in detail and provide an example of each, we should begin by defining a term that will be useful in outcome evaluation. The term *initial* is used to describe the status of the patient's medical condition at the time drug therapy is first *initiated* and goals of therapy are being established. This represents the beginning of therapy and allows the practitioner to determine the length of time required to achieve the observed clinical outcomes.

INITIAL   This unique outcome term is reserved to note the time (day) when pharmacotherapy was initiated to manage a patient's medical condition. Noting the initial date allows calculation of the total length of therapy as well as the time to reach goal.

> **Example**   A 56-year-old female has had elevated cholesterol and LDL over the past 18 months. She has changed her diet last year and started an exercise program 3 months ago. Today she is starting her statin therapy with atorvastatin 10 mg daily. The outcome status of her statin therapy today would be documented as *initial*.

It will be difficult to determine actual outcomes without a clear understanding of the initial status of a patient. Now we can describe each of the formal outcome terms.[5]

RESOLVED   The patient's desired goals of therapy have been successfully achieved, and drug therapy can be discontinued. The use of the term *resolved* is intended to represent a final positive patient outcome, and is most often applicable to acute medical conditions or illnesses. The action taken, in this case discontinuing the drug therapy, should be documented along with the clinical and/or laboratory evidence of the positive outcome.

> **Example**   Consider the case of a successful treatment of a community-acquired pneumonia in a 53-year-old male patient with a 10-day course of oral erythromycin therapy at a dosage of 500 mg four times each day. By the end of the 10 days of antibiotics, the patient's temperature is back to normal, he has stopped coughing, his white blood cell count is no longer elevated, and the infiltrates originally seen on his chest x-ray have cleared. He does not require any further antibiotics past the original 10-day course of treatment. No additional follow-up is needed as his pneumonia has *resolved*.

STABLE   The patient's goals of therapy have been achieved, and the same drug therapy will be continued to optimally manage the patient's chronic disease. This is most frequently the case when drug therapy is used to treat or prevent a chronic medical condition or illness. In these cases, stabilizing the patient's clinical condition and/or improving laboratory test results were the predetermined desired goals.

Example   In order to stabilize a 63-year-old female patient's blood pressure within a desired range of 110–120/70–80 mmHg within 2 months, the practitioner initiates pharmacotherapy with 25 mg of hydrochlorothiazide every morning, a sodium-restricted diet, and a low-impact exercise program. At the 60-day follow-up evaluation, the patient's blood pressure was 112/76 mmHg and her blood pressure was at goal; therefore, her hypertension was judged to be *stable* and no changes in hydrochlorothiazide dosage regimen were made. The next follow-up evaluation might be planned to occur in 90 days to reevaluate the continued success of the entire care plan.

IMPROVED   Measurable progress is being realized in achieving the patient's goals of therapy. Goals have not been completely achieved at this time; however, no changes in drug therapy will be implemented at this time because more time will be required to observe the full benefit from this drug regimen.

Example   Consider a 55-year-old male patient whose depressive signs and symptoms such as loss of energy and disturbances in sleep and eating patterns have improved following an initial 3 weeks of drug therapy with 100 mg daily of the antidepressant drug sertraline (Zoloft).

Although his depressed mood and ability to concentrate have still not fully responded, no changes in his dosage regimen will be instituted at this time. In this case, his depression is *improved* and an additional follow-up evaluation would be scheduled for 4 weeks.

PARTIAL IMPROVEMENT   The evaluation indicates that some positive progress is being made in achieving the patient's goals of therapy, but adjustments in drug therapy are considered necessary at this time in order to fully meet all of the goals of therapy by the next scheduled follow-up evaluation.

Example   A 47-year-old female patient whose arthritic hip pain has been somewhat relieved following 2 weeks of therapy with ketoprofen (Orudis) 12.5 mg four times daily, desires additional relief from her discomfort. The practitioner's evaluation is that her arthritis pain is *partially improved,* but indicates that greater effectiveness might be realized by increasing the total daily dosage of ketoprofen to 75 mg taken as 25 mg three times daily. The next follow-up evaluation is scheduled to occur in 2 weeks to determine if this adjustment in the dosage regimen of the nonsteroidal anti-inflammatory medication produces continued and/or additional relief for the patient without intolerable stomach irritation, headache, or fluid retention.

UNIMPROVED   The practitioner's clinical evaluation is that, to date, little or no positive progress has been made in achieving the patient's goals of therapy, but further improvement is still anticipated, given more time. Therefore, the patient's care plan will not be altered at this time. Thus, the *unimproved* status evaluation is dependent on the timing of the follow-up evaluation.

Example   An adult male patient who is allergic to penicillin is started on erythromycin 250 mg orally four times a day for the treatment of a localized soft tissue infection following a work-related injury to the right forearm. Twenty-four hours after initiating erythromycin therapy the patient experiences some nausea from the antibiotic, and the injured area on the arm is still inflamed and slightly swollen. The practitioner reassures the patient about the nausea and provides him with a suggestion as to how to minimize this undesirable side effect commonly associated with erythromycin, and documents an evaluation of the current effectiveness of therapy. The practitioner reports that although the arm is *unimproved* at this early stage in therapy, no dosage changes are indicated, and that 3 to 5 days would be an appropriate time to make another evaluation of the potential effectiveness of the erythromycin therapy.

WORSENED   The practitioner's evaluation describes a decline in the health of the patient despite an adequate therapeutic trial using the best-possible drug therapy for this individual. Because the goals of therapy are not being achieved, changes in the patient's drug therapies are necessary at this time. The drug dosage may need to be increased and/or additive or synergistic drug therapies might need to be added. A future follow-up evaluation should be planned to examine the status of the patient's condition once the changes in the drug therapy have been instituted.

Example   A 17-year-old athlete whose elbow stiffness and muscle pain have progressively become more bothersome over the past 4 days despite the use of acetaminophen 325 mg three times each day and ice packs. This *worsening* condition might call for increasing the acetaminophen dosage and/or adding a topical analgesic such as capsicum. Two days after increasing the acetaminophen dosage to 1000 mg three times a day and adding topical capsicum, the practitioner would follow-up again to determine the effectiveness in reducing the pain and stiffness in this varsity athlete.

FAILURE   The practitioner's evaluation indicates that the present drug therapies have been given at adequate dosages and for an adequate amount of time, yet they have failed to help the patient achieve the goals of therapy. Therefore, the present therapy should be discontinued and alternate pharmacotherapy initiated. In these situations, the desired outcomes have not been realized and the initial treatment is considered a *failure*.

> **Example**   A 37-year-old female patient whose symptoms of seasonal allergic rhinitis have not improved with 2 weeks of chlorpheniramine therapy at a total daily dose of 24 mg/day. The chlorpheniramine therapy is judged to be a *failure*. Therefore, it will be discontinued, and new drug therapy initiated such as loratadine (Claritin) 10 mg daily. The next follow-up evaluation is planned in 5 days to examine the effectiveness of loratadine in controlling the patient's symptoms of rhinitis.

EXPIRED   The fact that the patient dies while receiving drug therapy is documented in the record. Any important observations about contributing factors, especially if they are drug-related, should be noted.

Using this standard pharmacotherapy outcome status terminology is a powerful tool in analyzing and improving your ability to care for patients, maintain a viable practice, and communicate effectively with other practitioners. Deciding the status of a patient's condition is a necessary component in the care process. We use condition status to measure outcomes in patient care. After you have identified and documented a patient's drug therapy problems, you must evaluate and document the status of each of the patient's conditions. When evaluating the condition status, take into consideration both the patient's goals and drug therapy problems related to the condition.

To decide which status is appropriate you should ask yourself two questions:

1. Did we achieve the patient's goals of therapy for effectiveness and safety?
2. Were there any drug therapy problems? Did you change or adjust any drug therapies?

Table 8-7 describes the outcome status in terms of goals met.

Table 8-7 Outcome status in terms of goals met

Goals of therapy being met	Resolved: goals achieved, therapy completed
	Stable: goals achieved, continue same therapy
	Improved: progress being made, continue same therapy
	Partial improvement: progress being made, minor adjustments required
Goals of therapy not being met	Initial: goals being established, initiate therapy
	Unimproved: no progress yet, continue same therapy
	Worsened: decline in health, adjust therapy
	Failure: goals not achieved, discontinue current therapy and replace with different therapy

A clinical example of each status and when to use it is described below. These samples follow our patient RJ and show how we assigned his condition status for each encounter.

Clinical examples:

1. RJ is newly diagnosed with hypertension. During your appointment, you and RJ establish that his goals of therapy for hypertension are a blood pressure of less than 140/90 mmHg and no side effects from the medication. Together you decide that he needs additional therapy for an untreated condition and start lisinopril 10 mg daily.

    Condition status for hypertension would be *Initial* because it is a new diagnosis for the patient. You established goals today and initiated new therapy to resolve the drug therapy problem.

2. RJ returns for another appointment in 1 week and his blood pressure is down from 170/100 mmHg last week to 162/96 mmHg today without any side effects. Together, you decide to continue lisinopril 10 mg daily and follow-up in 1 month.

    Hypertension status would be *Improved* because you have made progress toward his goal BP of <140/90 mmHg, and you did not make any changes today (no drug therapy problem at this time).

3. RJ returns in 1 week, and his blood pressure is still 162/96 mmHg without any side effects. Together, you decide to continue lisinopril 10 mg daily and follow up in 1 month.

Hypertension status today would be *Unimproved* because you haven't made any progress yet toward RJ's goal blood pressure <140/90 mmHg but are not making any changes either (*no* drug therapy problem at this time).

4. RJ returns in 1 month and his blood pressure is 155/95 mmHg with no side effects. Together, you decide to increase to dosage of lisinopril to 30 mg daily and to follow up in 1 month.

Hypertension status today would be *Partial Improvement* because you have made progress toward goal BP of <140/90 mmHg but made a minor adjustment by increasing the dosage (drug therapy problem—dosage too low).

5. RJ returns in 1 month, and his blood pressure is 115/74 mmHg, and he describes feeling dizzy when he stands. He has fallen once due to dizziness. You attribute this to lisinopril and decrease his dosage to 20 mg daily and will follow-up in 2 weeks.

Hypertension status today would be *Worsened* because even though his BP goal of <140/90 mmHg was reached, his condition worsened due to side effects from the medication, and you made a change by decreasing his lisinopril dosage (drug therapy problem—adverse drug reaction).

6. RJ returns in 2 weeks, and his blood pressure is 144/94 mmHg. He describes having a dry cough that is annoying him. You attribute his cough to lisinopril. Together, you decide to change his lisinopril 20 mg hydrochlorothiazide 25 mg daily and will follow-up in 2 weeks.

Hypertension status today would be *Failure* because his BP goal is not at <140/90 mmHg and you discontinues current therapy due to an unmanageable side effect and changed to a new drug (drug therapy problem—adverse drug reaction).

7. RJ returns in 2 weeks and his blood pressure is 128/84 without any side effects. RJ reached his goals of BP <140/90 with no side effects. You decide to follow-up in 1 month.

Hypertension status today would be *Stable* because RJ reached all goals for hypertension and he will continue the same therapy without any changes (*no* drug therapy problem).

After reading these examples, some of the common mistakes should be clarified:

- Keep in mind that you are trying to achieve goals for effectiveness as well as for safety.
- Do not choose stable, improved, or unimproved if you found a drug therapy problem for the condition. Continuing the same therapy inherently means that you did not find a drug therapy problem today.

- Do not choose *initial* for a condition that is not new for the patient. If the patient has been taking medications for her hypertension for 5 years, and today is the first time you are meeting with her, the status cannot be initial.
- Do not be afraid to choose *failure*. It does not mean that you failed or the patient failed, it means that they drug therapy regimen failed to produce the desired outcome.
- Changing dosages are minor adjustments (*partial improvement, worsened*). Changing drugs is most likely *failure* or *partial improvement* in the case of an adverse drug reaction.

Carefully documented follow-up evaluations can provide important summary data to address vital questions such as "How long does it take for your patients with hypertension to achieve their goals and become stable on their new antihypertensive drug therapies?" or "Which of my patients receiving antidepressants are unimproved, or only partially improved, after 60–90 days of therapy?" Outcome data supporting the positive contributions of pharmaceutical care require person-to-person follow-up evaluations and systematic, explicit clinical decisions and documentation of patient outcomes over time.

Having command of this clinical outcomes vocabulary becomes noticeably important when one considers the complexity of patients encountered in practice. Some patients have acute or self-limiting conditions that might be expected to be totally resolved by appropriate drug therapy. Patients with acute bacterial infections represent common examples in which one might establish a realistic goal to *resolve* the infection within a certain time frame (10–14 days). However, the vast majority of patients suffer from chronic disorders such as hypertension, depression, hyperlipidemia, asthma, and/or arthritis for which patient's goals of therapy do not include the complete resolution, but rather include interim (surrogate) goals such as reducing blood pressure or blood glucose or improving the condition by reducing signs and symptoms, correcting abnormal test results, and/or improving the patient's endurance or ability to ambulate. In patients with chronic disorders, the status of *stable* (goals are being met and there are no drug therapy problems at this time) is often the best that can be expected.

In addition to individual laboratory outcome measurements, practitioners can make an overall clinical evaluation of the status of the patient's condition at each follow-up visit. The outcome status by condition can be used to track progress over time at achieving desired goals of therapy. These clinical outcome evaluations by the practitioners often require evaluating both quantitative (laboratory tests) and qualitative (questions about pain, cough, tiredness, sleeping and eating patterns) patient-specific data. The practitioner evaluates if the patient's drug regimen has achieved the desired goals of therapy or if measurable progress is being made toward the patient's goals.

Patient Data: Outcomes

As described earlier, practitioners use a standard set of terminology to (1) describe their pharmacotherapeutic evaluations of the patient's progress toward meeting the goals of therapy and (2) describe if an adjustment had to be made in the patient's drug therapy. In the patient data analyzed, the pharmaceutical care practitioner evaluated 33,273 individual medical conditions at least two separate times and the outcome status was documented for each.

KEY CLINICAL CONCEPTS

For those patients' medical conditions that were not at goal at their first visit (18,866), 54% of their conditions improved (10,195) with the identification and resolution of their drug therapy problem(s). This is strong evidence of the overall clinical value that pharmaceutical care practice can bring to our health care systems.

These practitioners worked directly with patients and their physicians to identify and resolve drug therapy problems, and thus make important progress in meeting patient-specific goals of therapy. More than one of every two medical conditions that was not at goal at the first visit was documented to be at goal by the latest documented pharmaceutical care visit.

Patients' clinical status declined in 26% of medical conditions (4837) and the status was unchanged (no measurable progress was made in achieving the goal of therapy) in 20% (3834). Therefore, in 74% of patients' medical conditions that were not at goal when the patient first visited the pharmaceutical care practitioner, their condition improved or remained the same (Figure 8-4).

Not all conditions can be improved to the extent of achieving the stated goals of therapy. However, by keeping comprehensive records of progress and lack of progress, practitioners can continue to make adjustments and manage the patient's drug therapies to maximize the benefits that the patient receives from his medications. Effective medication management requires constant vigilance and aggressive follow-up schedules to ensure that every patient's drug therapies are producing the desired outcomes.

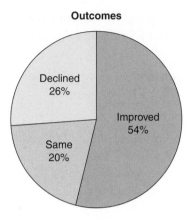

Outcomes

Figure 8-4 Outcomes of patients' medical conditions that were not at goal at the first visit (N = 18,866).

Patient Outcome Versus Practitioner Output

Dictionaries define *outcome* as the final result, or consequence. As applied to pharmaceutical care, outcomes refer to that which is a direct consequence of the collaborative efforts of practitioners and patients.

Much has been spoken and written about outcome evaluations and the positive outcomes that will result from various practitioners providing pharmaceutical care. However, much of this discourse is somewhat hollow. In fact, much of what is described as outcomes of drug therapy has little to do with patient outcomes at all. Much of this energy is misdirected toward counting and measuring *outputs* of practitioner activities. These practitioner outputs often include actions such as doses changed, the number of prescriptions substituted with a formulary approved generic product, or the percentage of time that prescribers agree with the recommendation of the pharmacist. These outputs may or may not have any measurable influence on the health and welfare of the patient. In fact, some of these activities may adversely affect the patient.

Patient outcomes do not include whether or not the prescriber followed the pharmacist's recommendation to change a dose. Patient outcomes do not include successfully substituting a less expensive drug product for another. It is also important to note that patient outcomes do not include implementing a protocol for a group of patients with a particular disorder, and outcomes do not include counseling patients on how to properly administer medications. Each of these well-meaning and frequently useful *interventions* may or may not have a positive impact on any given patient. To determine positive and/ or negative clinical outcomes, the effectiveness and safety of the patient's drug therapies must be evaluated and documented.

> **KEY CLINICAL CONCEPTS**
>
> There are no shortcuts to positive patient outcomes. Patient outcomes resulting from drug therapy cannot be determined from a distance. Outcomes cannot be measured from the boardroom, they cannot be measured from the hallway, and a computer program cannot generate them.

If one is truly concerned with the impact that drug therapies have on patients, there is no better method available to determine clinical outcomes than by personally contacting each and every patient at appropriately planned intervals and eliciting information describing the effectiveness and safety of pharmacotherapy. Only through the direct clinical approach can the impact of drug therapies be fully understood.

To fully accept responsibility for patient outcomes associated with drug therapy, the practitioner must be prepared to recognize not only the positive outcomes that can be anticipated, but also the negative. It is important to keep in mind that even the most carefully designed care plans and associated drug therapies cannot be expected to always result in positive outcomes. The performance of an appropriately scheduled, comprehensive, and continuous follow-up evaluation of effectiveness and safety is an essential responsibility within the practice of pharmaceutical care.

ASSESSMENT FOR NEW DRUG THERAPY PROBLEMS

Another purpose of follow-up evaluations is to identify new medical conditions that require treatment with drug therapy or determine if any new drug therapy problems have developed. This requires the application of the same skills used throughout the assessment step of the pharmaceutical care process.

A negative patient outcome at the follow-up evaluation is considered a new drug therapy problem and must be prioritized as such and resolved as expeditiously as possible. In pharmaceutical care practice, negative patient outcomes are resolved in the same way that other patient-specific drug-related needs are addressed.

For example, if your patient's major depressive disorder has not improved after the recommended 12 weeks of antidepressant therapy, then your patient's therapy has not resulted in a positive clinical outcome. If the clinical decision is that the outcome at this point would be considered a failure, then you would describe this new drug therapy problem as "the patient is receiving ineffective drug therapy for depression." You are now responsible to institute whatever interventions are needed in order to improve the patient's medication experience. Despite your best efforts, corrective action is required. You will need to discontinue the failed drug therapy and identify a new pharmacotherapeutic approach to manage this patient's depressive illness.

SCHEDULE FOR CONTINUOUS FOLLOW-UP EVALUATIONS

The last activity of a well-conducted evaluation is to establish the schedule and plan for continuous follow-up evaluations. The therapeutic relationship serves as the basis for providing continuous care and constantly improving the management of the patient's medications. Providing continuous care is an active process and requires a commitment to keep in contact with each patient throughout the entire course of therapy.

DOCUMENTING THE FOLLOW-UP EVALUATION

Documentation of the follow-up evaluation is required. The main objective when documenting your findings from a follow-up evaluation is to establish the association or connections between the patient's indication, drug therapy, and actual outcomes. It is essential that when you conduct a follow-up evaluation, you record the patient outcomes and your clinical evaluation of the patient's status while receiving drug therapy.

The outcome status is recorded using the standard outcome terminology of *resolved, stable, improved, partially improved, unimproved, worsened,* or *failure.* These terms represent your clinical judgment. Supporting evidence for that judgment can include improvements in clinical and/or laboratory values. These are balanced or compared to evidence (or lack of evidence) of adverse drug effects documented as undesirable changes in clinical and/or laboratory values caused by drug therapy (Appendix 3).

Recommended changes in drug therapy are documented at the follow-up evaluation, and the care plan is modified to reflect the new therapy. Changes in product, dose, interval, duration, and/or instructions need to be clearly and completely understood by the patient. The schedule for the next follow-up evaluation must be recorded.

You should place your signature on the evaluation record. This step, in essence, completes a circle of care. Furthermore, patients, other practitioners, and payers must be able to link the care provided with a specific practitioner or team. Care represents a people-process, so new practitioners should establish the clinical habit of signing all work.

SUMMARY

The follow-up evaluation supports and maintains a positive therapeutic relationship. It is the best method available to determine patient outcomes. Outcomes are what the patient experiences as a result of specific drug therapies and related drug information, advice, and other interventions. Follow-up evaluations are the critical points at which the effectiveness and safety of the patient's care plan and associated drug therapies are determined and balanced against one another, and where decisions concerning further adjustments in drug therapy are made.

There are several important activities and skills required of the practitioner in order to conduct an appropriate follow-up evaluation. During the follow-up evaluation, patient outcomes are observed and recorded, progress in meeting goals of therapy is appraised, effectiveness and safety of drug therapies are evaluated, and an assessment is made to determine whether new problems have developed since the last encounter. The connections the practitioner establishes throughout each follow-up evaluation include (1) the patient's medical condition, (2) the medication(s) used to manage that condition, (3) the clinical outcome at the time of the evaluation, (4) the practitioner's clinical judgment as to the outcome status, and (5) any changes in drug therapies that are necessary to improve the patient's medication experience.

In practice, patient outcomes are not always predictable and are not always positive. Practitioners must be willing to engage in critical, reflective reviews of all of their clinical decisions. Pharmacotherapy is a classic example of biology in which one introduces an exogenous chemical influence (drug) into a complex biological system (patient), and the result (outcome) is neither consistent nor universally predictable. Pharmaceutical care practice requires practitioners and patients to make decisions in areas of uncertainty.

The follow-up evaluation provides an ideal situation in which to grow as a practitioner. The best practitioner is on a constant quest to improve. This means that each practitioner can learn from every follow-up evaluation, gaining confidence from clinical successes and by recognizing failures or mistakes and work diligently toward improvement.

REFERENCES

1. Ernst FR, Grizzle AJ. Drug-related morbidity and mortality: updating the cost-of-illness model. *J Am Pharm Assoc* 2001;41(2):192–199.
2. Johnson JA, Bootman JL. Drug-related morbidity and mortality. A cost-of-illness model. *Arch Intern Med* 1995;155(18):1949–1956.
3. Johnson JA, Bootman JL. Drug-related morbidity and mortality and the economic impact of pharmaceutical care. *Am J Health Syst Pharm* 1997;54(5):554–558.
4. Heart Protection Study Collaborative Group. Randomized trial of the effects of cholesterol-lowering with simvastatin on peripheral vascular and other major vascular outcomes in 20,536 people with peripheral arterial disease and other high-risk conditions. *J Vasc Surg* 2007;45:645–654.
5. Cipolle RJ, Strand LM, Morley PC. *Pharmaceutical Care Practice.* New York, NY: McGraw-Hill; 1998.
6. Cipolle RJ, Strand LM, Morley PC. *Pharmaceutical Care Practice: The Clinician's Guide.* 2nd ed. New York, NY: McGraw-Hill; 2004.

Documentation in Practice

♀ KEY CONCEPTS

1 All patient care that is provided as medication management services must be documented to meet ethical, professional, and legal guidelines and standards.

2 The patient's Electronic Therapeutic Record is the basis for record-keeping for medication management services.

3 The Patient's Personalized Care Plan contains the information that is most useful to the patient and having this information allows the patient to actively participate in his care.

4 The Electronic Therapeutic Record provides physicians and other practitioners with unique, comprehensive, and useful information about all of the patient's medications, drug therapy problems, and recommendations to optimize the patient's medications.

5 The documentation of medication management services generates the data you will need to manage, expand, improve, and justify your service.

6 Governmental guidelines will require documentation systems used by pharmaceutical care practitioners to (a) meet meaningful use criteria, (b) communicate with other patient care systems, and (c) generate research data to improve patient care and population health in the future.

7 If you didn't document it, you didn't do it!

INTRODUCTION

It is the responsibility of all who provide direct patient care services to document three major categories of information: (a) the data used to make the decisions that fall within your scope of responsibility, (b) the decisions made for and with the patient, and (c) the actual outcomes that result from those decisions. Practitioners who provide medication management services are expected to meet this same standard. Documentation of patient care services is more than making a note or generating medication lists, it is recording the complete care process.

> **KEY CLINICAL CONCEPTS**
>
> The documentation not only must be useful to the pharmaceutical care practitioner, but needs to serve as the primary information resource for the patient, the patient's family, the patient's prescribers, and those who manage and evaluate the services provided.

THE ELECTRONIC THERAPEUTIC RECORD

Records used to document medication management services are called the "Electronic Therapeutic Record." Although it is possible to learn the practice of pharmaceutical care from a paper form of documentation, today it is nearly impossible and mostly impractical to manage a patient care practice with a paper system. This is why we refer to the "electronic" portion of this term. We call it a "therapeutic" record to differentiate it from the dispensing system output. Although information stored in an electronic dispensing system can be useful, it is quite limited in its value when managing a patient's medications. This record only includes prescription products; it only includes information about how the prescription was written, but not how it is actually being taken; and it does not accommodate recommendations made to change medications. The final word in the term is "record" because you will need a longitudinal record of the patient's care you provide. So, when medication management services are provided, we will refer to the documentation that follows as the patient's electronic therapeutic record.

We will discuss each of the documentation elements needed to provide quality care in detail, but first we need to clarify the term Electronic Therapeutic Record, for it is not the same as the Electronic Medical Record (EMR). The EMR is the record system used by most physician practices, hospitals, and other medical institutions to keep one consistent location for all medical, administrative, and billing information related to the care of the patient. Most EMRs were developed for administrative purposes (admissions, discharge, transfer, and billing). Their ability to support clinical services (laboratory, radiology, oncology, and all the other clinical support services) is still quite limited. This is the reason why there are many medical specialists who have developed their own clinical support systems that may or may not interface with the EMR being used in the practice or institution. This is certainly the case with pharmaceutical care practice. Because medication management services are new, most current EMRs do not support the practice other than providing a place to write notes. Although writing meaningful notes in the patient's chart can be important, this form of documentation does not meet any of the other needs, including patient reports and practice management data or management reports needed to demonstrate the clinical and economic value of the service. Therefore, the term Electronic Therapeutic Record refers to a clinical, administrative, and data analysis system that specifically supports the practice of pharmaceutical care (and the delivery of medication management services). This is necessary to deliver quality services in the era of technology. Such systems exist and perhaps the most advanced program is that of the Assurance System offered through Medication Management Systems, Inc (www.medsmanagement.com).

To be optimally effective, this record should interface with other clinicians' records (physicians, nurses, laboratory, consultants, pharmacies) so that you are able to obtain important information from their systems and you can provide others with new and useful information about the patient's drug-related needs, drug therapy problems, goals of therapy, and outcomes, over time. Your records need to be longitudinal because much of the care provided is chronic care over several months or years. Finally, documentation in medication management services needs to be current, kept up to date, and completed immediately following each patient encounter.

KEY CLINICAL CONCEPTS

The rule in health care is "your documentation needs to be completed before you go home today."

The documentation required to support medication management services is different from the documentation required to support a prescription dispensing business. Documentation is used here to refer to all the patient information that is recorded for long-term use and is related to the management of medications.

Documentation of a patient care service requires several different outputs to be routinely generated from the patient's electronic therapeutic record. The first set of information is the **Patient's Personalized Care Plan**. This care plan is printed and presented to the patient at each encounter. It is the tangible evidence that the patient is receiving medication management services. It contains several items of patient-specific information including (a) a comprehensive medication summary, (b) instruction on the proper use of each medication, and (c) any additional recommendations that the practitioner provides to optimize the outcomes of the patient's drug regimens.

The personalized care plan needs to organize information in a manner that is most useful to the patient (and/or the patient's care givers). Therefore, the personal medication summary, which is part of this Personalized Care Plan, is organized by medical condition, so the patient can understand that "these are the medications I use to control my diabetes," or the Personal Medication Summary can be organized by time of day, so the patient can understand "these are the medications I take in the morning and these are the medications I take at bedtime." Being able to provide physical, colored pictures of the patient's medications on her personal medication summary reduces confusion for patients taking numerous products each day.

Another vital capacity of any electronic therapeutic record is the ability to provide useful information and recommendations to physicians and others providing care for the patient. This **Medication Management Summary** must be designed to help physicians provide the best possible care for the patient. Therefore, it needs to contain any history of patient drug allergies, adverse drug reactions, and other alerts to prevent harm to the patient. Also, the patient's medication list must be comprehensive, that is, it must be able to include all of the drugs the patient is using to manage her medical conditions. This means the patient's electronic therapeutic record must contain all prescription medications, all nonprescription products used, any herbal, vitamin, or food supplements taken by the patient as well as why and how the patient is taking each (the indication). Providing other health care clinicians with a comprehensive medication summary that is organized by indication is of great value. All who provide care for the patient should be making decisions about the patient's drug therapies based on a single, universally available, electronic therapeutic record.

The third form of output that is needed to deliver quality medication management services, on a continuing basis, is the **Reports**, which we will call Management Reports. Just as the patient record helps the practitioner to manage the patient, the management reports help the practitioner to keep the practice viable and maintain its efficiency. The different management reports describe various aspects of your practice including workload, activity levels, patient needs, patient types, clinical outcomes, economic impact, payment levels, and quality indicator reports.

KEY CLINICAL CONCEPTS

Documentation of a patient care practice is so important that it is not an overstatement to suggest that if you do not have an appropriate method of documentation, then you do not have a practice.

The Electronic Therapeutic Record allows for both formative and summative documentation. Formative documentation refers to the recording of certain activities at the time they are performed and describes what is done when a physician, nurse, or pharmacist is caring for a patient. The medical or patient record is created in a formative manner. This document is a record of the information collected by the practitioner, the decisions made, and the actions taken at the time these events occur. It is created one patient at a time. This documentation is recorded at the same level it is used—at a patient-specific level. The output of this type of documentation is, optimally, the generation of a database describing the patient, drug, and disease information, decisions related to drug choice, dose determinations, modalities of administration, parameters for patient monitoring, and patient outcomes in terms of efficacy, length of treatment, incidence of side effects, toxicity, and other drug-related behaviors.

This type of documentation serves a formative function, which is to improve the care the patients receive and to develop the skills and knowledge of the practitioners through repeated practice and the collection and analysis of patient care information. It is performed concurrently with the pharmacist's activities and decisions, and accommodates changes when additional data become available. A distinct advantage of the formative type of documentation is the interactive nature of the process. Corrections can be made and adjustments recorded, which is consistent with any changing patient status. The documentation system also needs to be capable of doing summative reporting including practice management reports and these will be discussed later in the chapter.

Justification for the Electronic Therapeutic Record

The creation of a Patient's Electronic Therapeutic Record is important for many reasons. Perhaps the most obvious one today, and the one that comes to mind first, is legal liability. It is unfortunate, but truly the case that all activities performed on behalf of another person need to be documented so that if, in the future, legal action is brought against the practitioner, appropriate documentation is available. It is clearly the case that the more comprehensive the documentation, the "safer" the practitioner. But, let us concern ourselves with other, more patient-centered reasons for documenting the pharmaceutical care provided to patients.

We would like to think the most important reason for creating the Patient's Electronic Therapeutic Record is to provide quality care to the patient. Documenting patient care decisions and interventions is a vital responsibility of every practitioner providing pharmaceutical care. Documentation is essential because the patient's condition, needs, and outcomes are constantly changing. And, the amount of information required to provide pharmaceutical care is so voluminous as to necessitate recording the information.

No one is able to remember all the vital, clinically relevant information about an individual, and, as the practitioner sees the patient repeatedly, and the practice grows, it is unrealistic to think that quality care can be provided without complete documentation. In the practice of pharmaceutical care, you never see the "same patient" twice. Records must report decisions made, on a continuous basis, and reflect input from multiple practitioners. Each patient care decision made is based on accumulated results, and data derived from all of the previous decisions and outcomes. Therefore, patient care documentation must be a chronological record that can be constantly updated and evaluated to improve patient care. Also, it will seldom be the case that a practitioner works entirely alone. Technicians, support personnel, other pharmacists, physicians, and nurses will all require access to the written patient record. Therefore, it must be complete, consistent, easily retrievable, and kept up to date.

There are other reasons to record what is done in practice. It serves as the database for information provided to the patient. And, it serves as the database for learning to manage your practice. The Patient's Electronic Therapeutic Record is also important to the practice in the long term since it serves as the basis for payment and accountability. Any payer for health care services takes a similar position that "if it is not documented, it was not done."

KEY CLINICAL CONCEPTS

Payment and accountability are not possible without proper documentation.

The Content of the Patient's Electronic Therapeutic Record

We take up the strengths and weaknesses of different approaches to automated systems later in this chapter, but for now, suffice it to say that regardless of the type of documentation system (paper filing system with paper charts, an EMR, or a system that specifically supports medication management services), to function optimally, they all have to be structured to support the professional practice of pharmaceutical care. The following discussion is relevant to all methods of documentation.

The purpose of the Patient's Electronic Therapeutic Record is to record the results of the cognitive activities of the practitioner when completing the Pharmacotherapy Workup within the patient care process. Table 9-1 describes the three important components of practices: the description of the patient

Table 9-1 An integration of the patient care process, the cognitive process, and the documentation process

	The Therapeutic Relationship		
The Patient Care Process	Assessment of Drug Therapy	Care Planning	Follow-up Evaluation
The Pharmacotherapy Workup	Data collection Determine the patient's drug-related needs Identify drug therapy problems	Resolve drug therapy problems Achieve goals of therapy Prevent drug therapy problems	Determine effectiveness of drug therapy Determine safety of drug therapy Document outcome status
Documentation	Patient's Electronic Therapeutic Record		

care process, the description of the cognitive activities involved in the process (Pharmacotherapy Workup), and the description of what is documented as a result of the process.

The Patient's Electronic Therapeutic Record is intended to be the pharmacist's record of the patient-specific data, information, problems, decisions, activities, interventions, and results. It is important to keep in mind that this record is an instrument for the pharmacist(s) and should help the practitioner to provide care for numerous individual patients in an efficient and effective manner. The patient record is a living document and is continually updated with new or additional patient information, and therefore all entries need to be dated so that positive patient progress, or its absence, can be evaluated.

The Pharmacotherapy Workup prescribes the nature of the problem solving that must occur between the pharmacist and the patient. The pharmacist records what transpired during this interaction in the patient care record. During the workup, the pharmacist collects general and specific information and makes connections between the patient and his diseases and drug therapies. During the documentation process, the pharmacist records these connections.

Integrating the Patient's Electronic Therapeutic Record with Other Patient Care Providers

The information generated in the Patient's Electronic Therapeutic Record must be shared with the patients' other care providers. This can be done by interfacing with the EMR, which still remains costly and frequently is difficult to accomplish. The companies owning EMRs are reluctant to work with outside vendors. The alternative is for the Electronic Therapeutic Record to generate reports that can be sent to the EMR. The important point is that the results of pharmaceutical care practice must be shared, how this happens will continually evolve as technology advances.

The Patient's Electronic Therapeutic Record must be easily and quickly retrievable at all times. How this is implemented is institution specific because each institution has its own policy governing medical records. As most pharmaceutical care practices still establish a separate Electronic Therapeutic Record, this is the context in which documentation will be discussed.

THE PATIENT'S PERSONALIZED CARE PLAN

The patient is central to all therapeutic decisions and pharmacist interventions, therefore documentation must be able to support the patient's active participation in the care process. The Patient's Personalized Care plan must reflect this. The Personalized Care Plan is generated from the documentation system after each encounter with the patient so the patient is able to see what is happening with his drug therapy. This document represents the integration and culmination of the knowledge, experience, and skills of both the pharmacist and the patient applied for the benefit of the patient. The patient takes this document home and uses it to actively participate in his care.

The Patient's Personalized Care Plan is necessary because it:

- provides the patient with a summary of all of his drug, disease, and personal health information at all times. This information can be shared at all physician visits, dental visits, when the patient is on vacation and needs information, and if an emergency arises.
- provides the patient a place to record questions, observations, or findings related to drug therapy outcomes, so the patient can discuss them with the pharmacist, physician, or other health care provider.
- empowers the patient to become and stay actively involved in drug therapy decisions.

The Personalized Care Plan was designed after extensive examination of the information patients write down, carry with them, and use to keep their drug therapy safe and effective. This document is so useful and necessary that the United States federal government will soon be establishing standard format requirements for the document when distributing it to Medicare recipients who are receiving medication therapy management services under

Part D. Care should not be delivered without providing each patient with the information described below.

The Content of the Patient's Personalized Care Plan

Practitioners may construct a different formats for the Patient's Care Plan; however, because the practice must be consistent and practice standards continually met, the content of the care plan should always be the same. This will also help patients to know what to expect when they receive medication management services, regardless of where or who delivers the service (Table 9-2).

This printed document is often referred to by patients as their "list." It is quite common for patients to keep their "list" with them in their purse or wallet. Also, spouses who care for their mates and parents who care for children often keep their "list" to help them "keep everything straight." These

Table 9-2 Personalized pharmaceutical care plan

PERSONALIZED PHARMACEUTICAL CARE PLAN				
Name:		Address:		Date:
MEDICATION-RELATED NEEDS Special instructions for you Unique needs/preferences			Medication allergies	Adverse reactions
SUMMARY OF ALL OF YOUR MEDICATIONS				
Indication or Medical condition	Medications		Directions for use	Prescriber (source)
INFORMATION FOR EACH OF YOUR MEDICATIONS AND INSTRUCTIONS				
Medication	Goals of therapy	How to take this medication	Common side effects	Follow-up checkpoints
New Concerns/Questions/Expectations:				
Signature				Date:

lists not only contain what the patient is supposed to take, but many also contain what the patient is not supposed to take.

Medication-Related Needs

The Personalized Care Plan should also include a section on the *Medication Related Needs* that describes any unique patient needs or preferences that might influence drug therapy. Medication allergies and adverse reactions the patient may have experienced in the past and must be used to guide future drug therapy decisions should be noted. Information describing patient preferences such as liquid dosage forms or medications taken during the school day requiring an extra bottle with the school nurse can help patients receive the care they expect. Medication allergies on the Personalized Care Plan do not merely refer to the offending drug, but also include special instructions such as: allergic to penicillin and should avoid penicillin and related antibiotics such as amoxicillin, Amoxil, ampicillin, and Augmentin. Similarly, patients who are allergic to aspirin should be instructed to avoid other nonsteroidal anti-inflammatory drugs such as ibuprofen, Motrin, ketoprofen, Orudis, Clinoril, and sulindac.

Consistent with the Pharmacotherapy Workup, the Personalized Care Plan distinguishes adverse reactions to medications from true drug allergies. In the Personalized Care Plan, the patient can see that a past adverse reaction to a drug, such as nausea from erythromycin taken for acute bronchitis 2 years ago, might influence the choice of antibiotics in the future, but not necessarily rule out the future use of some other erythromycin product. Another example is sunburn associated with tetracycline therapy that can be avoided with proper precautions in the future. Such precautions would, of course, be noted and brought to the attention of the patient.

Summary of All of Your Medications

The Personalized Care Plan summarizes for the patient all of the medications she or he is taking and the medical conditions being treated or prevented.

The *Summary of All of Your Medications*, for the first time, puts all of a patient's drug therapies and their associated uses and directions for use in one place. This section connects four pieces of information for the patient: the indication or medical condition being treated, the medication, the directions for use and the prescriber or pharmacist who recommended the medication. The Personalized Care Plan can and should be continuously updated so that it can truly represent the patient's current therapies, indications, and directions.

If a patient is taking two of three medications for the same indication, all three are organized and related to the single indication. For instance, a patient taking Boniva, calcium supplements, and a multiple vitamin supplement for the prevention of osteoporosis would have all three of these therapies related to the same primary indication. Similarly, the Personalized Care Plan for a patient who is being treated for high blood pressure with lisinopril and hydrochlorothiazide would have these two medications related to the same "hypertension" indication.

All the information on the Personalized Care Plan should be clearly stated (avoid as much technical jargon as possible) and should be as "user friendly" as possible. The indications for drug therapy should be in terms the patient understands. If you have discussed hypertension in terms of *high blood pressure*, then the indication on the personalized pharmaceutical care plan should use the term "high blood pressure." Similarly, if the patient refers to episodes of gastritis as *heartburn*, then this term might best serve as the indication for the patient's Zantac. Allergic rhinitis might be recognized by the patient as *hayfever* or *seasonal allergies*.

There are no legal labeling requirements for the Personalized Care Plan. Thus, medications can be listed as generic, trade-name, or both, whichever is most helpful to the patient. The description and/or illustration of the tablet or capsule is often useful for the patient to distinguish one medication from another. For example, Prilosec (purple capsule), Augmentin (yellow round tablet), clarithromycin Biaxin (yellow tablet) serve as patient useful descriptions. The Directions for Use should represent how the patient is *actually* going to take the medication. In most cases the legal prescription requires the direction to read as the prescriber wrote, even if these directions are not clear, or directly relevant to what the patient is actually going to do. For instance, common prescription directions such as "Take 1 TID with meals and HS" might appear on the legal prescription label as "Take one (1) tablet three (3) times each day with meals and one (1) at bedtime." However, for the millions of people who do not eat the customary three meals a day, the directions for use on the Personalized Care Plan might read "Take one (1) tablet four (4) times a day. Take in the morning, midday, evening and at bedtime with some food to prevent stomach upset." In this situation the prevention of nausea with food is made explicit on the Personalized Care Plan, while it remains implicit on the legal prescription label. It is important that the Personalized Care Plan translates/interprets complex and often confusing directions into meaningful, comprehensible language and communicates a realistic attainable set of goals and directions to patients. In this sense the plan becomes a "cognitive map" for patients to locate solutions and follow pathways to effective drug therapy.

It might also be useful for drug therapies that the patient is no longer taking to be listed in a Personalized Care Plan. If the patient has been using an antihistamine preparation for several days with no relief for symptoms of the common cold, and is advised to begin therapy with a decongestant nasal spray to control nasal congestion, it might be very helpful to use the *Summary of All Your Medications* section of the Personalized Care Plan to remind the patient not to use the antihistamine for her cold.

Information for Each of the Medications and Instructions

The Personalized Care Plan not only contains the summarized information mentioned above, but for each medical indication for drug therapy the patient receives expanded, more detailed information. The medical condition is described including common terminology, signs and symptoms, causes, and common approaches to treatment. The Personalized Care Plan also includes other health advice the patient might find useful to assist in meeting expected outcomes. Advice about nondrug approaches, diet, exercise, foods or beverages to avoid, and methods to prevent the condition from reoccurring are useful forms of health information.

The more detailed information in the Personalized Care Plan describes the medication(s) for each medical condition or indication for drug therapy and describes the goals of therapy so the patient can understand what benefit to expect from the medications. Again, for each medication, specific, detailed instructions are written including times of day, length of therapy, and use with or without food are included for each drug product. Also associated with each medication are the common side effects of which the patient should be made aware. Here the judgment of the pharmacist is needed to keep the Personalized Care Plan useful to the patient and avoid making it just another long list of side effects that the manufacturer must list for medical legal purposes. Rather the contents of the Common Side Effects sections of the Personalized Care Plan reflect the discussion the pharmacist and the patient had about the patient's drug therapy.

KEY CLINICAL CONCEPTS

The therapeutic relationship between the patient and the pharmacist has a substantial influence on how much detail needs to be contained in any patient's Personalized Care Plan.

Different from a simple list of drugs a patient is taking, the Personalized Care Plan serves as a summary record of what the patient has agreed to undertake as personal responsibility for the care process (How to Take the

Medication), what should happen (Goals of Therapy and Follow-up check points), and what might happen (Common Side Effects).

A key section of the Personalized Care Plan is the description of the *Follow-up Checkpoints.* These include dates when the patient and/or pharmacist will have follow-up encounters to monitor progress. The Personalized Care Plan might suggest different follow-up checkpoints to monitor side effects as opposed to monitoring measurable improvement in the patient's health status. The follow-up check points not only list the agreed upon time and date, but they also describe what the patient should look for when evaluating the success or failure of their drug therapy. Conversely, the follow-up checkpoints should describe how the patient can tell if the drug is causing any unwanted side effects. Here the patient's information should be as detailed and useful as possible and indicate how patients can recognize that they are experiencing side effects.

New Concerns/Questions/Expectations

The Personalized Care Plan also includes a very important section to be used by patients to record concerns, questions, or other important issues that they want to discuss with the pharmacist or physician during their next visit. This section serves to not only allow but encourage patients to get all of their questions addressed. Often, patients think of additional questions or have new concerns after they have left the pharmacy or physician's office. This portion of the Personalized Care Plan makes it convenient to record these questions within the context of all of the patient's medical indications and associated drug therapies.

Finally, the Personalized Care Plan is signed by the pharmacist who prepared it for the patient, and dated in order to ensure that this individual can understand the content and its implications.

PHYSICIAN REPORTS

The electronic therapeutic record must also serve to effectively communicate with the patient's other care providers. The pharmaceutical care practitioner often needs to efficiently, but effectively, communicate with the patient's physician(s) about drug therapy problems identified and the recommendations to improve the patient's medication regimens. Below is the format for the report (Table 9-3). It is designed to be brief, organized, yet comprehensive. First the patient is identified by name, birth date, age, and reference number (or medical record #). The next information displayed is allergies and history of any severe adverse drug reactions. These data are presently early in the report to prevent any serious harm to the patient. Next, it is useful to provide the patient's alcohol, tobacco, and caffeine use if it will influence care decisions.

KEY CLINICAL CONCEPTS

The central portion of the physician report is the display of ALL of the patient's medications arranged by medical condition.

For many physicians, this is the first time they have been presented with a comprehensive list of their patient's drug therapies organized in a way that makes sense to a physician. Note that the pharmaceutical care practitioner's most recent evaluation status is included for each condition being managed with medications. These data inform the physician if the patient's drug therapy has achieved or is achieving the goals of therapy. Many physicians are unaware of all of the medications being provided to the patient by other prescribers, pharmacists, and family members, so the total number of conditions, medications, and daily doses are summarized. This provides an estimate of the complexity of the patient's medication regimens. Also, estimates of the total monthly costs of all of the patient's medications can be informative.

Drug therapy problems are clearly described using the seven categories with the common causes (see Chapter 5). This includes the drug(s) involved and the medical condition(s) being affected. Then the pharmaceutical care practitioner's recommendations are the last section. Up to now, all of the information in this physician report is generated directly from the documentation and is in the form of coded data. Therefore, all of this report becomes data. Only the written text of the recommendations and any additional comments are free text. Remember free text does not create data, and therefore is not very useful in summary reports needed to manage busy practices.

In summary, the physician report is formatted to (1) identify the patient, (2) present allergy/alert information, (3) organize all drug therapies used to manage conditions according to the medical condition, (4) identify drug therapy problems and causes, and finally (5) provide the recommendation to improve the patient's outcomes (Table 9-3).

There is a tendency on the part of new practitioners to write lengthy notes describing all they know and/or learned about the patient and the patient's drug therapies. Our experience and the feedback we repeatedly receive from physician colleagues are that the pharmaceutical care practitioners report

Table 9-3 Physician report for medication management services

Medication Management Service Address Phone #				
Patient Name	Date of Birth	Age	Gender	Reference #
History of Drug Allergies				
Medication		Allergic reactions		Date verified
Adverse Drug Reactions				
Medication		Adverse reactions		Date verified
Alcohol use				Special alerts
Tobacco use				
Caffeine use				
Activity				
Conditions Managed with Drug Therapy				
Condition		Drug therapy evaluation status (date)	Medication, use and prescriber	
Number of conditions	Number of active medications	Total number of daily doses	Estimate of month cost	
Drug Therapy Problems Addressed				
Drug Therapy Problem		Drugs Involved	Condition	
Pharmacist Evaluation and Recommendations				
Signature:			Date:	

needs to be as brief as possible, include all of the patient's medications, and end with the "bottom line" of your recommendation to improve the drug therapy for this patient.

PRACTICE MANAGEMENT REPORTS

Because medication management services are new to most health care systems, it will be vital to justify, expand, and improve those services with evidence and data. The documentation of the services provided to patients must also serve as the data their managers use to evaluate the quality of the service. Therefore, you will have to combine and summarize patients' Electronic Therapeutic Record data into practice-wide summary data to make useful management reports.

Summative, or practice-level documentation is created by combining the formative patient care records described above and summarizing various aspects of the practice for the purpose of improving the overall care for all patients in the practice. This type of documentation usually takes on the form of Management Reports. The Management Reports will focus on such issues as how many patients are seen daily? How long do practitioners spend, on average, with patients? What types of problems are most common in the practice? What types of resources are most frequently required for patient care? These types of issues can be addressed from the data generated from summative documentation, and are essential to the effective management of any practice.

Most Management Reports represent work and services performed in the past and reflect the interventions or outcomes of several individuals providing care for many different patients. Therefore, summative data, in the form of Management Reports, are not used for the purpose of caring for an individual patient. However, summative data recorded as Management Reports are often useful to assist practitioners to improve the way they deliver care to all patients or subpopulations of patients.

KEY CLINICAL CONCEPTS

Management Reports can be used to determine which services are most effective and should be continued, and which are less valuable and should be modified or discontinued.

The quality of the Management Reports generated and the validity of the data gathered will depend entirely on the quality of the data entered by the pharmacists when they care for the individual patients. It is certainly a case of "garbage in, garbage out." This is just one more reason to consist on complete and quality documentation at the time the care is provided.

Management Reports are necessary to answer the following types of questions (and more):

- How efficient and effective are your professional and technical personnel at managing the patient workload?
- What are the right type and amount of resources (professional, physical) to effectively and efficiently care for our patients?
- How financially successful is our practice at this time?
- How can we best expand our practice in the future?

The information you will need documented in order to create these Management Reports is described below.

The Content Required to Generate Management Reports

The capacity to integrate patient data from selected groups or populations with similar characteristics to make management, protocol development, marketing, staffing, and staff development decisions, is essential to the provision of quality pharmaceutical care. The patient variables and combination of patient variables frequently used to select patient "populations" for this type of summative management report include:

- age, body weight, gender, pregnancy, race, marital status
- tobacco use, alcohol use, caffeine use
- insurance carrier, employer, occupation
- address
- indication for drug therapy (*ICD-9* code, *ICD-10* code, Systematized Nomenclature of Medicine—Clinical Terms (SNOMED))
- the medication classification, drug product (NDC), pharmacological class
- number of drug therapy problems (the types and causes of the problems)
- monitoring parameters, values and time frames (laboratory values, patient assessment questions, patient satisfaction questionnaires)
- patient outcomes, goals of therapy met and not met, patient status at first and last follow-up evaluation
- complexity of the patient drug therapy needs, service date(s)
- service billing amount(s)

The information listed about is necessary to conduct population data analyses on the practice to constantly evaluate and improve the pharmaceutical care provided. Both aspects of documentation, formative (patient specific) and summative (population, management), are important to the provision of quality pharmaceutical care.

SOFTWARE PROGRAMS FOR THE DOCUMENTATION OF MEDICATION MANAGEMENT SERVICES

Early in the development of the practice of pharmaceutical care described in this text, we found that in order to care for many patients on a continuous basis, paper records could not adequately support the pharmacist or provide the useful summative reports to manage busy practices. To aid pharmacists participating in the Minnesota Pharmaceutical Care Project,[1] we worked to develop a computerized pharmaceutical care documentation system now marketed worldwide as the Assurance System. This computerized documentation system is based on the practice of pharmaceutical care as described in this text and is designed to assist pharmaceutical care practitioners who provide care to many patients over time. The Assurance System is presently used by pharmacists in several countries and is used to teach pharmacy students in many institutions across North America. In addition, all of the patient data analyses presented in this text were made possible because of this software. The software can be previewed and more information about it can be found at www.medsmanagement.com.

If you are interested in using a paper system to learn the practice or to begin to learn to document the practice, you can find a copy of the Pharmacotherapy Workup Notes in Appendix 3.

The pharmaceutical care documentation system specifically developed to support the practice uses a relational database to create and maintain a patient-centered, longitudinal record of the patient's drug-related needs, care provided, and patient outcomes. Being patient-centered means the patient's records are always kept together as a whole record with the patient as the central identifying unit (rather than the drug or the disease). The relational database allows the practitioner to relate, compare, or contrast any patient, drug, and disease information. This can be accomplished within an individual patient, among a selected group of patients, or across the entire patient population.

All commonly used billing mechanisms must be supported by the pharmaceutical care software. These include the ability to generate standardized forms such the CMS 1500 (Centers for Medicare and

Medicaid Services), the resource-based relative value scale (Clinical Procedural Terminology—CPT codes)[2] as well as individualized invoices for private, self-pay patients and payers.

Evaluating Software for Use in Practice

Although it is almost impossible to provide pharmaceutical care without computer support, we have found that a large number of pharmacists are still recording what is done on paper. The significant amount of patient, drug, and disease information required, the changing of this information over time, and the task of billing for services mandates an automated process. In addition, written communication with patients and other health care practitioners, the generation of personalized pharmaceutical care plans for patients, and access to drug information all make computerization essential. Instead of specifically focusing on one commercial software product, we will discuss the most important characteristics and capabilities of pharmaceutical care software programs. Pharmacists and managers need to evaluate software as to how best it can support their patient care services, ensure that appropriate billing records exist, and generate required manage reports.

Unlike commonly used dispensing computer systems, in which the primary concerns are speed and simplicity of data input, patient care systems should be primarily evaluated on their output capacities. In this context, output capacities include the patient care records or charts for the pharmacist's use, Personalized Care Plans for the patient's use, and Management Reports used by managers. Pharmaceutical care software systems should also facilitate communication between pharmacists, physicians, dentists, nurses, and other health care practitioners. Furthermore, pharmaceutical care software systems must have the capacity to generate clinical quality measure reimbursement information and billing for private pay patients, commercial third-party payers, pharmacy benefit management companies, and governmental agencies.

Following is a list of important questions to be asked when evaluating software to support the practice of pharmaceutical care.

- Does the software system really support the practice of pharmaceutical care or does it force the pharmacist to perform activities or gather patient information simply because the software requires it?
- Is the pharmaceutical care software system sufficiently comprehensive to support the care that you will provide for numerous patients with diverse medical conditions, diseases, and illnesses?

- How much free text input is required? Remember, free text input is time consuming and is not very useful when combined or integrated into summative management reports.
- Can the software system support continuously adding data and updating patient records required to provide continuous care to patients with chronic medical conditions?
- Can the pharmaceutical care software system support the implementation of drug therapy protocols from numerous sources such as physician clinics, health maintenance organizations, insurance carriers, pharmacy benefits management companies, the pharmaceutical industry, governmental agencies, and research institutes?
- Does the program use a relational database to support the association of each drug product with its unique indication, drug therapy problems, resolutions, interventions, and outcomes?
- Does the program's database permit integrating data from numerous patients into useful management reports?
- Can the program support searching patient records by multiple patient, drug, and/or disease characteristics?
- Can the software support several practitioners in different practice settings?
- Can the software system integrate large sets of patient data from numerous practices into a single large databank to support network, franchise, or chain pharmacy operations?
- Does the software system have on-line tutorials and help screens to facilitate new employees as they begin to use the patient care documentation system?

Because many pharmacies have computerized their prescription dispensing systems, it would seem logical to try to interface the pharmaceutical care documentation system and the prescription dispensing system. The primary objective would be to reduce the need for double entries for data such as patient name, address, insurance information, and so on. Also, an interface might reduce some double entries for prescription medications. This can easily be achieved with an interface program between the Patient's Electronic Therapeutic Record and the dispensing system in the pharmacy or the PBM (pharmacy benefits manager). Also, an interface with laboratory information systems is needed to support the evaluation of effectiveness and safety of many drug therapies. Just as our Electronic Therapeutic Record uses standard terminology and coding for drugs, drug therapy problems, interventions, and outcomes, the laboratory systems use standard coding for tests such as blood glucose, hemoglobin A1c, thyroid-stimulating hormone, and cholesterol. Although interfacing all of these functions is ideal, it is important not to wait for this to happen before you start caring for patients. The important thing is to take care of as many patients as possible, and document it—but do not wait for the perfect solution in order to begin.

MEANINGFUL USE FOR HEALTH INFORMATION TECHNOLOGY

It is well known that fragmentation within most health care systems has led to numerous problems and inefficiencies. In a direct attempt to improve and standardize information gathering and exchange within the U.S. health care systems, the Centers for Medicare and Medicaid Services (CMS) have created policies to ensure "meaningful use" for electronic health records (EHRs). The plan is to encourage the use of health information technology (HIT) in the United States to improve the quality, safety, and efficiency of health care. The meaningful use initiative was contained in the Health Information Technology for Economic and Clinical Health (HITECH) Act, which was part of the American Recovery and Reinvestment Act of 2009. It defines criteria that must be met including the electronic exchange of health information and the submission of clinical quality measures. The Act contained financial incentives for systems to achieve the meaningful use guidelines. "No outcome, no income" became the slogan associated with this Act. There are three stages involved in the implementation and evaluation of meaningful use of health information technologies.[3]

> Stage 1 (years 2011–2012) focus on basic elements of health information technologies and quality including the capture of information in a coded format and using that information to track progress for selected key conditions and reporting of clinical quality measures.
> Stage 2 (years 2013–2014) expands into areas including medication management, clinical decision-making, and bidirectional communication among health care agencies, and patient access to their health information.
> Stage 3 (years 2015 and beyond) will focus on improvements in quality and safety with the goal of improving population health outcomes.

There are several core objectives for Stage 1 of the meaningful use initiative that relate directly to documentation standards for pharmaceutical care practice and medication management services. Table 9-4 illustrates the meaningful use objectives, the relationship to the practice and how the Electronic Therapeutic Record achieves them.

The "Meaningful Use" initiative has provided these general guidelines for electronic health information in Stage 1. Stage 2 will directly impact the

Table 9-4   Meaningful use objectives* (stage 1) and the Electronic
Therapeutic Record

Objective	Description	Electronic Therapeutic Record (Assurance System)
Computerized physician order entry	Orders directly entered by any licensed health care professional	Direct order entry by physicians, pharmacists, nurses, laboratory personnel with proper credentials. Also patients can add information into their records.
Drug–drug and Drug–allergy checks	Drug interactions checked based on drug database used	Drug interactions can be checked and verified as any new drug is added or is discontinued. Also, allergy and history of adverse drug reactions can signal safety warnings. Clinical rules are used to identify high-risk medications in specific patients with risk factors.
Maintain up-to-date problem list	Diagnoses and other indications need to be coded (*ICD-9-CM* or SNOMED CT)	All medications are electronically linked to an appropriate clinical indication and goals of therapy are established for each indication.
Maintain active medication list	Focuses on prescribed medications. Indicate "none" if the patient is not currently prescribed any medication	All drugs the patient is taking (prescription, nonprescription, vitamin, food and herbal supplements) are included in the record. Every drug is associated with an indication. A history of discontinued medications and the reason they were discontinued is maintained.
Maintain an active medication allergy list	The threshold is to have 80% of patient records include medication allergy information	All patient records contain medication allergy information coded by specific product and/or drug class. Clinical rules function verifies that allergy information is documented.
Record demographics	Patient gender, race, ethnicity, date of birth, and preferred language	Comprehensive patient demographic information is gathered in coded formats including gender, race, age, language, patient preferences, occupation, employer, weight, height, BMI, address, contact phone numbers, and e-mail address.

(Continued)

Table 9-4 (*Continued*) Meaningful use objectives* (stage 1) and the Electronic Therapeutic Record

Objective	Description	Electronic Therapeutic Record (Assurance System)
Record changes in vital signs	Height, weight, blood pressure, calculate BMI	Vital signs are coded and dated similar to all laboratory values including blood pressure, pulse, respiratory rate, and weight, height, gender, and calculated BMI are displayed.
Record smoking status	For patients 13 years or older	Smoking history and current smoking exposure is coded and dated. Levels of tobacco use are coded. Patient desire to participate in smoking cessation program noted. Also, alcohol and caffeine use also coded as dosage or exposure level.
Incorporate clinical lab-test results in patient record	Threshold is to have at least 50% of lab test results that were ordered documented in the patient's record	All laboratory values used to evaluate the effectiveness and or safety of the patient's medications are documented, and dated, including normal, high and low ranges for therapeutic decision-making. Clinical rules function notifies practitioner of labs that should be obtained, but have not been documented. Lab results are color coded to signify out of range (high or low) values. Details of lab values over time are associated with medical conditions and drug therapies to evaluate progress in meeting goals of therapy.
Generate list of patients by specific conditions	To be used for quality improvement, reduction in disparities, research, and outreach	Continuous 24/7 access to patient lists by indication, disease (ICD-9) codes, including medications or by excluding certain medications. Patient lists can be selected by age, gender, disease, drug, drug therapy problem, intervention, outcome, or any combination. Patient lists can be printed or exported into standard computer (excel) files.

(*Continued*)

Table 9-4 *(Continued)* Meaningful use objectives* (stage 1) and the Electronic Therapeutic Record

Objective	Description	Electronic Therapeutic Record (Assurance System)
Report ambulatory quality measures to CMS or to the State	To be electronically submitted in 2012	All CMS requirements for Medicare Part D plans are reported out at year-end. Paper copies or electronic reports can be generated. Patient eligibility by month throughout the covered year is maintained and recorded for CMS audit purposes.
Send reminders to patients	For preventive care, threshold is that 50% of patients included	All patients eligible to receive preventive care or any other services are notified in writing, by telephone, and/or by e-mail. Follow-up contacts are tracked, coded, and dated.
Implement clinical decision support rules	Implement up to five clinical support rules and have ability to tract compliance with the rules	Clinical rules functionality supports application of unlimited rule tracking over time. Rules can include disease parameters, lab values, date of service records, drug therapy selections, dosage, outcomes, cost data, and/or financial impact. Clinical rules are controlled at the practice level, therefore can be implemented and reviewed for any selected time period.
Check insurance eligibility	Be able to verify eligibility for public and private payers	Service eligibility checks in place and verified at each service date. Clinical rules can be applied as per payer/plan agreements.
Submit claims electronically	Submit to both public and private payers	Service bills submitted according to rules established by any payer (private and/or public). CMS 1500 format available electronically or on paper forms. Standard service invoicing performed electronically also. Billings and billing history can be sorted by dates, payers, practitioner, place of service, eligibility criteria, and/or billing amounts.

(Continued)

Table 9-4 *(Continued)* Meaningful use objectives* (stage 1) and the Electronic Therapeutic Record

Objective	Description	Electronic Therapeutic Record (Assurance System)
Provide patient with copy of health record	Including diagnostic test results, problem list, medication lists, and allergies	The Patient's Personalised Care Plan contains all indications for drug therapies (can include pictures of drug products), instructions, allergy and alert information. Therapy detail reports illustrate changes in laboratory values over time for each medical condition being managed with drug therapy.
Capability to exchange key clinical information among providers	For example: problem lists, medication list, allergies, diagnostic test results	All medication, disease, indication, lab test, drug therapy problem data are coded in a standard format and can be electronically shared with any provider or any patient authorized entity. Medication lists can be organized by indication, by drug class, or by drug administration time schedule. All patient and all physician reports are electronically exportable in coded formats as text or pdf files.
Provide summary care record for transition of care and referrals	Provide summary of each patient visit	Every patient encounter is documented and dated, so it can be shared electronically with any other provider. Referrals are tracked to ensure patient actually seen by the other provider. Referral can be shared with individual providers or clinics. Medication reconciliation functionality supports transition of care.
Protect electronic health information	Use certified HER technology with appropriate capabilities	All patient health information is protected from access or view by unauthorized individuals. No patient health information is stored on local computers. All data are coded and encrypted when sent to other providers. Multiple levels of security in place including patient access and restricted access by support personnel.

* https://www.cms.gov/EHRIncentivePrograms/30_Meaningful_Use.asp

requirements for medication management services and how we document and interact with patients and their EHRs, but nothing has yet been published to clarify exactly what is expected. Stage 3 has yet to be further delineated as well. This document should be monitored for it will impact the way the practice is documented for many years to come.

GUIDELINES FOR DOCUMENTING PHARMACEUTICAL CARE

The standards for documentation are described throughout the patient care process (see Chapters 6–8); however, a few general suggestions as to how to improve your skills are discussed here. Although it takes time to document well, the benefits of a complete and timely patient care record far outweigh the effort.

KEY CLINICAL CONCEPTS

Documentation of patient care is not optional in our health care system. It is mandatory. Patient care cannot be provided, ethically, without a written record of what occurred.

Be timely   Learn to document a patient's care as soon as possible after providing the care. This is only logical in that critical information can be forgotten or confused with the passing of time. Also, other people may need to use the information you have about a patient for the patient's benefit, making it necessary to have the information available as soon as possible.

Practitioners themselves usually document the care they provide; however, if resources are available, it is possible to dictate the information to be included in the patient chart or to have technical personnel complete the documentation. Whichever approach is taken, make documentation a priority. The quality of your care depends upon information being available where and when you need it.

Be precise   The care of your patient will depend upon details about laboratory values, clinical signs and symptoms, descriptions of your patient's preferences, and much more. It is important that you report exact values, specific impressions, and clear descriptions. Do not guess, do not estimate, and do not be inconclusive about your judgments. Other practitioners may have to make decisions based on what you record—be precise.

Be concise   It is important to be short, to the point, and not waste words. It takes time to read written or computerized material. Therefore, chose your words carefully, and make each word communicate something specific and unique. This will take practice.

Be complete   Costly mistakes are caused by missing information. When information is missing, practitioners may assume that information is either normal or not relevant and both assumptions could be costly to your patient.

A comment about the use of SOAP notes to document pharmaceutical care practice   The question is frequently asked as to why Subjective-Objective-Assessment-Plan (SOAP) notes are not included in the documentation system developed for pharmaceutical care practice. This question results from the use of SOAP notes in other approaches to pharmacist activities and their somewhat extensive use in the practices of nursing and medicine. There are a number of reasons why they are not encouraged in pharmaceutical care practice:

1. There is no common understanding of what patient-specific information is considered S—subjective, and O—objective referred to in the acronym. This often leads to confusion and inconsistency in the information contained in these two sections.
2. Because SOAP notes are written in long-hand and there is no standardization, they can ramble, be difficult to read, and not contribute unique information to the care of the patient.
3. The common practice is to SOAP the medical problem. There is no reason for one more practitioner to SOAP the same medical problem being managed by physicians and nurses. In pharmaceutical care, there is no reason to SOAP the medical problem. The only item that would be rational to SOAP is the drug therapy problem, but the system described in Chapters 5 through 8 deals with drug therapy problems in a much more direct manner and requires more extensive management than what a SOAP note allows.
4. The data in SOAP notes cannot be consolidated and retrieved because they are written in long-hand (text). SOAP notes do not create data. Therefore, they cannot be evaluated, summarized, or reported in any standardized format.

The experience of medicine and nursing with this approach suggests that SOAP notes are not as effective or as efficient as they were originally envisioned to be. Even Weed, the creator of the SOAP note suggests that the concept should be rethought.[4] Subjective has become a pejorative term implying that what patients tell us is *all in the mind,* whereas the data that we clinicians capture is often biased and anything but *objective*.[5] A lesson to be learned from this example is that we should think about what we are doing and not follow blindly where others go. There are better ways to document medication management services. Be true to the professional practice as you determine how you will document what you do.

SUMMARY

The computer program is not your practice. It is important not to let the computer system you may be using dictate what is your practice and how you practice it. The computer system should only dictate how you record what it is you are doing when you care for patient.

The skills needed to provide quality pharmaceutical care to patients are numerous and include high-quality documentation. This chapter has described both the input and the output needed to achieve quality care. At the beginning of this chapter we emphasized the importance of differentiating between the description of the patient care process, the cognitive activities within the process, and what is recorded in the practice. The greatest risk comes from pharmacists who confuse a computer system they use to document practice with the practice itself. The computer software program is merely an aid to support practice; it is a means to an end. When the pharmacist allows the software to define or to drive what the practitioner does for a patient, the practice is certain to be ineffective and short lived.

On the other hand, it is essential to keep in mind that the patient care documentation system represents the evidence or your practice. If you do not document it, you did not do it. As with all documentation systems considerable effort may be required to enter new patients, but in the practice of pharmaceutical care, a patient is only new once and it is not always necessary to gather all possible patient, drug and disease information at the very first patient encounter. The pharmaceutical care documentation system must represent a "living document" that changes, grows, and improves with your patients.

REFERENCES

1. Cipolle RJ, Strand LM, Morley PC. *Pharmaceutical Care Practice.* New York, NY: McGraw-Hill; 1998.
2. Abraham M, Ahlman JT, Boudreau AJ, Connelly JL. *CPT 2011 CPT/Current Procedural Terminology.* Chicago, IL: American Medical Association; 2011.
3. Jacoby R, Berman B, Nash DB. No outcome, no income CMS's "Meaningful Use" initiative. In: *Health Policy Newsletter.* Philadelphia PA: Jefferson School of Population Health; 2011:1–2.
4. Weed LL. New connections between medical knowledge and patient care. *BMJ.* 1997; 315(7102):231–235.
5. Wyatt JC. Clinical data systems. Part 1. Data and medical records. *Lancet.* 1994; 344:1543–1547.

chapter ten

Acquiring and Applying the Knowledge and Clinical Skills Required to Manage Drug Therapy

---

♀ KEY CONCEPTS

1 The practice of pharmaceutical care requires the integration of information about individual patients, their medical conditions, and their drug therapies.

2 The dimensions of the patient that become most important include the personal medication experience, living environment, and physiological status, including medical conditions or illnesses that need to be managed with drug therapy.

3 The disease information that becomes most important includes the characteristics, prognosis, and natural course of the disease, and the goals of therapy that are achievable with drug therapy.

4   Pharmacological information that is central to all patient cases includes the characteristics of the drug, its pharmacology, mechanism of action, toxicity, pharmacokinetic and pharmacodynamic properties, and the effectiveness and safety that can be expected for a patient.

5   The Pharmacotherapy Workup serves as the conceptual framework to gather, organize, evaluate, and learn new patient, disease, and drug information.

6   In a generalist's practice, common things are common, meaning that the most frequently encountered medical conditions, drug products, and drug therapy problems represent a majority of the information needed to be mastered.

7   The most valuable clinical skills you learn are those needed to be reflective in practice—it is the best way to improve yourself as a practitioner.

8   The pharmacotherapy case presentation has a specific format that facilitates the successful communication among practitioners who share the responsibility for managing medications.

ACQUIRING THE KNOWLEDGE NEEDED TO PRACTICE

In this chapter, we focus our attention directly on those who wish to become pharmaceutical care practitioners, be they students or pharmacists who intend to change their focus from prescriptions to patient care.

KEY CLINICAL CONCEPTS

The contribution of a pharmaceutical care practitioner is measured by her ability to apply a unique body of knowledge to identify and resolve drug therapy problems for patients.

This unique knowledge focuses on pharmacology and pharmacotherapy and is applied to resolve and prevent drug therapy problems and optimize the patient's medication experience.

However, the mere accumulation of knowledge is not sufficient; the key is applying this knowledge to help patients. Caring for patients and resolving drug therapy problems require that you integrate patient, disease, and drug knowledge, and then apply it to a specific patient. There are often other practitioners such as physicians or nurses who will know more than you do about a specific patient or a disease, but no other patient care practitioner will know more about the drug therapy.

Becoming Familiar with What You Need to Know

Learning all that is required may seem like an enormous task, but there are three basic concepts that will help to make it manageable:

1. The knowledge that you must learn, integrate, and use in practice can be classified into three broad categories: knowledge about *patients*, knowledge about *diseases*, and knowledge about *drugs*. All three categories of knowledge are equally important; however, your unique expertise will lie in drug therapies. Because you will be using this knowledge to make patient-specific decisions, you will always think about and apply it in a specific order:
   - understand the *patient* and the patient-specific variables that will influence your decision
   - understand the patient's *disease*, illness, or medical condition, so you can think about treatment appropriately
   - understand the *drug therapy* used to treat the medical condition in enough detail to make meaningful decisions about initiating it, dosing it, and monitoring its effectiveness and safety. Learning and continually applying this order of thinking will make everything easier.

   Patient ⇔ *Disease* ⇔ *Drug Therapy*

   As pharmacists, we are used to starting with the prescription or the medication list. This approach "skips" the two most important categories of information you will need in order to make the most optimal decisions for and with a patient.

2. Although it will be necessary to gain knowledge in a number of different sciences, the foundation of your knowledge will be how drugs work (pharmacology), how drugs are used to treat and prevent diseases (pharmacotherapy), and how we apply this knowledge to help individual patients (pharmaceutical care practice). Focus on these content areas.

   Pharmacology ⇔ *Pharmacotherapy* ⇔ *Pharmaceutical Care Practice*

As pharmacists, we have traditionally been taught that accumulating knowledge about drug therapy is a laudable end in itself. However, as direct patient care providers, knowing the information is only of equal value to applying this knowledge to help another person. Knowing something without using it to better another human being is wasted knowledge in patient care practice.

3. It will be prudent to begin your learning with those patients, diseases, and drug therapies that are most commonly encountered in practice. For example, start your learning agenda with the top 10 diseases, drug therapies, and drug therapy problems. Do not try to learn everything immediately, start with the drug therapy problems that patients experience most frequently. Data from over 500,000 patient encounters are now documented. These data allow a learning agenda to be created based on the medical conditions and drug therapies most frequently encountered in practice (these will be presented throughout this chapter).

KEY CLINICAL CONCEPTS

The practice of pharmaceutical care generally—and the Pharmacotherapy Workup specifically—is the framework in which to learn the patient, disease, and drug knowledge you will need to apply in practice.

An organizing theme used throughout this book is that the more comprehensively you understand pharmaceutical care practice, the easier it will be to acquire, remember, and apply all of the new information needed about patients, diseases, and drugs to become a successful practitioner. The practice process will provide you with the appropriate questions to ask, and then the challenge is to have or find the appropriate answers.

As you might imagine, becoming a competent practitioner is quite an extensive process. You can become qualified through your formal educational process within pharmacy and experiential training in practice. At this time, the formal educational process is only beginning to teach the practice of pharmaceutical care in a way that can be helpful. There are still few experiential training sites that provide and teach pharmaceutical care. Therefore, the more active role you play in your learning process, the more quickly and extensively you will learn.

Your success will depend on your ability to take control of your learning agenda, your commitment to learning the pharmaceutical care process, and your dedication to provide pharmaceutical care.

Understanding the Important Relationships: Patient–Disease–Drug Therapy

Schools and colleges of pharmacy have continuously expanded the amount of knowledge that pharmacy students require for graduation. However, acquiring knowledge is only a portion of what is necessary to practice pharmaceutical care. First, you must determine that you are acquiring the appropriate knowledge, and second, you must learn and apply this knowledge for the specific purpose of identifying, resolving, and preventing drug therapy problems.

Traditionally, patient, disease, and drug information have been taught as though they can be learned in isolation. Pharmacology is often taught as drug actions on cells or organ systems. Disease knowledge is often presented as though there is a single, predictable course for every patient. Similarly, patient characteristics are studied as though they are static and independent of disease and drug. In clinical practice, it quickly becomes evident that for a specific patient, the status of her medical condition and the impact of drug therapy all influence how the patient will respond to drug therapy decisions, advice, and instructions.

> **KEY CLINICAL CONCEPTS**
>
> The integration of patient, disease, and drug therapy knowledge must occur from the beginning of the learning process and then continue throughout your career, in a consistent manner.

Knowledge You Need About the Patient

The patient is central to pharmaceutical care practice. You must know your patient. You must discover your patient's wants, needs, and concerns, and understand how she will respond to your information and advice.

Table 10-1 describes the patient information required to understand patients in general and each patient individually.[1]

There are a number of important points to be made about the information in this table. First, you have to not only gather the patient-specific information that is contained in the physiological category, which includes a patient's signs and symptoms, allergies, and risk factors for illness, toxicity, or treatment failures, but you must first place the patient into her social and cultural context in order to understand the physiological information. This includes the environmental factors that can influence your patient's drug-related needs including living conditions, employment, and cultural background.

Table 10-1   Patient information needed for practice

Timeframe	Dimensions		
	Personal	**Environmental**	**Physiological**
Present	Health concerns Expectations of treatment outcomes Understanding of disease and drug therapies	Living situation Who lives with the patient Who cares for the patient	Indications for drug therapy Diagnosis, conditions Signs and symptoms Medications
History of present condition	Change in mood or behavior Change in habits Change in mental outlook	Change in living situation Change in physical environment	Change in signs and symptoms Change in physical condition Change in medications
Background	Personality traits Coping mechanisms	Socioeconomic status Cultural influences Job/employment Insurance benefits Personal relationships	Risk factors Allergies/alerts Family history Hereditary factors Cultural traits

This table will be helpful to you on two different levels. First, it describes the scope of information you will need from each of your patients, and it also shows you how to organize the information about a specific patient in order to care for her (refer to the assessment step of the patient care process described in Chapter 6). Second, it describes how to organize knowledge about patients, as you acquire it. For example, content from a medical sociology course and content from a laboratory course all *fit* into this organizational framework. You should use this table as a map of knowledge you will need about patients to practice pharmaceutical care. Understanding the scope and finding a *place* for newly acquired knowledge will facilitate its recollection in practice when it is needed.

Knowledge You Need About the Patient's Medical Conditions

The practitioner must also have a standard set of knowledge related to commonly encountered diseases in order to provide pharmaceutical care. In pharmaceutical care practice, one of the first decisions the practitioner must make is whether the indication for the drug is clinically appropriate. You must know the primary indication for each drug your patient is taking, and your patient should understand this as well.

The indication and its presentation (clinical signs and symptoms) serve as parameters that are used to establish goals of therapy. That is, reducing or eliminating the presenting signs and symptoms often becomes the goal of therapy. The status of these signs and symptoms will be evaluated at follow-up and thus serve to determine the effectiveness of the drug therapy.

> **KEY CLINICAL CONCEPTS**
>
> The patient's unique presentation of her reason for needing medication dictates the goals of therapy, and achieving the goals of therapy determines the outcomes of drug therapy.

The association between the presenting signs and symptoms (documented in the assessment), the goals of therapy (agreed upon and documented in the care plan), and the patient outcomes (documented at each follow-up evaluation) serve as the core set of data used by the pharmaceutical care practitioner to make clinical decisions at every encounter. An organizational structure illustrating the scope of knowledge regarding medical conditions used by pharmaceutical care practitioners is shown in Table 10-2. This table displays the knowledge you will need about each medical condition you encounter.[2,3]

It should be emphasized that you do not need to know all the information described in this table for all medical conditions, but use this table to help find the necessary information when you encounter a medical condition with which you are unfamiliar.

It is almost overwhelming to think that you will need to understand all of this information about all the diseases experienced by patients in practice. Therefore, it will be helpful to approach this challenge with a manageable goal. The most logical method is to begin with common medical problems. This is achievable because pharmaceutical care has been provided to enough patients so the most common medical problems are well known and represent a relatively manageable number of medical conditions. These are presented below.

Common Conditions are Common

In a generalist practice such as pharmaceutical care, the practitioner encounters numerous patients with common medical conditions, who are treated with commonly used medications. Therefore, the learning curve of a generalist practitioner can be steep. It is important to realize that being reflective and

Table 10-2   Disease information for pharmaceutical care

	Dimensions
Characteristics of the disease	Definition of the disease: 　Presentation of the disease 　Structural abnormalities including disturbances of the normal 　　anatomic and/or biochemical conformation of the body 　Functional abnormalities including disturbances in the normal 　　performances and actions of cells, tissues, and organs 　Results including clinical presentation or signs, symptoms, 　　and laboratory abnormalities Epidemiology: 　Frequency and distribution of causes 　Incidence—rate at which a disease occurs (numbers/time) 　Prevalence—total number of cases in existence at a given time Causes/etiology: 　What brings about the condition or produces the effect Natural course of the disease: 　Onset 　Severity/intensity 　Prognosis
Intent of treatment	Specify: 　Pharmacotherapy 　Nondrug therapy For the following purposes: 　Curative 　Preventive 　Palliative 　Diagnostic
Goals of therapy	Clinical (physiological): 　Resolution of signs and symptoms, laboratory abnormalities Improvement in: 　Physiological activities 　Quality of life Behavioral (psychological) 　Patient satisfaction 　Adherence Economic (cost savings) 　Avoid unnecessary clinic or office visits 　Reduce drug costs 　Reduce employee sick days 　Reduce missed days of school 　Prevent emergency department visits 　Prevent admissions to long-term care facility 　Prevent hospitalization

Table 10-3 Ten most common indications for drug therapy in patients in pharmaceutical care practices

1.	Hypertension	6.	Osteoporosis treatment/prevention
2.	Diabetes	7.	Depression
3.	Hyperlipidemia	8.	Secondary prevention of myocardial infarction/stroke
4.	Vitamin supplements/nutritional deficiency	9.	Pain-generalized
5.	Esophagitis (gastroesophageal reflux disease)	10.	Allergic rhinitis

learning the most you can from every patient encounter accelerates learning. More will be said about these skills later in the chapter.

The more efficient you are at dealing with the most common problems, the more time and effort you can spend meeting the less common drug-related needs of your patients. This process of rapidly recognizing and dealing with common patient needs and constantly expanding your ability to deal with more complex patient needs is the foundation of becoming a competent practitioner.

The results we have generated from over 500,000 pharmaceutical care encounters from numerous community-based practices provide an informative description of the common medical conditions encountered. Table 10-3 lists the 10 most commonly encountered clinical indications managed with drug therapy in pharmaceutical care practice, while Table 10-4 lists the 10 diagnoses most frequently encountered by Family Practice physicians.

Table 10-4 Top 10 reasons for visits to a typical family physician's practice*

1.	Throat symptoms	6.	Stomach and abdominal pain
2.	Cough	7.	Hypertension
3.	Medication refill	8.	Headache
4.	Back symptoms	9.	Congestion or coryza
5.	Earache or ear infection	10.	Diabetes

* Data from National Ambulatory Medical Care Survey, 2000. http://www.cdc.gov/nchs/about/major/ahcd/ahcd1.htm

Table 10-5   Top 10 reasons for physician visits in Canada*

1.	Hypertension	6.	Upper respiratory infection (acute)
2.	General medical examination	7.	Normal pregnancy supervision
3.	Diabetes	8.	Hyperlipidemia
4.	Depression	9.	Unknown cause of morbidity (illness)
5.	Anxiety	10.	Contraception

* Adapted from IMS Health, Canadian Disease and Therapeutic Index (2009).

A comparison of Tables 10-3, 10-4, 10-5, and 10-6 reaffirms the concept that this is a generalist practice in that the medical conditions seen by pharmaceutical care practitioners in the community are similar to the most common medical conditions resulting in visits to primary care medical practitioners in Canada and the United States. Of possibly greater interest to the student practitioner are the following facts:

1. *What you need to learn is known.* A limited number of medical conditions and illnesses represent a large portion of the information that you will need to understand in order to become a successful practitioner. The top 10 medical conditions consistently represent over half of all indications for drug therapy. There are national and international guidelines available to guide the treatment of the majority of the most common conditions.[4–12]
2. *The data you will need are available.* Much is known about virtually all of these common medical conditions, so you can easily find information concerning etiology, presenting signs and symptoms, diagnostic

Table 10-6   Top 10 reasons for physician visits in United States*

1.	Hypertension	6.	Neoplasm (cancer)
2.	Upper respiratory infection (acute)	7.	Normal pregnancy supervision
3.	Arthritis	8.	Generalized pain (muscular/skeletal)
4.	Back pain	9.	Otitis media
5.	Diabetes	10.	Heart disease (excluding ischemia)

* Ambulatory Care 2006 excluding routine infant and gynecological visits. National Health Statistics Reports, #8, from The 2006 National Ambulatory Medical Care Survey; August 2008.

criteria, effectiveness of various treatments, and recommended follow-up procedures.[13–15]

3. *You will have numerous, effective solutions available for your patients.* There are several very efficacious drug therapies available to treat and/or prevent these common medical conditions giving you numerous therapeutic alternatives (prescription, nonprescription, herbal remedies, dietary supplements) from which to select in order to meet the individual needs of your patients.[16–21]

The most useful advice to the new practitioner is to acquire knowledge when you discover you need it (take control of your learning process), and practice providing pharmaceutical care at every opportunity you have.

Knowledge You Need About the Patient's Drug Therapies

There are well-defined, standard categories of therapeutic information that a practitioner must be able to integrate and apply in order to meet patients' drug-related needs. In practice, having command of therapeutic information in a format that can be applied to individual patients with unique clinical conditions is essential. Patients, other practitioners, and colleagues expect the pharmaceutical care practitioner to possess a level of understanding of pharmacotherapy and the ability to apply clinical pharmacological principles that is the highest among all patient care clinicians. Your colleagues will expect you to have a command of in-depth and expansive pharmacotherapeutic knowledge in order to identify, resolve, and prevent drug therapy problems regardless of patient, disease, or drug products involved. And, this information has to be available to solve problems in all types of patients with multiple comorbidities and multiple medications.

As described throughout this text, the rational, well-reasoned, problem-solving approach, which is at the core of pharmaceutical care practice, is nothing less and nothing more than a structured method to assess the drug-related needs of individual patients through the application of accepted clinical pharmacological principles.

KEY CLINICAL CONCEPTS

The pharmaceutical care practitioner repeatedly cycles through problem solving in the areas of indication, effectiveness, safety, and adherence.

Most clinical pharmacology knowledge is developed and reported in the following four areas.[21]

1. **Indication**—Therapeutic uses or intent for the drug or drug products due to the known pharmacological actions of the active ingredient(s).
2. **Efficacy**—Desired pharmacological action resulting in the somewhat predictable benefit of a medication in a patient population with a specific disease or illness. *Efficacy* is used to describe benefits to a population, while *effectiveness* describes benefits to individuals.
3. **Safety**—Side effects, toxicology, and other undesirable pharmacological actions that the drug is known to exhibit at the doses used to treat patients.
4. **Adherence**—Onset and duration of action (pharmacokinetic and pharmacodynamic characteristics) of the drug product and their influence on the instructions for use by patients.

Table 10-7 describes the knowledge you will need about each medication you evaluate in practice.[2] The information you will need is always the same, regardless of the specific medication being assessed. Knowing what you need to know and how you need to apply the knowledge will let you be in control of your learning agenda as you begin to care for patients.

Practitioners train themselves to make decisions based on the series of questions described below. These questions serve as the basis for every assessment of each patient's drug therapy regardless of the patient, disease, or drug therapy involved. The information you gather during this process will become the database and clinical experience you will use to form your own drug-related knowledge base.

1. Are all of my patient's medications appropriately indicated at this time? (*Indication*)
2. Are all of the patient's clinical indications for drug therapy being appropriately treated or prevented with medications at this time? (*Indication*)
3. Are the drug product(s) that my patient is taking producing or likely to produce the desired outcomes for each medical condition? (*Effectiveness*)
4. Are the dosage regimen(s) that my patient is taking producing or likely to produce the desired outcomes for each medical condition? (*Effectiveness*)
5. Are any of the drug products causing or likely to cause my patient to experience an adverse reaction? (*Safety*)
6. Are any of the dosage regimens causing or likely to produce toxic side effects? (*Safety*)
7. Are the instructions for all drug therapy regimens understood and can my patient incorporate them into his or her daily life as recommended? (*Adherence*)

Table 10-7 Pharmacotherapeutic knowledge needed for pharmaceutical care practice

	Dimensions
Characteristics of the drug	Description of the drug
	Efficacy for an indication
	Dosage regimen for the drug
	Dose (initial, adjustments, maximum)
	Dosing interval
	Frequency
	Duration
	Pharmacology (actions of the drug)
	Mechanism of action
	Sites of action
	Toxicology
	Contraindications
	Adverse effects
	Precautions
Activity of the drug in the patient	Pharmaceutical process
	Bioavailability
	Physiochemical properties
	Formulations and dosage forms
	Methods of drug administration
	Pharmacokinetic process
	Absorption
	Distribution
	Metabolism
	Elimination
	Pharmacodynamic process
	Impact of the drug on cell, tissue, or organs
	Time course of the effects
The outcomes of drug therapy	Therapeutic process
	Effectiveness: The therapeutic effect–expected beneficial pharmacological effects of the drug on the course of the patient's disease or illness
	Improvement in signs, symptoms, and/or laboratory findings
	Safety: Detrimental pharmacological effects of the drug on the patient
	Undesirable or harmful effects and adverse drug reactions

This is a good time to point out the relationship between the practice of pharmaceutical care and the principles of the discipline of clinical pharmacology. The need for pharmaceutical care practice is not new. Over 25 years ago, Goodman and Gilman described the need for the clinical application of pharmacological principles primarily to avoid therapeutic failures and unnecessary adverse effects. They called for the *rational use of drugs* and stated that the practitioner

> ...is advised to examine each therapeutic effort in a systematic manner, questions similar to the following; Is there a valid indication for this drug? Is it the agent of choice? Are its effects modified by the patient's illness or concurrent medications? Is the dosage schedule appropriate? Is ancillary medication indicated? What is the therapeutic objective and what evidence of efficacy and potential adverse effects should be monitored? Is the patient adequately informed and instructed about the medication and can his/her compliance be expected?[21]

In this concise description of a rational process for thinking about a patient's drug-related needs, these pharmacologists established the scientific framework for what has eventually become the practice of pharmaceutical care. This framework is a well-reasoned thought process based on established clinical pharmacological principles, beginning with a critical assessment of whether the patient has a valid *indication* for each drug she is taking. The practitioner must then work with the patient to establish measurable goals of therapy, evaluate *effectiveness* of therapy as well as the *safety* of those therapies, finally working with the patient to ensure the best understanding and *adherence* possible.

It is noteworthy that the rational thought process, which is at the foundation of the Pharmacotherapy Workup and pharmaceutical care practice, has its roots in the discipline of clinical pharmacology. The role of the clinical pharmacologist was to narrow the gap between the quantity of available scientific information on drugs and their safe and effective use in practice. Pharmaceutical care practice is intended to accomplish this same goal one patient at a time, in a way that is scalable to all patients and all practitioners.

KEY CLINICAL CONCEPTS

Pharmaceutical care can be described as the practical application of well-reasoned, clinical pharmacology principles in the primary care setting in order to ensure effective and safe drug therapy for every patient.

Understanding the pharmacology of a drug is essential. How the drug affects the body at the organ, cell, and even biochemistry level is the basis for understanding what and how the drug will affect your patient. Understanding in the pharmacological sense really means being able to predict, based on scientific knowledge, what effects the drug's action will have on your patient, given your patient's unique characteristics (age, gender, renal function, mental status, etc.) and disease or illness (diabetes, depression, hyperlipidemia, peripheral artery disease, rash, breast cancer, etc.).

KEY CLINICAL CONCEPTS

The pharmaceutical care practitioner, who accepts the responsibility for the outcomes (good and/or bad) of a patient's drug therapies, must possess a comprehensive and in-depth knowledge of the drug's actions or potential actions.

This responsibility can only be met by coming to each patient's case with a pharmacological database that ensures that you know (can reasonably predict) what benefit the patient will experience and what risk (toxicity, side effects, adverse reaction) your patient might experience. Most benefits from drug therapies are a direct result of the pharmacological action of the drug on the patient. Also, most toxicities, side effects, and adverse reactions are a direct result of the pharmacological actions of the drug on the patient. Therefore, by understanding all of the drug's pharmacology (desirable actions and undesirable actions), you can manage and sometimes, even control, the effects that drug therapies will have on your patients.

Understanding the drug's pharmacology is more than knowing that simvastatin can lower cholesterol. Everyone knows that. That superficial level of drug information can be found in Wikipedia, Google, from your local barber and/or hairdresser. Statins have several pharmacological actions. It is necessary for the practitioner to understand the influence that 3-hydroxy-3 -methylglutaryl coenzyme A (HMG-CoA) reductase inhibitors, or statins, have on the metabolic pathways of mevalonic acid and the effects this can have on patients. Primarily, they are used because they inhibit the rate-limiting step in the conversion of HMG-CoA to mevlonate, which results in less cholesterol being synthesized.[22] However, there are several "downstream" effects of this inhibition including inhibition of isoprenoid intermediates and altered cellular signal transduction. These pleiotropic effects of statins can have positive or negative effects on any patient who takes a statin. (Statins are among the most widely prescribed drugs in the world.) At lower concentrations, they seem to be proangiogenic (increase the formation of new blood vessels from existing vasculature), and at higher concentrations, statins have antiangiogenic effects. The effect that a statin will have on your patient can differ depending on the underlying disease(s) present. Simvastatin can promote angiogenesis in response to hypoxic conditions (ischemia associated with stroke and/or myocardial infarction), and it inhibits angiogenesis medicated by inflammation (diabetic retinopathy and some forms of cancer).[22,23]

For the practitioner, it is also instructive to know that you will need to treat 16 patients with peripheral artery disease (PAD) for 5 years in order to prevent one patient from having her first peripheral vascular event (myocardial infarction, stroke, or coronary death).[14] Also, if you understand that simvastatin and other HMG-CoA reductase inhibitors cause apoptosis (cell death) in human skeletal muscle cells, then you can understand that (and how) these drugs cause myositis and rhabdomyolysis and even why physical exercise can aggravate these skeletal muscle effects.[24]

Learning your pharmacology is a life-long endeavor. Practitioners are constantly challenged with new drugs, new information about drugs, and new information about old drugs. Simplistic concepts like "drug of choice" do little to support rational decision-making within pharmacotherapy. Case in point propoxyphene which has been prescribed to millions of patients since its introduction in the U.S. in 1957, was once a "drug of choice" for the treatment of mild and moderate pain. It was removed from the U.S. market in November 2010 because clinical data demonstrated propoxyphene puts patients at risk of potentially serious or even fatal heart rhythm abnormalities. In 1999, Premarin (conjugated estrogen) was the most frequently prescribed product in the U.S. and was considered the "drug of choice" for managing postmenopausal symptoms. Today, we understand that hormone replacement therapies can increase the risk of breast cancer and ovarian cancer, so they are seldom prescribed for this indication. In 2010, Premarin had fallen to number 28th on the list of most frequently prescribed products.

The information about drugs and drug products changes very rapidly, and the sources of reliable information vary over time (books, manuscripts, Internet), so the practitioner is challenged to constantly broaden his or her scope of drug knowledge. You have to be in the best possible position to contribute positively to meeting each patient's drug-related needs. If you want to help people get the maximum from their drug therapies without causing undue harm, the lesson continues to be:

"Learn your pharmacology, learn your pharmacology, and learn your pharmacology."

The drug knowledge required to provide pharmaceutical care goes well beyond pharmacology and includes a thorough understanding of pharmaceutical, pharmacokinetic, and pharmacodynamic processes (Table 10-7). Pharmaceutical processes describe how a drug gets into the patient. The application of pharmacokinetic principles to predict and control drug concentrations at the drug's site of action is also important. Pharmacodynamic processes describe the intensity and the timeframe of the effects that the drug has on the patient.

Clearly, the practitioner's clinical judgment is most influenced by the therapeutic processes (Table 10-7). These include most notably how to determine if the desired therapeutic outcome did in fact occur (effectiveness) and if the patient experienced any detrimental effects from drug therapy (safety). Effectiveness and safety are the two primary processes that practitioners must assess and evaluate continuously in each patient, for every disorder, and at every patient–practitioner encounter. Learning the process of identifying, resolving, and preventing drug therapy problems, rather than simply finding *answers* to questions is what will make the pharmaceutical care practitioner useful to patients well into the future.

Organizing Evidence-based Information

It became clear quite early in the implementation of the practice that current resources were not organized in a comprehensive manner that allows a practitioner to make all the decisions required in delivering pharmaceutical care to patients. The most common resources used by practitioners are national consensus guidelines, textbooks, and published clinical trials. Although each of these resources is unique and has its place in practice, there is no single resource that helps the practitioner to make all the decisions necessary to care for a patient. By examining the uses and limitations of each type of resource, practitioners can better understand how each resource can best be used in practice and see how the information relates to the practice of pharmaceutical care.

National Consensus Guidelines

National guidelines are consensus documents that recommend the best evidence-based approach to treatment or prevention. Each set of guidelines is focused on a medical condition and is created by a number of experts who specialize in that medical condition. These experts rely on published clinical trials and extensive clinical experience to construct treatment or prevention guidelines and algorithms.

National guidelines are considered current practice until clinical trials provide sufficient data to create new national guidelines. For example, national guidelines for the treatment of hyperlipidemia were created in 2001 by the National Cholesterol Education Program. The guidelines stated, "since [Adult Treatment Panel] ATP II, a number of controlled clinical trials with newer cholesterol lowering drugs have been reported. These trials demonstrated remarkable reductions in risk for CHD, in both primary and secondary prevention. Their results enrich the evidence base upon which the new guidelines are founded."[10]

Although useful in creating a general approach to treatment or prevention, there are a few drawbacks to national guidelines. One drawback is guidelines can be long documents with somewhat complicated recommendations. The Seventh Report of the Joint National Committee (JNC) on the Prevention, Detection, Evaluation, and Treatment of High Blood Pressure (JNC 7) recognized this stating the "decision to appoint a JNC 7 Committee was predicated on four reasons: (1) publication of many new hypertension observational studies and clinical trials; (2) need for a new, clear, and concise guideline that would be useful for clinicians; (3) need to simplify the classification of blood pressure; and (4) clear recognition that the JNC reports were not being used to their maximum benefit."[8]

The most important drawback to the majority of national guidelines is they are not "stand-alone" documents that practitioners can use to determine effectiveness and safety of a patient's drug therapy and create a care plan. Guidelines may serve as an outline for a general approach to treatment, though it is nearly impossible to include recommendations for every clinical situation or specific patient case. Most guidelines will explicitly state they are not intended to replace clinical judgment for individual patients. Therefore, a national guideline, like ATP III or JNC 7, must be supplemented with information about the medical condition and specific drug information on efficacy and safety. Only then is a practitioner able to make rational drug therapy decisions and construct a pharmaceutical care plan with and for a patient.

The Use of Textbooks in Pharmaceutical Care Practice

Textbooks are another common resource used by practitioners. Textbooks are valuable for learning more about a patient's condition and the specifics about a patient's drug therapies. Textbooks used regularly to learn more about a patient's medical condition include Harrison's Principles of Internal Medicine,[13] Griffith's 5-Minute Clinical Consult,[25] Pharmacotherapy,[14] Handbook of Nonprescription Drugs,[17] and Applied Therapeutics.[26] Although pharmacists do not normally serve as the diagnostician, it is important to have a basic understanding of the medical condition including presenting signs and symptoms, risk factors, frequency/incidence, and diagnostic tests. Presenting signs and symptoms and diagnostic tests may aid in developing goals of therapy and in monitoring drug therapies. Along with signs and symptoms, risk factors and frequency/incidence help in identifying potential undiagnosed patients.

To understand more about a patient's drug therapies, practitioners may use textbooks such as Lexi-Comp's Drug Information Handbook,[19] Goodman & Gilman's The Pharmacological Basis of Therapeutics,[21]

Therapeutic Choices,[16] Handbook of Clinical Drug Data,[27] Handbook of Nonprescription Drugs,[17] and Pharmacotherapy.[14] Specific drug information can be used to determine if a drug regimen is effective and safe for a patient and when to follow-up with a patient.

Textbooks can be valuable to learn about patients' medical conditions and drug therapies, but they have some drawbacks. The main drawback of textbooks is that each book has a narrow scope. Practitioners would have to draw from many of the books mentioned above to develop a comprehensive care plan for a complex patient. Each book may provide unique information about a patient's medical condition or drug therapy, but it is difficult to identify one book that completely presents a framework to help make rational drug therapy decisions and develop a patient's entire care plan. Another drawback is that many of the textbooks do not include current treatment approaches either because the book becomes out-of-date or because treatment approaches are not within the scope of the book.

Published Clinical Trials

For those who deem textbooks as ancient history, clinical trials may become their primary resource. Some common journals where clinical trials are published include Pharmacotherapy, the New England Journal of Medicine, and the Journal of American Pharmacists Association. These publications provide practitioners with the most up-to-date information regarding the latest treatment modalities. Most journals are now available online to supplement the printed version. Online access allows practitioners to use this information at any practice site without going to the library or carrying around multiple journals.

Practitioners generally use these clinical trials to enhance and to "fine tune" their knowledge. A clinical trial explores a single facet of a medical condition or treatment modality and assumes the practitioner has a general basis for understanding. This can be a drawback for practitioners who are faced with a medical condition or treatment with which they are not familiar. The practitioner may need to use other resources to understand the meaning of the clinical trial.

Practitioners are challenged daily to make rational drug therapy decisions and to create pharmaceutical care plans for their patients. Clearly national guidelines, textbooks, and published clinical trials provide useful information, but often it is not in the form with which a practitioner can apply it in the care of an individual patient.

Using evidence from clinical research trials, review articles and meta-analyses to make drug therapy decisions for individual patients can be difficult. Often your patient is not similar to the patients treated in the trial, or the trial did not report the same outcome you want to achieve. The statistics reported can be confusing and there is a tendency to only report positive results. However, a fundamental understanding of a few terms will be helpful. Suppose that in a randomized controlled trial, two treatments are used and that the probabilities of demonstrating a positive outcome are reported as 0.10 for the new treatment and 0.05 for the control treatment. The absolute risk reduction is 0.05 (0.10–0.05). In other words, in 100 patients, there are on average of five more responders in the new treatment group.[28] Other measures to describe benefit of a new treatment are the relative risk, the relative risk reduction, and the number needed to treat (NNT) can be calculated.[29]

- *Absolute risk reduction*: Difference in event rates for two groups, usually treatment and control groups.
- *Relative risk*: Risk for achieving an event or outcome with treatment in the treatment group relative to the control group. Can also describe preventing an event with prophylaxis.
- *Relative risk reduction:* Reduction in events with treatment compared with control. This number is often expressed as a percentage.
- *Number needed to treat:* Number of persons who must be treated for a given period to achieve an event (treatment) or to prevent an event (prophylaxis). Calculated as the reciprocal of the absolute risk reduction.

The number needed to treat (NNT) is an expression of the benefit of the new treatment compared to the control (or placebo) treatment. The NNT is defined as the inverse of the absolute risk reduction, so in the above example, NNT is equal to 20 (1/0.05) and would be interpreted as 20 patients would need to be treated with the new treatment for one patient to benefit compared to the control patients. NNT for treatments should be small, for example, from two to four. There are other restrictions to the direct application of the NNT described elsewhere.[29] For example, the NNT for *Helicobacter pylori* eradication with triple or dual therapy is 1.2. The NNT for prophylaxis will be larger. For example, as secondary prophylaxis, the use of aspirin to prevent one death at 5 weeks after myocardial infarction had an NNT of 40. However, the use of aspirin for primary prevention, for every 1000 subjects treated with aspirin, 3 cardiovascular events would be prevented and 2.5 major bleeding events would occur in women. In men, four cardiovascular disease events would be prevented and three major bleeding events would occur.[30] These findings supported the 2009 update of the Antithrombotic Trialists' Collaboration meta-analysis and suggest that unless your patient has coronary or cerebrovascular disease, the available data do not justify routine use of aspirin in patients based solely on a moderate risk level.[31]

The number needed to treat data is often used to compare treatments. For example, randomized controlled trials, which compare ranitidine and omeprazole with endoscopic healing of erosive reflux esophagitis after 8 weeks revealed that the overall number needed to treat for omeprazole compared to ranitidine was 3.3. This means that for every three patients with erosive reflux esophagitis treated with omeprazole, one will be healed who would not have been healed if they had been treated with ranitidine. These types of comparative data are useful, not only in making original drug selection decisions but are also helpful in understanding the effort required to actually improve on existing therapies.

Use of the Pharmacotherapy Workup as a Conceptual Framework to Organize Knowledge in Practice

It became clear as we were developing the practice of pharmaceutical care that we would need a better resource than just guidelines, textbooks, and clinical trials to make rational decisions about drug therapy. Although all contribute to the work that needs to be done, there remains many "holes" in the knowledge needed to provide quality care. With time and experience, it became clear that the Pharmacotherapy Workup is an ideal conceptual framework for organizing knowledge in practice for a number of reasons (see Appendix 3 for the complete Workup). First, it describes what information is needed to make the necessary decisions. Secondly, we can describe the thought processes and actual decisions that need to be made with this information. Thirdly, the Workup organizes information in the order that a practitioner would use it to manage a patient's drug therapy.

It seemed a fairly straightforward exercise to extrapolate this framework to that of a comprehensive care plan for practice. The Pharmacotherapy Workup was used to develop a standard outline of information needed each time a practitioner develops a care plan for a patient receiving pharmaceutical care. This standard outline was developed from the decisions made during the Workup and follows the logical evaluation process to ensure, first, appropriateness of each medication, then, effectiveness, then safety, and finally, the convenience of the regimen for the patient so that adherence is possible. We called this new tool the Pharmaceutical Care Plan Reference.

The standard outline for the Pharmaceutical Care Plan References was developed by Christina Cipolle, Rae'd Abu-Ghazeleh, Robert J. Cipolle, Linda M. Strand, and Michael J. Frakes in 2004 at the Peters Institute of Pharmaceutical Care in the College of Pharmacy at the University of Minnesota. This standard outline was then used to develop specific Pharmaceutical Care Plan References for six common diseases requiring management with drug therapy. This sounded simple at first, but after creating six different care plan references, we tallied up the time and number of references (textbooks, guidelines, articles) needed to construct a useful care plan reference. It requires a minimum of 30 references and approximately 100 hours to identify the information needed and then reorganize it into a more useful format for each care plan! The basic outline for each care plan reference is in Table 10-8. To date, we have constructed care plan references for Type I diabetes, Type II diabetes, hyperlipidemia, osteoporosis, hypertension, and depression. These care plans require constant updates and maintenance to be useful. With this outline, you can construct the care plans that are most useful for you.

Common Drugs Are Common

There are thousands of drug products available to treat and prevent diseases. The Food and Drug Administration approves a new drug product for use in the United States approximately every 15 days. Learning all that is required about them can seem like a formidable task for the student practitioner. There is much to be learned. Learning the characteristics listed in Table 10-7 for classes of drugs can be helpful but sometimes confusing. We have tricyclic antidepressants, which are grouped based on their chemical structure but used in practice for numerous indications other than depression (enuresis). Antihistamines are grouped based on their mechanism of action. There are histamine H_1-receptor antagonists. We also have a category of relatively nonsedating antihistamines grouped because of a lower incidence of a side effect. H_2-blockers act at another histamine site of action but are not generally referred to as antihistamines. Nonsteroidal anti-inflammatory drugs are grouped based on a chemical structure that they do not possess. Grouping of drug products by similarities in chemical structure, mechanism of action, or selected indication does not yield mutually exclusive categories, and therefore can cause some confusion for the early learner. It is important to understand all of a drug's actions on your patients, not just the intended or marketed actions, as advertised.

There is an efficient way to begin or to expand your pharmacotherapy learning process. Create a personal learning agenda that begins with the drug products you will encounter most frequently. The 25 most common prescription products selected for use by practitioners are listed in Tables 10-9 and 10-10. In 2008, there were 2.4 billion generic drug products prescribed in the United States, and there were 1.4 billion brand-name products prescribed that year, so these top 25 medications will need to be managed frequently.

Patients also use numerous nonprescription products to self-medicate and manage their drug-related needs. Patients frequently ask their pharmacist for recommendations for selection, use, effectiveness, and safety of nonprescription drug products. The most common nonprescription product categories are listed in Table 10-11. Also included is the size (in million of dollars)

Table 10-8   Care plan reference outline

INDICATION	*Definition*

	Includes an explanation of:
	    the condition described in this care plan both
	        generally (e.g., hyperlipidemia) and specifically
	        (e.g., hypercholesterolemia)
	    how patients contract the condition (idiopathic,
	        hereditary, etc.)
	    possible complications during the course of the disease
	        (e.g., heart attack, end organ damage, etc.)

	Presenting signs and symptoms Define key terms

	Frequency and incidence
	Include information that is relevant to the condition
	    total number of people with the condition
	    number of diagnosed vs. undiagnosed people with
	        condition
	    number of new people diagnosed each year
	    age groups
	    men vs. women
	    ethnic groups
	Also include evidence related to the morbidity and mortality
	    of the condition

	Risk factors Include genetic and lifestyle risk factors

	Unique diagnostic criteria
	Tests, exams, or lab values that determine a diagnosis
	Short explanation of what the test/exam entails.
	    For example, fasting plasma glucose >126 mg/dL.
	    Fasting is defined as no caloric intake for 8 hours.
	Explain whether the test/exam is an x-ray, scan, blood,
	    or other test

	Assessment checklist
	You are not diagnosing but need to assess what the state of
	    the patient's condition is. Include information needed to
	    establish goals of therapy and to evaluate effectiveness
	    and safety on a consistent basis. (e.g., signs and
	    symptoms, recent lab values, medication experience)
	Why/how the value may be used. For example, "current
	    weight and height for BMI and normal growth
	    development"

(Continued)

Table 10-8 *(Continued)* Care plan reference outline

EFFECTIVENESS	*Short-term goals of therapy (timeframe)* Each goal must include a parameter, value, and timing. These goals of therapy are related to the patient's drug therapy
	Long-term goals of therapy Includes prevention of complications/end organ damage and/or risk reduction.
	Therapeutic alternatives The standard approach to the treatment (or prevention) of the indication Synopsis of the current guidelines for initial drug selection in patients without complications Rationale when adding or changing drug therapies Rationale The reasoning behind the order used to list the pharmacological classes and the drugs within each class is explained

	Pharmacological class
	Pharmacology:
	Efficacy:
	Dosage guidelines:
	Subclass of drugs if applicable (e.g., loop diuretics)
	Pharmacology: if applicable
	Efficacy: if applicable.
	Dosage guidelines:
	Generic drug name (brand name if only available in brand)
	   Initial dosage:
	   Adjustments: include intervals and dosage changes
	   Maximum dosage:

SAFETY	*General safety concerns for the condition that apply to all patients are explained.* *Pharmacological class* Contraindications: The contraindications and warnings. If there is a pregnancy contraindication, give the risk category (e.g., risk category X) *Consider discontinuation of drug:*
	Adverse drug reactions: Percentage is used when possible Dose-related toxicity: If it is dose-related for therapeutic doses (not overdoses), it is described here

(Continued)

Table 10-8 (*Continued*) Care plan reference outline

ADHERENCE	*General patient instructions*
	Effectiveness: The positive outcomes patients should expect to see and when
	Safety: Safety concerns that all patients should be aware of regardless of the drug therapy they are taking. For example, with hypertension, what patients need to know about hypotension (There may be some repeat from the "SAFETY" section.)
	Pharmacological class
	Take with meals.
	Avoid alcohol (increased risk of hypoglycemia).
	Self care
	Includes additional instructions that the patient can follow to optimize the therapeutic response and prevent progression of the disease (exercise, nutrition, quit smoking, check blood glucose regularly).
	What the patient should do, for how long, what the activity entails, and how it will affect their condition (lower blood pressure 2–4 mmHg)
	Therapeutic lifestyle changes are described here
DRUG THERAPY PROBLEMS	*Drug Therapy Problem Category (%)*
	Unnecessary drug therapy
	Additional drug therapy needed
	Ineffective drug
	Dosage too low
	Adverse drug reaction
	Dosage too high
	Nonadherence
FOLLOW-UP EVALUATION	*Effectiveness*
	Follow-up when the patient is not at goal. Include parameter, value, and timing
	Follow-up when the patient has met goal and is stable. Include parameter, value, and timing
	Safety
	Pharmacological class: listed by class in the same order as in "EFFECTIVENESS" and in "SAFETY."
	Evaluate: For each class, the parameters (exams, lab tests) that the practitioner should evaluate and when to evaluate them are described here
REFERENCES	All appropriate and up-to-date references will be listed here

Table 10-9   The 25 most frequently dispensed prescription drugs (generic) in the United States (2009)*

1.	Hydrocodone/Acetaminophen	14.	Metoprolol tartrate
2.	Lisinopril	15.	Sertraline
3.	Simvastatin	16.	Zolpidem tartrate
4.	Levothyroxine	17.	Metoprolol succinate
5.	Amoxicillin	18.	Oxycodone w/Acetaminophen
6.	Azithromycin	19.	Prednisone
7.	Hydrochlorothiazide	20.	Citalopram
8.	Amlodipine besylate	21.	Ibuprofen
9.	Alprazolam	22.	Fluoxetine
10.	Metformin	23.	Gabapentin
11.	Omeprazole	24.	Warfarin
12.	Atenolol	25.	Tramadol
13.	Furosemide		

* Data from Drug Topic Resource Guide, Top 200 Drugs: A 5-year compilation. (Originally published, June 1, 2009 online edition of Drug Topics).

Table 10-10   The 25 most frequently dispensed prescription drugs (Brand) in the United States (2009)*

1.	Lipitor	14.	Prevacid
2.	Nexium	15.	Diovan HCT
3.	Plavix	16.	Actos
4.	Singulair	17.	Flomax
5.	Lexapro	18.	Seroquel
6.	ProAir HFA	19.	Levaquin
7.	Synthroid	20.	Tricor
8.	Crestor	21.	Yaz
9.	Advair Diskus	22.	Vytorin
10.	Diovan	23.	Viagra
11.	Cymbalta	24.	Celebrex
12.	Effexor XR	25.	Lantus
13.	Klor-Con		

* Data from 2009, www.drugs.com/yop200.html

Table 10-11 Most frequently purchased nonprescription drug products

Rank	Treatment category	Sales (in $ millions)*	Most frequently recommended products by pharmacists (2010)[†]
1.	Cough/cold	$4172	Adult cold—Robitussin Antitussive—Delsym Pediatric cough—Delsym Expectorant—Mucinex Antihistamines—Claritin Pediatric antihistamine—Children's Claritin Decongestants oral—Sudafed Decongestant topical—Afrin Pediatric decongestant—Children's Sudafed liquid Multisymptoms—NyQuil Pediatric multisymptoms—Children's Dimetapp Nasal saline—Ocean Nasal irrigation—Simply Saline
2.	Analgesics (internal)	$2486	Adult headache—Tylenol Menstrual pain—Advil Migraine—Motrin IB Osteoarthritis oral—Tylenol Pain with sleeplessness—Tylenol PM Pediatric analgesic—Children's Advil
3.	Heartburn	$1277	Episodic heartburn—Pepcid AC Frequent heartburn—Prilosec OTC Upset stomach/nausea—Emetrol
4.	Laxatives	$822	Fiber—Metamucil Nonfiber—Dulcolax Stool softener—Colace Hemorrhoidal—Preparation H
5.	Sunscreens and blocks	$499	Sunscreen—Neutrogena Minor burns—Solarcaine
6.	Antismoking	$493	NicoDerm CQ
7.	Eye care	$474	Allergy—Zaditor Artificial tears—Refresh Eye wash—Collyrium Vasoconstrictors/decongestant—Visine

(Continued)

Table 10-11 (*Continued*) Most frequently purchased nonprescription drug products

Rank	Treatment category	Sales (in $ millions)*	Most frequently recommended products by pharmacists (2010)[†]
8.	Lip remedies	$408	Canker sore—Orabase, Anbesol Cold sore—Abreva Lip balms—Carmex
9.	Foot care	$334	Athlete's foot—Lamisil AT General foot care—Dr. Scholl's Nail antifungal—Fungal Nail
10.	Acne remedies	$333	Benzoyl peroxide—Clearasil, ProActiv Salicyclic acid—Clean and Clear

* Data source: The Nielsen Company, Consumer Healthcare Products Association, www.chpa-info.org/pressroom/Sales_Category.aspx
† Pharmacy Today, OTC Supplement, February 2011.

of the U.S. market for each of the categories and the products most frequently recommended by pharmacists.

Because half of all consumers purchase herbal supplements to manage their health care needs, it is important to know which are the most common. Table 10-12 displays the top-selling herbal supplements in 2008.

The days of drug information being the "property" of physicians, pharmacists, and nurses are long past. Direct to consumer advertising of both prescription as well as nonprescription products, coupled with the almost uni-

Table 10-12 Top-selling herbal supplements (2008)*

Cranberry	Green tea
Soy	Evening primrose
Garlic	Valerian
Saw palmetto	Horny goat weed
Ginkgo	Grapeseed
Echinacea	Elderberry
Milk thistle	Bilberry
St. John's wort	Ginger
Ginseng	Horse chestnut seed
Black cohosh	Yohimbe

* Data from More than half of all U.S. consumers' use supplements (2008 Nielsen Global Online Survey) Drug Topics, September 2009.

Table 10-13 Most frequently viewed drugs at PrescriptionDrug-Info.com

1.	Oxycodone (OxyContin)	6.	Vicodin (hydrocodone + acetaminophen)
2.	Alprazolam	7.	Dilaudid (hydromorphone)
3.	Clonazepam	8.	Percocet (oxycodone + acetaminophen)
4.	Acetaminophen	9.	Suboxone (buprenorphine)
5.	Tramadol	10.	Hydrocodone

Data from www.prescriptiondrug-info.com/top_prescription_drugs.asp (March 2011 views).

versal availability of the Internet, has made information (good and bad) about medications available to everyone. Your patients have ample opportunity to gather information on their own. Table 10-13 lists the products associated with some of the most common drug-related inquiries made by consumers.

KEY CLINICAL CONCEPTS

The most efficient learning method is to begin caring for patients, under supervision. Care for as many patients as possible. The best practitioners in any field are the busiest practitioners.

Busy practitioners must be effective and efficient at providing care. The best way to become effective and efficient is to learn first how to care for patients with common problems. Building upon this base of core clinical knowledge will allow you to eventually help patients with more complex and/ or less commonly encountered problems. This appears inconsistent with the way referrals are often made in that referrals usually involve more complex patients. This emphasizes the importance of acquiring clinical experience in a generalist practice prior to establishing a practice of your own where referrals will be a key to your success.

ACQUIRING THE CLINICAL SKILLS YOU NEED TO PRACTICE

The practice of pharmaceutical care requires the mastery of a number of clinical skills. The four sets of skills that are used on a continuous basis are:

1. gathering information about your patient's medical conditions and drugs
2. evaluating and applying information to meet your patient's specific needs

3. communicating information to patients and professional colleagues
4. learning from your experience for the purpose of improving through reflective practice.

Because the information practitioners need and use can be complex, and is often technical, special skills are required to master this unique body of knowledge.

The first skill set requires that practitioners learn to retrieve, *gather*, and assemble patient, disease, and drug information from patients. You will need observational, interview, and physical assessment skills to accomplish this. The patient's medication experience is central for this skill set. Frequently, the patient will present with a medical condition that is unfamiliar, a drug therapy that is new, or a unique set of circumstances that requires you to gather information from books, the literature, colleagues, or the Internet. Retrieving information in an effective manner will improve your ability to care for patients.

The second set of clinical skills comprises those required to *apply* the knowledge you have accumulated to the patient for whom you are caring. This will allow you to generate hypotheses, solve problems, and make rational and logical decisions about the patient's pharmacotherapy. These skills rely on the practitioner's inquiry, discovery, and creativity abilities. The Pharmacotherapy Workup is central for this skill set. It is often the case that information from guidelines or protocols must be interpreted and/or modified in order to apply the decision rules to your patient's situation.

The third skill set includes the ability to *communicate* what the practitioner knows and the decisions she has made. A practitioner's communication skills often determine the level of success in practice. Both written and verbal communication skills are important and communication with patients as well as with other practitioners is required to be successful. The Pharmacotherapy Case Presentation Format is central for this skill set. Written communication, in the form of documentation in the electronic therapeutic record and medical record, is also a skill that must be mastered.

The fourth category is the skills required to *be reflective* in practice, so that you can learn from each patient care experience. Reflective skills allow you to convert clinical experience into clinical knowledge. Summaries or reports of your practice that can be generated from your documentation system are central for this skill set. This skill set allows the practitioner to reflect on a patient encounter to determine what went well and why, what did not go as expected and why, and what must be changed in the future. These skills help you to learn on a daily basis from both your patients and your colleagues. Reflective skills are powerful as they allow practitioners to learn from both successful and unsuccessful experiences.

Although these skills are discussed frequently in the nursing and medical literature, pharmacy programs have not uniformly developed these skills in their student practitioners. The basic skill of being reflective in practice will have a significant impact on how quickly you become a competent pharmaceutical care practitioner.

KEY CLINICAL CONCEPTS

Clinical skills are like any other skill set. To master them requires training, practice, and reflection.

The student practitioner can work to develop these skill sets in stages. Although all are required to provide pharmaceutical care for a patient, it is useful to focus on one set at a time while you are developing your clinical skills.

For the new practitioner, there is no substitute for practice. The more patients you see and provide direct care for, the more proficient you will become. New practitioners should avail themselves of every possible opportunity to provide pharmaceutical care to patients. Internalizing the clinical skills and decision-making processes necessary to perform at a level dictated by the standards of practice requires considerable time and a variety of patient cases for a new practitioner to become effective and eventually efficient.

Obtaining Clinical Information From Your Patient

KEY CLINICAL CONCEPTS

Eliciting relevant information from your patient is not only the first skill you should have, but it is one of the most important when providing care.

The quality of the information you elicit will determine the quality of the care you can provide. This skill set integrates observational, interview, and physical assessment skills.

Observational Skills
The first skill to learn is gathering information from observation. Although the amount of physical effort involved in this skill is minimal, the amount

Table 10-14 Information obtained from observational skills

Patient variable	Examples of values to document
Age	Approximate age in years or decades for older patients Example: A gentleman who appears to be in his 80's
Height, weight	Approximate height and weight Example: Normal weight, slightly obese, very obese
Gender	Male, female
Overall health status	Assessment of physical/mental health Example: Excellent, good, poor
Physical grooming and personal hygiene	Example: Neat, clean, unkempt, disheveled
Posture and general ability to ambulate	Level of physical activity No difficulty ambulating Difficulty ambulating Example: good posture, poor posture
Ability to communicate	Language ability, use of hearing aid
Outward signs of illness	Normal or pallid skin tone Energetic, lethargic Example: Well nourished, malnourished
Apprehension, fear, agitation	Example: Anxious, distressed, preoccupied
Willingness and ability to participate	Cooperative, uncooperative Example: Good historian, quiet

of insight and sensitivity required to optimize the information you elicit through observation can be substantial. Observational skills require you to collect information with your eyes and your powers of deduction. Table 10-14 describes the information you can often elicit with these skills, and the table includes suggestions as to how you might document this information in the pharmaceutical care record.

Improving your observational skills first requires you to become conscious of the variables that will have an impact on your care plan. If you teach yourself to be aware of these items, you can save yourself and your patient a significant amount of time and effort. Becoming sensitive to nonverbal clues will help you throughout the Pharmacotherapy Workup.

Respect the power of keen observational skills. You can collect this information in the first moments of your assessment. Simply make mental notes of the data you collect before you begin your assessment interview so that it does not get lost or overlooked. You will want to record this information in writing as soon as it is appropriate. After you have taught yourself to be effective at observation, then you are ready to develop your listening skills.

Assessment Interview Skills

You will gain most of your information from your patient during the assessment. The assessment consists of primarily patient-specific information collected using the process described in Chapter 6. The assessment interview is a purposeful conversation, which differs from casual or friend-to-friend conversations.

KEY CLINICAL CONCEPTS

An effective assessment interview requires that the practitioner becomes skilled at using open-ended inquiries to elicit patient responses and then explores the topic more extensively through pointed questioning.

Learning these assessment interview skills requires practicing to be an active listener. Active listening means taking the time and energy to hear and understand what your patient has just told you. As a student practitioner, you will want to practice listening to patients' stories about their medication experiences and the impact that drug therapies have had on their lives.

Student practitioners tend to ask the patient a question and then immediately start to think of what the next question should be. Experienced practitioners approach the assessment interview much differently. Skilled practitioners listen very carefully to the patient's response, and after fully hearing and understanding what was said, formulate the next logical question. The next question in an effective assessment interview should be related to the patient's response to the previous question.

Therefore, you will not know what the next best question should be until you have understood what your patient is telling you. Listen, then listen more, and then listen even more. If all you hear is your voice, change your approach.

Take your time to formulate questions. If it requires a few moments, that is not a problem. The time you take to formulate your next question may seem like an uncomfortable lull to you, but the pause usually does not bother patients. Students often feel nervous and hurried when conducting their first few assessment interviews. Remain calm, and proceed in a relaxed manner. Let your patient know about how long you anticipate the assessment will take, and let her do most of the talking. Establish and maintain good eye contact and be conscious of your posture and body position. Sit up straight in the chair or stand without leaning, and avoid nervous repetitive movements.

Listen with an open mind   When you first begin to develop your assessment skills, you may not feel you are adequately prepared to deal with some of the issues that patients present to you. Some practitioners may feel that the sexual, psychiatric, or interpersonal problems the patient discusses may be beyond their scope to manage in an assessment interview. However, this information may have a direct impact on the course of action your patient is willing to pursue, and it may impact the outcome of therapy, so it is important that you obtain the relevant information.

> **Example**   The topic of sexual activity is often thought of as a *private matter*, and is too often avoided. Interviewing a patient about sexuality and sexual problems can be a complex and difficult dimension of the Pharmacotherapy Workup. In a world in which human immunodeficiency virus, acquired immunodeficiency syndrome, and numerous other sexually transmitted diseases cause significant morbidity and mortality, practitioners must understand these conditions and develop the ability to obtain appropriate information during an assessment. Drug therapy is an essential form of treatment and prevention of many sexually transmitted illnesses. Practitioners need to inform the patient of the need to ask some questions about her sexual life. Questions of how her illness has affected her sexual life can be helpful in evaluating the effectiveness of drug therapy. Similarly, inquiring as to how the patient feels that her drug therapy has impacted sexual activity can identify adverse drug reactions that require adjustment in pharmacotherapy.[32]

Listen with empathy   Demonstrating empathy for your patient's emotional situation can be comforting for her. Being empathetic—having the ability to imagine yourself in your patient's position—will positively impact the relationship you establish with the patient. The challenge of learning empathic skills lies in learning the primary approaches of reflecting and legitimating and then integrating an interpersonal style that feels genuine to you and is likely to be perceived as genuine by the patient. *Reflecting* refers to the practitioner describing the emotional experience of the patient.

Example   "I can see that you are upset by this."

Legitimating confirms that the emotion is understood and accepted.

Example   "I can understand why that would make you upset."

Your patients will want to know that you intend to be supportive of their needs. Skillfully explaining that they can depend on your assistance is reassuring. This can be accomplished by explaining: "I would like to work together with you to develop the best possible treatment plan once we have agreed on what goals we will try to achieve."[32]

It is not necessary to wait until the end of an assessment interview to summarize. By summarizing what you have heard and your interpretation of that information, you can get immediate feedback as to whether you and your patient have the same understanding. Summarizing is also an effective method of regaining control of the conversation and redirecting it as you feel is necessary.

Did you miss anything important? This question perplexes new practitioners during their first few assessment interviews. The best method to be confident that you did not omit an important area is to give your patient ample opportunity to respond to: "Is there anything else you feel I should know?" After you share your summary of the assessment with the patient, make certain that the patient has ample opportunity to add information that may not have been mentioned. This technique helps the patient feel that you have done your best to understand his or her needs or problems.

Becoming efficient at collecting patient information   You must first become *effective* at conducting a comprehensive assessment of a patient's drug-related needs before you attempt to become *efficient*. Efficiency is effectiveness over time, and therefore an ineffective approach to patient assessment will never result in an efficient process. As a student practitioner, take your time, and learn how to get it right. Most patients appreciate someone spending sufficient time to fully hear their story.

Collect only the information you will use   During the assessment process, you should only gather information that you will use to make your clinical judgments and decisions. It is often difficult for student practitioners to know what information will be necessary and/or useful. As you become more experienced in patient assessment, you will find that you can select the most useful and important questions within each assessment. You will feel more confident that you have a clinically sound idea of your patient's drug-related needs and can identify her drug therapy problems. Experts use surprisingly few pieces of key data to make their initial clinical judgments, and then proceed to gather more facts in order to verify or refute their initial decisions.[32,33]

There are no shortcuts to collecting patient, disease, and drug information, and knowing specifically what information is needed and when. You will not find effective recipes for care. Patient care does not provide a list of necessary ingredients (information) and a formula (knowledge) of how to combine them. The best way to learn what information you need to gather in order to make clinical decisions is to gather it, then decide if it was actually helpful to you when you made the decision. If it was, you have learned how that particular information can be applied to make patient-specific clinical decisions about drug therapies. If you find that the information you gathered did not help, then you will have learned from that as well.

Physical Assessment Skills

Pharmaceutical care practitioners primarily use physical assessment skills to evaluate the effectiveness and safety of their patient's medications. The physical assessment skills used within the diagnostic process far exceed those required for the pharmaceutical care process. However, physical assessment skills are essential to determine if your patient is experiencing positive or negative effects from her drug therapies.

The follow-up evaluation in the pharmaceutical care process calls for the collection of clinical and/or laboratory parameters necessary to determine if the patient's drug therapies are being effective and/or causing any harm. Drug effectiveness is often determined based on the improvement of clinical signs and symptoms. The practitioner uses physical assessment skills to detect side effects caused by medications.

There are a number of basic physical assessment skills that student practitioners need to acquire and understand in order to provide pharmaceutical care. The specific techniques are beyond the scope of this text but are described in detail in textbooks used by medical, nursing, pharmacy, and other students of the health sciences.[13,17] As an example, the core set of physical assessment skills would include measuring the patient's vital signs.

Vital signs   Measurement of vital signs includes the patient's blood pressure, heart rate, respiratory rate, and temperature. These basic clinical parameters are essential to determine the effectiveness and safety of a great majority of medications commonly used today. A sphygmomanometer is commonly used to measure your patient's blood pressure, a thermometer is required to determine temperature, and a functional timepiece is helpful to accurately measure a pulse rate, but no other equipment or expense is involved in obtaining a patient's vital signs.

Hypertension is among the most common indications for the use of prescription medications. The effectiveness of antihypertensive drug therapy and much of the evaluation of its safety are based on the measurement of blood pressure. This is a skill that every pharmaceutical care practitioner will use throughout her career.

Temperature is the hallmark sign of most infectious processes. Antibiotic drug therapies are evaluated based on the improvement of signs, symptoms, and laboratory parameters. The patient's temperature often serves as the primary clinical indicator of effectiveness. Numerous techniques and innovative technologies are available to obtain the patient's temperature, and familiarity with their application is a useful clinical skill.

The patient's pulse or heart rate can be greatly influenced by drug therapies.

Most cardiovascular agents increase or decrease the pulse when used at pharmacologically active dosages. Drugs that slow the heart rate can put patients at risk of becoming dizzy or losing consciousness due to lack of blood supply to vital organs including brain.

> **Example**   The pulse rate is one of the common parameters used to evaluate the safety of digoxin dosing in patients with heart failure or cardiac dysrhythmias, and beta-blockers such as atenolol and metoprolol used to manage patients with angina pectoris or hypertension.

Improving the patient's breathing symptoms is frequently a goal of drug therapy. The respiratory status of the patient includes the rate, rhythm, depth, and effort of breathing, all of which can be observed and easily counted. Respiratory rates are often essential in determining the effectiveness of drug therapy to manage asthma, pneumonia, bronchitis, congestive heart failure, chronic obstructive pulmonary disease, and cystic fibrosis.

Retrieving Information

No matter how experienced you become as a practitioner, you will always have to retrieve information from books and the literature. Pharmacotherapy changes continually and it is virtually impossible to remember everything you need to know to practice pharmaceutical care. Your ability to retrieve necessary information at the right time is an important skill.

As student practitioners begin to develop their clinical skills, subscribing to one important guideline can be helpful: *Look it up now.* If you come across information you need to retrieve from a book, a study or a guideline, find the answer immediately. Retention of newly acquired knowledge is easier and more efficient when that new knowledge is placed in a clinically appropriate context, that is, the care of a patient. If you stop and put forth the effort to retrieve these data when you need to apply them to identify or resolve a patient's drug therapy problem, you will retain that new knowledge.

Student practitioners and experienced practitioners tend to use different sources as references because they generally have different needs. Students, especially early in their studies, are best served by texts containing full descriptions of pharmacological actions, disease processes, and pharmacotherapeutic approaches. References with this level of detail and comprehensive explanations are useful to provide new practitioners with the necessary overall understanding of the topic. And, although there are a number of references available and each has its strength, there are a few that no practitioner should be without. This list includes the following:

- *The Pharmacological Basis of Therapeutics,* Goodman and Gilman[21]
- *Pharmacotherapy: A Pathophysiological Approach*[14]
- *Handbook of Nonprescription Drugs*[17]
- *Applied Therapeutics: The Clinical Use of Drugs*[26]
- *Principles of Internal Medicine*[13]
- *American Hospital Formulary Service Drug Information*[34]
- *Natural Medicines Comprehensive Database*[35]

Busy practitioners already have a general and often thorough understanding of the topic, but they need a small piece of data to support a specific decision that has to be made. Therefore, while students need comprehensive pharmacology, pathophysiology, and pharmacotherapy textbooks at their disposal, experienced practitioners tend to make better use of reference handbooks from which they can quickly retrieve a single piece of data needed to complete the clinical decision-making process. Following is a list useful reference handbooks best utilized by experienced practitioners:

- *Facts and Comparisons*[20]
- *Clinical Drug Data*[36]
- *Drug Information Handbook*[19]
- *Therapeutic Choices*[16]
- *Griffith's 5-minute Clinical Consult*[25]
- *Geriatric Dosage Handbook*[37]
- *Pediatric Dosage Handbook*[38]
- *Tyler's Honest Herbal: A Sensible Guide to the Use of Herbs and Related Remedies*[39]
- *The Top 100 Drug Interactions: A Guide to Patient Management.*[40]

There are many texts in these areas, and the selection of an appropriate one can be confusing. New practitioners must be certain that the books they use to establish their reference library will be the most useful. It is useful for students to choose an example topic and examine that section in a book before it is purchased. Did it answer your questions? Can the topic be understood? How the text is indexed is especially important because you will often need to refer to the index to identify and learn new material quickly and effectively.

Some references deal only with products licensed for use in one country; some contain information on products only available without a prescription. Other references focus on herbal and natural products. Students may need several references just to learn about all of the medications that patients take.

In order to look up information for a patient taking an herbal product, two prescription medications, and a commonly used nonprescription drug product, a student may use three separate texts. Efficiently using these references requires an understanding of how each reference organizes and presents information.

Some references list drug information alphabetically by generic names, some organize the drug information by therapeutic class, and some organize information by the primary pharmacological actions of the drug. The use and retrieval of primary literature sources is a skill that every practitioner must possess in order to continue learning. Because it often requires 1 to 3 years to bring a new reference book to publication, professional journals are considered the best source for contemporary information, controversial topics, alternative approaches, and comparison studies.

Many drug information sources are now available on computers, smart phones, and personal digital assistants. These sources, including Lexicomp, Micromedex, Medscape, iPharmacy, and WebMD, have the advantages of being mobile and accessible wherever Internet access is sufficient. They are also updated frequently with new product information and warnings. These sources of drug information tend to be general and population-based, and therefore the practitioner must be able to interpret this information in the context of a specific patient and decide if it is appropriate.

Contemporary topics such as multiple sclerosis or pain management are best researched using the primary literature. Also, individual case reports and unusual or rare events are most frequently published in primary sources and can be helpful to verify whether your patient's outcome has been reported in other patient cases. Searching for information from the primary literature has become extremely efficient through the Internet. Many professional journals make the full text of articles available on their websites. Obtaining information from the Internet can be the most efficient method to obtain access to the current literature and information. Remember, how-ever, that it is important to verify that you are using only reputable sources. Learn how to critically evaluate information from websites you might use as well as those your patients might use. Some of the value we contribute lies in helping patients to sort the accurate from the inaccurate information about medications.

In general, the information explosion that has occurred in pharmaco-therapy knowledge over the past few decades is well served by the capacity and timeliness of the Internet. For example, many of the major pharma-ceutical firms provide open access to the current understanding of the pharmacology, efficacy, and safety of their products. Additionally, infor-mation about new products that are still in the developmental process can be researched via the Internet. There are many sites on the World Wide Web that provide useful information about diseases or drug therapies. A common advantage of these sites is that the explanations and descriptions are written with terms that can be understood by patients. For example, visit www.medicinenet.com, www.webmd.com, www.mayoclinic.com, www.diabetes.org, and www.americanheart.org.

COMMUNICATION SKILLS

This text is not intended to teach you to master the basic skills involved in human communication. There are a number of other useful texts for that purpose.[32,33,41,42] We begin with the assumption that those who have been successful at securing a position in a professional education program have a basic command of the skills required to communicate verbally and in writ-ing. Therefore, this is not intended to be a basic or theoretical discussion of communication skills. Instead, we want to present the unique aspects of communicating with patients and other health care professionals about drug therapy issues in pharmaceutical care practice.

Patient-focused Communication

KEY CLINICAL CONCEPTS

Communication with patients brings together many of the dimen-sions of pharmaceutical care practice. At the center of communica-tion is the relationship between the patient and the practitioner.

The nature and ethical framework of the relationship that is required to practice pharmaceutical care dictates the specific guidelines for the communication that occurs between patient and practitioner (see Chapter 3 for a discussion of the ethical dimensions of pharmaceutical care and Chapter 4 for a discussion of the therapeutic relationship).

The key to building a therapeutic relationship as well as successfully communicating with patients is to create an environment for the patient that has the right conditions for fostering good communication. Empathy, positive regard, and congruence define these conditions. Empathy is the process of communicating to patients the feeling of being understood; it is putting yourself in the patient's situation. Positive regard is the process of communicating support to the patient in a caring and nonjudgmental way; it is communication that is genuine, unthreatening, and unconditional.

Communicating congruence involves the honest expression of the practitioner's own thoughts and feelings; it requires that the caring professional will respond honestly to the patient and attempts to be genuine in the relationship with the patient. As a pharmaceutical care practitioner, you have three primary objectives or reasons to communicate with the patient: (1) to elicit necessary information from the patient to make your decisions, (2) to negotiate the terms of the goals of therapy and the patient's role in achieving them, and (3) to educate the patient about the drug therapy she is receiving and/or taking.

A significant amount of space in this text has been devoted to explaining the assessment interview skills required to practice pharmaceutical care (see Chapter 6 for a detailed discussion of the assessment process). We will not repeat this information but focus on the skills required to educate patients about their drug therapy. Educating the patient about drug therapy is most beneficial if you first understand the patient. You will be most effective if you establish with the patient:

1. what your patient *wants* to know
2. what the patient *already knows*

The best way to recognize this difference is to: (a) determine the preferred language of the patient, (b) determine the level of comprehension best suited to the patient—this will determine the vocabulary/terms that are familiar to the patient and (c) identify any cultural or religious issues that are relevant to communicating with the patient.

The following material should be conveyed to all patients, unless you have identified a patient-specific reason for not sharing this information. This is considered to be the basic information about the patient's medication that will help her to actively engage in the care plan and be compliant with her medications. You will want to explain the following to the patient:

1. The reason for taking each medication (Indication).
   - Explain how the medication works, what it will do for your patient
   - Use pictures and diagrams whenever possible
   - Provide patients with information and labeling to take home with them that ties the reason for taking the medication to the drug product, to the directions for administration to the goals of therapy, and to a time-frame for meeting the goals.
2. The specific instructions of how to take the medication explained in a manner the patient can understand.
   - Use the same terms from one encounter to the next
   - Use phrases that are familiar to the patient so they are not misunderstood (twice a day, dissolved in water, with food)
   - Start from your patient's point of reference (when do they eat, what time do they go to bed).
3. A description of how the patient will know that the medication is working well (Effectiveness).
   - Describe how the patient's symptoms will change and when to expect these improvements
   - Create an understandable system for complicated terms (clinical parameters or laboratory values)
   - Include specific values that will serve as endpoints
   - Communicate how confident you are that the patient's pharmacotherapy will be effective.
4. Explain the undesirable effects that might be expected (Safety).
   - Be specific about when adverse reactions are most likely to occur.
   - Provide the patient with clear instructions of what to do if any problems arise with the medication.
5. Be clear about what the patient should do if a dose of the medication is missed or if she takes an extra dose of the medication (Adherence).
6. Inform the patient of when and how you intend to follow-up to evaluate effectiveness and safety of the medication.
7. Provide the patient with a way to contact you if the medication is not working within the timeframe you discussed.

Care must be taken when communicating this much information. Be sure to speak slowly, as much information about medications may be new to the patient. It may also be the case that the practitioner's first language is not the patient's first language. Be sure to evaluate the extent of understanding by your patient when you are finished communicating this information. Provide her with written information whenever possible to reinforce the major points made during the discussion.

Written correspondence with patients It can be reinforcing to correspond with the patient in writing. Written correspondence might be used to provide your patient with literature about the medication being taken or a reminder about an appointment. This activity can be important in achieving the desired goals of therapy for a patient. It is worth remembering that written correspondence of all types (letters, email, drug information brochures) is a reflection on you as a professional and a practitioner. You will always want to proofread this correspondence well.

When communicating with a patient in writing, be sure to print the material in a size that the patient can easily read. Everything we discussed for optimizing verbal communication with your patient applies to written communication. Before communicating with your patient in writing, be sure you have determined how much information your patient wants and what the patient already knows. Your purpose for communicating is always the same, to fill the gap between what the patient wants to know and already knows in a way that a particular patient can best understand (see Chapter 9 on documentation). It is not helpful to give the patient more information than is needed or wanted.

Practitioner-focused Communication

KEY CLINICAL CONCEPTS

Practitioners use a specific practice vocabulary, and it should be employed when communicating with other health care practitioners, whether verbally or in writing.

We have emphasized the use of the glossary in this book for this very reason (see Appendix 2). You should not create new definitions for practice terms or use practice terms differently than intended. All practitioners have an obligation to learn and to use standardized terms so that communication is facilitated at all times.

Your purpose for communicating with colleagues usually involves patient care. You may be asking for help with the care of a patient or providing help to a colleague who is caring for a patient. You may be sharing the care of a patient with a coworker or sharing your knowledge more generally with colleagues and students in the practice setting. All of these clinical situations require effective communication.

It is important that you be precise when discussing a patient's care because confusion can precipitate costly errors on your part. Be concise when you talk with colleagues because neither you nor your colleague has time to waste. You must be complete because anything not mentioned is assumed to be normal, and this could lead to significant misunderstanding. Going back to "fill in" information for a colleague can be very time consuming.

The Pharmacotherapy Patient Case Presentation Format, which is presented later in this Chapter, presents the standard format for how pharmaceutical care practitioners present patient cases for the purpose of seeking help or provide help to colleagues. It is the format that should be used for discussing a patient case with a colleague, whether verbally or in writing.

Written correspondence with other practitioners   Corresponding with health care practitioners in writing (letters, medical records, email communications) requires the same attention described for verbal communication with practitioners.

You will be communicating with practitioners in writing most frequently about the care of a specific patient. Identify for your colleague the patient to whom you are referring early in your correspondence. You often will be providing recommendations for specific changes in a patient's drug therapy or initiation of drug therapy. There are a few rules that might be helpful. Always state the drug therapy problem clearly and always try to provide your colleague with two different options from which to choose. However, make sure both options are acceptable to you before presenting them as alternatives. Make clear which of the options you recommend and why you believe this to be the better of the two. When you explain your rationale always compare and contrast effectiveness and safety evidence. You may want to explain to the practitioner under which conditions the second option would be better.

Make your written correspondence to other practitioners precise, concise, and complete so they do not have questions at the conclusion (see Chapter 9 on documentation). If the practitioner has to contact you with questions or is confused by your correspondence, you have created more work, not less.

Your purpose should always be to facilitate the care of a patient, not interfere with it. Only provide information that is necessary for the practitioner to make a decision or to be informed. Reading written correspondence takes time, as does responding to written correspondence. Therefore, whenever possible, provide the practitioner with a quick and easy way to respond. Perhaps checking off or initialing an approval box and returning it is a good alternative.

Learning to be Reflective in Practice

Self-improvement must be a goal of all patient care practitioners. Drug knowledge is constantly expanding, and health care is too complex to know everything all the time, obligating practitioners to establish an active learning routine. There are two important skills you will have to develop to become actively engaged in the self-improvement process: (1) learn how to be reflective in practice to learn the most you can from every patient experience and (2) become proficient at presenting patient cases so you can learn from your colleagues. We will now focus on how to become reflective and the remainder of this chapter will discuss how to present patient cases.

> **KEY CLINICAL CONCEPTS**
>
> Each interaction with a patient is an opportunity to gain new knowledge.

To turn every patient experience into the most valuable learning situation that is possible, new practitioners need to develop a few reflective skills. Always take a moment and recollect your thoughts and feelings about the encounter you just had with the patient. These reflective skills take only a few moments but can dramatically enhance learning, knowledge, and confidence.[43]

As the term implies, reflecting upon what just occurred between you and your patient simply requires a few moments immediately after each patient encounter to critically examine a few key ideas:

- How do you feel about the last patient encounter?
- What went well during the patient visit and why?
- What did not go as well as you would have liked and why not?
- What would you do differently?
- What did you learn from this experience?

Critical reflection is the hallmark of adult learning. Kitchener and King claim it is the seventh stage of learning that only develops in a person's late 20s and early 30s.[44] This would help to explain why students in the professional program often do not demonstrate this skill without prompting and are slow to internalize the process to make it part of their routine learning agenda.

These skills can be developed when they are taught, expected, modeled, and reinforced. However, because faculty and mentors must be reflective to teach these skills, there is not as much teaching of reflective skills as is necessary. Therefore, student practitioners need to make these skills a learning agenda item in their own active learning process. Many different strategies have been suggested to develop the skills required in reflection.

One of the most useful is the strategy described by the acronym **LEARN**. These steps can be implemented by you in any practice setting for all types of patients. This strategy combined with the work of Atkins and Murphy helps to create a comprehensive understanding of the skills required to promote reflection in practice. The results are described in Table 10-15 next to each of the skills required to promote reflection.[45]

This skill is so important that you will want to look for opportunities to develop it whenever possible. Selected strategies for stimulating reflection include writing and reading journals, constructing professional portfolios, conducting small group discussions, and performing self-assessments. The reflective process needs to be applied to each patient you care for, from your very first to the very last. Self-improvement needs to be the goal of all patient care practitioners.[46] One of the best ways to be reflective is to review the patient cases you have seen each day. In order to do this efficiently, you will need a structure for thinking about patients, talking about patient cases, and writing up patient cases. Fortunately in pharmaceutical care practice, there is one structure that meets all these needs.

PRESENTING PATIENT CASES: THE PHARMACOTHERAPY PATIENT CASE PRESENTATION FORMAT

A practitioner is judged by peers according to how well she cares for patients. Interestingly, practitioners usually do not directly observe their colleagues as they provide care, yet all practitioners develop opinions regarding who is skilled and who is not. Have you ever considered how practitioners develop these opinions? Opinions are formed when practitioners present patient cases to other practitioners.

Patient cases are presented to colleagues on a daily basis for three primary reasons. First, one practitioner needs another to assume responsibility for a patient when leaving a shift, taking a vacation, or sharing responsibilities. Second, a practitioner needs advice from a colleague concerning the care of a patient. Third, and most frequently in the case of student practitioners, the purpose is to present patient cases to a mentor/practitioner when learning to care for patients. You will be expected to present patient cases throughout the remainder of your career, so it is important to learn the skills to do this properly as early in your career as possible.

Table 10-15 Skills to promote reflective learning

Skill	Definition	Strategy to promote reflection
Self-awareness	An honest examination of feelings How did this experience affect me? How is this experience important to me?	**L**ook back at an experience or event that happened in your practice recently. Review it in your mind as if you were watching a video.
Description	Accurate recall of experiences in detail. What happened including thoughts and feelings?	**E**laborate and describe, verbally or in writing, what happened during the event. How did you feel, and how do you think others felt? What were the outcomes? Were you surprised by what happened during the event, or did it turn out as you expected?
Critical analysis	Examining all expects of the experience including: Challenging assumptions- identifying current knowledge, seeking alternatives. What sense can I make of this experience? What are the significant aspects of this experience?	**A**nalyze the outcomes. Review why the event turned out the way it did. Why did you feel or react the way you did, and why did others feel/react the way they did? If the event or outcomes were not what you expected, consider how you could improve on them next time. This is an opportunity to question your beliefs and assumptions, and ask yourself what the experience reveals about what you value. It is also a great time to ask for feedback from others.
Synthesis	Integration of new and current knowledge to creatively solve problems and predict consequences. How will I apply this to another experience? What will I change or complement in my practice?	**R**evise your approach based on your review of the event and decide how, or if, you will change your approach. This might involve asking others for ideas for dealing with the situation next time or how to work on a learning-need. With your new learning, you may decide to try a new approach, learning more about the subject, or decide that you handled the situation very well.

(Continued)

Table 10-15 (*Continued*) Skills to promote reflective learning

Skill	Definition	Strategy to promote reflection
Evaluation	Making value judgments using criteria and standards. How has this experience changed my values, my beliefs? How do I think about others?	New trial. Put your new approach into action. This may require anticipating or creating a situation in which you can then try out your new approach.

Need for a Specific Format

All practitioners present patient cases to their colleagues including physicians, nurses, dentists, and veterinarians. The specific format for the case presentation is dictated by each practitioner's primary function. The physician presents patient information for the purpose of arriving at a diagnosis of the medical problem and planning treatment approaches. The nurse focuses on presenting nursing care problems and the dentist on dental problems. Therefore, the context of the case presentation for each practitioner is slightly different from the others, but the format is generally the same. This is also true for the pharmaceutical care practitioner.

KEY CLINICAL CONCEPTS

The case presentation format in pharmaceutical care practice is structured to present patient information for the purpose of identifying, resolving, and preventing drug therapy problems.

Sharing information about a patient requires skill and proficiency, but it starts with knowing your role and responsibilities. The case presentation is a specific speaking format that allows efficient transfer of information that can be technical and complex.[47,48] The Pharmacotherapy Case Presentation Format is such a structure. In pharmaceutical care practice, a case presentation should consist of selected and processed data from the Pharmacotherapy Workup and must be delivered in a lucid, precise manner. The oral presentation of a patient's case is usually an abbreviated effort. It includes all of the important positive findings and a few pertinent negative findings; however, information that you may have gathered but did not use to make decisions or provide care for the patient are not included in your presentation.

> **KEY CLINICAL CONCEPTS**
>
> All pharmacotherapy case presentations begin with a brief description of the patient. They contain the same core information, including the indication for drug therapy (medical conditions), drug therapy problems, associated drug therapies goals of therapy, the plan for care, and resulting outcomes.

All case presentations end by summarizing the information you feel is most relevant to your understanding of how to optimize the patient's medication experience.

You will always use the same order for the presentation because both the presenter and the practitioners listening to the case follow the same structure. The listeners are prepared to listen a certain way. They expect you to describe the patient's case using a specific format. The best way to organize your case presentation is the same way you conduct the work, according to the Pharmacotherapy Workup. Table 10-16 describes the major components of the pharmacotherapy patient care presentation in detail.

Colleagues will expect you to have done your work in order to present your patient's case. It will be unfair to present a patient for whom a comprehensive Pharmacotherapy Workup has not been completed. Therefore, if there are any aspects of the Workup you have not completed, this must be made known during the case presentation.

During a case presentation, your decisions are described and your rationale is explained. Drug therapy problems are a good example. During the presentation of your patient's case, you will need to describe which drug therapy problem your patient has and how you decided to resolve it. Case presentations are not like novels or mystery stories for your listeners to try to solve. You have already completed the assessment, identified drug therapy problems, constructed care plans, and may have evaluated your patient's outcomes. The case presentation tells the story of what you found, what you did, and what happened.

Some case presentations are designed for the purpose of obtaining assistance from a colleague. You might need help in determining what your patient's drug therapy problem is or what might be the best approach to achieving the goals of therapy. In either situation, your presentation should inform your colleague what help you need.

Table 10-16 Pharmacotherapy patient case presentation format

ASSESSMENT	Brief description of the patient (age, gender, appearance)
	Primary reason for the patient encounter or visit
	Additional patient background/demographics
	The medication experience as reported by the patient (wants, expectations, concerns, understanding, preferences, attitudes, and beliefs that determine the patient's medication-taking behavior)
	Comprehensive medication history (allergies, alerts, social drug use, and immunization status)
	Current medication record: description of all medical conditions being managed with pharmacotherapy with the following associations made:
	Indication–drug product–dosage regimen–result to date
	Relevant past medical history: outcomes of past medication use
	Review of systems
	Identification of drug therapy problems: description of the drug therapy problem, medications involved, and causal relationships
	Prioritization of multiple drug therapy problems
	Summary of the assessment
CARE PLAN (for each indication)	Goals of therapy
	Clinical and laboratory parameters used to define the goals of therapy
	Observable, measurable value and timeline for each
	How you plan to resolve the patient's drug therapy problems
	Therapeutic alternative approaches considered
	Rationale for your product and dosage selections
	How you plan to achieve the goals of therapy
	Nonpharmacologic interventions
	Prevention of drug therapy problems
	Schedule for follow-up evaluation
FOLLOW-UP EVALUATION	Clinical and/or laboratory evidence of effectiveness of drug therapies for each indication
	Clinical and/or laboratory evidence of safety of every drug regimen
	Evidence of compliance
	Evaluation of outcome status
	Changes required in drug therapies
	Schedule for future evaluations
	Summary of case

Example   "I have not been able to determine why my patient is not responding to her drug therapy. I would appreciate your opinion about what the drug therapy problem might be in this case."

Listening to the presentation of a patient case, one can tell if the presenter knows her patient's drug therapy problems and can properly process and organize data. Even the most complicated case should be presented in a minimum amount of time. The story becomes lengthy when the student is not confident or skilled in identifying the clinically relevant information. The more thought and organization that goes into it, the shorter the presentation becomes. When the story rambles on and on, it often means that the presenter cannot organize the clues, data or thoughts, make decisions, or solve the patient's problems.

Your First Case Presentation

Case presentations employ a unique format, contain new vocabulary, and often involve patients, diseases, and drug therapies that are new to student practitioners. Therefore, the first time a new practitioner is asked to present a patient case to a group of colleagues or faculty can be quite intimidating. To become proficient at case presentation skills, start with the fundamentals. Do not feel as though you need to master all of these new skills and all of the new information during your first attempt.

Your first few attempts need not display your pharmacotherapeutic prowess, but rather these initial presentations are best used to practice organization, communication, and decision-making skills. To get started, focus on a few key steps of the process. These include a brief description of your patient, the primary reason for the encounter, and your patient's active medical conditions with associated drug therapies. Be clear about the drug therapy problem(s) you decide your patient has. For each care plan, describe the goals of therapy, the changes you recommend in your patient's drug therapy, and your plan and schedule for the next follow-up evaluation.

Note that all of these fundamental items inform your audience of who your patient is, what illnesses are presently being managed with medications, what you are attempting to achieve, and when you will know if your plan is working. Note also that the drug therapies and interventions you recommend are only one portion of your case presentation. Although these *answers* may seem important, learning the case presentation structure is the focus of your first presentations.

It is useful to present your first few cases as though you are asking a colleague for advice in determining the nature of your patient's drug therapy problem.

Example "I would like your help in identifying my patient's drug therapy problem. G.W. is a 57-year-old…" This presentation can continue through the first three fundamental steps and end with "what do you think my patient's drug therapy problem might be?"

The primary purpose is to practice clearly describing the patient, by organizing the patient's information about medical conditions and/or illnesses being managed with drug therapies, and their effectiveness up to now. This can be a considerable amount of information to have gathered, analyzed, researched, and organized within your Pharmacotherapy Workup. Presenting this much of a patient's case for the first few times lets you become comfortable with the structured format of a pharmacotherapy case presentation.

Future case presentations can focus on determining a clinically appropriate care plan and follow-up evaluation schedule. The focus of these case presentations is planning the timing to determine the effectiveness and safety of all of the patient's drug therapies.

Any advice you intend to request from a colleague, instructor, mentor, or practitioner concerning one of your patients must be asked for within the Pharmacotherapy Case Presentation Format. For instance, if you are asking your colleague whether an unusual side effect can be caused by a certain drug your patient is taking, you will ask it in the context of your patient's case.

Example "Dr. Johnson, I would like to know if you have ever heard about or seen a patient who has had this side effect from a medication. My patient is a 59-year-old male taxicab driver who weighs about 150 lb and has presented with a new complaint of swelling and edema of both ankles and feet which he thinks started shortly after he began taking a new drug treatment for his back pain…"

In order to become comfortable, competent, and confident at making case presentations, you need to practice. However, repetition alone is not sufficient. Repeating mistakes and bad habits can slow your development as a competent practitioner. As a student practitioner, you need to take full advantage of every opportunity to obtain feedback on your ability to make case presentations. There are numerous methods to obtain the necessary help in developing your case presentation skills. Students, instructors, and/or mentors can listen to your presentations and provide constructive feedback. Student colleagues can help one another by providing honest feedback. Videotaping yourself while making case presentations can be especially instructive in the areas of nonverbal communication skills as well as revealing speech habits that you may not be aware that you use. The sections of the Pharmaceutical Care Case Presentation format follow.

Assessment of the Patient's Drug-related Needs

Brief Description of the Patient

All case presentations begin with a brief description of the patient. This provides your colleagues with a mental picture of this individual.

Practitioners need to *see* the patient in order to care for her. This should be simple, straightforward, and include how the patient appeared to you (physically, emotionally, and health-wise). Your introduction of the patient should include age, gender, and physical description (height, weight, and ethnic origin if it is germane to the care this patient). Be sensitive to the words you use and how you say them. Patient names and other patient identifiers (address, telephone numbers) are seldom appropriate in a case presentation, as you are responsible to always maintain patient confidentiality. An exception to this is if you are formally transferring or referring a patient to another practitioner. In these situations, you will give the patient's full name to your colleague. Your goal is to provide your audience with a mental picture of a person they may not have met. Consider the following three patients (M.J., Mr. W. and B.L.).

> **Example**   M.J. is a 23-year-old female who is 5 ft 3 in. tall and weighs 132 lb.
>
> Mr. W. is a 71-year-old Caucasian male who is approximately 6 ft tall and of average weight.
>
> B.L. is a 55-year-old, 6 ft 3 in. 220-lb male construction worker who appears very uncomfortable due to his recent work-related injury to his right hand.

Reason for the Patient Encounter

The next item discussed is the description of the patient's reason for the encounter with the practitioner. Your description should focus on the patient's initial request or the precipitating event. It is most helpful to use the patient's own words when describing her initial request for care. Therefore, your description may include direct quotations from the patient describing her perceptions of need. This might include items the patient does not understand, expressed concerns, or expectations that are unrealistic. Using the patient's own words avoids adding your own bias or interpretation onto the patient's description of her primary concern.

When presenting a description of the patient's original reason for the encounter, be certain to describe *the primary reason for the visit* or the *chief complaint* that directed your assessment interview. You may also need to include the patient's presenting signs, symptoms, or illness behavior and a description of the patient's general health.

Example   M.J. presented to our pharmaceutical care clinic with a cough that has "kept me awake for the past two nights."

Mr. W. was referred to me by Dr. Samuelson for assessment and continued follow-up of his anticoagulant therapy. Mr. W. explained that he has "been taking these pills for over 6 years, and I don't know why they keep taking blood samples."

B.L. asked us to contact his primary care physician and obtain "a new drug that will work" to relieve the pain and inflammation in his injured right hand.

The patient background summarizes the context in which the patient lives. The intent is to provide your colleagues with a more complete image of your patient as an individual. In order to fully understand your patient's drug-related needs, you may need to describe her employment, family support, and socioeconomic status. Lifestyle, living conditions, occupation, and family (or other care-givers affected by the person's illness) can all impact the patient's medication-taking beliefs, behaviors, and outcomes. A patient's functional capacity (physical, emotional, and social) should also be included here.

The last portion of the background will include a description of any special needs she has. Language barriers, physical limitations (hearing or sight, walking restrictions), or diverse cultural backgrounds (beliefs, religion, traditions) should all be noted if they impact the drug therapy decisions that will be made. It is important to be respectful of individual differences and sensitive when describing patient characteristics that represent beliefs or lifestyles that differ from your own.

Example   M.J. has a history of animal allergies and has recently begun taking care of her partner's three cats.

Mr. W. lives alone in a gated retirement community. He uses a cane to assist with walking and requires large print books and newspapers to read due to his failing eyesight.

B.L. recently moved from Mexico and speaks very little English. His oldest daughter accompanied him to help as an interpreter.

Medication Experience Reported by the Patient

The patient's medication experience includes a summary of the relevant events in a patient's lifetime that involve drug therapy. This summary will include the patient's attitudes, beliefs, and preferences about drug therapy that have been shaped by the patient's experiences, traditions, religion, and culture. This information is most useful when it, too, is presented in the patient's own words. The focus of this portion of your presentation is to describe how your patient makes decisions about using medications.

The patient's medication experience is important because it forms the context in which to understand the remaining information in the case. This information helps you to understand the *whole* person and will be necessary as you try to identify common ground on which to develop the care plan.

> **Example** M.J. explained that this type of cough has occurred "at least three or four times in the past, whenever my partner brings her cats to my apartment. I think it is because of the cats, but I really like animals."
>
> Mr. W. has been meticulously observant of all his appointments to have his international normalized ratio (INR) measured and his warfarin dosage adjusted. He keeps a record of all his past INR results in his wallet.
>
> B.L. asked his daughter to ask why he had to see a physician, just to get some more pain medication. In his hometown in Mexico, that was not required. He could purchase most medications his family needed at any pharmacy.

Now that your audience has a fairly complete description of the patient as a person, the reason for the encounter, and an understanding of the medication experience, it is necessary to focus on the patient's medication history and current medication record. A comprehensive description of your patient's medications involves several important areas. These include allergies, alerts, immunization records, and social drug use that may impact your decisions about medications as well as all of your patient's current medical conditions or illnesses and pharmacotherapies used to manage them at this time.

Comprehensive Medication History

Allergies and alerts/social drug use/immunization record To describe a complete medication history and to include all the information required to prevent drug therapy problems, it is necessary to describe any allergies (and associated allergens) or adverse reactions to previously taken drug therapy. In your case presentation, it is important to clearly differentiate drug allergies from adverse drug reactions that your patient may have experienced in the past. To do this, you will want to include the nature of the reaction, the timing of the reaction relative to the specific drug therapy, and the consequences of the episode. Describing how the episode was treated is often useful. It is also important to describe your interpretation of future risk to the patient should she be exposed to the drug.

Tobacco use, alcohol, and recreational drug use can all influence your patient's risk for certain diseases and drug therapy outcomes. Therefore, a clear and honest description of this information is necessary, as well as a determination of the consequences it can have on this patient's care. It should be emphasized that patient confidentiality and consent should be assured as they relate to reporting recreational drug use. Your responsibility is to emphasize the association between sensitive information and the drug therapy decisions being made that you choose to share with your colleagues.

Prevention is one of the primary responsibilities in pharmaceutical care. Therefore, the patient's immunization history is an essential aspect of the Pharmacotherapy Workup and case presentation. This is especially true in vulnerable populations such as children, immune-compromised patients, and the elderly. The degree to which your patient's immunization status is current is an important part of every pharmacotherapy case presentation. Plans to provide necessary immunizations can also be included.

Up-to-date information should be reported, and when it is not available, it should be sought.

> **Example** M.J. reports no drug allergies, but is allergic to animal dander and some forms of nuts, which manifest as severe itching and rash that respond to Benadryl (diphenhydramine) and cool compresses. She has never used tobacco and drinks one or two alcoholic beverages only on social occasions.
>
> Mr. W. indicated he was allergic to codeine. He reported that he had to go to the emergency department because he developed angioedema shortly after he took his first dose of Tylenol with codeine for a dental procedure in 1998. He quit smoking cigarettes after his wife died in 1991. He reports no use of alcohol of any type.
>
> B.L. reports no history of any drug or food allergies. He describes his alcohol use as *"two beers after work"* and does not smoke cigarettes or cigars.

Current Medication Record: Indication–Drug Product–Dosage Regimen–Outcome

An essential portion of every pharmacotherapy case presentation is the patient's current medication record. Pharmaceutical practitioners add substantial and useful information to every patient's case by gathering and analyzing patient, disease, and drug data, and creating new information in the format of indication–drug therapy–outcome.

The Pharmacotherapy Case Presentation Format calls for a specific approach to describing your patient's current drug regimens. This format uses a comprehensive method to describe each drug the patient is taking. First, the indication is described, then the specific drug product, then the dosage regimen the patient is taking and how long she has been taking it at that dosage, and finally, the response she has exhibited or described that has resulted from that drug therapy. Recall that the framework for your Pharmacotherapy Workup asked you to assess the relationships between indication, drug product, dosage regimen, and outcome. This same unique framework is applied to the method you use to describe your patient's medication usage.

> **Example** M.J. is presently treating tendonitis of the right elbow with ibuprofen 600 mg taken three times each day for the past 5 days. She is satisfied with the relief of both the pain and stiffness and has not experienced any gastrointestinal side effects.
>
> Mr. W., who has long-standing atrial fibrillation, is presently taking warfarin 2.5 mg orally each morning for prevention of a stroke or myocardial infarction. His most recent INR was 2.2 last month, and he has not experienced any bleeding; therefore, no dosage adjustments were made at that time.
>
> B.L. injured his right hand, and for analgesia, has been taking aspirin, 325 mg two times each day, for the past 3 days with no relief of his pain or inflammation of the right hand.

The medication record is organized by therapeutic indication. When your patient is taking several medications for one indication, all of them are described together.

> **Example** Mr. W., who has longstanding atrial fibrillation, is presently taking warfarin 2.5 mg orally each morning for prevention of a stroke or myocardial infarction. His INR last month was 2.2, and no dosage adjustments were made at that time. His heart rate and rhythm have been successfully controlled for the past three years with digoxin 0.25 mg orally every day, furosemide 20 mg each morning, and oral potassium supplement of 20 meq daily. A review of systems revealed that Mr. W. has not experienced any adverse reactions from his drug therapies.

The medication record is complete when you describe the patient's overall understanding of the medications she is taking and the patient's ability and willingness to comply with instructions.

Past Medical History and Associated Drug Therapies

Next you may need to describe the pertinent portions of the patient's past medical history. Keep in mind that this is a pharmacotherapy case presentation and not the presentation of a patient's complete medical workup. Therefore, present only the information and experience you used to make current drug therapy decisions. Past medical history is used most often to describe those experiences in the patient's past that suggest a risk factor or contraindication to drug therapy. These situations may include: serious illnesses, hospitalizations, surgical procedures, accidents and injuries, pregnancies, deliveries, and complications to any medical treatments.

> **Example** M.J. was diagnosed with exercise-induced asthma at 7 years of age but has not needed any drug therapy or other medical care for that condition for the past 8 years.
>
> Mr. W. had dental surgery last April at which time his warfarin was discontinued for 7 days and then restarted without incident.

Providing any evidence of success or failure of past attempts at treating or preventing an illness can be a very informative portion of your case presentation. If you discover that a specific form of drug therapy had failed to produce the desired response in your patient in the past, then explaining that finding can clarify why you have chosen certain other forms of pharmacotherapy.

Similarly, if you know that a drug product or a dosage regimen was effective at treating the same problem your patient has at this time, then that information becomes essential to include in your pharmacotherapy case presentation.

> **Example** M.J. is presently treating tendonitis of the right elbow with ibuprofen 600 mg taken three times each day for the past 5 days. She is satisfied with the relief of both the pain and stiffness. The week prior, she attempted to treat her tendonitis by taking 200 mg twice daily but felt no relief.
>
> M.J. also reported that she attempted to treat a similar cough with dextromethorphan last spring, but "that medication did not help much and it upset my stomach."
>
> In 1999, Mr. W. was instructed to take 2.5 mg of warfarin every other day, alternating with 5 mg, but he could not keep track of his dosing schedule. He was seen in clinic on two occasions that year with bleeding from the nose. He reported that his INR was "way too high because I was taking too much medicine."

Review of Systems

There are several situations in which you will need to present positive or negative findings from your oral review of systems:

- To establish the relationship of a finding to a drug therapy your patient is taking. This is either evidence of the presence or absence of a side effect or adverse drug reaction. "The verbal review of systems revealed that the patient was not nauseous or agitated and has not experienced headache or dizziness and showed no other side effects from her fluoxetine."
- To identify additional drug therapy needs of the patient that were not discovered during your assessment interview. "The review of systems revealed that the patient has experienced excessive bruising over the past 3–4 months thought to be related to…"
- To present your interpretation of any abnormal or unexpected findings. "The review of systems revealed that the patient experienced a feeling of fullness in the abdomen, which subsided when she started her ranitidine therapy."

The report of the review of systems represents a systematic review of physical findings, descriptions, and experiences offered by the patient and laboratory values not already associated with a specific medical condition (and reported earlier). The review of systems must be presented in a concise and useful manner. Only the important positive and pertinent negative findings and laboratory tests should be reported.

> **Example** An oral review of systems was unremarkable except for his report of intermittent nausea over the past 2 weeks, which the patient feels is a result of his new diet.

Always make the association between the finding and drug therapy for the listener. If you have a series of values to report, presentation of the data in a flow sheet or graph may be preferable.

Summary of the Assessment

The summary of the assessment should include a brief review of your clinical judgment regarding the patient, her active medical conditions, associated drug therapies, and any drug therapy problems identified. Your summary should report your judgment as to whether you think that all of your patient's drug therapy is appropriately indicated, the most effective available, as safe as possible, and whether the patient is taking it as intended.

This summary informs your colleagues where you are in the course of the case presentation.

> **Example** "The summary of my assessment of M.J. is that she is a healthy 23-year-old female who is bothered by coughing in the evening, which is disrupting her sleep and is felt to be a manifestation of her allergies to cat dander. We will need to provide drug therapy to control these symptoms, as she will be in contact with cats for the next 2 weeks."

The summary needs to be only be a few sentences, as you are only including the most important data that were used to make your clinical decisions.

Drug Therapy Problem Identification

Problem–Drug Therapy–Cause and Effect
If drug therapy problems have been identified, they must be stated clearly during your presentation of the patient's case.

> **KEY CLINICAL CONCEPTS**
>
> There is a specific format used to describe a patient's drug therapy problems. This format has three parts that must be described together: (a) the medical condition associated with the drug therapy problem, (b) the drug therapy involved, and (c) the relationship (cause and effect) between the medical problem and the drug therapy.

It must be clearly stated so your colleagues can understand your clinical decision.

> **Example** "The patient's ibuprofen dosage of 200 mg twice a day was too low to provide effective relief of her tendonitis."
>
> "The patient requires potassium supplements to prevent diuretic-induced hypokalemia."
>
> "The patient has developed orthostatic hypotension due to the excessive dosage increase of her enalapril."
>
> "The patient prefers not to take his cefuroxime suspension for pharyngitis because of the poor taste."

Remember, this represents one of the most important clinical decisions you make. The identification of the patient's drug therapy problems is to the pharmacotherapy case presentation what the diagnosis is to the medical case presentation. The drug therapy problems should be prioritized based on the patient's needs, and those being addressed currently should be differentiated from those to be addressed in the future.

In addition, if your patient has any risk factors for specific drug therapy problems that need to be prevented at this time, this should also be stated here.

The Care Plan

Identifying your patient's drug-related needs, as well as resolving and preventing drug therapy problems, requires an organized care planning process. Therefore, presenting the care plans you have constructed for your patient also requires organization. The care plan should be organized and prioritized by active medical conditions being managed with drug therapy. The problems should be presented in order of risk, severity, and importance to the patient.

The care plan is complete when you can describe how to manage the medical condition with drug therapies and other nondrug interventions. For each medical condition, you will need to present your plan to resolve any drug therapy problems associated with that medical condition, a clear description of the goals of therapy, and the interventions you intend to make to achieve the goals of therapy and prevent any drug therapy problems from occurring in the patient.

> **Example** "Our goal is to eliminate the orthostatic hypotension by holding her enalapril for 1 day and then reducing the daily dosage regimen of enalapril to 10 mg twice each day, beginning on Tuesday."

When describing the goals, be certain to include the timeframe in which you expect to achieve each goal.

> **Example** "The goal of therapy is to reduce and then maintain her blood pressure at a systolic of 120–130 mmHg and a diastolic of 70–80 mmHg within the next 4 weeks."

Generally, therapeutic alternatives to resolve drug therapy problems are only presented if controversial, if you are still uncertain about your decision, or if your mentor needs to know that you have considered all of the reasonable therapeutic choices. When presenting the therapeutic alternatives considered and the drug therapy selected, be sure to explain the rationale for your choice. When describing pharmacotherapy rationale, always explain both the efficacy and safety considerations for each alternative. What is the comparative efficacy, and what is the comparative safety of the multiple products you considered? Additional considerations (cost and convenience) can be described here too, but efficacy and safety are always the required minimum.

Interventions are complete if they include who is responsible for the activity: you, the patient, or another practitioner. The final information you will present in your care plan section of the presentation is the schedule for follow-up meetings with the patient. This plan should also include the parameters you intend to use to evaluate the effectiveness of your plan and the parameters you plan to use to evaluate the safety of your patient's drug therapies.

> **Example**   "The patient will take her own blood pressure every morning and record it on her medication diary. She will also record any feelings of dizziness or lightheadedness. I will evaluate these records at the next appointment on August 23. I will evaluate renal function using blood urea nitrogen, serum creatinine, and potassium determinations at that visit. I will also inquire to determine if she has developed a cough from her enalapril therapy."

Follow-up Evaluation

Some case presentations focus on a single, recent follow-up evaluation.[47] In these situations, your presentation generally follows the above outline with respect to briefly describing the patient, the main conditions, and the drug therapies involved. For presentations of the follow-up evaluation, your focus is on the evidence of success or failure of past care plans and interventions.

The presentation of a follow-up evaluation generally has three sections. First, you must briefly review the patient and what you were trying to achieve at previous visits. This generally focuses on resolution of drug therapy problems and achieving goals of therapy. Second, you will describe what happened to the patient (patient outcome) since the last visit. You will need to compare the patient's outcomes to what was intended (goals of therapy). This comparison is based on clinical and/or laboratory findings used as evidence of effectiveness and safety of drug therapies and patient compliance. Third, you present your clinical judgment (evaluation) of the patient's progress toward achieving the goals of therapy as of the date of the follow-up presentation being described. It is most useful to be consistent in your use of outcome terminology. The terms to describe pharmacotherapy outcome status include *resolved, stable, improved, partially improved, worsened, and failure.* It is important to be clear in your use of these outcome status categories (see Chapter 8). Finally, report any new drug therapy problems the patient may have developed since the previous evaluation.

> **Example** "As you will recall, we had reduced this patient's dosage of enalapril 4 weeks ago, due to episodes of orthostatic hypotension. I think we have successfully resolved that drug therapy problem.
>
> Today, she reports one episode of slight dizziness that diminished within 2 minutes. She has no other complaints including no cough associated with her drug therapy. Her renal function tests have not changed over the past month and all remain within normal limits. Her blood pressure readings over the past month have steadily declined to a daily range of 124–130 over 75–80 mmHg, which are within the planned goal of 120–130 over 70–80 mmHg. My evaluation at this visit is that her blood pressure control has improved, and no changes should be made in her drug regimen at this time. She has no new problems to report at this time. I plan to reevaluate her hypertension pharmacotherapy in 3 months."

Summary of the Case

The case presentation ends with a brief summary of the most cogent points. Be sure to summarize the drug-related needs of the patient, the resolution and prevention of drug therapy problems, as well as evidence of effectiveness and safety of the patient's pharmacotherapy.

COMMON CHALLENGES IN THE CASE PRESENTATION

Because case presentations are indicative of your capacity to process data and solve clinical problems, some common errors should be mentioned.

Items frequently omitted from student practitioner case presentations include the primary reason the patient sought care, the original reason for admission to the hospital or clinic, the nonprescription medications or herbal supplements being used as self-care and their indications, evidence of the patient's ability to understand and adhere to the medication instructions, and evidence that the drug therapy is being effective. Such deficiencies invariably lead to confusion and questions that interrupt the case presentation. For complex patients, be sure to organize the information by medical condition (i.e., for her diabetes, my patient is presently taking...)

The terminology used in patient case presentations will communicate your preparedness, your experience, and your standard of care. Be sure to use appropriate practice vocabulary and be precise in the words you choose. It is also important to be as concise as possible because you are either seeking help or providing it, and the listener's time is valuable. The objective of the patient case presentation format is to make the presentation of the case efficient. This depends on your organization of the patient information, your clinical decisions, and the patient responses. Be complete, but do not include any information that is not directly relevant to the objective for presenting the case. Remember that omitted information is the source of the most confusion in case presentations.

The strength of the case presentation format is its simplicity. Be sure not to negate this by being confusing, long-winded, or making the case appears complex when it is not. These are the most common problems encountered by new practitioners.

Written Case Summaries

Written case presentations are very similar in format to the verbal presentations described in this chapter. The outline and contents are the same, but a few differences exist. A written case presentation, often referred to as a *write-up*, should include headings or subheadings for major sections (description of patient, current medication record, drug therapy problems) to help the reader locate information. It is necessary to use quotations when using the patient's own words. Write-ups often include tables to summarize multiple drug therapies and/or laboratory results.

Your write-up may become part of the patient's permanent record, so attend to the accuracy and concise nature of the words you include. Always sign your work and indicate how others can contact you if they have questions.

Example of a Pharmacotherapy Case Presentation

The following is an example of a pharmacotherapy case presentation. The sections are listed on the left side of the table, while the example information that would be presented is illustrated in the right column (Table 10-17).

Table 10-17 Example of a pharmacotherapy case presentation

Brief description of the patient	M.J. is a 23-year-old female who is 5 ft 3 in. tall and weighs 132 lb.
Primary reason for the encounter	She presented to our pharmaceutical care clinic concerned about cough that she explained has "kept me awake for the past two nights."
Additional patient background	M.J. has a history of animal allergies including cat dander and has recently been taking care of her partner's three cats. She feels the cough is related to the cats but would like to continue to care for the cats until her partner returns in 2 weeks.
Medication experience	She has not attempted to treat this episode of the cough, but she did attempt to treat a similar cough last spring using dextromethorphan. M.J. described that she prefers not to take dextromethorphan again, as it caused her to "feel nauseated and it did not help much".
Comprehensive medication history	She reports no drug allergies and does not use tobacco. She uses alcohol only on special social occasions, which averages two to three times per month. She is up to date with her immunizations and received her annual influenza vaccine at her place of employment last month.
Current medication record	M.J. is presently treating an episode of tendonitis of the right elbow with ibuprofen 600 mg three times daily for the past 5 days. She originally tried 200 mg twice daily, but found no relief. The increased dosage of ibuprofen is providing satisfactory relief, and she reports no gastrointestinal upset from this therapy.
Relevant past medical history	M.J. describes herself as being in excellent health with no chronic medical conditions. She has a history of exercise-induced asthma at age 7 but has not needed any drug therapy or medical care for the past 8 years.
Review of systems	A brief review of systems revealed no cardiovascular, renal, or gastrointestinal problems. As for her respiratory status, she reported only the cough and no shortness of breath or wheezing. M.J. is not pregnant.
Summary of the assessment	The summary of my assessment of M.J. is that she is a healthy 23-year-old female who is bothered by coughing in the evening, which is disrupting her sleep and is felt to be a manifestation of her allergies to cat dander.

(Continued)

Table 10-17   (*Continued*) Example of a pharmacotherapy case presentation

Drug therapy problem	Her drug therapy problem is that she requires additional drug therapy to relieve the symptoms (cough) she is experiencing secondary to her animal allergies. M.J. agreed with this assessment.
Care plan	Relief of symptoms associated with allergies to cat dander.
Goals of therapy	We discussed goals of therapy and agreed that achieving a restful night of sleep tonight and for the next two nights without the constant coughing would be most desirable. During the day, she is at work and leaves the cats alone in her apartment, and the cough is not a problem at work.
Therapeutic alternatives	We discussed several alternatives including cough suppressants (codeine and dextromethorphan, which was not effective in the past) and antihistamines such as diphenhydramine, chlorpheniramine, and less sedating agents such as loratadine.
Pharmacotherapy	M.J. was started on diphenhydramine HCl (Benadryl) 25 mg orally in the afternoon after work and 25 mg at bedtime. She agreed that if it caused her to feel drowsy, that might be beneficial in her case. She will also make her bedroom off-limits to the cats in an attempt to minimize her exposure to allergens. She will also continue taking 600 mg of ibuprofen three times each day for tendonitis.
Follow-up evaluation plan	I plan to follow-up and evaluate her new therapy next Tuesday and will evaluate effectiveness in terms of restful sleep and to make certain that she is not bothered with early morning drowsiness from her diphenhydramine therapy.

SUMMARY

It may seem as though there is an impossible amount of information that must be mastered by the pharmaceutical care practitioner. It is true that patients can be complex with multiple medical conditions and we have an ever-expanding array of medications at our disposal, with an enormous variety of dosage forms and products. However, using the Pharmacotherapy Workup as your context for learning new information and for evaluating evidence of effectiveness and safety makes the challenge possible and enjoyable. Learning from every one of your patients requires the skill of being reflective in your practice. Take a moment after each patient encounter to examine what went well, what you could improve, and what you have learned. Finally, learning from your colleagues requires the skill of making effective, well-organized pharmacotherapy case presentations. Others will judge you not from what you have learned, but how you can demonstrate what you have learned when you apply it to the care of patients.

REFERENCES

1. Norman DD. *Perceptions of the Elderly Regarding the Medicating Experience: A Discourse Analysis of the Interpretation of Medication Usage*, in *Social and Administrative Pharmacy*. Minneapolis, MN: University of Minnesota; 1995.
2. Cipolle RJ, Strand LM, Morley PC. *Pharmaceutical Care Practice*. New York, NY: McGraw-Hill; 1998.
3. Cipolle RJ, Strand LM, Morley PC. *Pharmaceutical Care Practice: The Clinician's Guide*. 2nd ed. New York, NY: McGraw-Hill; 2004.
4. Blumer I. *Canadian Diabetes Association 2008 Clinical Practixe Guidelines for the Prevention and Management of Diabetes in Canada: Executive Summary.* Canadian Diabetes Association; 2009:1–15.
5. Chou R, Fanciullo GJ, Fine PG, et al. Clinical guidelines for the use of chronic opioid therapy in chronic noncancer pain. *J Pain*. 2009;10(12):113–130.
6. National Heart, Lung, and Blood Institute. *Guidelines for th Diagnosis and Management of Asthma: Expert Panel Report 3*. National Institutes of Health Publication number 08–4051;2007.
7. Chobanian AV, Bakris GL, Black HR, et al. Seventh report of the joint national committee on prevention, detection, evaluation, and treatment of high blood pressure. *Hypertension*. 2003;42(6):1206–1252.
8. Jones DW, Hall JE. Seventh report of the joint national committee on prevention, detection, evaluation, and treatment of high blood pressure and evidence from new hypertension trials. *Hypertension*. 2004;43(1):1–3.
9. North American Menopause Society. Management of osteoporosis in postmemopausal women: 2010 postition statement of the North American menopausal society. *Menopause*. 2010;17(1):25–54.
10. NIH. *Detection, Evaluation, and Treatment of High Blood Cholesterol in Adults (Adult Treatment Panel III)*. US Department of Health and Human Services, Public Health Service, National Institutes of Health, National Heart, Lung, and Blood Institute, NIH Publication No. 01–3305;2001.
11. NIH. *Prevention, Detection, Evaluation, and Treatment of High Blood Pressure*. US Department of Health anc Human Services, National Institutes of Health,, National Heart, Lung, and Blood Institute, National High Blood Pressure Education Program; 2003.
12. Vaidya B, Pearce SH. Management of hypothyroidism in adults. *BMJ*. 2008;337:a801.
13. Kasper KL, Fauci AS, Longo DL, Braunwald E, Hauser S, Jameson JL. (eds) *Harrison's Principles of Internal Medicine*. 16th ed. New York, NY: McGraw-Hill; 2005.
14. Dipiro JT, Talbert RL, Yee GC, Matzke GR, Wells BG, Posey LM. *Pharmacotherapy: A Pathophysiologic Approach*. 7th ed. New York: McGraw-Hill; 2008.
15. Weiss BD, *Primary Care: 20 Common Problems*. New York, NY: McGraw-Hill; 1999.

16. Gray J. *Therapeutic Choices*. 4th ed. Ottawa, Ontario: Canadian Pharmacists Association; 2003.

17. Berardi RR, Ferreri SP, Hume AL, et al. *Handbook of Nonprescription Drugs*. In: Young LL, ed. Washington, DC: American Pharmaceutical Association; 2009.

18. Glassman PA, Garcia D, Delafiel JP. *Outpatient Care Handbook*. 2nd ed. Philadelphia, PA: Hanlelyl & Belfus; 1999.

19. Lacy CF, Armstrong LL, Goldman MP, Lance, LL, *Lexi-Comp's: Drug Information Handbook*. 17th ed. New York: McGraw-Hill; 2010–2011.

20. Facts and Comparisons Publishing Group, *Drug Facts and Comparisons*. St. Louis, MO: Wolters Kluwer Health; 2011.

21. Hardman JG, Limbird LE (eds) *Goodman & Gilman's the Pharmacological Basis of Therapeutics*. 10th ed. In: Gilman A, Hardman JG, Limbird LE, eds. New York, NY: McGraw-Hill; 2001.

22. Gonyeau MJ, Yuen DW. A clinical review of statins and cancer: helpful or harmful? Pharmacotherapy. 2010;30(2):177–194.

23. Heart-Protection-Study-Collaborative-Group. Randomized trial of the effects of cholesterol-lowering with simvastatin on peripheral vascular and other major vascular outcomes in 20,536 people iwth peripheral arterial disease and other high-risk conditions. *J Vasc Surg*. 2007;45:645–654.

24. Sacher J, Weigl L, Werner M, Szegedi C, Hohenegger M. *Delineation of myotoxicity induced by 3-hdroxy-3-methylglutaryl CoA* reductase inhibitors in human skeletal muscle cells. *J Pharmacol Exp Ther*. 2005;314(3):1032–1041.

25. Dambro MR, ed. *Griffith's 5-Minute Clinical Consult*. Philadelphia, PA: Lippincott Williams & Wilkins; 2003.

26. Koda-Kimble MA and Young LY. *Applied Therapeutics : The Clinical Use of Drugs*. 7th ed. Baltimore, MD: Lippincott Williams & Wilkins; 2001.

27. Anderson PO, Knoben JE, Troutman WG. *Handbook of Clinical Drug Data*. 10th ed. New York, NY: McGraw-Hill; 2002.

28. Lesaffre E. *Number Needed to Treat*, in *Encyclopedia of Statistics in Behavioral Scinece*. Everitt BS, Howell DC, eds. Chichester: John Wiley & Sons, Ltd; 2005:1448–1450.

29. McQuay HJ, Moore RA. Using numerical results from systematic reviews in clinical practice. *Ann Intern Med*. 1997;126(9):712–720.

30. Krantz MJ, Berger JS, Hiatt WR. An aspirin a day: are we barking up the wrong willow tree? *Pharmacotherapy*. 2010;30(2):115–118.

31. Antithrombotic Trialists's Collaboration, Baigent C, Blackwell L. Aspirin in the primary and secondary prevention of vasculare disease: collaborative meta-analysis of individual participant data from randomized trials. *Lancet*. 2009;373:1849–1860.

32. Cole SA, Bird J. *The Medical Interview: The Three-function Approach*. Schmitt W, ed. St. Louis, MO: Mosby, Inc; 2000.

33. Lipkin MH, Putman SM, Lazare A. *The Medical Interview: Clinical Care, Education, and Research*. New York: Springer; 1995.

34. McEvoy GK, American Society of Health-System Pharmacists. *AHFS drug information essentials*. Bethesda, MD: American Society of Health-System Pharmacists; 2004:v.

35. Jellin JM, Batz F, Hitchens K. *Natural Medicines Comprehensive Database*. Stockton, CA: Therapeutic Research Faculty; 1999:v.

36. Anderson PO, Knoben JE, Troutman WG. *Clinical Drug Data*. 11th ed. New York, NY: McGraw-Hill Medical; 2010:1336 p.

37. Semla TP, Beizer JL, Higbee MD. *Geriatric Dosage Handbook*. 16th ed. Cleveland, OH: Lexi-Comp Inc; 2011.

38. Taketomo CK, Hodding JH, Kraus DM. *Pediatric & Neonatal Dosing Handbook*. 18th ed. Cleveland, OH: Lexi-Comp Inc; 2011.
39. Foster S, Tyler VE. *Tyler's Honest Herbal: A sensible Guide to the Use of Herbs and Related Remedies*. 4th ed. New York, NY: Haworth Herbal Press; 1999. xxi, 442 p.
40. Hansten PD, Horn JR. *The Top 100 Drug Interactions*. H & H Publications; 2011.
41. Coulehan JL, Block MR. *The Medical Interview: Mastring Skills for Clinical Practice*. 4th ed. Philadelphia, PA: F.A. Davis Company; 2001:155–169.
42. Isetts.BJ, Brown LB, *Patient Assessment and Consultation*, in *Handbook of Nonprescription Drugs: An Interactive Approach to Self-Care*. Washington, DC: American Pharmaceutical Association; 2009.
43. Isetts BJ. Evaluaiton of pharmacy students' abilities to provide pharmaceutical care. *Am J Pharm Education*. 1999;63:11–20.
44. Kitchener KS, King PM. *The Reflective Judgement Model: Transforming Assumptions About Knowing. Fostering Critical Reflection in Adulthood*. San Francisco, CA: Jossey-Bass; 1990.
45. Atkins S, Murphy K. Reflection: a review of the literature. *J Adv Nurs*. 1993;18(8): 1188–1192.
46. Schon DA. *The Reflective Practitioner: How Professionals Think in Action*. Basic Books, Inc; 1983.
47. Billings JA, Stoeckle JD. *The Clinical Encounter: A Guide to the Medical Interview and Case Presentation*. Chicago: Year Book Medical Publishers, Inc; 1989.
48. Smith RC. *The Patient's Story: Integrated Patient-Doctor Interviewing*. Boston, MA: Little Brown and Company; 1996.

chapter eleven

Managing Medication Management Services

🔑 KEY CONCEPTS

1 The most important factor in building a successful pharmaceutical care practice is the preparedness of the practitioner.

2 Understanding the service you provide and articulating that service to patients and other practitioners is essential.

3 Find a supportive environment in which to practice.

4 Do not expect the practice site to change for you—teach them how to accommodate your new practice.

5 Recruit new patients through referrals, other patients, and collaborative practice agreements.

6 A network of qualified pharmaceutical care practitioners could be your most important asset.

7 Be realistic in your expectations. Commit 2 years to building your practice.

8 Know how to charge for your service using on the resource-based relative value scale.

9 The best marketing plan is to provide high-quality patient care.

10 Learn to write a business plan—your practice depends upon it.

UNDERSTANDING THE PRACTICE MANAGEMENT SYSTEM

Introduction

This chapter focuses on issues associated with establishing a practice. This chapter is not intended to provide you with the scope and detail you will need to become a good manager; that knowledge and experience should be gained from schools of management and experienced management personnel.

Pharmaceutical care is still new enough that there are relatively few practices that have been established long enough from which to learn. Therefore, it is necessary to learn from other patient care practitioners who have built successful practices, namely, nurse practitioners, physicians, dentists, and veterinarians. These practitioners have been building practices that are well managed and successful from both the professional and financial perspectives for many years. A number of resources are available from these practice areas.[1–5]

The key to a successful practice is to add new patients continually so the practice can become financially viable, and survive over the long term. Providing care to more than one patient, on a repeat basis, requires an efficient and effective organization. To accomplish this, a practice management system that can facilitate the work—in this case, provide pharmaceutical care, must be developed.

Just as it is necessary to have an orderly, systematic approach to patient care, which is described as the patient care process in Chapters 6 to 8, it is also necessary to have an orderly, systematic approach to managing a practice when providing pharmaceutical care. This requires a practice management or support system that is consistent with one's practice.

KEY CLINICAL CONCEPTS

A practice management system includes all the support required to provide a service to patients in a proficient and productive manner.

Most simply stated, the practice management system includes

1. a clear understanding of the mission of the practice (a clear description of the service provided); this mission defines the standards and expectations for the service.
2. all the resources required to deliver the service (it includes physical, financial, and human resources; it includes documentation and reporting aspects, and appointment processes, among others).
3. the means by which the service can be evaluated, in the short term, to represent patient-specific experiences, and in the long term to represent the quality of the service. Therefore, the evaluation processes must measure the practitioner's ability to manage the patient, and the ability of the practitioner, or in some situations a manager, to manage the practice. Both aspects will contribute to the outcomes described above.

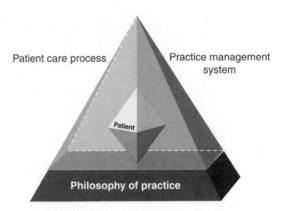

Figure 11-1 The Practice of Pharmaceutical Care.

4. the means to reward the practitioner, and financially support the longevity of the practice (payment mechanisms). This represents the value of the service to the patient in the short term and to the payer and society in the long term.

It is necessary to place the practice management system in the context of the practice. Figure 11-1 indicates that the practice management system has as its foundation, the philosophy of practice.

We can see from the figure that the patient care process and the management system directly impact each other, on a constant basis. This is expected because the patient care process represents the work that must be accomplished, and the practice management system facilitates that work. So, as we learned, the patient care process changes minimally with the practice setting, but it is the practice management system that will adapt to the setting where the practice is being delivered. Therefore, the patient care process stays essentially the same and it is the practice management system that changes with the physical, social, political, and economic environments. Even when we look at different countries in Chapter 12, the practice will be universally the same and the delivery of the service changes based on the factors surrounding the service.

ESTABLISHING A SUCCESSFUL PRACTICE

Establishing a successful pharmaceutical care practice is not a simple task. Although there are relatively few established, new practices are being built every day and we are learning from them. The magnitude of the change from a dispensing mission to a patient care mission is tremendous, so it is frequently difficult for pharmacists to imagine what is needed to support a patient care practice separate from dispensing. Other practitioners such as physicians, dentists, and nurses have made substantial changes in their practices, but none have had to completely change the focus from a product to patient care. A change of this scope requires an evolutionary change on the professional level, and on the individual practitioner level, it requires a personal, revolutionary change. Only if you are prepared for this, will you find the energy required to build a practice. However, it can be done, it has been done, and with the guidance that follows, should be significantly easier than it appears at first glance.

We will present the principal steps that we have used to build hundreds of such practices to date.[1,2,5]

The material presented here will be applicable for building a practice in any ambulatory practice setting, specifically the clinic-based practice, medical home-based practice, assisted living facility, or home visit–based practice. It is applicable to a commercial retail pharmacy setting *only* if dedicated space is identified in the pharmacy and the service is managed as a separate, independent, identifiable, service physically and financially separated from the dispensing business. This physical space, usually from 100 to 250 square feet, along with a dedicated pharmacist practitioner and appropriate support staff, must be regarded as separate from the rest of the pharmacy operation. There is a direct conflict of interest for a pharmacist to provide patient care services if he will benefit directly from the sale of the drug product in the commercial retail pharmacy. Pharmacists must be conscious of this conflict and manage it successfully or they run the risk of losing the opportunity.

There are fundamental steps to building a new pharmaceutical care practice. There will be a natural tendency to want to start this process at other places than at the beginning. We would like to warn against this. Pharmacists usually want to begin with payment because they are very focused on their financial concerns. However, this is last step in the process! Starting anywhere other than the beginning will lead to a short-lived, failed experiment. It is also necessary to complete each step before moving on to the next. And, you will have to complete the entire process if you hope to succeed. We repeat, success will be highly unlikely unless the work described here is accomplished in the order that it is presented and unless all the steps are completely finished. Obviously, the time frame required to complete each step will vary with individuals. So, it is the order, and the completeness, not the time frame, we wish to emphasize. Let us begin the process of building a successful, sustainable pharmaceutical care practice. We will identify the essential steps necessary to accomplish this.

Preparing Yourself

Become a Competent Practitioner

KEY CLINICAL CONCEPTS

The single most important variable in a new patient care practice is the quality of the practitioner providing the care. The success of the practice depends upon how knowledgeable and skilled the practitioner is and the level of commitment the practitioner has to patient care.

In health care, the best practitioners are the busiest practitioners. Therefore, to assure your highest level of success in practice you want to gain experience with qualified colleagues until you are confident of your ability to function independently. *"It is easy to start a practice if you know how to take care of patients."*

Pharmacists frequently "assume" they know how to provide pharmaceutical care because they have worked in or near patient care settings. We have found that frequently this is not the case. Because pharmacists have not traditionally been taught a specific philosophy of practice or been required to apply a specific patient care process, they are not aware of what they do not know. It is very important to learn the terminology, internalize the philosophy and utilize the same patient care process in order to be competent in practice. If a pharmacist has not received formal preparation in the practice of pharmaceutical care after graduation from pharmacy school, it is highly recommended that a course be completed.

Being partially or inadequately prepared will only prolong the time until a successful practice can be realized. In fact, the greatest advantage you can give yourself when starting a new practice is to ensure that you can provide care that meets the standards defined for the practice. These standards can be found in Appendix 1. In any patient care service, the practitioner is the *"product"* that is marketed.

It is commonly understood in practitioner circles that it is impossible to become a skilled practitioner on your own. You are going to need the help of colleagues. Identify qualified practitioners in your geographical area and schedule routine meetings to present patient cases, and to exchange information, questions, concerns, and experiences related to patient care. This network of practitioners may become your greatest asset.

Take care of enough patients to become very good at it. This takes constant practice. You will need to add a minimum of two to three new patients each day to your practice in order to become competent at practicing pharmaceutical care. Remember, it will take 700 to 1500 patients to become financially viable so this is a good rate at which to establish your practice.

Understand and Describe Your Service and the Mission of Your Practice

Pharmaceutical care practice is the first new patient care service to be introduced into the health care system in many decades. Therefore, it will be new to everyone who comes in contact with you. You will have to describe this new service over and over again before physicians, nurses, and patients clearly understand what you will be doing. You should not get frustrated or interpret their questions as a lack of interest or support. Do not expect people to demand a service that they do not understand or have never experienced.

KEY CLINICAL CONCEPTS

The most effective way to introduce new health care service is to provide it.

Providing the service will show patients what they can expect and how they can benefit from the service. Realize that new behaviors have to be learned by everyone involved in the health care system and this will take time.

Getting started means the pharmacist must understand clearly, and define explicitly, the service that will be offered to patients. This is the most important step and impacts all subsequent decisions. It sounds simple enough, but to do this well most pharmacists must change the way they think about their business enterprise. And, remember, the patient needs to hear what you are going to do for her in terms she will understand so you will not want to describe for her your professional practice, you want to describe the service she is about to receive.

The service is the aspect of the practice that the patient experiences and remembers at each interaction, so it is very important to "get it right." Because pharmacy as a profession has been product focused for so long, you will have to work to change the expectations the patient has of the pharmacist. Keep in mind, the expectations patients have today are the direct result of what has been done to/for them in the past. The expectations they develop in the future will be a direct result of what is done for them today. The fastest way to change patient expectations is to provide services that patients want and need. The pharmacist has to establish that she has something to offer of value beyond the product. The quickest way to do this is to provide a valuable service that the patient wants and needs.

Although this sounds uncomplicated and often is, it can be confusing because in the case of a professional practice generally, and drug therapy specifically, the patient needs the pharmacist to help identify the patient's drug therapy needs. Often, the pharmacist is able to best determine what service the patient needs, but the patient is best at determining how the service should be delivered. Both are essential for a quality service.

A quality service can accomplish the following:

- attract new patients
- increase patient loyalty and the retention of existing patients
- increase the retention of service-oriented personnel
- decrease liability
- increase a practice's attractiveness for group or network affiliation.[1]

Moreover, because the quality of the care provided will ultimately determine if a patient returns or not, we include clinical rationale for a quality service. A quality service will

- lead to improved identification, resolution, and prevention of drug therapy problems.
- improve adherence with treatment regimens.
- facilitate quality clinical outcomes.
- increase the opportunity for continuity of care.[1]

With these basic concepts as the foundation or the starting point, we must create a mission for our practice, a description of the service to be offered, which is clearly stated, and can be communicated explicitly. We suggest the following:

> *The mission of this organization (or the service to be provided) is to meet the individual drug therapy needs of our patients, in a compassionate, caring, and professional manner, and to execute the services required as effectively, comprehensively, and efficiently as possible.*
>
> *The pharmacist will accomplish this mission by ensuring that the medications you are taking are appropriate, as effective as possible, the safest available and that they are able to be taken as intended. This will be done to optimize your medication experience and to help you to achieve the outcomes you want from your medications.*

It is important to create wording that is meaningful to you while remembering that pharmacists must be applying the same professional practice to deliver consistent patient care services, regardless of practice setting, patient type, medical problem or specific drug therapy being used. This will ensure recognition and acceptance in the shortest time frame.

Focus on Your Patient

KEY CLINICAL CONCEPTS

Practitioners build practices. The pharmacist will neither make it happen, or be the rate-limiting step.

The manager, the physical plant, the pharmaceutical industry, computer systems, and third-party payers do not build practices. They can certainly facilitate, or make it very difficult, for a practitioner or group of practitioners to build a successful practice. The practitioner has to place the patient's interests first to build a successful practice. It means the answer is always "yes, I can help." The most important concept we strive to communicate to the neophyte pharmaceutical care practitioner is the following:

Strive to discover your patients' priorities and value system and integrate their desires with your broad knowledge of drug therapy to develop a care plan which is in your patient's best interest and your practice will flourish.[4]

Providing a financially viable service means giving people what they need, the way they want it. Let patients know that they, as individuals, are the most important aspect of your practice and that meeting their needs and desires is central to your service. This is so important that it may be appropriate to prominently display a sign with the following message:

Our goal is to provide the very best care, support, and information, you need for a healthy life.

However, before posting this signage, it is important to know patients and their drug-related needs, and to be providing the service that will meet these needs. This sounds obvious and simple. Neither is the case.

Pharmacists are not taught, nor are they accustomed to, looking for a patient's drug-related needs. Therefore, it is uncomfortable, unusual, and certainly "risky" on everyone's part for the pharmacist to start a practice. The patient and her drug-related needs will "drive" the entire practice. How effectively this happens depends on the ability of practitioners to create the "right" patient experience.

Creating the right experience for the patient can be difficult because we usually begin with the practitioner, which is the wrong starting place. Even more menacing is to begin by focusing on the physical plant because it is tangible and much easier to address, than attitude, culture, or communication. It may be useful to walk into someone else's practice, as a patient, and ask yourself the following questions:

- Does the patient know where to go to receive the service?
- Is the space well signed so the patient is not confused from the start?
- When a patient enters the practice, is it clean, neat, professional, quiet?
- Is the person meeting/greeting the patient pleasant, and focused on the patient first?
- Is there appropriate space for the patient (and her children) to wait to see the pharmacist and to receive the service?
- Is there private/semiprivate space available for the patient to discuss her care with the pharmacist?
- Does the flow of the work focus on the patient and her needs and not the pharmacist first?
- When the telephone rings, is it answered professionally to reinforce that the patient comes first?
- If the pharmacist is interrupted, is it done professionally, and with the respect of the patient foremost?
- Does the patient always come first?
- Does the patient have access to what she needs while in your practice?
- Can patients sit comfortably?
- Do the children have what they need?
- Are there educational materials available?
- Are there facilities for patients with disabilities?
- Is the lighting sufficient?
- Are there interruptive noises where the patient receives care, from paging systems, computer printers, modems, or radios?
- Can the patient have a positive, therapeutic experience receiving your service?

Each aspect of the patient's experience while in your presence requires consideration, down to the smallest detail. For example, does your name-tag encourage patients to relate to you on a personal, informal manner, or is it intimidating? Can it be read from a distance? Pharmacists, managers, and support staff are often too close to the practice to see clutter, mess, poor signage, messy notes hanging on walls and counters, as well as notices to staff attached to doors, desks, and shelves. Therefore, it is necessary to ask patients what *they* see, what *they* hear, and what *they* experience in your practice. Such feedback is

Table 11-1   Continuum of methods of patient inquiry

Formal				Informal
Focus groups	Suggestion	Patient	Exit	Walk around
In-depth interviews	boxes	advisory	interviews	and talk with
Surveys		boards		patients

Data from reference 1.

very important, and must be constant. Patients constantly transform a practice as they also change, so we must constantly adapt to provide the quality service that will contribute to the development of a positive practice environment.

To stay close to the patient you must find out what the patient thinks of the service you provide. This cannot be done immediately. You must provide the service first, and learn how to be efficient and effective at its delivery. For the next 6 to 9 months, you must engage in a complete process of inquiry. This means that you ask patients for their opinions about your service. In addition to this, you must listen, empathize, and respond to their opinions. This is especially important when a new service is introduced.

There are a number of methods to use when asking patients for their opinions about the quality of the service you provide. It is easiest to categorize these methods from the most formal to the least formal. Table 11-1 presents a number of options.

The most appropriate method(s) will depend on you, your specific situation, the patient population you are caring for and the financial and human resources you have available. The important message is that you ask your patients what they want, and how they want it, and indicate to them that you are prepared, formally, to receive and act on the feedback.

Select a Supportive Environment

The challenge of starting a new patient care practice in an existing health care system, is a significant undertaking. Therefore, identify a practice setting that is conducive and friendly to your goal. Several decades of experience suggest that the retail, commercial pharmacy does not facilitate patient care, so this may not be the best place to start a patient care practice. The "business" of patient care requires a professional, clinical setting, dedicated scheduled time with the patient, proximity to other patient care providers and a payment structure for patient care services. The retail pharmacy does not provide these basic requirements and in addition presents a number of challenges. The number of prescriptions that need to be filled keeps increasing, staffing is continuously decreased to make the business more profitable, workplaces become busier and more noisy, and pharmacists are not able to provide care and improve their knowledge and skills each day. In contrast, working next to the physician and nurse in an ambulatory care clinic or medical home structure provides many of the necessary resources to be successful.

Therefore, choose your practice site carefully. The major criteria to consider are whether patients feel comfortable and whether high-quality pharmaceutical care can be provided in this setting. Be certain that the personnel with whom you work are supportive, friendly, and encouraging.

Understand the Resources You Will Need to Be Successful

You will need a number of resources to get started. The major categories include (1) competent practitioner(s), (2) good space that facilitates the delivery of a quality service, (3) access to professional manuscripts/books/guidelines, (4) support systems such as appointments, documentation, clinical decision rules, reporting, billing, (5) access to patients, and (6) access to the patients' health care providers. Most of these categories speak for themselves and are dealt with in other sections of this book. However, to put them in order of priority, the most important resource (as we have mentioned previously) is a well-qualified practitioner. Your practice will go nowhere unless you have someone who can provide a high-quality service. The second most important resource is access to patients, for without patients, you have no practice. The best access can be gained through physicians. Referrals are the most productive avenue to patients, especially at the start of your practice before patients are familiar with the service. The third most important resource will be your documentation system. If you choose well, your documentation system will allow you to make appointments with your patients, apply clinical decision rules, generate written documentation for your patient and the patient's prescribers, provide reports on your progress, and electronically bill for your services. Most electronic medical records are not able to perform these functions for the common medical services much less newer services like medication management. You will have to select a system that is specifically designed to support this practice.

Accommodate the Organization So It Can Help

You will probably build your service within an existing organizational structure. Although a number of pharmacists envision independent practices, it is unlikely that this structure can be supported as the health care system evolves to the medical home structure. All patient care practices are based on having access to patients, so your success will depend on being part of a clinic, a medical home, or a care facility of some type. This is not to say that independent practitioners cannot be successful; however, the key to starting a practice is to start where things are the easiest, where you are the most likely to succeed.

There are already a number of challenges to starting a "new" patient care service, so be sure to introduce as few additional challenges as you can. Utilizing existing structures will certainly facilitate your success.

Do not expect people to change to meet your needs—you are the *new* practitioner. The health care system has not accommodated a new practitioner very recently or very often, so do not expect it to change for you. Nurse practitioners have had to travel this same road. Some physicians may ignore you, nurses may prefer that you not be in their space, but neither of these reactions should be taken personally or interpreted as a negative reaction to pharmaceutical care. Physicians and nurses are busy, and they have important responsibilities. New personnel or new procedures interrupt their already complex schedule.

It will be necessary for you to understand the organization in which you practice so you can teach the personnel (physicians, nurses, support personnel) what they need to do in order to accommodate your work. You will save everyone a significant amount of time if you think through what impact you will have on each person's routine and prepare those involved.

KEY CLINICAL CONCEPTS

Expect to teach patients and other personnel what you do, over and over again.

You and your service are new to the health care system—they may have no intuitive knowledge of the practice because it has never existed before. Patients and health care personnel do not know what to expect and this makes people uncomfortable and defensive. This is not a reflection on you or pharmaceutical care, but is related to the difficulty people have accommodating change. Physicians, nurses, and patients already have their own ideas of what a pharmacist does and how a pharmacist works within the health care system. Becoming a pharmaceutical care practitioner changes this. You will need to change their fixed idea of what you do and how you can contribute. This will take continual effort on your part. Remember that all behavior in health care is learned through experience. Therefore, providing the service to *show* others what is involved is much more effective than talking about the practice.

The ultimate success of any practice will depend on the quality of the service delivered. Service is provided by people. Nothing will have greater impact on that service than the people who provide it. The commitment, cooperation, and participation of all practice personnel are essential for success. By practice personnel, we are referring to; the practitioner (pharmacist) who provides the care, the support staff (clerks, technicians, secretaries, etc.) who support the practitioner and make things happen on a day-to-day basis, and the practice manager who makes things happen usually on a long-term basis. Depending on the size of the practice, as well as the specific nature of the practice, the number and specific type of personnel may vary.

Many different factors concerning the practice personnel can influence the success of your practice, but none so much as communication. Both the ability to communicate and the willingness to communicate, with each other, and with patients, will be the best predictor of whether a practice will succeed. *Care means communication. Quality service means quality communication.*

A number of different sources present tips to communicate well.[1-3] All of these references are useful, but we would like to emphasize a few suggestions that are most relevant to building a pharmaceutical care practice.

- Make the technical content of your explanations appropriate for the receiver.
- Check with the receiver to determine that your intended message is being received.
- Do not be afraid of softer words that show emotion.
- Ask questions in a manner that facilitates answers with meaning.
- Answer questions effectively.
- Use the skills of empathy, listening, and managing conflict frequently.

These ideas appear too simple to be helpful. However, we have found that if these behaviors are stated explicitly and expected by all practice staff, they can have a significant impact on the success of your practice.

It takes all practice personnel to provide a quality service. A good place to begin is to make certain all personnel first understand the mission of the organization, or the service they are expected to deliver. Second, each person must understand her own role and the role of all others in the practice. The pharmacist practitioner is responsible for the day-to-day, moment-to-moment, decision-making concerning direct patient care and all that is associated with this responsibility. No other staff is allowed to interfere with the completion of these responsibilities.

The support staff is responsible for facilitating the patient care process including patient flow, work flow, meeting any other needs the patient might have, such as questions concerning hours of operation, access to services, eligibility for services, costs, billing procedures, scheduling, and other general information. The clear definition of responsibility and work flow will serve you well as you expand your practice.

Understanding the Demands of a Financially Viable Practice

Know the Costs of Doing Business

The following sections will address the two most fundamental questions asked by pharmacists when planning, designing, implementing, and evaluating medication management services:

1. What do I have to invest to get started?
2. What can I expect to get in return for providing these services?

We will answer these questions based on our experience of starting practices in many different settings. First, What do I have to invest to start providing pharmaceutical care?

It is often tempting to discuss the readily apparent tangible investments required to begin providing pharmaceutical care, but in practice, it is more useful to begin by recognizing and planning for the intangible investments. These can include substantial personal energies and commitments to change attitudes, mindsets, and priorities. Redirecting oneself from a product-dispensing–focused business to a patient-centered, need-focused activities can require substantial investment in personal time, thought, self-reflection, honesty, critical analysis, humility, and training. Although these personal investments are difficult to quantify, they are real and must be recognized, monitored, and supported throughout the initial implementation process.

A substantial investment in innovative thinking and risk taking must also be available during the initial implementation phase of pharmaceutical care services. New ideas, a clear vision of the practice and the service, plus the ability to communicate this new vision to others is essential in the implementation of this service. This direction must come from the practitioners providing that service. Waiting for a governmental agency, or regulating body to give their approval to start or waiting for a professional association to take the lead in patient care activities will not be effective.

Enthusiasm is another essential ingredient required to successfully begin providing medication management services. Again, initial enthusiasm to help patients identify and meet their drug-related needs must come from the individual practitioners. This enthusiasm will be apparent to patients, their families, colleagues, and other health care practitioners.

In addition, time and monetary investment in training is required to continually learn to better care for patients. As with all new patient care services, practitioners and patients must both learn how best to communicate, trust, and work together to ensure that all drug-related needs are being met.

The time and energy required may be even greater for the first few practitioners who decide to begin to offer pharmaceutical care in a given community. This is often the case because there are still numerous unknowns when trying something innovative in a new setting. Once the first generation has invested sufficient time and energy, and discovered the most effective methods to deliver medication management services, practitioners who follow can learn from these experiences and can begin more efficiently.

There are also several tangible investments that must be made. The first to be considered is personnel. Pharmacists and support personnel must be available to support the initiation of these services. In addition to pharmacists investing time in patient care activities, they must also plan to invest time to establish new professional relationships with local physicians, nurses, dentists, and other health care practitioners who need to be aware of the new service in order to refer patients to the pharmacist practitioner. Describing pharmaceutical care and medication management services to health care administrators in a particular geographic area will also require an initial investment of time. Local businesses and other employers should be contacted to inform them, their employees, and their families, of the availability and benefits of the new services.

The amount of direct face-to-face patient care time invested by the pharmacist(s) during the early stages of the new service will depend to a great extent on the goals and objectives set forth in the initial planning stages. Obviously, if the initial objective is to provide medication management services for all patients who present, it will require a much greater initial investment of the pharmacist's time than it will if the initial objective is to provide pharmaceutical care for two new patients each day. It is essential that when first offering medication management services the pharmacist must be provided sufficient opportunities to practice and improve patient care skills. The busiest patient care practitioners are the best.

The practice learning curve requires seeing and caring for a sufficient number of patients to continually develop and improve clinical skills. "Practice requires practice" should be the pharmaceutical care practitioner's mantra. Limiting the scope of medication management services too severely in the beginning can paradoxically slow or even prevent the service from becoming a success. Starting slowly in order to minimize pharmacist time investment will end in frustration and failure because the pharmacist will not make adequate progress on her learning curve, and patients will not be satisfied with the new service. Fewer than two to four patient encounters per day do not provide sufficient practice opportunities for pharmacists, and will represent a poor initial investment.

Other initial tangible investments that must be considered include computer hardware to support required patient care documentation as well as drug and medical information programs available through CD-ROM and Internet technology. Pharmaceutical care software license fees and support fees also need to be considered when initiating medication management services. Additional telephone line(s) may be required to support patient follow-up evaluations, computer modem, Internet access, or fax machines. Other initial tangible investment that may not already be available in an existing operation include current reference texts, signage to direct patient flow, a desk for the pharmacist's work space, and chairs for patients and pharmacists to use during consultations. Although a number of references are now available via the Internet, there is still a need for quick access to contemporary information. Chapter 10 lists the reference texts and handbooks and Smartphone applications we have found to be useful for practitioners.

The physical resources that must be considered are physical plant or space, furniture, telephones, computers, software programs, medical equipment, reference material, and any photocopy or fax machines you will need. The physical plant must meet all of the expectations suggested above for the "right" patient experience.

In order to effectively plan workable physical space to provide pharmaceutical care it is useful to consider how you want to deal with several requirements. These include

a. a semiprivate, quiet area for patient and pharmacist to meet. Keep in mind that for busy practices, each pharmacist providing pharmaceutical care will need a semiprivate area to practice. Providing some fully private space to meet with patients with very special needs is also important. However, most patients prefer a comfortable, open, yet semiprivate area in which others cannot directly view or overhear conversation. Some patients prefer to remain standing if the interaction with the pharmacist is only going to require a few minutes, but some patients need to sit, or prefer to sit, during this encounter.

b. a neat, clean surface in the patient–pharmacist meeting area. Be mindful to avoid leaving clutter, stacks of paper, office supplies, in the semiprivate patient care area. These will be distracting to patients and diminish the patient's confidence that the pharmacist's full attention is on the patient. A clock is useful to help both patients and pharmacists keep track of time spent in consultation. Also having paper and pen available for the patient to use is helpful and often reassuring for patients to feel that you really want them to understand, remember, and participate.

c. a desk and work space for the pharmacist. This space will be necessary to research patient questions, access drug information, and complete documentation.

d. computer system for patient care documentation with full printing capabilities. This system should also provide CD-ROM capabilities for drug information and medical information software and provide Internet access to medical, drug, and other health-related information.

e. consideration should be given to the space provided for patients when they are waiting to meet with the pharmacist. This space can be useful to display samples of health-related information available from your service, educational videotapes, samples of self-care diagnostic procedures, products, and references concerning herbal, nutritional, and other forms of alternative therapeutic approaches to patient needs.

The major criteria to be considered in designing your physical plant in your particular setting is whether your patients feel comfortable, and whether you are able to provide quality pharmaceutical care in this setting. If you can accomplish these two objectives, then you have the correct physical space.

The second question commonly asked about starting a practice is, what level of payment can be expected, or, is this practice financially viable? It certainly takes time and effort to establish a practice that is financially viable. It can take up to 2 years to work into a full-time practice capable of supporting a practitioner, depending on the rate at which patients are added to the practice. Let us consider more specifically what is required to be successful financially.

Building a Stable Revenue Base

KEY CLINICAL CONCEPTS

In order to be successful, you will eventually need to provide care to a minimum of 10 to 15 patients per day.

This activity represents a combination of new patients and established patients for follow-up evaluations. A single practitioner with this volume of service would have between 2400 and 3750 patient encounters annually, which represent a practice of approximately 1500 to 2000 patients at any time. This volume of patients is a full-time commitment to patient care.

In a patient care service, the primary method for generating revenue is to provide care to patients. However in a new practice, a significant amount of work is required to recruit new patients. Obviously, each patient will need to learn what you have to offer, and the patient will have to learn how she can benefit from the service.

There is a natural tendency to want to print brochures, send mailings, or create posters to announce the service. Although these marketing approaches may help along the way, this is not the usual way a patient care service successfully expands. Patient care is too personal for these generic approaches.

> **KEY CLINICAL CONCEPTS**
>
> The most effective way to expand your service is to provide the care and allow the patients themselves to market you through word of mouth and reputation. This is how most medical services become successful.

You are the "*product*," and your patients will be the most effective means for "*selling*" you to others. This takes some time, so be realistic in your expectations.

Physician referrals help to recruit patients at a faster rate if you are in a clinic or hospital setting. Physician referrals can introduce you to patients who are in need of the service in a more efficient manner. However, there are a number of "rules" you must be aware of with regard to physician referrals.

1. Referrals are a two-way street. Professionals function by depending upon each other. When a practitioner refers a patient to another, it is expected that patients are also referred back to the original practitioner. This is the only way a referral system is maintained.
2. Physicians will refer patients who are more severely ill, more complicated, and more challenging than the average patient. You will have to plan for this. The workload associated with referred patients is usually greater than patients who identify the need for the service themselves. Referrals on average will take more time and require more follow-up.
3. Referrals can seldom be relied upon as the sole source for new patients. Referrals take some control out of your practice, and you must plan accordingly. Referrals are unpredictable. Therefore, it is important to recruit a steady, consistent clientele that is supplemented by referred patients. For this reason, it is probably not a good idea to build an entire practice around referrals if you are a generalist practitioner. However, referrals can become more predictable and stable if you are in a practice situation that involves collaborative practice agreements or joint practices with specific physicians.[6] Collaborative practice agreements, which

are becoming very common in practice today, help to identify groups of patients that will be referred to you as a portion of their comprehensive care.

Recruiting patients is probably the most time- and energy-consuming activity required to establish a new practice. This activity can be made more manageable if you are successful at contracting for services to a specific patient population. There are a number of additional mechanisms to recruit patients. One is to provide incentives to patients. This might include waiving a copayment for the service or offering a discount for the initial assessment. Or, you may be in a situation where you can provide care for a captive audience, such as all of the employees of your company, or a self-insured population.

When you begin your practice, it will be helpful if you establish a specific date on which you will begin. Establish hours for your service and commit to them. It is necessary for patients and colleagues to know where you will be so they can refer patients to you. You can begin by establishing *clinic hours* for 2 to 3 days a week, and as the service expands, add extra hours as needed.

Determine the number of patients you will need to maintain a viable practice and how long will it take to get there. The key to a successful practice is to add new patients continually so the practice can become financially viable over the long term. Providing care for numerous patients on a continuous basis requires an efficient and effective organization.

REALIZE THE REWARDS

It is impossible to provide care to patients long term unless payment for the services is realized. In some cases a pharmacist is paid a salary and medication management services are defined as a responsibility of the position. However, more frequently the pharmacist has to justify the addition of the service and requires payment for the service just as physicians and dentists do. Recognition and payment for these services have been relatively slow and challenging. However, in the United States now both the federal and state governments are paying for the service, as are a number of private insurance programs and employers. As soon as medication management services become a standard of care for patients the issue of payment should be resolved. We trust this day is not far away.

Payment Mechanisms

The primary mechanism for a practitioner to generate revenue is to provide direct patient services. Therefore, the time you spend on other activities such as *administrative functions* will interfere with becoming financially viable. Successful practitioners delegate all activities other than patient care to someone else, so that their time is dedicated to seeing patients and generating revenue.

Providing a financially viable service means providing people with the service they need, the way they want it. It means getting paid for that service. You will need a mechanism for billing. Patient care providers are reimbursed in very structured predetermined ways. The most widely used approach to health services billing in the United States is the resource-based relative value scale (RBRVS).

The issue of payment becomes much simpler once patient care is separated completely from the drug product. It is then possible to critically examine the approaches being used by other health care providers who are being paid for patient care services. However, in order to do this, it is necessary to first establish the objectives that the "optimal" reimbursement mechanism must meet. The following objectives for the "ideal" reimbursement system will:

- reimburse the pharmacist for *all* the work performed, regardless of whether or not a prescription is involved.
- be based on the complexity of the patient and not the practitioner.
- include all practice settings, allow for payment in community, hospital, long-term care, or wherever pharmaceutical care may be provided.
- be consistent with the practice so that the philosophy of practice and the philosophy of reimbursement do not interfere with each other.
- be consistent with the approach used to pay other health care practitioners for patient care.

With this as a conceptual framework, all available approaches which could possibly meet these objectives, were considered. Three candidates were identified: the fee-for-service system, the capitation method, and the RBRVS approach. We will discuss each and explain why the RBRVS approach was selected as the most appropriate payment mechanism for the practice of pharmaceutical care.

Fee-for-Service

The fee-for-service system is a traditional, well-established approach that has been in use for many years. A practitioner is paid based on the number and type of services provided. Each time a service is delivered, a charge is generated. The decision to provide a service is based on decisions made by the practitioner, for a specific patient. Payment has traditionally been made with the expectation that a service is performed only if it is necessary, and appropriate, and therefore justified.

This approach has a number of limitations associated with its use. First, every effort is currently being made to eliminate this system of payment because it has proven to be a very expensive method and encourages practitioners to provide more services than necessary in order to receive higher levels of payment.

It is somewhat short-sighted to select a reimbursement system that has gone out-of-favor, and would appear to have a short life. It is difficult to argue for reimbursement of a brand new service, using an inefficient payment system.

Another limitation of the fee-for-service system is that it does not meet a number of the objectives outlined above. For example, if all the work of the pharmacist is to be reimbursed, then each and every activity of the pharmacist has to be argued as a reimbursable service. This appears to be a tremendous task, especially in the politicoeconomic environment of cost cutting and service minimization. Nor does fee-for-service focus on what the patient needs; instead, the focus is on what the practitioner does. We know that this is not the direction the health care system is moving, so a system that promotes practitioner-driven reimbursement has little chance of surviving in the long term.

It is less clear as to whether fee-for-service is able to accommodate the practitioner in all practice settings. Because practitioner-driven activities are quite dependent on practice setting, especially in the traditional sense of pharmacy, it is likely that this would require approval of activities performed at one practice setting at a time.

The philosophy of pharmaceutical care centers on the patient and her drug therapy needs, not the practitioner. This is inconsistent with the fee-for-service approach. Caring requires we bring whatever resources are necessary to meet a patient's needs, regardless of whether they are on the reimbursement list of services or not. Moreover, pharmaceutical care involves a list of practitioner activities that have little history, thus each one would have to be negotiated on its own merit. This is a difficult challenge for a completely new service.

Finally, as was previously mentioned, this approach is being used less and less by other health care providers. Whether it is managed care organizations or the federal government, the majority of decision makers in the health care industry today are trying to minimize the services paid by fee-for-service. We should also reiterate here that pharmacists have had a long history of not succeeding with negotiating this form of reimbursement for its services. One can reasonably conclude that this does not appear to be a viable alternative for pharmaceutical care.

The Capitation Method

Capitation payment is an increasingly popular approach with which to purchase health care services. This payment method awards the provider a predetermined amount of payment, for a pre-set level of services, paid out on a per patient basis, for a fixed period of time. For example, a dentist may be paid $10.00 per month, per patient, for preventive care, to be re-negotiated after 12 months. Usually, the capitation payment method has significant financial risk built into the contract, for both the provider and the purchaser. For example, the dentist would be paid the fixed amount for all patients, whether they used few services (less than $10.00 per month), or many services (greater than $10.00 per month). The risk to the provider is that too many patients would request more services than the $10.00 per month would reimburse, and money would be lost. The risk to the payer is that too few patients would request so few services that the payer would be purchasing services not received. Usually both the loss and the profit are shared by provider and payer. The specific risk assumed by each is negotiated on a contract specific basis.

This payment method appears to meet many of the objectives outlined earlier in this chapter. All of the activities, in this case those associated with preventive dental care, are reimbursed by the payer. In addition, payment focuses on the patient and not on the practitioner's activities. Therefore, pharmaceutical care would appear to be accommodated by this payment system. The practice setting has little to do with a "per patient" method of reimbursement, and more and more practitioners are being paid with a capitation method. Why not select the capitation method of payment for pharmaceutical care?

Although pharmacists may be paid on a capitation basis in the future, there is presently too much risk associated with this method. A successful capitation system requires that the pharmacist be familiar with all the costs associated with providing the service, the usage rates for the service, the variability in usage rates, and the impact the service can have on the patient. Ultimately, data generated in practice, gathered from the documentation system, will provide the information necessary to design a successful capitation system for pharmaceutical care; but in the mean time, a different system is required.

The Resource-based Relative Value Scale System

The method of payment based on the RBRVS became widely known and used in January of 1992 when it became the new Medicare physician payment system.[7] The federal government now uses this system to pay for a broad range of services.

The basic principles underlying the RBRVS are not new. Physicians and insurers have been using this system since the first relative value scale was developed by the California Medical Association in 1956. In an RBRVS, services are ranked according to the relative costs of the resources required to provide them. For example, if Service A consumed twice as many resources (time, overhead expense, difficulty) as Service B, then Service A would have a relative value of twice as much as Service A. The relative value scale then must be multiplied by a dollar conversation factor to become a payment schedule.[8,9]

The data that led to OBRA 89, (the Federal legislation that enacted the Medicare physician payment reform provisions) were generated in a national study that began in 1985 at Harvard University. The study funded the development of RBRVS for almost 30 physician specialties (in two different phases of the study). The American Medical Association (AMA) was intimately involved in this study, under subcontract from Harvard, to facilitate general medicine's "buy-in" to the system. The AMA eventually accepted the results of the study and backed the development of a national system of payment for physician services based on an RBRVS system. This system comprises three components: (1) the relative physician work involved in providing a service, (2) the practice expenses, and (3) practice liability insurance costs.[9]

There are other factors that were built into the provision. For example, a 5-year transition period was accepted (beginning in 1992), geographic differences were taken into account when calculating practice expenses, specialty differentials in payment for the same service were eliminated, and a process for determining the annual update in the conversion factor was defined. Suffice it to say that a tremendous amount of time, energy, research, and discussion went into the development of this system for physician payment. This system has been broadly applied to include payment for nonphysician practitioners' services, including

- physical and occupational therapists;
- physician assistants;
- nurse practitioners and clinical nurse specialists in certain settings;
- certified registered nurse anesthetists;
- nurse midwives;
- clinical psychologists; and
- clinical social workers.

RBRVS applied to pharmaceutical care

In 1993, the RBRVS system was adapted to pharmaceutical care to determine both practitioner workload and reimbursement amounts.[11,12] The pharmaceutical care reimbursement grid was developed and is described in

Figure 11-2. This use of the RBRVS system for medication management services is based on a "crosswalk" between the workload (patient complexity) values for each patient encounter and the Current Procedural Terminology (CPT) (time-based) codes approved in 2005 for use by pharmacists in billing for medication management services.

These CPT codes were the result of a request by the Pharmacist Services Technical Advisory Coalition, to the AMA, the organization that establishes and approves billing codes for practitioners in the United States.[13] Medication therapy management (MTM) codes have been assigned CPT numbers that pharmacists can use for billing, and are included in the AMA's CPT manual since 2008.[14] It is noteworthy, that the definition of the service used in this national billing guide requires that MTM services be separate from commercial, dispensing functions. The CPT manual published by the AMA[14] defines MTM services as:

> "medication therapy management services describe face-to-face patient assessment and intervention as appropriate, by a pharmacist upon request. MTMS is provided to optimize the response to medications or to manage treatment related medication interactions or complications. MTM includes the following documented elements: review of the pertinent patient history, medication profile (prescription and non prescription), and recommendations for improving health outcomes and treatment compliance. These codes are not to be used to describe the provision of product specific information at the point of dispensing or any other routine dispensing related activities."

The MTM codes provided for MTM are:

99605 MTM service(s) provided by a pharmacist, individual, face-to-face, with patient, with assessment and intervention if provided; initial 15 minutes new patient

99606 Initial 15 minutes, established patient

+ 99607 Each additional 15 minutes, list separately in addition to code for primary service. Use 99607 in conjunction with 99605 and 99606.

In the Medication Management RBRVS grid (Figure 11-2), there are five levels of payment, similar to other RBRVS systems. The resources required, the complexity of the patient's case, and the levels of reimbursement are determined by three components:

- Number of medical conditions being managed with pharmacotherapy
- Number of drug therapy problems identified and resolved
- Number of medications involved

Medication therapy management services: Resource-based relative value scale					
Level of service provided	Level #1	Level #2	Level #3	Level #4	Level #5
Assessment of drug-related needs	Problem-focused 1 Medication	Expanded problem 2 Medications	Detailed 3-5 Medications	Expanded detailed 6-8 Medications	Comprehensive ≥9 Medications
Identification drug therapy problems	Problem-focused 0 Drug therapy problems	Expanded problem 1 Drug therapy problem	Detailed 2 Drug therapy problems	Expanded detailed 3 Drug therapy problems	Comprehensiv ≥4 Drug therapy problems
Complexity of care planning & follow-up evaluation	Straightforward 1 Medical condition	Straightforward 1 Medical condition	Low complexity 2 Medical conditions	Moderate complexity 3 Medical conditions	High complexity ≥4 Medical conditions
CPT codes	99605 initial encounter with a new patient (or 99606 for all follow-up encounters)	99605 (or 99606) and 99607	99605 (or 99606) and 2 × 99607	99605 (or 99606) and 3 × 99607	99605 (or 99606) and ≥4 × 99607
Face-to-face time	15 minutes	16-30 minutes	31-45 minutes	46-60 minutes	≥60 minutes
Amount initial follow-up	$52 $34	$76 $58	$100 $82	$124 $106	$148 $130

Figure 11-2 The pharmaceutical care reimbursement grid based on RBRVS.[11,12] Reimbursement amounts ($) based on the Minnesota Medicaid Program.

Across the top of the grid are displayed the five *levels of complexity.*

Payment by the RBRVS is calculated at one of these levels. The payment level in this system is based on documented patient need and is calculated to be at the lowest level where all the key components are met. The levels of need vary from *straightforward* at Level 1 to the *high complexity* at Level 5. The quantitative criteria are described on the grid.

Example When a patient is taking two medications, has no drug therapy problems, and one medical condition, the encounter is designated as Level 1.

Remember, the level of complexity of the encounter depends on the documentation and is designated at the lowest level where *all three criteria* are met. The variables that go into the calculation of the level of patient need are presented down the left hand side of the grid in Figure 11-2. Let us discuss how these variables integrate to create the level of patient need.

Example   When a patient has four medical conditions that require six medications and who had two drug therapy problems that were identified and resolved, the encounter is designated as Level 3. One of the strengths of the RBRVS is that it is self-auditing.

Example   If the practitioner documents that a patient has seven medical conditions and is taking nine drugs, and one drug therapy problem is identified and resolved, then the patient's needs are designated at Level 2.

This scale always yields a patient need at the lowest level of the three documented criteria. This internal logic promotes comprehensive documentation, yet rewards efficiency. If the practitioner documents a patient's needs to be two medical conditions and two drug therapy problems involving two prescription medications, the patient's needs would be Level 2. However, if this same patient also was taking daily aspirin to prevent a myocardial infarction and the practitioner documented this additional preventive pharmacotherapy, then the patient's needs would be increased to Level 3.

The pharmaceutical care practitioner, at each of the five complexity levels, provides a different intensity of work, but the nature of the work is the same at *all* levels. The *work* includes the following:

- Assessment of drug-related needs
- Identification of drug therapy problems
- The nature of the risks and complexity reflected in care planning and follow-up evaluation.

We will discuss each of the components of the work. This work and the relative resources required to provide the service are what creates the five levels of care.

Determining the assessment of drug-related needs

The RBRVS recognizes five different levels of work. A major criterion determining the different levels is the number of medications the patient is taking. This affects the amount of information necessary to provide pharmaceutical care and the amount of data integration required. The most straightforward workup is a *problem-focused workup* and involves a single form of drug therapy. The next level is an *expanded problem-focused workup* and is appropriate when one or two medications are required. With three or four active medications, the practitioner must conduct a *detailed workup*, with five to eight, an *expanded detailed workup.* Finally, when a patient requires nine or more medications *a comprehensive workup* of drug therapy is required.

KEY CLINICAL CONCEPTS

The RBRVS system is based on the documented patient need as determined by each patient's diseases, drug therapy problems, and medications.

It is not specific to any particular disease state or drug product. The five levels of service encompass the wide variation in skill, effort, time, responsibility, and knowledge required for the prevention and resolution of drug therapy problems. In the medical system of RVRBS, the key components in selecting the appropriate level are history, examination, and medical decision-making (diagnosis). In the pharmaceutical care system of RBRVS, the key components in selecting the appropriate level are the number of medical conditions being managed with drug therapies, the number of drug therapy problems resolved, and the number of medications involved in both.[11,12] The specific values for the number of medical conditions, drug therapy problems, and drugs involved for each level of service on the pharmaceutical care reimbursement grid were based on the findings from the Minnesota Pharmaceutical Care Project.[11]

Example Examine a case involving a 52-year-old female patient who was being treated with sertraline (Zoloft) for major depression, was managing her hypothyroidism with levothyroxine (Synthroid), had long-standing hypertension controlled with metoprolol and hydrochlorothiazide, and was also taking aspirin daily to prevent a stroke or heart attack. If the practitioner identified and resolved two drug therapy problems for this patient (dose of sertraline was too low to provide effective control of depressive symptoms, and patient required potassium supplements to prevent hypokalemia), then this would represent a Level 3. This patient's needs were determined based on four medical conditions (treatment of depression, hypothyroidism, hypertension, and prevention of MI/stroke), six medications (sertraline, levothyroxine, metoprolol, hydrochlorothiazide, potassium chloride, aspirin), and two drug therapy problems. Note that if the practitioner had documented that this patient was hypokalemic, the case would contain five medical conditions, but would not change the RBRVS level.

If the practitioner did not decide that this same patient needed daily potassium supplementation, then the case would represent Level 2 (four medical conditions, five medications, one drug therapy problem). If at the next follow-up visit, the practitioner evaluated the patient's hypertension and depression and found them both to be stable, but did decide that the patient required additional drug therapy in the form of daily potassium chloride supplements to treat hypokalemia, then at this later visit the case would represent Level 2 (three medical conditions evaluated, involving four medications, and one drug therapy problem).

Examine this same patient at her third follow-up evaluation, if the practitioner documents that her depression and hypertension are stable, her preventive aspirin continues to be effective, her hypokalemia is improved, and she has no drug therapy problems at this time, it would be Level 1 (four medical conditions, five medications, and no drug therapy problems).

Determining complexity: number of drug therapy problems

The complexity of the assessment process follows the same descriptive categories as presented above for the levels of the workup. However, the variable of interest is the number of drug therapy problems identified and resolved. Each drug therapy problem requires a sophisticated decision-making process for its identification and resolution (see Chapter 5).

Determining the nature of the risks reflected in care planning and follow-up evaluation

The number of active medical conditions or illnesses managed with drug therapies determines the level of risk associated with the care of the patient. Clearly, number and type of medications in addition to the number and type of drug therapy problems also represent risk, but these contribute in their own way to the level of reimbursement.

Therefore, this variable depends on the number of active medical problems experienced by the patient and requiring pharmacotherapy. Each medical condition will require that the practitioner establish the goals of therapy and establish an appropriate care plan with the patient to accomplish the goals. In addition, it will be necessary to evaluate the outcomes at a follow-up visit.

Time: determining the amount of face-to-face time spent with the patient

Time is not a major criterion used in most RBRVS calculations. Whenever time is described within the RBRVS system, it is considered to be an *average* of the face-to-face time required to provide that level of service by the *average* practitioner. In the case of MTM services in the United States, the CPT codes associated with the various levels of service are proportioned based on 15-minute (face-to-face) time intervals. Data generated from widespread provision of these services will be required to eventually determine the relative resources required for each level of medication management services.

> **Example** If the RBRVS estimate for Level 2 was 15 minutes, and you can provide that level of service in 10 to –12 minutes, it reflects your efficiency. If that same level of service requires 18 to 25 minutes of face-to-face time, this also reflects on your efficiency. In some situations, time estimates are useful because practitioners can document special situations when excess time was required and thereby increase the service level by one. In these unusual circumstances, a *modifier* is used and additional documentation is necessary[10]. The specific times associated with each level of payment are averages representing a range of times, which may be higher or lower depending on actual practice circumstances, and the skill level of the practitioner.

It is important to note that time refers only to *face-to-face* time. Face-to-face time is defined as that time the practitioner spends with the patient and/or family. This includes the time in which the practitioner performs such tasks as making an assessment, identifying drug therapy problems, preparing a care plan, and providing the patient with individualized information.

Practitioners will also spend time doing work before and after the face-to-face encounter with the patient, performing such tasks as reviewing records and tests, arranging for follow-up services, and communicating with other professionals. This time is not included in the face-to-face time estimate component of the RBRVS.

Calculating the reimbursement amount

The reimbursement dollar amount is calculated based on the variables described above, and reflects the resources required to provide documented care at each level. The actual dollar amount assigned to Level 2 is the sum of all the resources used to deliver care at this level. The data for calculating this amount is presently unique to each practice site until enough practices are established to develop a national database. Figure 11-2 includes reimbursement amounts ($) from the Minnesota Medicaid Program. Since being approved, the average patient encounter has been billed out for approximately $90–$100 using this RBRVS billing grid.

Table 11-2 Distribution of patient complexity using the Resource-based Relative Value System

Complexity level	Number of patient encounters	Percentage of patient encounters
1	15,264	30.4
2	13,623	27.2
3	9,066	18.1
4	6,527	13.0
5	5,662	11.3
Totals	**50,142**	**100**

RBRVS as a workload measurement tool

The RBRVS has been functioning since 1993 and has been used to generate charges for care delivered to over 100,000 patients. In this edition of the text, we have been illustrating clinical and management points based on data from the Assurance Enterprise Database, which included 22,694 patients with 50,142 documented encounters. In addition to a billing structure, the system functions as a workload measurement tool. Because each level of care demands and consumes different amounts of resources, it is important to be aware of the distribution of patients by complexity of their drug-related needs within your practice. Table 11-2 is the distribution by level of complexity of 50,142 patient encounters for medication management services.

It is important to realize that the majority of patients seen in a generalist practice are Levels 1, 2, and 3. It should be emphasized here that a patient with no drug therapy problems still requires an assessment by the pharmaceutical care practitioner to ensure that all goals of therapy continue to be met and that positive outcomes are achieved. Its corollary is the dentist who sees patients every 6 months to assure good oral hygiene is being maintained and that no dental problems have developed.

PROFESSIONAL SATISFACTION

In almost all cases, pharmacists' job satisfaction immediately improves, once they actively and directly become involved in patient care. Taking care of patients and experiencing with them improved outcomes, enhanced health status, and increased patient loyalty are important positive rewards realized from the provision of pharmaceutical care. Because many of the pharmacist's activities are clinically engaging practitioners feel that they are contributing in a meaningful way to their patients' quality of life.

Professional recognition from peers, colleagues, physicians, nurses and other health care providers is also enhanced through the practice of pharmaceutical care. Through the provision of pharmaceutical care, physicians recognize the improvement in patient care as well as patients' understanding of their drug therapies. This leads to a new more professionally satisfying relationship between prescribers and pharmacists. When both consider their primary responsibility to be the improvement of the patient's health, teamwork and collaboration logically follow. Rather than numerous phone calls and questions concerning refill authorizations, product availability, generic substitutions and formulary regulations required in the dispensing operation, pharmaceutical care requires a different interaction between prescriber, pharmacists, and other health care professionals. The patient's drug-related needs become the "nucleus" of all questions, comments and inquiries, for those actually providing care.

> **KEY CLINICAL CONCEPTS**
>
> Practitioners providing services to patients discover that physician and nurse colleagues will refer patients to them in order to be confident that all of the patient's drug-related needs are being met and that drug therapy problems are being identified, resolved, and prevented.

WRITING THE BUSINESS PLAN

It takes time to build a practice, for many reasons: (1) you will not be very efficient at first; (2) patients need to learn what your practice is and what it can do for them; (3) you need to earn the trust of colleagues; and (4) you will have to learn how to make the patient care system work for you. Physicians and dentists require 2 to 3 years to build a clientele of significant size. Because pharmaceutical care is a new service in an existing health care system, you can expect that it may take even longer. One of the quickest ways to ensure that your expectations for your practice are realistic is to write a business plan for your practice.

Establishing a new practice is similar to starting a business, and there is a specific, clearly delineated process involved. In addition to a number of legal steps that must be taken, there are a number of planning activities that must occur. Developing the business plan is one of the first steps in starting a new practice. It describes the service, the product, the market, the people, and the financial needs. The business plan is an important step because it helps the practitioner determine the feasibility and desirability of pursuing the steps necessary to start a practice. If it is necessary to seek outside financing for the new service, then the business plan is an important sales tool for raising capital from outside investors.

Most of today's medical and nursing practitioners have not had to take the time and energy to create a business plan because their *new* practices were extensions of existing group practices. However, because developing a pharmaceutical care practice is truly a new service, a business plan is required to improve the likelihood of success. It is most likely that you will join a medical practice or create a joint practice with other practitioners. A business plan will communicate your vision of the practice to those with whom you wish to work. It is the most common way to communicate your ideas concisely, for the purpose of establishing a new practice.

Business plans vary but contain a core structure that describes the service, the competition, the economic benchmarks, and the expected return on investment. The list below represents the basic sections of a typical business plan for the new service.

1. Executive summary
2. General description of the service
3. Marketing plans
4. Operational plans
5. Management and organization
6. Structure and capitalization
7. Milestones
8. Financial plan

There are many references, consulting groups, and computer software programs that can help you construct your business plan, but the plan must be yours: you must write it and you must *own* it. It is often helpful to have a professional assist you once you have drafted your plan. However, you must be able to describe your business plan to someone else within a moment's notice. Business plans represent a value proposition. Therefore, you need to consider what patients and/or colleagues value. The following outlines the major contents of a business plan to introduce a new service.[15] Most business plans include a one to two page executive summary describing the major components of the plan.

Executive summary

- Description of the service you will be offering
- Description of the problem you will be solving
- The market potential
- Why your service is the best answer to the problem
- Major milestones for growth of your service
- Financial summary

General description of the service

- Fundamental activities and nature of the service you offer
- The mission statement
- The problem you are addressing
- The objectives of your service
- Who is your client?
- Where will you offer the service?
- How is your service used?
- What are the unique features of the service?
- In what stage of development is the service? How ready is it for operation?

Marketing plans

- What are the factors that establish demand for your service?
- What are your relevant target markets?
- Which markets are of primary importance?
- What marketing strategies will be employed?
- How will you organize and implement your marketing plans?
- How will you make your service available to your clients?
- What is your pricing structure?
- What advertising and/or public relations campaign is needed?
- What is the impact of regulation and laws on your service?
- What are your forecasts of market share and growth?

Competition

- What is the relevant competition to your service?
- What are future sources of competition for your service?
- What impact will competition likely have?

Barriers to entry

- Do any legal, copyright, trademark, license barriers exist?
- Do you have consultants available in pharmaceutical care practice?
- What is the lead time to initiating the service?

Operational plans

- How will your service remain state-of-the-art?
- What continued development efforts are planned?
- What are the capital requirements to provide the service?
- What are the labor requirements to provide the service?
- What suppliers are required to support the service?

Management and operations

- What is the background of the key individuals in your organization?
- Who will be the key employees and/or support staff?
- Who will direct the service?
- What key advisors will be available?
- Develop an organizational chart
- Develop a policy statement of how support staff will be selected and trained

Structure and capitalization

- What legal form will this service company take?
- How much capital is needed?
- Describe the manner of financial participation or investment

Milestones

- Describe the first test market
- Calculate break-even performance
- Quantify expansion steps

Financial plan

- Describe the set of assumptions on which projections are based
- Project income statements for 5 years
- Project detailed cash flow statements for 2 years

The executive summary of your business plan is important because it serves as the primary document that others will evaluate. The content of the business plan serves to support what is presented in the executive summary. Business plans are similar to care plans in that both are proposals designed to achieve a specific set of goals. Your plan should clearly describe the value others are going to place upon your service. Be specific about the problem your service solves for people. Is it drug therapy problems? Is it minimizing confusion about drug therapies? Is it increasing confidence in the effectiveness and safety of medications?

Why does your customer, client, or patient need your service? What are the top three benefits of your service? What are the top three objections to the service? Market research can help identify what your intended clients want and what they may not want from your service. The time and energy spent in researching, planning, and writing a business plan is a valuable investment to help ensure the success of your new patient care service.

GET STARTED

Discussions, planning, and worrying, do not take care of patients. There is really only one way to change a practice paradigm, and that is to actually begin to take care of patients' drug-related needs and stick with it. Every pharmacy practitioner who has successfully changed her practice can point to a day of change, that is, the day in which she actually started providing pharmaceutical care and accepted the responsibility for patient outcomes.

Choose a day. By this time you will have described the new mission, planned with staff, and acquired at least some of the necessary primary resources, such as semiprivate patient care area, and a documentation system.

Let all the staff know that it will be an important day. This first day will serve not only as the beginning for accounting and management purposes, but everyone involved will constantly use the first day as a comparison with future developments and improvements. Attempts to identify progress usually begin here.

Begin by providing pharmaceutical care for a minimum of two new patients each day. This will provide a constant stream of new patients required to build a practice and provide the direct patient experience necessary for growth. As in all new endeavors, practice requires doing something over and over in order to gain mastery. It is very important to remain committed to providing care for at least two new patients every day. During this early stage of development it is often tempting to "skip" a few patients, or a few days because "things are hectic." Such temptation must be resisted. Continuity of care begins with a fundamental understanding of sustained effort.

After much consternation, many pharmacists begin where they are most comfortable, with patients with whom they are most familiar. However, it must be emphasized here that if the patients are frequent visitors to the pharmacy or clinic, then they may be complex individuals with many medical conditions and a large number of drug-related needs. This is not always the best place to start. When first developing pharmaceutical care skills, it is reasonable to begin with uncomplicated medical conditions and uncomplicated drug therapies. Usually the best rule is, just start.

Two to four new patients each day represents a rapidly growing workload due to the follow-up evaluations required for every patient. Some patients will require numerous follow-up evaluations even for acute problems and those with chronic disorders (the majority of patients) will require constant, repeated, follow-up evaluations on a long-term basis. This has a direct impact on practice workload. It is important to keep good, clear, and concise documentation, as the work of a practice can grow exponentially.

Let new patients know how much they will be charged for this new service. There are several ways to accomplish this. First, by charging them directly the same way other general practitioners have done for decades. Without a charge, services are always undervalued. The practitioner should present new patients with an invoice for the service. Some practitioners feel they should not require reimbursement until they have developed their new skills, and so they display the value on the invoice and "zero it out" indicating that it will usually cost $120.00, but this time there will be no charge. By displaying the usual and customary fee, you are changing patients' expectations of payment. People pay for services that they consider valuable and important to them.

After 2 to 4 weeks of active practice, it is important to meet with all of the staff, and discuss how they think the new service is being accepted by patients, and solicit their suggestions. Review patient care documentation to see that it is complete and concise. If the practice has multiple pharmacists, discuss the problems and successes of each individual. Collaboration with staff is important and group meetings can lead to the exchange of important information. As areas of improvement are identified, staff activities can be directed to better support the provision of pharmaceutical care. This process is repeated at week 8 and week 12.

After 12 weeks of building a practice, a summary of data should be presented to all staff. This should easily be accomplished through your documentation system. It will help everyone to understand the number of patients receiving care, the age distribution, the most common indications for drug therapy, the number and types of drug therapy problems identified and resolved. Additionally, a summary of the number of drug therapy regimens that have been changed, as well as the number and costs of unnecessary clinic visits, nursing home admissions, or hospitalizations that have been prevented should be completed. These data, although very preliminary, provide the essential feedback for evaluating progress and making changes where necessary.

Starting a new practice with a new service and probably a new practitioner is not easy. It will take a significant amount of time and effort, commitment, dedication, and just plain hard work. It will be worth it, though. Patients who need medication management services are everywhere and the service works. It is our responsibility to learn to provide quality services and to learn how to deliver them effectively. We hope this book has helped toward that end.

SUMMARY

After developing the practice of pharmaceutical care, teaching it and establishing practices to provide the service throughout the past 25 years, we have made a number of observations.[16] We thought that as a summary of this chapter, it would be fitting to share these observations with you. Building, managing, and growing a new patient care service within existing health care systems requires that a number of things must change. Some old beliefs are discovered to no longer apply.

Following is the list of items we consider to be "truisms" because of the extensive evidence available to support the observations. We hope the list is helpful as you develop your own practice.

What we have learned about the *practice*:

- There can be only one universal patient care practice for the profession of pharmacy.
- All practitioners are judged by the number of patients cared for and by the clinical outcomes achieved in their practice.
- Patient care is delivered and evaluated based on clearly described practice standards.
- The closer the pharmacist works with the physician, the more successful the practice.
- The dispensing (technical) functions must be completely separate from the patient care practice functions.

What we have learned from *patients*:

- Patients love this practice—they consistently rate the practice favorably—98% of the time.
- Patients have to "learn" how to engage in a new practice such as pharmaceutical care.
- Patients are not the primary cause of nonadherence.
- A majority of nonadherent behavior is valid (ineffective/unsafe medications).

What we have learned about *pharmacists*:

- Pharmacists must be explicitly taught the practice of pharmaceutical care—complete with the philosophy of practice, the patient care process, and the practice management system, it is not intuitive nor do pharmacists "already know it."
- Pharmacists are not familiar with the "rules" of patient care. The "rules" of patient care are written by physicians, they are non-negotiable and pharmacists have to practice by them to participate in patient care.
- The key to training is learning the practice of pharmaceutical care first, therapeutics second.
- Pharmacists cannot become great practitioners alone. A "community of practitioners" is required to provide the needed collaboration and feedback.
- Pharmacists who learn to manage patients with the 10 most common medical conditions are able to care for over 50% of the drug therapy problems seen in practice.
- Preparing pharmacists is the rate-limiting step to pharmaceutical care being practiced on a large scale.
- Pharmacists have to understand and learn to apply the principles of pharmacology well enough to manage patients' drug therapies.
- The busiest practitioners are the best practitioners.

What we have learned from *physicians*:

- Physicians recognize and endorse the comprehensive practice of pharmaceutical care.
- Physicians want to know who is competent to deliver it and how they gain access to the service for their patients.
- Physicians agree with the recommendations made by pharmacists who provide pharmaceutical care over 90% of the time.

What we have learned from *payers*:

- When pharmacists deliver a service that meets the standards of patient care, payers will recognize and pay pharmacists for patient care.
- The pharmacist must add unique value (measurable) to the care of the patient.
- Drug therapy problems are the currency of the future.
- Documentation in practice is the key to almost everything (workload, quality, reimbursement).
- Pharmaceutical care practice saves or avoids three to five times more than it costs to deliver the service.

The past 25 years have been enlightening, challenging, at times frustrating and always rewarding. Most of all, however, we have seen patients' lives changed forever after receiving medication management services. This is why we started those many years ago and why we are certain that a new standard for medication use will soon be in place.

REFERENCES

1. Bradford V. *The Total Service Medical Practice: 17 Steps to Satisfying Your Internal and External Customers.* Chicago, IL: Irwin Professional Publishing; 1997.
2. Joseph SR. Developing a marketing plan. In: *Marketing the Physician Practice.* Chicago, IL: American Medical Association; 2000.
3. Koch, WH, *Chiropractic—The Superior Alternative.* Calgary AB, Canada: Bayeux Arts Inc; 1995.
4. Silker EL. *Dentistry: Building Your Million Dollar Solo Practice.* Lakeshore, MN: Silk Pages Publishing; 1995.
5. Nicoleti B. *Five Strategies for a More Vital Practice.* 2004; www.aafp.org/fpm.
6. McDonough RP, Doucette WR. Dynamics of pharmaceutical care: developing collaborative working relations between pharmacists and physicians. *J Am Pharm Assoc.* 2001;41(5):682–692.
7. AMA. *Medicare Physician Payment Reform: The Physicians' Guide.* Vol. 1. Chicago: American Medical Association; 1992.
8. Lee PR, Ginsburg PB, LeRoy LB, Hammons GT. The physician payment review commission report to congress. *JAMA.* 1989;261:2382–2385.
9. Hasio WC, Bruan P, Yntema D, Becker ER. Estimating physicians' work for a resource-based relative-value scale. *N Engl J Med.* 1988;319:835–841.
10. AMA. *Medicare RBRVS: The Physicians' Guide.* Chicago, IL: American Medical Association; 2000.
11. Cipolle RJ, Strand LM, Morley PC. *Pharmaceutical Care Practice.* New York, NY: McGraw-Hill; 1998.
12. Cipolle RJ, Strand LM, Morley PC. *Pharmaceutical Care Practice: The Clinician's Guide.* 2nd ed. New York, NY: McGraw-Hill; 2004.
13. Isetts BJ, Buffington DE. CPT code-change proposal: national data on pharmacists' medication therapy management services. *J Am Pharm Assoc: JAPhA.* 2007;47(4):491–495.
14. Abraham M, Ahlman JT, Boudreau AJ, Connelly JL. *CPT 2011 CPT/Current Procedural Terminology.* Chicago, IL: American Medical Association; 2011.
15. Schaffer CA. *A Guide to Starting a Business in Minnesota.* St. Paul, MN: Minnesota Department of Trade ad Economic Development; 2001.
16. Strand LM, Cipolle RJ, Morley PC, Frakes MJ. The impact of pharmaceutical care practice on the practitioner and the patient in the ambulatory practice setting: twenty-five years of experience. *Curr Pharm Des.* 2004;10(31):3987–4001.

The Global Perspective

INTRODUCTION

In this, the final section of the book, we are pleased to present perspectives from around the world. These perspectives are presented by individuals with a firsthand knowledge of developments in their respective countries. Moreover, they have contributed to their "national dialogue," and have actively participated in the development of medication management services. Their observations serve to remind us that it will take a global effort to establish the urgency of the problem at hand and demonstrate the central role to be played by pharmacy in meeting the universal need for medication management services. Pharmaceutical "misadventuring" is a growing problem that requires immediate attention. The content of these reports reveals that consciousness is increasing and pharmacy is poised to participate with other health care professionals to address the problem with the necessary knowledge and analytic skills to make a significant contribution to human health and the economic consequences of drug-related morbidity and mortality.

The reports included here are not to be seen as a random selection, nor are the observations generalizable to other countries within the same geopolitical region. Rather, they are "samples of convenience" in that they represent a number of individuals with whom we have worked or are known to us as pharmacists committed to the development and implementation of medication management services in their countries. In sum, these reports provide a "snap shot" of activities that are being conducted outside of and in the United States to serve as a reminder that in many places pharmacists are extending their knowledge and practices into the health care system. Of course, this does not mean that there is an absence of challenges, conflicting professional expectations, or competing ideologies. Struggles abound! But, what comes out of this dialogue is clear evidence that there is a strong resolve to further develop pharmacy as a health profession, and move its members toward full participation, in collaboration with other health professionals, in the team work necessary to meet patient need and improve their therapeutic outcomes.

In Australia, for example, we find that consumer discontent played a large part in the formulation of the National Medicines Policy. Here, the government provided a comprehensive framework for the development of strategies to meet consumer demand. With a government mandate and consumer legitimation, the pharmacy profession, through the Pharmacy Guild of Australia and the efforts of individual pharmacists and academics, promotes a movement toward pharmacists playing a major role in primary health care. Home health visits appear to be the first recognized and reimbursed service for pharmacists here.

Moving to New Zealand we find that policy makers are focused on the need for "greater integration and collaboration" in the health care system. As with Australia, primary health care is central to health care provision for the pharmacist. Also, central is the issue of payment and the necessary divorce from dispensing. What is clear in both Australia and New Zealand is that government and regional health boards have taken an active interest in health care reform and propose greater teamwork to address all health-related problems. Suffice it to say, the pharmacists clearly have numerous opportunities, in both countries, to further develop strategies and practices for their contribution to the medication management responsibilities.

The Asian context also offers a mix of opportunities and challenges. In China, for example, we learn that pharmacy education focuses on pharmaceutical sciences. Pharmacy practice is almost entirely focused on "compounding, dispensing, pharmacy administration, and laboratory experiences." Licensing is as recent as 1994, but is not required for all areas of pharmacy practice. Clinical pharmacy, at this time, subsumes all efforts of pharmaceutical care and medication management. The government has mandated that all hospitals develop clinical pharmacy programs to address drug-related problems and provide rational drug use. Developments moved forward in an important manner when in 2002 the Ministry of Health gave legal status to clinical pharmacy and required hospitals to establish "the patient-centered model of medication therapy management." China appears to be moving toward significant reform, and in doing so, opening the door for pharmacists to participate in further clinical roles, in spite of the small number of practices established to date.

The East Asian country of Korea is also poised to introduce major reforms in health care services. Clinical pharmacy began in the 1980s. Clinical pharmacy services such as therapeutic drug monitoring, anticoagulation services, and nutritional support services paved the way. Interestingly, clinical pharmacists (heavily influenced by the U.S. model) began to teach pharmaceutical care. More recently, hospitals have undertaken projects in medication management. A significant number of pharmacists have expressed interest in this service, but there is no strong governmental support for medication management services or the extended role of pharmacists. Professional associations appear to have taken the lead and now require further governmental legitimation and direction. However, there is reason for optimism and Korea is a strong case of pharmacists taking the initiative to broaden their responsibilities and expand those into the integrated health care system.

India is a complex country. With 1.21 billion people, great ethnic and linguistic diversity, and a vast geographic area, it offers countless challenges for those who are drawn to its cultural depth and its social contrasts. It is, in many ways, a giant very much in the process of waking and shaking off the mantel of its earlier experiences with colonial rule. It is the largest democracy in the world and faces all the challenges and perplexities that this entails. Perhaps the most worrisome challenge is the struggle with health care access and delivery, which is described in this contribution as "failing." Government expenditure is low and private responsibility is high. Access, in the main, depends on ability to pay. India has a National Drug Policy and Essential Medicines List (similar to those generated by the World Health Organization). Any medicine is available over-the-counter without a prescription "even those legally mandated as prescription-only medications." Numerous other problems are found in regulating medications. It seems that there is no reference to pharmacy as a health profession in any governmental policy related to health and pharmaceuticals. As found in many other contexts, clinical pharmacy and the concept of pharmacy practice derives from the efforts of clinical pharmacologists and academics. In the 1980s, western influence impacted both hospital practices and educational development. From approximately 1993 to the present change has occurred in both practice and education. The impetus toward pharmacy's role in patient care has gained momentum and in 2008 the PharmD program became a reality. The vision and exemplary hard work of numerous individuals has been rewarded. This is not to say that their work is over. It would seem that the regulatory framework does not yet recognize "the need for clinical pharmacists" and there are few positions available in hospitals for such individuals. However, this report also ends on a note of optimism. The Indian government and professional associations are working to implement pilot projects to engage pharmacists in health care initiatives. The challenges are great but we are confident that pharmacy will progress and take its place in the delivery of pharmaceutical care and medication management.

Like India, the Arabic-speaking Middle East is a complex area. In the report presented here nine countries are selected. Egypt, Jordan, Kuwait, Lebanon, Oman, Qatar, Saudi Arabia, Sudan, and the United Arab Republic Emirates. In the case of Egypt, pharmacy education has been dominated by "traditional chemistry-based courses and clinical application of pharmaceutical knowledge on the part of pharmacists has been limited." Change began in the 1980s at Tanta University, influenced by the clinical pharmacy program at the University of Tennessee. Since that time there has been a slow growth of "traditional" clinical pharmacy particularly in private universities. At a governmental level there has been a reluctance to accept an extended role for pharmacists. Some attempts were made to establish clinical pharmacy departments at the Egyptian Drug Authority and the Ministry of Health, providing the governmental authority to establish a place for clinical pharmacy practice. Physicians have not been particularly supportive of such measures and consider clinical pharmacy to be "trespassing" on their "pitch." Additionally, pharmacists are not overly enthusiastic to engage in anything approximating pharmaceutical care until there is legislative support that defines both the scope and "terms of reference" of practice. With budgetary support and legislative mandates, there are signs that there will be positive developments in the future. Jordan rarely sees pharmaceutical care and medication management, but concerned practitioners and academic leaders are showing substantial interest and are engaged in a dialogue that promises to lead to positive developments.

In Kuwait, as in Jordan, it is the younger pharmacists who are taking the lead and creating new services. This is a generational issue we find elsewhere. Inpatient pharmacists appear to be the "trial" context of innovation. The faculty of pharmacy at Kuwait University was granted the right to offer a PharmD degree in 2012. This could be the opportunity to further develop pharmacists for a role in medication management.

Lebanon, while quite advanced in its education development, has an economic crisis that prevents governmental support for any reimbursement scheme and pharmacists' job satisfaction is low. Clinical pharmacy and medication management are at early stages of development and as elsewhere is more widely found in the hospital context.

In the United Arab Emirates, an oil-rich federation, the economy is sound but there is a lack of payment for services and a shortage of "qualified staff." Also, there is no legislative framework to legitimize pharmacy as a health profession. Clearly, the relationship between supportive governmental regulation and the development of pharmacy is an important one. Once again, we see more progress being made in the hospital setting rather than in the community. Of particular interest is the drafting of standards of practice being undertaken by colleges of pharmacy. This important step may well usher in a new generation of pharmacists who will settle for nothing less than full membership in the health care community.

Qatar has no "autonomous professional pharmacy association or society that regulates the practice of pharmacy" or, for that matter, promotes it. Qatar's only pharmacy program is at Qatar University and is the newest in the region. Qatar has a PharmD program that has been accredited by the Canadian Council on Accreditation of Pharmacy Programs, so this small country promises to further the development of pharmaceutical care and clinical services. Indeed, the college mission statement states that its purpose is to promote such activities in the region. Medication management, as a consequence of pharmaceutical care practice, is to be an educational priority.

Saudi Arabia and Sudan both embrace, in general, the concept of pharmaceutical care practice. The former, however, equates this with the more traditional notion of clinical pharmacy, and the latter is presently in a more analytic mode attempting to develop a "pharmaceutical roadmap" for the profession. In Sudan, we find that a small group of community pharmacists has established a pharmaceutical care practice independent of any government or association initiative. This positive development, even if it is small, holds promise for the further evolution of medication management services. This will take time, but the path is becoming clearer as leaders in the profession advance educational and regulatory reforms.

The Arabic-speaking Middle East is undergoing major educational and professional change within health care generally and pharmacy in particular. Most importantly, the area has the economic resources to develop and implement medication management services. Educational and governmental collaboration will test the resolve of all concerned. We expect to see growth in medication management as an essential service in this area.

In Europe, we find that there is widespread recognition of the need for medication management services. In Germany, for example, the pharmacist is operating under "increasing economic pressure" and consumer demand to provide limited "cognitive services." The government is also voicing support but seems less than enthusiastic to implement laws mandating cognitive services. Studies of the effectiveness of the pharmacists' extended roles have been recommended, but, as the report indicates, little has been done to date. The authors raise an important issue regarding the development of patient-centered services when they note that Germany has to "find its own way" to develop medication management services. While the clinical method used to solve adverse drug events receives universal appeal there remains the challenge of "tailoring" the particulars of any medication management system to the actual sociopolitical, legal, and cultural context of the country in question. These factors will play a highly significant role in shaping the nature of any medication management system.

Of particular interest in the German context, is the role of technicians. In Germany, technicians are considered professionals with a 2.5-year preparation. It is indeed an advantage to delegate a significant portion of the dispensing process to qualified technicians thereby freeing the pharmacist from this time-consuming task and facilitating her commitment to the more cognitive dimensions of pharmaceutical care, leading to medication management services. The role of technicians is central to the full utilization of the pharmacist's knowledge and problem-solving role. However, the question remains as to whether the retail commercial environment will support a comprehensive patient care service.

In the Netherlands, pharmaceutical care has emerged as the central model of practice for community pharmacy. Indeed, we find that while clinical pharmacy began within the hospital context, pharmaceutical care owes its origins to community pharmacy and its highly motivated pharmacists. Within this context there is a commitment to the expansion of patient-centered activities. During the late 1990s, there was a concerted effort to implement a software documentation system for patient consultations. Norms and standards also received attention and ongoing refinement. Numerous studies are discussed to explore the role of the pharmacist and pharmaceutical care in improving the quality of life of patients. The Netherlands is an interesting case of community pharmacy playing a leading role in the development of pharmaceutical care. Numerous studies were conducted to test the viability and effectiveness of this practice, and now the question is to what extent this research has resulted in practice changes. The study results are most encouraging. Reimbursement for pharmaceutical care services has been recently approved by the Dutch government and health insurance companies. Indeed, it would appear that the preconditions for the implementation of medication management services are in place and will continue to develop.

Spain does not have widespread medication management services, and there is a limited number of practitioners who have been involved in projects with a view to developing them. While pharmaceutical care has been discussed and examined since the mid-1990s this was largely of interest to community pharmacists. Hospital pharmacists largely followed the U.S. example of clinical pharmacy in hospital settings.

While pharmaceutical care was initially enthusiastically embraced it would appear that many pharmacists abandoned it due to the extra work, increased responsibility, and lack of compensation. In Spain, we find the discussion revolving around the terminology related to drug therapy problems. For example, it is thought that "negative clinical outcomes" is more precise than "drug therapy problems." Such terminological issues have created an interesting linguistic issue, but failed to motivate individuals to develop services. Part of the linguistic problem may very well be that "negative clinical outcomes" is far from precise when the problem is specifically drug-related. As, to a large extent, language defines reality; it is not surprising to find practitioners moving in a universe of some confusion. This might be a small thing but it has large consequences.

The Spanish case is difficult to assess. While there are minimal medication management services offered, pharmaceutical care is the topic of constant debate. Indeed, it is safe to say that discussion of medication management services enjoys a similar presence. This is surely a case where theoretical discourse is yet to be translated into widespread meaningful practice.

Scandinavia, consisting of Norway, Sweden, and Denmark, are largely democratic welfare states with a strong commitment to the general well-being of their citizens. Thus, while major organizational differences are found in the distribution and level of services, and legislative frameworks, there is a clear recognition that health care is a human right. This is the cultural, sociolegal, and ethical framework wherein health care is defined and operationalized. For those skeptical of any form of welfare state it is important to emphasize that this concept defines basic values embraced by the very people served. Thus, it is no utopian dream, but rather simply a reflection of societal norms and values. In this regard, it is useful to explore the health care dynamics of Scandinavian countries and compare them with the so-called "free-market" approach to health care organization and delivery. Doing so provides a valuable insight into political ideology and social values as these become foundational to a health care system.

Iceland shares similar values with the Scandinavian countries. In 1262, Iceland fell under Norwegian rule, and in 1380 Iceland and Norway became Danish possessions. Independence from Denmark occurred in 1918 and in 1920 a new constitution was formed. It is hardly surprising then, that a great many values are shared by all these countries. Of course, there are many cultural differences, but specific human values remain intact. The reader will note that pharmaceutical care, as value, is recognized in all Scandinavian countries. How it is delivered, standardized, and at an individual level practiced, show significant differences. Iceland has clearly embraced pharmaceutical care, but as yet there is no standard concept of this in practice. Medication management services are limited and policy makers need to more fully recognize the value of this practice before further development can occur.

Throughout Scandinavia and Iceland more research must be done to demonstrate the personal and economic value of pharmaceutical care and medication management. Here, as elsewhere, this will probably occur within the hospital setting. Within emerging educational programs, there is a clear commitment to medication management and the pharmacists' role in its provision.

The United Kingdom has a long history of nationalized health care, since 1948. This system has "strengthened the patient's perception that it is doctors who are solely responsible for the management of their treatment in terms of appropriateness, effectiveness, safety, and compliance." The pharmacist continues to be regarded as largely responsible for dispensing. Medication reviews, medicines use review are terms used to describe the pharmacist's extended role in patient care. And, as the author of this report notes, these activities appear to conform to basic concepts of medication management.

Generally, the United Kingdom has many pharmacists providing aspects of pharmaceutical care, "but it appears to be sporadic with little consistency and little documentation or follow up." Perhaps the best example of emerging medication management services is found in Scotland. Here, the Scottish Chronic Medication Service is very progressive and has excellent individualized care as its primary objective. Moreover, it is constructed within a "collaborative national contractual framework with general practitioners (GPs) and patients." Possibly the Scottish model will become the standard that defines comprehensive medication management within the United Kingdom as a whole.

Brazil is a very large country that constitutes 47% of the landmass that is South America. With a population of 190,732,694(2010), it is the world's fifth most populous country. A former Portuguese colony it is now an independent, rapidly developing country with all the socio-economic problems that growth entails.

This section explores the many issues of health care reform and the author critically examines the future and promise of pharmacy as it struggles to establish its place in the emerging health care systems—public and private. Health care in Brazil is a constitutional right and it is the state's duty to provide the necessary services to meet this commitment.

While public and private schools of pharmacy continue to increase their numbers (in 2008 there were 321 and this has grown since hen) there is little evidence that pharmaceutical care and standards of practice are emphasized. There are few clinical faculty and the basic and pharmaceutical sciences have achieved control over curricular development. Of course this is not unique to Brazil, but it does present serious challenges to reform. Essentially the "fit" between the health care needs of the populace and the focus of college preparation is somewhat weak. This is also not unique to Brazil. The author sees educational reform as an essential prolegomenon to the development of pharmaceutical care and medication management services. Such change, as seen elsewhere, is slow and encounters numerous forms of resistance from both the profession of pharmacy itself and other health care professionals. It seems that "turf wars" will always be a universal part of this story as it unfolds.

This section provides a useful focus where pharmacists lend their voice to the debate. Some 28 pharmacists provide their observations and insights into pharmaceutical care as they attempt to develop, implement, and practice it. We need more studies of pharmacists in situ as they work to provide care. The dynamics of such enterprise will be most instructive, and the reality of practice will be presented in context rather than left to those who fail to move beyond the abstract, disengaged, dimensions of policy. To this end this paper places educational reform and critical thinking at the forefront of change. There is a lesson here: we cannot allow politics and the appeal to tradition to bury the essential truth that education and the free expression of ideas is the foundation of all positive change in society. To ignore this maxim is to retreat from reason and ignore the needs of those who deserve the best treatment possible.

In Canada's public health system, government payers have become increasingly interested in paying for pharmacy services that deliver the best patient care value. For the past few years, negotiations have been taking place between provincial government representatives and pharmacy representatives. The focus of these negotiations is on increased transparency in drug pricing to drive drug costs down, and subsequent reinvestment of some savings into payments for high-value services such as comprehensive medication management.

Canadian pharmacists and provincial health systems are at varying stages of development and implementation of comprehensive medication management initiatives across the country. Critical success factors for these, and future initiatives include realistic funding models, practice change support for frontline pharmacists, operational reorganization of the pharmacist's workspace and workday, effective interprofessional relationships, realistic patient expectations, pharmacist confidence and readiness to change, pharmacist willingness to change (overcoming change fatigue), pharmacist access to clinical tools, support for pharmacists from pharmacy management, linkages and integration with existing health programs, and trust and collaboration between stakeholders.

Work continues in earnest across the country to ensure Canadian pharmacists have the support and systems they need to provide comprehensive medication management to Canadian citizens so they can achieve optimal drug therapy outcomes.

In the United States, medication management as pharmaceutical care has been evolving since 1990. More than anywhere else this country has engaged in serious critical reflection and practice development in both hospital and community settings. The documentation of drug-related morbidity also has a long history and a plethora of research papers that identify the seriousness of the problem. In short, there is general agreement (evidence-based) that the problem of drug-related morbidity and mortality is of a sufficient high order to warrant a critical rethinking of our approach to pharmacotherapeutic intervention. Indeed, we could argue that it is time for a significant paradigm shift! Certainly the American experience calls for no less. As the author of the United States' report correctly states, a rational medication-use system is a powerful response to an urgent problem.

The United States' case reflects the importance of legislative support and legitimation. Whether it is the Minnesota Pharmaceutical Care Demonstration Project of 1993–1997, or the broader dimensions of Congressional initiatives of the mid-1990s, we find that legislative support is of paramount importance. This we have seen within the context of other countries. The most recent example of governmental initiative is found in the Part D Prescription Drug Benefit of the Medicare Program.

It is reasonable to argue that great progress has been made in the United States. But, as the report indicates, there is still much to do. Future developments will necessarily demand more trained pharmacists, attitude changes on their part, substantial economic resources, educational changes (curricula), and a significant move away from distribution/dispensing roles. In sum, the United States faces many challenges similar to those found elsewhere.

In summary, the papers presented in this chapter provide a critical examination of the changes, challenges and possibilities confronting those committed to the promulgation of pharmaceutical care and medication management services. The countries examined have their own socio-cultural-political issues to contextualize such developments. But, there are common themes and common values that should not be overlooked. Perhaps the most important of these is the desire to offer the sick and the suffering the best possible care available. This means that pharmacists have highly valued knowledge to put into practice and thereby play a significant role in any health care system. The problems of drug therapy are many and we are confident that solutions can, and will be found and offered to those in need.

AUSTRALIA

Geoff March, BPharm, PhD
Quality Use of Medicine and Pharmacy Research Centre
Sansom Institute for Health Research
University of South Australia
Adelaide, South Australia

Understanding the Practice Context

Australia spends a significant amount of money on health. In 2007–2008, health expenditure was $103.6 billion, exceeding $100 billion for the first time, equaled 9.1% of gross domestic product with the various levels of government funding almost 70% of that health expenditure. Successive Australian governments have put in place a range of policy initiatives including universal access to health care (Medicare) and a scheme to provide access to necessary medicines for the general public and veterans at affordable prices (the Pharmaceutical Benefits Scheme or PBS).

In 2011, there were approximately 26,000 registered pharmacists, of which 21,000 work in community (retail) pharmacies and 4000 work within the public and private hospital system. There are an estimated 5000 community pharmacies throughout Australia and approximately 1300 hospitals (public and private).

In analyzing the current and future role of pharmacists in Australia, an understanding of the context of practice is helpful. There is an overarching framework that guides the health of all Australians provided by the Australian government's National Health Strategy, of which a National Medicines Policy is one component but which holds particular relevance as a tool for change in pharmacy. The role of governments in Australia in setting the agenda for health is traditionally a strong one. Australian governments, whether Commonwealth or state governments, are the largest funders of health services. The private sector has a relatively more minor role; generally limited to providing a private hospital alternative and insuring for a number of services (e.g., dentistry, physiotherapy outside of the public hospital system, alternative health practitioners) that are not funded or subsidized by government.

The Policy Framework

The National Medicines Policy arose from consumer discontent in the late 1980s surrounding the level of harm associated with the use of medications, coupled with the inaction of the health professions and successive governments to confront this issue. Perhaps the need for change was exemplified in the statement written in the first of 12 National Health Strategy (1991) issues papers:

> *"...widespread concerns of those in the health field that achieving optimum health outcomes for Australians in the future requires a reassessment of the way the components of the system are structured and incentives which operate between the various parts"* (p. 6).

It was toward the end of the 1980s that the community demanded that all health professionals, including pharmacists, assume responsibility for outcomes associated with medication use.

The Australian government responded, in part, by introducing the National Medicines Policy, which included the National Strategy for achieving the Quality Use of Medicines (QUM), with the objective of better meeting the medication-related needs of the Australian community.

The underlying philosophy is the primacy of satisfying the needs of the individual, and for the partners—governments, health practitioners, health educators, medicine suppliers, health care consumers, and the media—to work together to achieve this aim.

Of particular interest is the fourth policy arm of the National Medicines Policy, namely achieving the QUM. QUM is defined as follows:

- *Judicious selection of management options.* This involves consideration of the place of medications in treating illness and maintaining health. It may mean that a nondrug option, or no treatment, may be the appropriate management choice.
- *Appropriate choice of medicines.* Where a medicine is considered necessary the most appropriate medicines are chosen, taking into account factors such as the clinical condition being treated, the potential risks and benefits of treatment, dosage, length of treatment, and cost.
- *Safe and effective use.* Ensuring patients have the knowledge and skills required to achieve the goals of therapy, and that systems exist to prevent medication-related problems.

The key partners in achieving the aims of QUM include

- those who take or consider taking medicines
- those who prescribe, provide, and monitor the use of medicines
- those who assist people in learning more about health issues and health care through information, education, and discussion
- those who provide health services within hospital and community settings
- those who develop, make, market, distribute, and sell medicines

- those who produce, report, publish, and broadcast information about medicines and health matters
- those in both the public and private sectors who fund and/or purchase the range of health services within which medicines play an important part
- the governments who, acting in the public interest, assess and register medicines, monitor their safety, and provide equity of access to them.

This requires the involvement of consumers and their carers; health practitioners; health educators; local, state, and commonwealth governments; health and aged care facilities; media; the pharmaceutical industry; and health care funders and purchasers. There are six building blocks that support QUM:

1. Policy development and implementation
2. Facilitation and coordination of QUM initiatives
3. Provision of objective information and ethical promotion
4. Education and training
5. Provision of services and appropriate interventions
6. Strategic research, evaluation, and routine data collection.

What does this policy framework mean for health practitioners? An example is the issue of harm associated with the transfer of health consumers across health settings and health providers. Researchers had found a number of systems' errors around medications management that could lead to harm for the patient. These included.[1]

- on admission to hospital, up to one in two patients had an incomplete medicine list provided, resulting in a medicine not being administered during the hospital stay.
- 1.6% of hospital admissions are associated with the occurrence of an adverse medicines event, and medicines are considered to be the causal agent of 10% of all adverse events experienced in hospitals.
- 78% of GPs were not directly informed that their patient had been admitted to hospital and 73% did not directly receive a discharge summary.
- 12% of patients had an error in their discharge prescription.
- omission of medicine from the discharge summary list sent to community health care professionals was associated with an increased risk (by a factor of 2.3) of hospital readmission or adverse medicine event.

A further QUM issue has been the timely access to medicines following discharge from hospital. Hospitals commonly only provided patients with

7 days (or less) of medications, expecting that the person would visit their own medical practitioner and get new prescriptions for their changed medications. Roughead et al.,[2] in a retrospective data analysis of the Department of Veterans Affairs' claims data, indicated that the median time to first pharmacy visit was 6 days (interquartile range 2–14) and 12 days for a GP visit (interquartile range 4–31). In addition, community pharmacists are not routinely advised of hospitalization or sent discharge plans. Consequently, a number of patients were not seeing their medical practitioners in a timely manner to get prescriptions for the new medications (even if the medical practitioner had received postdischarge information) and so were not taking their new medications.

In line with the QUM principles, the Australian government consulted widely with key stakeholders via the Australian Pharmaceutical Advisory Council to develop a set of guidelines around continuity of management in 1998, and after evaluation, redrafted the guidelines in 2005.[1] These now form the basis of a major multigovernment initiative across Australia to reduce the level of harm around medication management as people transfer between health settings and health practitioners. The guidelines cover two components of this change; the first covers the organizational obligations of leadership, responsibility and accountability for medication management within the organization, and the second relates to the specific patient care activities required to ensure continuity of care. The two tiers of government have agreed to fund these changes in the health system.

Hospital pharmacists will be expected to be a part of the team that ensures accurate medication histories are taken at admission (including liaising with community pharmacists and medical practitioners) including adverse drug events and allergies, chart medication review, warfarin and aminoglycoside therapeutic drug monitoring, participation in the process of a medication action plan, patient counseling prior to discharge, review and reconciliation of discharge prescriptions (compared to medication plan), and participation of discharge summary to relevant health care professionals. Data relating to performance for each of these are required to be collected and analyzed to produce an indicator, which is then used as a component of the quality assurance process. The use of indicators is designed to ensure the required activities are applied consistently across hospitals throughout Australia.[3]

Evolution of Pharmacy Services

Since the 1970s, educators within the Australian University pharmacy schools focused primarily on developing pharmacists with a sound knowledge of clinical pharmacy skills. Australia has not had a history of drug development and manufacturing, and therefore, the need to produce graduates specializing in pharmaceutical sciences is not as strong as in a number of other countries. Consequently, Australian pharmacy schools produce pharmacy graduates who are generalists but with a strong clinical pharmacy foundation and who have an expectation to be able to use these skills.

Within the hospital system, clinical services include the collection of detailed medication histories at admission, medication review while an inpatient, patient counseling, clinical reviews, therapeutic drug monitoring, adverse drug reaction monitoring, selection of drug therapy, the provision of drug information to other health professionals of the care team and involvement in quality assurance programs around medication management. A number of pharmacists employed within the hospital department are allocated to work fulltime on the ward as a member of the health care team. However, there is not one consistent practice model around patient care that is routinely applied across all hospital sites.

Community pharmacy practice is dominated by the drug supply model where between 50% and 70% of income for community pharmacy owners is derived from dispensing PBS prescriptions. This dispensing component of current pharmacy services has its genesis in the establishment by the Australian government in the late 1940s of the PBS where drugs were listed and subsidized by the government, which ensured equity of access to expensive medicines for all Australians. Community pharmacy consequently developed work systems and pharmacy layouts that ensured the efficient dispensing of these subsidized prescriptions in order to maximize income.

By the early 1990s, some community pharmacists began to realize that they were both over-qualified for the tasks they undertook and under-utilized by the health system. A number of community pharmacists became disillusioned with the community pharmacy model. A number of practice variants were postulated as a method of re-professionalization including consultant pharmacy and enhanced patient counseling where the design of the pharmacy was altered to enable the pharmacist and patient to easily interact with each other.

Although the QUM strategy was promulgated in the early 1990s and could have been used as a sign post toward re-professionalization, the significance of this was not grasped until Helper and Strand described a systematically applied patient care process whereby medication-related problems could be solved by a pharmacist. Indeed, the aims of QUM strategy and pharmaceutical care were for all intents identical in terms of reducing medication related harm–in Australia the QUM policy needed a practice model for the profession and pharmaceutical care was that model. Both approaches arose from a social need; in Australia the public "drove" the process complaining about the level of harm associated with medicines and the lack of response from governments and health practitioners, and for Hepler and Strand, identification and resolution of drug-related problems and their associated social and economic cost. The motivation for change was primarily public policy rather than the profession per se. The QUM strategy provided an environment in which pharmaceutical care could be practiced.

One objective of the QUM strategy highlighted the need for health practitioners to work together. A project was funded to explore new models of practice for community pharmacists using pharmaceutical care[4] while a second project explored improving collaboration between medical practitioners and pharmacists around the provision of medication management.[5] In the first study, community pharmacists provided patient care directly to patients at risk of medication-related harm; assessment, care planning, education, follow-up, and documentation of the service. Pharmacists provided pharmaceutical care either within the community pharmacy environment or in the person's own home. A key feature of this process was that the pharmacist conducted a case conference face to face with the person's medical practitioner to discuss what was found and how to address the medication-related problems. The pharmacists then monitored the patient to ascertain outcomes of the process. <u>Ultimately, the difficulties for pharmacists working in a community pharmacy to provide pharmaceutical care proved insurmountable.</u> The Australian government decided to fund the provision of this service in the person's own home with the establishment of the Home Medicines Review (HMR) program. A separate funding pool was also provided for accredited pharmacists to provide medication chart reviews in aged care facilities.

The Home Medicines Review Program

Based on the results of the research described above, in 2001, the Home Medicines Review (HMR) program was established to fund community pharmacists and medical practitioners to work collaboratively with the patient, the patient's caregivers and, when appropriate, other health practitioners to address issues with the use of medicines.

The objectives of the HMR program are as follows:[6]

- Achieve safe, effective, and appropriate use of medicines by detecting and addressing potential medication-related problems that interfere with desired patient outcomes,
- Improve the patient's quality of life and health outcomes using a best-practice approach that involves a collaborative effort between the GP, pharmacists, and other relevant health professionals, the patient, and where appropriate their carer,
- Improve patients' and health professionals' knowledge and understanding about medications,

- Facilitate cooperative working relationships between members of the health care team, in the interests of patient health and well-being,
- Target people living at home who may be at risk of medication misadventure.

Service Elements The HMR process, as approved by the Australian government, is outlined in Figure 12-1. The medical practitioner is required to assess the need for an HMR and then makes a referral either to the patient's community pharmacy (this was a requirement from 2001) or directly to a pharmacist credentialed to provide the service (this referral option was introduced in 2011). The community pharmacy is required to engage an accredited pharmacist to provide the service when a community pharmacy referral is made. The accredited pharmacist is (1) provided with patient information from the GP and the patient's community pharmacy, (2) visits the person's home and undertakes a systematic review of that person's medication and use, and then (3) provides a report (generally written but occasionally face-to-face) to the person's medical practitioner outlining issues and possible solutions. The medical practitioner then devises a medication management plan that is discussed with the person (or carer) at a follow-up appointment with the medical practitioner.

Service Providers A registered pharmacist is required to complete a credentialing and certification process to become an accredited pharmacist before being permitted to seek payment for conducting HMRs.

However, the administrative process surrounding this service is quite complex. The provision of HMRs by community pharmacy is governed by a set of business rules.[7] The business rules set out in detail the responsibilities of the community pharmacy and the accredited pharmacist in providing an HMR service, as well as those of the Australian government's Health Insurance Commission that administers the payment. Payment for the service is provided either to the community pharmacy proprietor or the accredited pharmacist depending on where the referral from the medical practitioner is sent.

An HMR can only be initiated by the medical practitioner after consulting with the patient. Once the HMR has been completed, the accredited pharmacist either visits the referring medical practitioner or sends a written report to the medical practitioner who then devises or revises a Medication Management Plan in conjunction with the patient. The community pharmacy may then have further involvement in the implementation of the Medication Management Plan if the plan is relayed to the community pharmacy by discussing the patient's progress in implementing the plan whenever they visit the pharmacy.

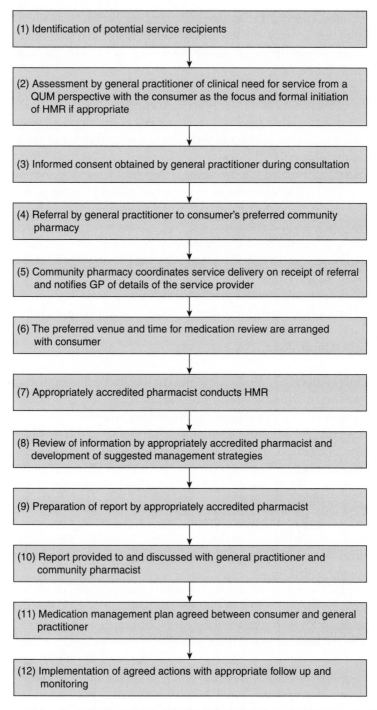

Figure 12-1 The HMR process (Source: Data from Health Insurance).

Credentialing Process   Pharmacists are required to be credentialed to be able to be remunerated for conducting HMRs. There are two methods of achieving credentialing: the first is passing the examination offered by the USA-based Commission for Certification in Geriatric Pharmacy, and the second is completing a certification and credentialing program offered in Australia by the Australian Association of Consultant Pharmacy (AACP). The AACP program is more popular and involves a two-step process.

The first step is a preparatory program that is process-orientated whereby the pharmacist is required to demonstrate the ability to establish therapeutic relationships, interact with other health professionals effectively, and understand the pharmaceutical care process (including identifying appropriate patient-specific outcomes and follow-up procedures). The second step requires the pharmacist to have completed 40 points of Continuing Professional Development (CPD) in the previous 12 months, complete a communications module and answer 12 multiple choice questions (MCQ), and submit a portfolio of experience where the pharmacist is required to reach 100 points from the following tasks:

1. A 500-word written description of an activity related to a patient clinical intervention. 20 points are allocated per activity, with a maximum of three activities allowed to be claimed (60 points).
2. A 500-word literature review or drug information query. 20 points are allocated per activity, with a maximum of two activities allowed to be claimed (20 points).
3. A referee report on skills (10 points).
4. Publication worth 20 points. Maximum of two publications (20 points).
5. Reflective writing on a particular area of practice that relates to the communication module. 500 words with a maximum of two pieces worth 10 points each (20 points).

Reaccreditation involves an annual submission of a CPD log and a clinical assessment every third year.

Pharmacist Participation in HMR Program   By 2011, about 8% of all registered pharmacists had completed the accreditation process required for the provision of HMRs. According to the Australian Association of Consultant Pharmacists (www.aacp.com.au), there is a range of reasons given by pharmacists wanting to become accredited. These include:

• For an employee community pharmacist, accreditation makes him more attractive to potential employers,

- For pharmacy owners, the HMR services is an alternative income stream and a way to differentiate them from their local competitors,
- Other owners saw the program as a means of improving consumer loyalty and is a means of "selling" other income-generating pharmacy services such as the provision of dose administration aids,
- Both owners and employees liked the idea of a funded pharmacy service outside the "drug supply" system,
- Younger pharmacists in particular see the program as a means of utilizing and extending their clinical knowledge.

A number of online HMR software tools have been developed to support accredited pharmacists; however, to date these have not undergone evaluation.

Uptake of HMRs   Over 300,000 claims for the provision of HMRs have been processed since the start of the program in 2001. In 2010, there were 52,201 claims for HMRs. Over three quarters of these interactions (76.3%) were with people aged 65 years or older who made up 16.3% of Australia's population. The bias toward providing this service to older people is in recognition of the level of harm occurring with increased medication use associated with multiple chronic illnesses. Of people over 65 years of age, 90% have two or more chronic health problems, and 90% of this group will have at least one medication-related problem. In 2010, just 1.6% of this "at-risk" population of older Australians received an HMR. While the number of HMRs has increased by 19% between 2008 and 2010, the percentage of older Australians receiving an HMR decreased 1.7% in 2008 indicating the rapid growth of the ageing Australian population and the underutilization of this service by the health professions.

Evaluation of HMR Program   The HMR program has undergone several evaluations since its inception.

In the first review of the HMR program it was found that all parties saw the HMR program as "addressing genuine and ongoing community needs, as delivering benefits for consumer health and wellbeing."[8] However, some significant issues were raised. In the first 4 years of the program, the level of HMR referrals from medical practitioners was less than anticipated, yet the numbers of accredited pharmacists were not sufficient to meet demand. The time and cost involved in achieving and continuing accreditation was not seen to be commensurate with the income generated. Evaluation of data relating to patient outcomes was problematic. Firstly, the medication management plan devised by the medical practitioner may not be relayed to either the accredited pharmacist or community pharmacist. Secondly, accredited pharmacists or the community pharmacists rarely follow up the patient to determine if any changes to their medications had been made by the medical practitioner, and if the patient's problems were resolved or well managed.

A second program evaluation was completed in 2008.[9] It found that those most at need of the service; certain patients after hospital discharge, indigenous people from both culturally and linguistically diverse backgrounds, palliative care patient and noncompliant consumers, were least likely to receive the service. In addition, the ongoing lack of documenting patient outcomes resulted in medical practitioners not being convinced that HMRs are effective in improving the outcomes for patients. The medical practitioner is the motivation for the service, for without the referral, the service cannot be provided.

The report also identified a number of barriers to the uptake of the service in addition to HMR access. These included: (1) the rigidity of the business rules around the provision of HMRs that negatively influenced the willingness of medical practitioners and pharmacists to become or maintain their involvement, (2) both the lack of team work and effective communication between health professionals including between pharmacy owners/managers and contracted accredited pharmacists, and (3) the lack of knowledge about the service by consumers. The consumers who had experienced the service valued it but would not necessarily request the service from their medical practitioner even after receiving it.

This is not to say that the value of the HMR service is negligible. Roughead et al.[10] found that the provision of HMRs in a population with heart failure was effective in delaying the time for hospitalization with a 45% reduction in the rate of hospitalization. It is remarkable that these barriers continue to retard the "roll out" of the program, even in the face of evidence from practice-based research. The risk of medication misadventure crosses boundaries between primary and secondary/tertiary levels of care. If pharmacists are going to assume responsibility for medication use, and in doing so become part of the care team, then pharmacists should become active participants in this program.

In Australia, one in three hospitalizations for older people are medicines-related; 40% of patients with multiple chronic illnesses are hospitalized at least once a year (with hospital stays being expensive); 10% will experience an error in their care while in hospital; and for medication-related admissions, between 25% and 75% are preventable.[11] It has also been found that 50% of medical practitioner referral letters for patients entering hospitals included a medication list that was inaccurate in terms of medication or dose of medication. The time taken to provide an HMR initiated directly with the accredited pharmacist at the time of hospital discharge was halved compared with the HMR process took using the usual rules.[12] Hospitals are explicitly excluded from the HMR program under current rules, although at the time of publication, this was being reviewed in light of concerns about the time taken for HMRS to be organized and completed postdischarge[13] with the view of allowing hospital initiated HMRs to occur.

Shifts in Hospital Pharmacy Practice

The role of clinical pharmacists is defined as a multidisciplinary team member working to optimize QUM for patients.[14] Their role is to participate in the management of individual patients, contribute their knowledge and skills when working with other members of the health care team, provide education to patients, carers, and other members of the health care team, identify and address risks associated with the use of medications, and be involved in research.

Clinical pharmacists are involved in six areas when undertaking this role: generate patient-specific data, identify clinical problems, establish therapeutic goals, evaluate therapeutic options, individualize therapy and monitor outcomes. A set of clinical activities are also defined and allocated to each of these six areas. A set of procedures accompanies each clinical activity. A clinical pharmacist is able to self-assess his practice using these standards.

In hospital practice, significant changes are occurring with increasing numbers of clinical pharmacists being employed in some states of Australia. Over the years, evidence of the value of clinical pharmacists has been accumulating, but convincing funders (State Governments in Australia) to fund clinical pharmacists on all wards as a matter of routine has been difficult, especially in the climate of reducing government spending. State governments have the responsibility for funding the public hospital system, and the Commonwealth government has responsibility for other areas of health funding, including Medicare (universal health insurance covering free access to public hospitals and subsidized medical practitioners) and access to subsidized medicines (PBS). This political structure has caused disharmony between the state and commonwealth governments primarily around cost shifting where the States and the Commonwealth governments try to reduce costs in their respective health budgets, especially in the area of expensive cancer medicines. The Commonwealth government met with the states and introduced a policy of Pharmaceutical Reforms, whereby the Commonwealth government would fund the provision of a month's supply of medications for outpatients and discharged patients. Interestingly in the state of South Australia, following the development of a business plan by hospital pharmacists to link the pharmaceutical reforms with the APAC guidelines, the South Australian government is now funding 35 extra clinical pharmacist positions, allowing hospitals to have a clinical pharmacist on each ward.[15] However, this approach is not uniform across Australia, with the result that clinical pharmacist numbers have increased little or not at all in other states. As part of the agreement with the South Australian government, clinical pharmacists will be required to comply with a competency-based quality assurance process, a tool for which is in the developmental stage. In this process, each clinical pharmacist undertakes a self-assessment using the competency tool, and then works with a clinical pharmacist mentor who observes, and provides feedback and education in an ongoing reflective process to develop the knowledge and skills of each clinical pharmacist.

Developing Pharmacy Practice

There are a number of initiatives designed to iteratively shift the practice of pharmacy toward more patient-oriented care. In the hospital sector, some of those changes have already been described. The South Australian approach of linking two government reform initiatives with clinical pharmacy services and an evaluation process has resulted in the state government being willing to fund more clinical pharmacy positions in their public hospitals. Having service performance indicators and a quality improvement process for pharmacists will provide evidence for the value of clinical pharmacy to the funders and the general public.

Community pharmacists have traditionally been involved in the preparation, storage, and supply of medicines. As remuneration for community pharmacists is based primarily on a fee for the supply of medicines through the PBS, community practice evolved around the efficient dispensing of medicines. However, to satisfy the aim and objectives of the National Medicines Policy, it has become apparent that pharmacists would need to contribute more than dispensing medicines and episodically providing advice on their use.

A mechanism available to facilitate practice change is the Government–Community Pharmacy Agreement process. Since 1991, the Pharmacy Guild of Australia (the organization that represents community pharmacy owners) and the Australian Government have negotiated a series of 5-year agreements (called the Community Pharmacy Agreement) that relates to the funding of community pharmacies to supply medicines under the PBS. Consecutive Agreements have broadened the focus from a mechanism for negotiating issues around the supply and payment for dispensing Pharmaceutical Benefit Scheme medications in the initial two agreements to include funding of community pharmacy based patient care services on a trial basis over the last three agreements. HMR is an example of a service funded under the Agreements. In the 2010 Agreement, approximately $600 million was allocated to develop a range of pharmacy related services.[16] A schedule and outline of these programs can be found under Appendix 1 in the Agreement document. Of interest is the payment of practice incentives covering six priority areas (as agreed between the Pharmacy Guild of Australia and the Commonwealth

Government). These include the provision of Dose Administration Aids, Documentation of Clinical Interventions, Provision of Staged Supply, Primary Health Care activities, Community Services Support, and Working With Others. Community pharmacy owners will be paid for providing these services, but payment will be linked to performance standards that have been developed for each service, and to ongoing provision of the service in a manner that is not episodic. If a pharmacist is not committed to providing a service, the practice incentive payments will be ceased.

A number of the leading pharmacy organizations have formed a coalition to lobby for changes in pharmacy practice, the Pharmacist Coalition for Health Reform. These include the two peak professional organizations, the Pharmaceutical Society of Australia and the Society of Hospital Pharmacists Australia and the Association of Professional Engineers Scientists and Managers, Australia. They have formed the coalition to address the need for a whole-of-pharmacy approach in negotiating pharmacy's role in the National Health Reform agenda. The Australian Government's health reform agenda is based upon the understanding that the current model of health care in Australia will not be viable by 2050 in the face of an ageing population with greater complexity of chronic illnesses and a smaller workforce. The reform agenda is designed to shift the focus of health care from hospitals to the primary care setting.

The aims include having pharmacists:

- involved in health care teams to provide integrated care for patients in medical practices, clinics, hospitals and rehabilitation and aged care facilities,
- providing follow up support to patients discharged from hospitals,
- able to consult with patients in pharmacies and in their own homes to improve medication management at the individual level,
- being part of the team working through Medicare Locals. (Regional primary care organizations established to identify and address gaps in local health services, utilize team arrangements around health care, make it easier to navigate the health system for patients and carers, and link with local hospital networks to facilitate safe and efficient transition between the levels of care.)

The Pharmacy Guild of Australia has also recognized the need to look to the future with the publication of their vision for community pharmacy.[17] They will be using their close relationship with the Commonwealth government to expedite their vision of necessary changes, and see that using the current and future Community Pharmacy Agreements as the process for achieving changes they believe are important.

In addition, the Pharmaceutical Society of Australia is following the lead of England, Canada, and New Zealand in producing a vision for the whole of pharmacy with the aim of having a vision document ready by 2012.

However, it would appear that these approaches still have not clearly defined what the "practice" of pharmacy is. Both the Pharmacy Guild of Australia's Roadmap document and the Pharmaceutical Society of Australia's Vision draft document do not clearly define this practice. The South Australian hospital clinical pharmacist practice is perhaps the closest, where the pharmacist's responsibilities are clearly defined, utilizing a set of standards that are measurable for the individual practitioner and having a set of indicators that can be used for evaluation purposes. The issue of being responsible for the outcomes in patients for whom they have been caring is a challenge for pharmacists working in the acute sector as generally, length of hospital stays are relatively short. Under the new arrangements, it will be the responsibility of the clinical pharmacist to ensure that relevant medication-related information is transferred as part of the discharge planning process.

At the practitioner level, there have been recent examples of pharmacists working in medical clinics working with other health professionals and also providing direct patient care around mediation management without being involved in the traditional medicines supply function.[18] It is these pharmacists who appear to challenge the orthodoxy and are developing a practice independent of traditional pharmacy. However, they have yet to achieve independent practitioner status by having their own Medicare number as other health practitioners have. That may come in the future.

In addition to these path-finding pharmacists, the rise of the independent HMR pharmacist working collaboratively with the medical practitioner and being paid directly for that service provides some foundation for the belief that at some stage in the future there will be a number of pharmacists working either independently or perhaps more likely part of a medical clinic providing pharmaceutical care, and that these pharmacists will also be providing care across the various health care sectors in a coordinated way that will benefit the patient.

REFERENCES

1. Australian Pharmaceutical Advisory Council. *Guiding Principles to Achieve Continuity in Medication Management.* Canberra: Commonwealth of Australia; 2005.
2. Roughead EE, Kalisch LM, Ramsay EN, Ryan P, Gilbert AL. Continuity of care: when do patients visit community health care providers after leaving hospital? *Intern Med J.* 2011;41(9):662–667
3. Continuity in Medication Management. *South Australian APAC Key Performance Indicators for Hospitals Participating in Pharmaceutical Reform.* SA Health, Government of South Australia; 2010.

4. March G, Gilbert A, Roughead E, Quintrell N. Developing and evaluating a model for pharmaceutical care in Australian community pharmacies. *Int J Pharm Pract.* 1999;7:220–229.

5. Chen T, Crampton M, Krass I, Benrimoj S. Collaboration between community pharmacists and GPs–the medication review process. *J Soc Adm Pharm.* 1999;16:145–156.

6. Home Medicines Review. http://www.medicareaustralia.gov.au/provider/pbs/fifth-agreement/home-medicines-review.jsp (Accessed July 17, 2011).

7. Home Medicines Review: Terms and conditions. http://www.medicareaustralia.gov.au/provider/pbs/fifth-agreement/files/4718-mmr-terms-and-conditions.pdf (Accessed July 17, 2011).

8. Urbis Keys Young. Evaluation of the Home Medicines Review Program: Pharmacy component. Prepared for the Pharmacy Guild of Australia;2005. http://www.guild.org.au/iwov-resources/documents/The_Guild/PDFs/CPA%20and%20Programs/3CPA%20General/2004-526/2004-526_fr.pdf (Accessed June 15th,2011)

9. Campbell Researching and Consulting. 2008. Home Medicines Review Program Qualitative Research Project Final Report. Canberra: Department of Health & Ageing Medication Management & Research Section http://www.health.gov.au/internet/main/publishing.nsf/Content/hmr-qualitative-research-final-report.

10. Roughead EE, Barratt JD, Ramsay E, Pratt N, Ryan P, Peck R, Killer G, Gilbert, A. The effectiveness of collaborative medicine reviews in delaying time to next hospitalization for heart failure patients in the practice setting: results of a cohort study. *Circ Heart Fail.* 2009;2(5):424–428.

11. Roughead EE, Semple SJ. Medication safety in acute care in Australia: where are we now? Part 1: a review of the extent and causes of medication problems 2002–2008. *Aust New Zealand Health Policy.* 2009;6:18.

12. Schoen C, Osborn R, Doty MM, Bishop M, Peugh J, Murukutla N. Toward Higher-performance health systems: adults' health care experiences in seven countries. *Health Aff (Millwood).* 2007;26(6):w717–w734.

13. Angley M, Ponniah A, Spurling L, Sheridan L, Colley D, Nooney V, Bong XJ, Padhye V, Shakib S. Alternative pathways to post-discharge home medication reviews for high risk patients: Investigating feasibility and timeliness. *J Pharm Pract Res.* 2011;41(1):27–32.

14. Society of Hospital Pharmacists Australia. SHPA standards of practice for clinic pharmacy. *J Pharm Pract Res.* 2005;35(2):122–146.

15. SA Health, 2011. Pharmaceutical Reforms. http://www.sahealth.sa.gov.au/wps/wcm/connect/public+content/sa+health+internet/about+us/safety+and+quality/medication+safety/pharmaceutical+reform (Accessed July 12, 2011).

16. The Fifth Community Pharmacy Agreement between the Commonwealth of Australia and the Pharmacy Guild of Australia. 2010. http://www.guild.org.au/iwov-resources/documents/The_Guild/PDFs/Other/Fifth%20Community%20Pharmacy%20Agreement.pdf (Accessed July 18, 2011).

17. Pharmacy Guild of Australia. 2010. The roadmap–the strategic direction for community pharmacy. http://www.guild.org.au/iwov-resources/documents/The_Guild/PDFs/News%20and%20Events/Publications/The%20Roadmap/Roadmap.pdf (Accessed June 18, 2011).

18. Akermann E, Williams IE, Freeman C. Pharmacists in general practice--a proposed role in the multi-disciplinary team. *Aust Family Physician.* 2010;39(3):163–164.

NEW ZEALAND

Lynne M. Bye, DipPharm, PG DipHlthMngt
Senior Tutor, School of Pharmacy
Faculty of Medical and Health Sciences
The University of Auckland, New Zealand

Chair, Pharmacy Advisory Group
Waitemata District Health Board
Auckland, New Zealand

Introduction

New Zealand is a small country in the South Pacific with an estimated population of 4.4 million.[1] There are currently 944 community pharmacies that are an integral part of primary health care delivery in New Zealand[2] and 31 hospital pharmacies with onsite pharmacist services. In New Zealand, prescribed medicines are subject to significant government subsidies and administratively the country is split up into 20 District Health Boards who are crown entities whose main function is to provide health and disability services to the population in their area. Primary Health Organizations (PHO) are essentially a group of health care providers (mainly doctors) who receive a set amount of funding from District Health Boards to provide a range of primary health care services for the people they have enrolled with them. Pharmacy services currently funded by all District Health Boards (DHB) are defined in the National Framework for Pharmacists Services as "Base Pharmacy Services" which are largely based on the supply function for example; dispensing of medicines and "Broad Specialised Pharmacy services" for example; pharmacy methadone services for opioid dependence, monitored therapy medicine services for patients taking clozapine, ascetic pharmacy services for the provision of prefilled syringes for syringe driver devices.[3] All District Health Boards are obliged to ensure that these services are available to their populations.

In New Zealand practicing pharmacists are required to hold an annual practicing certificate regardless of the number of hours they practice each year and be registered with the Pharmacy Council of New Zealand in the "Pharmacist Scope of Practice." As part of the application process for an annual practicing certificate, pharmacists must also provide details that enable the Pharmacy Council of New Zealand to assess; (1) a pharmacist's fitness to practice, (2) the area of practice they are practicing in and (3) their participation in an approved continual professional development recertification program. After gaining a Bachelor of Pharmacy (4-year degree) if a graduate wishes to practice as a pharmacist they must complete the Preregistration

Training Programme of the Pharmaceutical Society of New Zealand and register with the Pharmacy Council of New Zealand in the "Intern Pharmacist Scope of Practice." An intern pharmacist must always practice under the supervision of a registered practicing pharmacist. The Board of Health Workforce New Zealand has recently accepted the Pharmacy Council of New Zealand's application for designated prescriber rights for pharmacists. Additional qualifications will be required by pharmacist prescribers before they can register in the "Pharmacist Prescriber Scope of Practice," however, changes to legislation are required and these are not expected to be introduced until 2012. As at June 2011 there were 3,223 practicing pharmacists on the Pharmacy Council register of 4,444 with 221 recorded as having the "Intern Pharmacist Scope of Practice" and 996 having retained their registration but are recorded on the nonpracticing register.[4] The majority (76%) of pharmacists with a current annual practicing certificate practice in the community pharmacy setting while 12% practice in hospital pharmacies.[4]

The Pharmacy Council of New Zealand's Competence Framework

Assessment against a set of competency standards for the pharmacy profession was first introduced in 1997. When the Health Practitioners Competency Assurance Act was implemented in 2003 it became a requirement for practicing pharmacists to register in the "Pharmacist Scope of Practice" and hold an annual practicing certificate. The Pharmacy Council of New Zealand currently has two frameworks that outline the competency standards required for the provision of various pharmacist services within the Pharmacist Scope of Practice.[5] When the "Pharmacist Prescriber Scope" of practice is introduced in the near future, pharmacists will be required to meet separate competencies and qualifications to register in this separate scope of practice.

1. The Competency Framework for the Pharmacy Profession; the standards against which all practicing pharmacists must maintain competence for the "pharmacist Scope of Practice." The seven broad areas of competency are: practice pharmacy in a professional and culturally competent manner; contribute to the quality use of medicines; Provide primary health care; apply management and organization skills; research and provide information; dispense medicines; and prepare pharmaceutical products.

2. The Medicines Management Competency Framework; the standards against which accredited pharmacists must meet when providing patient-centered services that improve medicine-related health outcomes. The five broad areas of competency are: interpret medicines review services in the context of the New Zealand health care system; practice effective

working relationships; manage the service; maintain service quality; and practice medicines review.

New Zealand has two Schools of Pharmacy; the School of Pharmacy at The University of Auckland which produces on an average 95 Bachelor of Pharmacy graduates annually and the National School of Pharmacy at Otago University with approximately 115 students graduating annually.[4]

Historical Development of Medication Management Services in New Zealand

In the late 1990s, a clinical pharmacy role, which was established in hospital pharmacy practice, began to emerge in the primary health care setting in New Zealand. These services were known as Comprehensive Pharmaceutical Care (CPC) and Pharmaceutical Review Services (PRS). Pharmaceutical Review Services received some government funding for a period of time via the community pharmacy services contract. Various medication review services and pilots around New Zealand were implemented; however, the uptake of the model of pharmaceutical care in the community pharmacy setting was relatively low, reflecting international experience.[6] Following are some examples of medicines management services which utilized CPC or PRS services and consequently informed the implementation of the Medicines Management Competency Framework in 2006 and the development of the National Framework for Pharmacist Services which was launched by the District Health Board New Zealand in 2007.

- Canterbury DHB Medicine Management Pilot was a service provided through community pharmacies for people living in the community who were deemed to be at risk of an adverse drug outcome.
- South East and City PHO Medication Management Service (Capital & Coast District Health Board) was a "seamless medication management" program for the enrolled population in primacy care and community settings.
- Porirua Health Plus PHO service is provided for people who have diabetes, cardiovascular, and other chronic diseases.
- South Wellington Pharmacy service is provided for people who have chronic diseases and are receiving multiple medications.
- Hutt Valley District Health Board discharge Pharmacist service provided a smooth transition from hospital to home for people with high health needs.
- Kowhai Health Trust Service provided medicines management services for people enrolled in the Primary Health Organizations in the Hutt

Valley DHB who have chronic diseases and are receiving multiple medications.

- Taranaki District Health Board medication review service is provided for people who are at risk of medication-related problems.
- HealthWest PHO CarePlus Medicines Review is for people enrolled in CarePlus who are prescribed multiple medicines and are considered to not be coping with their medication regimens.
- Older People at Risk Project provided Comprehensive Pharmaceutical Care service to people over the age of 65 living in Central Auckland who had multiple comorbidities and were considered not to be coping well in their homes.

In 2003, the Pharmaceutical Society of New Zealand, now a voluntary organization that represents pharmacists from all sectors, commissioned a Pharmacy Sector Action Group to develop and consult on a *Ten year Vision for Pharmacists in New Zealand: 2004–2014*. The aims of the 10-year vision document were to provide a clear vision for the pharmacy profession, identify the major goals in achieving the vision, and provide guidance for the profession in reaching the vision.[7] It contains 24 vision statements covering 12 key areas, such as patient focus, relationships with other health professionals, alignment with government health strategies, and so on. Within the range of services described in the key areas, the vision document explicitly sets out an expectation that pharmacist will provide a range of enhanced medicine management services, each with its own training/proficiency requirements, within the scope of practice of accredited pharmacists, and tailored to local patient and community priorities.[8]

Pharmacy Council of New Zealand
Medicines Management Framework

In 2006, the Pharmacy Council of New Zealand ratified the *"Pharmacy Council of New Zealand Medicines Management Competency Framework"* and the *"Medicine Use Review Competencies Standards"* and accredited the training course in 2007. It was envisaged that the same process could continue for the Medicine Therapy Assessment and Comprehensive Medicines Management services. In 2008, the Pharmacy Council of New Zealand resolved to hand over the reasonability for developing standards for Medicine Therapy Assessment and Comprehensive Medicines Management to professional organizations. Pharmaceutical Society of New Zealand took up the responsibility of developing the Medicine Therapy Assessment standards and consulted on the proposed Medicine Therapy Assessment during the later part of 2010. What is expected to be adopted by the

Pharmacy Council of New Zealand sometime in 2011 are five generic Medicines Review Standards with specific schedules that relate to Medicine Use Review, Medicine Therapy Assessment, and Comprehensive Medicines Management. The five generic Medicines Review Standards are based on the Pharmacy Council of New Zealand Medicine Use Review competency standards. The schedules contain education, training, assessment, accreditation, and recertification requirements for the particular medicines management service. The Comprehensive Medicines Management schedule is yet to be developed.

New Zealand National Pharmacist Services Framework

With the specific aim of better utilizing pharmacist skills, District Health Boards invested in the development of the National Pharmacist Services Framework in 2007 that sought to standardize the extended services being provided by pharmacists. The framework and its accompanying service specifications describe existing dispensing services funded by District Health Boards and provided by community pharmacies, and additional five new services in two main themes:[3]

1. Information services.
   - Health education to patients. For example, pharmacist health education services provided to individuals or groups of patients on specified health areas, such as immunization and smoking cessation. These services are provided by pharmacists working in the community pharmacy setting and also in Primary Health Organizations.
   - Medicines and clinical information support to practitioners (this includes Clinical advisory Pharmacist and Pharmacist Facilitation roles). For example, evidence-based, specialized pharmacist information services with a focus on information provision to health care providers to facilitate optimization and effective utilization of medicines. These services are provided by pharmacists generally working in Primary Health Organizations.
2. Medicines review services.
   - Medicines Use Review and Adherence Support, where the pharmacist works with the patient to review their understanding of their medication and supports them to self-manage their medication over a 12-month period. This service is provided by pharmacists working in the community pharmacy setting.
   - Medicines Therapy Assessment, where the pharmacists undertakes a full review of all the medication the patient is taking and works with prescriber to optimize the therapy for that patient. This service

is ideally suited in the long-term residential care setting and occurs over a 12-month period in partnership with the prescriber. Pharmacists providing this service are usually working in conjunction with a community pharmacy that has a specific contract to provide services to a long-term residential care facility, with a hospital pharmacy or Primary Health Organization.

- Comprehensive Medicines Management are case based, more comprehensive reviews used in specialized areas such as mental health.

Medication Management Services Delivered in New Zealand

The Pharmacy Council of New Zealand's definition of Medicines Management is:

> *"A range of patient-centred services that improve medicines-related health outcomes"*[9]

The Pharmacy Council of New Zealand's Medicines Management Competency Framework outlines four levels of medicines management services, the specific competency standards for the specific level plus the qualification, training, accreditation, and recertification requirements for each level of service (see Figure 12-2).

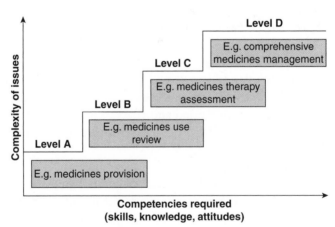

Figure 12-2 Levels of medicines management services. Reproduced from the Pharmacy Council of New Zealand © 2006, Medicines Management, Competence Framework (Pharmacy Council of NZ Medicines Management Competence Framework page 2), ratified July 2006 http://www.pharmacycouncil.org.nz/cms_show_download.php?id=124.

Levels A, "Medicines Provision," includes the product-oriented services via the traditional dispensing and medicine supply roles of pharmacists. The levels B, C, and D medicines management services are all patient-centered care services.

Medicines Use Review

The definition of the Medicines Use Review (Level B Medicines Management service) is:

> *"Medicines Use Review is a structured, systematic, documented and consultation-based service undertaken by an accredited pharmacist. Medicines Use Review aims to improve the patient's understanding of their medicines-related health outcomes by identifying access, adherence, and day to day management issues a patient has with their medicines and setting goals with the patient to resolve these issue."* [10]

The Medicines Use Review service, commonly referred to as MUR in New Zealand, aims to improve the patient's medicines-related health outcomes by identifying issues they have with their medicines in relation to access, adherence, and day-to-day self-management. The service is intended to help the patient find out more about the medicines they are taking, identify any problems they may be experiencing, and improve the effectiveness of the medicines being taken. This service includes complementary medicines and relevant lifestyle issues. A therapeutic relationship is developed between the pharmacist and the patient. The pharmacist actively elicits the patient's perspective and there is mutual agreement between the pharmacist and the patient in determining the recommendations and any changes arising from the Medicines Use Review service. They are agreed to by the patient. The service may take place with or without full access to the patient's medical information from the health care team; however, the pharmacist must have full access to the patent's medicines record. The patient must be present during the initial and follow-up consultations that may take place in a consultation room in a pharmacy or in the patient's home depending on the circumstances and wishes of the patient.

The competency standards required by the pharmacist providing Medicine Use Review services are outlined in Table 12-1. [9]

Key components of the Medicine Use Review service are summarized in Table 12-2.

Medicines Therapy Assessment

The definition of the Medicines Therapy Assessment service is:

> Structured and systematic, consultation-based reviews of all medicines currently prescribed for an individual patient, provided as part of multidisciplinary health team. For the provision of this service the accredited pharmacist will have access

Table 12-1 Medicines Use Review Competence Standards

Medicine Use Review 1	Understand Medicines Use Review in the Context of Medicines Management Services. 1.1 Differentiate between the levels of Medicines Management Services 1.2 Describe the principles, aims and scope of the Medicines Use Review service 1.3 Describe the place of Medicines Use Review in the wider context of national and local health care goals.
Medicine Use Review 2	Establish and Maintain Effective Working Relationships 2.1 Understand the principles of privacy and consent 2.2 Build a relationship with the patient 2.3 Build a relationship with the health care team 2.4 Communicate effectively with the patient 2.5 Communicate effectively with the health care team
Medicine Use Review 3	Document the Service 3.1 Develop effective recording systems 3.1 Maintain patient records
Medicine Use Review 4	Maintain Ongoing Quality 4.1 Undertake professional development 4.2 Maintain peer support 4.3 Implement a quality improvement procedure

Data from reference 6.

to full clinical notes and will proactively interact and/or intervene with both the patient (and/or their care giver) and their prescribers. Interactions are planned and do require the active participation of both the patient (and/or their care giver) and his prescriber(s), in an effort to optimise the outcomes from his medicines and improve the patient's understanding and management of his medicines and his health.[3]

The Medicine Therapy Assessment service is ideally suited for patients in the long-term residential care setting; however, it can also be provided to patients living independently in the community. These services aim to optimize health outcomes for individual patients by promoting the safe, effective, rational, and economic use of medicines. They focus mainly on the appropriate choice of medicines and dosing regimens for the patient with regular and efficient monitoring of the impact of medicines on the patient's health. Pharmacists providing Medicine Therapy Assessment services work as part of a multidisciplinary team and have full access to patients'

Table 12-2   Components of the Level B Medicine Management Service—
Medicines Use Review

Medicines Use Review	• Patients living in the community. • Utilization of a private area for the consultations. • Formal referral into the service by patient, family, caregiver, pharmacist or health practitioner (e.g., nurse or doctor). • The physical presence of the patient at the initial consultations plus 2 or 3 formal follow-up consultations over a period of 12 months. • Review of the use of all current medicines. • Formal referral and report to other health professional of issues identified as beyond the Medicine Use Review pharmacists scope of practice. • Patient education about current medicines and to promote appropriate self-management of medicines. • Provision of a patient held medication record • Removal of out of date medicines and medicine that are no longer required. • Reporting of suspected adverse medicine effects • Liaising with prescribers to align and streamline the patient's medication regimen. • Documenting of services provided. • Pharmacist peer review/support.
Adherence Support	• Ongoing monitor of patients utilization of medicines • Provision of support/tools to encourage appropriate medicines utilization • Appropriate documentation of services provided.

medical records. Accredited Medicine Therapy Assessment pharmacists will have: (a) at least 2 years of appropriate patient-oriented experience in a hospital, community, or primary care setting after initial registration in the Pharmacist Scope of Practice, (b) be Medicine Use Review accredited, and (c) have completed a Postgraduate Certificate in Pharmacy (Medicines Management).

Key components of the Medicine Therapy Assessment service are summarized in Table 12-3.

Table 12-3 Components of the Level C Medicines Management Service—
Medicines Therapy Assessment

Medicines Therapy Assessment	• Patients can be living independently in the community or in long term residential care facilities. • Utilization of a private area for the consultations. • Physical presence of the patient whenever possible. • Formal referral into the service from other health care practitioners. • Service includes initial consultation plus quarterly follow-ups over a 12-month period. • Pharmacist may be involved in weekly rounds or multi-disciplinary team meetings. • Assessment of all therapy to identify and evaluate actual or potential medicine therapy problems. • Reporting of suspected adverse medicine effects • Assistance with and monitoring of medicines. • Formulate, document and implement a pharmaceutical care plan • Formal referral and report to other health professional of issues identified as beyond the Medicine Therapy Assessment pharmacists scope of practice. • Documenting of services provided. • Pharmacist peer review/support.

Comprehensive Medicines Management

The definition of the Comprehensive Medicines Management service is:

> Accredited pharmacist Comprehensive Medicines Management services are autonomous advanced case-based management of all current and potential treatment for individual patients to improve therapeutic effectiveness and health outcomes. For the provision of this service the accredited pharmacist will have access to full clinical notes and will proactively interact and/or intervene with both patient (and/or their caregiver) and his prescriber(s). Interactions are planned and do require the active participation of both the patient (and/or their care giver) and his prescriber(s) in an effort to optimise the outcomes from medicines and improve the therapeutic effectiveness and health outcomes for the patient.[3]

The Comprehensive Medicines Management service is expected to be undertaken as part of specialist pharmacy service where the Comprehensive Medicines Management accredited pharmacist is referred to as a practitioner who is an expert in a particular area of clinical services, for example, mental health or renal. The Comprehensive Medicines Management service mainly focuses on the accurate and timely assessment of a person's need for medicines, the appropriate choice of medicines and dosing regimens, and the regular and efficient monitoring of the impact of medicines on a patient's health. This service is initiated via a referral from a member of the patient's health care team that may include a pharmacist providing Medicine Use Review and or Medicine Therapy Assessment services. The Comprehensive Medicines Management service involves an initial consultation and quarterly follow-ups over a 12-month period. Accredited pharmacists providing Comprehensive Medicines Management services have had; (a) at least 2 years of appropriate patient-orientated experience, the same requirement for the provision of the Medicine Therapy Assessment service and, (b) in addition, holds a Postgraduate Diploma in Clinical Pharmacy or higher qualification.

The key components of this service include all of those listed in Table 12-3 plus the service encompasses specialized clinical or therapeutic roles and liaising with prescribers and community pharmacists with potential referral to the Medicine Use Review service. There is the potential for this service to be provided in a variety of settings such as mental health clinics, Primary Health Organizations, and general practice surgeries and "Integrated Family Health Centres" which are starting to be developed in the primary health care sector in New Zealand.

Providers of Medication Management Services in New Zealand

In order to be able to deliver Level B, C, and D medicines management services in New Zealand, a pharmacist has to: (a) be registered in the Pharmacist Scope of Practice in New Zealand (b) hold a current Annual Practicing Certificate without conditions and (c) be assessed as competent against the relevant medicines management competency standards by an accredited education provider organization. Once accredited, there is a requirement for pharmacists to be actively involved in a peer review/support program, continual professional development, and a recertification program. On an annual basis, all pharmacists must declare, when applying for their Annual Practicing Certificate, the number of learning outcome credits from the continual professional development they have gained during the last year. This process is auditable and Pharmacy Council of New Zealand annually audits a sample of pharmacists from the register of pharmacists with Annual Practicing Certificates who must submit their continual professional development and recertification portfolio of evidence for audit.

There is a requirement that pharmacists providing Medicine Therapy Assessment and Comprehensive Medicines Management services will have;

(a) at least 2 years' appropriate patient-orientated experience in a hospital, community, or primary care setting after initial registration in the Pharmacist Scope of Practice, and (b) have active professional affiliations with relevant special interest groups in New Zealand or recognized groups internationally. Pharmacists providing a Medicine Therapy Assessment service would have as a minimum, a Postgraduate Certificate in Pharmacy (Medicines Management), and those providing Comprehensive Medicines Management services, a Postgraduate Diploma in Clinical Pharmacy.

Currently the New Zealand College of Pharmacists is the only training organization that is accredited to provide training and accreditation for Comprehensive Pharmaceutical Care and Medicine Use Review medicines management services. Both of the Schools of Pharmacy teach pharmaceutical care, care planning, and the provision of medicines management services in their 4-year undergraduate Bachelor of Pharmacy programs. During their Bachelor of Pharmacy program all students undertake medication reviews as part of their experiential learning programs in both the community pharmacy and hospital pharmacy settings. Both Schools of Pharmacy also deliver full postgraduate programs that provide the foundation training for pharmacists wishing to provide Medicine Therapy Assessment and Comprehensive Medicines Management level services, and in 2012 will jointly offer a post graduate certificate in pharmacist prescribing.

Current Status of Medication Management Services in New Zealand

Patients have experienced the benefit of patient-focused medication management services in particular the Medicine Use Review service as District Health Boards and Primary Health Organizations around New Zealand implement the National Pharmacist Services Framework. There are currently 11 of the 20 District Health Boards regions that have contracts in place to fund Medicine Use Review services and there are a small number of contracts in place to fund Medicine Therapy Assessment and Comprehensive Medicines Management services; however, there is currently no accurate data available on the number of pharmacists providing Medicine Therapy Assessment or Comprehensive Medicines Management services. There is also the option for patients to self-fund a Medicine Use Review, Medicine Therapy Assessment, or Comprehensive Medicines Management service; however, the "user pay market" in the pharmacy sector in New Zealand is relatively small.

There are currently 268 Medicine Use Review accredited pharmacists in New Zealand with a further 600 in the process of completing training and accreditation requirements.[11] Many pharmacists have been keen to undertake the training, however, find the accreditation process a challenge. In some areas, a number of pharmacists have undertaken the training; however, the District Health Board or Primary Health Organizations in the region do not offer contracts for the funding of medicines management services. This situation has resulted in quite a large number of pharmacists not completing the accreditation process.

The Medicine Therapy Assessment competency standards and training and accreditation requirements are expected to be adopted by the Pharmacy Council of New Zealand in late 2011–early 2012. It is expected that these competency standards will provide a pathway for more formal development of Medicine Therapy Assessment services, particularly in the long-term residential care settings. One of the large District Health Boards is currently funding a pilot service where a hospital pharmacist is engaged to provide full medication reviews to patients in long-term residential facilities in the district. It is expected that a number of pharmacists who had previously trained in Comprehensive Pharmaceutical Care will become accredited to provide Medicine Therapy Assessment Services once the standards are ratified by the Council.

Acceptance of Medication Management Services in New Zealand

A study conducted in 1999 sought to determine New Zealand community pharmacists' views on pharmaceutical care in order to inform the implementation and development of Comprehensive Pharmaceutical Care and Pharmaceutical Review services.[6] This study concluded that community pharmacists expressed a willingness to implement pharmaceutical care into their practice but identified a number of barriers to successful implementation, which was consistent with those identified by pharmacists internationally.[6]

A postal survey to randomly selected community pharmacists and general practitioners was undertaken in 1998 and repeated in 2002 to examine whether the perception of the role of a community pharmacist may be a barrier to greater involvement in medicines management.[12] This study reports a significant ($P < 0.01$) and positive change in the perceptions of the general practitioners between 1998 and 2002, which suggests a growing acceptance of a role for pharmacists in providing medicines management services; however, it revealed a gap in perceptions regarding the current role of community pharmacists.[12] There was general acceptance in terms of the technical roles of community pharmacists but less agreement with the more clinical focused roles, such as medication reviews.[12] This study highlighted barriers such as a mandate, legitimacy, adequacy, and effectiveness that need to be addressed for community pharmacists to become more involved in medicines management services.[12]

Following the General Practitioner-Pharmacist Collaboration study, which was conducted between 2002 and 2004, perceptions of the clinical medication reviews undertaken by community pharmacists were sought from both general practitioners and pharmacists.[13,14] The pharmacists reported satisfaction in building better rapport with patients and approved of the opportunity to make a difference and help people. They all considered that medication reviews would be part of the future of pharmacy. However, pharmacists also commented on; (a) the challenge of incorporating an extra service into the normal dispensing and supply function of a community pharmacy, (b) lack of confidence in clinical and personal skills, and (c) the need for peer support.[14] General practitioners reported finding the recommendations made by the pharmacists following the medication reviews as useful and acknowledged the usefulness of an outside perspective on the patient's use of their medicines and the opportunity to stop or change medicines.[13] General practitioners in New Zealand are primarily a fee-for-service business, and there is a strong view that general practitioners should be funded when spending time with pharmacists talking about patients that have received a medication review. It is interesting to note that general practitioners participating in the General Practitioner-Pharmacist Collaboration Study generally commented that they did not find the medication reviews threatening or encroaching on their territory. They also felt that having a professional relationship with the pharmacist was very important.[13]

A study undertaken in 2008 found that all Medicine Use Review pharmacists believed the service as being "highly valuable" or "valuable to patients"; however, this study did not seek data on patient outcomes as the Medicine Use Review service was only just starting to be delivered.[15] This study suggests that the earlier experience of Comprehensive Pharmaceutical Care and Pharmaceutical Review Service collaborative medication review services appear to have fostered the development of Medicine Use Review services in New Zealand.[15]

Delivery of Medication Management Services in New Zealand

In the primary care setting, the delivery of the Medicine Use Review, Medicine Therapy Assessment, and Comprehensive Medicines Management services are a face-to-face consultation-based services with an initial consultation and formal follow-ups at quarterly intervals. Patients are generally enrolled in these services for a period of 12 months. There is an informed consent process and patients are registered to receive the service.

Where the actual consultation takes place is generally the patient's choice with most pharmacists undertaking some Medicine Use Review services in the patient's homes, and some in consultation rooms in the community pharmacy. With a trend toward co-location of community pharmacies in General Practice buildings, some pharmacists are delivering medicines management services from these premises.

A small number of pharmacies have focused on the long-term residential care market and have dedicated pharmacists providing Medicine Therapy Assessment services in the long-term residential care institutions. There are a handful of pharmacists who have specialized in the mental health area who provide Comprehensive Medicines Management services for mental health clients both in the community setting and in mental health facilities.

Funding of Medication Management Services in New Zealand

The New Zealand National Pharmacist defines all the pharmacists' services that may be funded by District Health Boards. Medicines Management services in New Zealand as "new value-added services" that are in addition to the base mandatory pharmacy services and the existing extended services defined in the current pharmacy service agreements funded by the government via the District Health Boards. Medicines management services are not compulsory in terms of District Health Boards' funding or pharmacist provision and can be funded according to local District Health Boards' need and availability of funding. Currently, 11 of the 20 District Health Boards are funding the Medicine Use Review service; and a number of the Primary Health Organizations are funding the Medicine Use Review service and some Medicine Therapy Assessment and Comprehensive Medicines Management services. There are some regions in New Zealand where there is no government funding for these services. There is the option for patients to self-fund these services; however, in reality in the New Zealand health environment this is rare. At this stage medical insurance companies have not included medication management services in their schedules of benefits for medical insurance policies.

Remuneration for Medicine Use Review services by District Health Boards uses a capitated funding model where the community pharmacy that holds the contract for the service is paid a fee for providing the service to the patient for 1 year. This fee varies from contract to contract with a range of $150 to $200 NZ dollars per patient per annum, with the majority two-thirds of the fee paid after the initial consultation and implementation of the care plan and the remainder of the fee paid after the follow-up consultations have occurred.

A considerable number of long-term residential care institutions are receiving some sort of medicines management service as part of their contractual arrangements for the supply of medications for their patients.

These are usually level C–Medicine Therapy Assessment services. However, there is no current accurate information available as to the number of pharmacists providing these services or the number of institutions who are purchasing these services. There is no current accurate information available on the specific remuneration for these services as they tend to be bundled into complex commercially sensitive contracts involving the provisions of medicines and long-term residential care staff education.

Future Direction

In New Zealand, policymakers are calling for greater integration and collaboration in the health care sector in conjunction with a population health focus and strategic focus on "Better Sooner More Convenient Care" in the community for all New Zealanders.[16,17] One of the key objectives in the Medicines New Zealand strategy is "to optimize the quality use of medicines" and it highlights the central position of pharmacists in assisting patients to understand their medicines better, to use them appropriately, monitor side effects and adverse reactions, and to optimize therapeutic outcomes through medicines use and adherence.[18,19]

With the expanding and different health needs of New Zealand population groups, such as the increasing burden of long-term conditions, there is a view that better utilization of the pharmacist workforce through medicines review services will support both the patient and the prescriber to achieve better quality use of medicines; improve patient health, well-being, and health outcomes; gain efficiencies; reduce the volume of wasted medicines; and prevent medicine-related hospitalizations.

Pharmacists in New Zealand are generally positive about becoming involved in providing new and enhanced services and making a shift form product to patient-centered care.[20] In particular, young pharmacists who have been trained in the principles of pharmaceutical care and care planning are keen to deliver medicines management services. Although the reform of New Zealand primary health care has provided the opportunity for some pharmacists to provide medicines management services, a number of barriers need to be addressed to achieve a greater implementation and better utilization of the pharmacist workforce. A key barrier is a lack of adequate remuneration, which requires District Health Boards to realign funding models, which facilitate integration and collaboration amongst key primary health care providers such as GPs, nurses, and pharmacists, and removes the requirement for pharmacy to sell product in order to deliver services. Pharmacists may have to adopt a more user-pay approach to the services they provide than they have done in the past and become less reliant on government funding.

REFERENCES

1. Statistics New Zealand: *National Population Estimates: March 2011 Quarter.* http://www.stats. govt.NEW ZEALAND/browse_for_stats/population/estimeates_and_projections/National PopulationEstimates-HOTPMar21qrt.aspxz.
2. Campbell L. Personal Communication. Pharmacy Licensing Co-ordiantor, Ministry of Health, Wellington, New Zealand, June 2011.
3. District Health Board New Zealand Pharmacy Advisory Group. *New Zealand National Pharmacist Services Framework.* Wellington, New Zealand: District Health Boards New Zealand; 2007.
4. Pharmacy Council of New Zealand. *Pharmacy Council of New Zealand Workforce Demographics as at 30 June 2011.* Wellington, New Zealand: Pharmacy Council of New Zealand; 2011.
5. Pharmacy Council of New Zealand. *Competence Standards for the Pharmacy Profession.* Wellington, New Zealand: Pharmacy Council of New Zealand; 2011.
6. Pharmacy Council of New Zealand. *Medicines Management.* Wellington, New Zealand: Pharmacy Council of New Zealand; 2006.
7. Pharmacy Council of New Zealand. *Medicines Use Review (MEDICINE USE REVIEW).* Wellington, New Zealand: Pharmacy Council of New Zealand; 2006.
8. Dunlop JA, Shaw JP. Community pharmacists' perspectives on pharmaceutical care implementation in New Zealand. *Pharm World Sci.* 2002;24(6):224–230.
9. Scahill S, Harrison J, Carswell P, Shaw JP. Health care policy and community pharmacy: implications for the New Zealand primary health care sector. *N Z Med J.* 2010;123(1317):41–51.
10. Pharmaceutical Society of New Zealand. *Focus on the Future: Ten Year Vision for Pharmacists in New Zealand: 2004–2014.* Wellington, New Zealand: Pharmaceutical Society of New Zealand; 2004.
11. Buckham B: Personal Communication. Manager New Zealand College of Pharmacists, Wellington, New Zealand; June 2011.
12. Bryant LJM, Coster G, Gamble GD, McCormick RN. General practitioners' and pharmacists' perceptions of the role of community pharmacist in delivering clinical services. *Res Social Adm Pharm.* 2009;5(4):347–362.
13. Bryant LJM, Coster G, McCormick RN. General practitioner perceptions of clinical medication reviews undertaken by community pharmacists. *J Prim Health Care.* 2010;2(3):225–233.
14. Bryant LJM, Coster G, McCormick RN. Community pharmacist perceptions of clinical medication reviews. *J Prim Health Care.* 2010;2(3):234–242.
15. Lee E, Braund R, Tordoff J. Examining the first year of Medicines Use Review services provided by pharmacists in New Zealand: 2008. *N Z Med J.* 2009;122(1293):26–35.
16. Ministry of Health. *New Zealand Primary Health Care Strategy.* Wellington, New Zealand: Ministry of Health; 2011.
17. Ministry of Health: Better, Sooner, More Convenient Health Care in the Community. Wellington, New Zealand: Ministry of Health; 2011.
18. Ministry of Health. *Medicines New Zealand.* Wellington, New Zealand: Ministry of Health; 2007.
19. Associate Minister of Health, Minister of Health. *Actioning Medicines New Zealand 2010.* Wellington, New Zealand: Ministry of Health; 2010.
20. Scahill S, Harrison J, Sheridan J. The ABC of New Zealand's Ten Year Vision for Pharmacists: awareness, barriers and consultation. *Int J Pharm Pract.* 2009;17(3):135–142.

CHINA

Siting Zhou, PhD
Research Analyst, HealthCore, Inc.
Wilmington, Delaware

Traditional Pharmacy Education in China

Modern higher education in pharmacy in China began in the Qing Dynasty in 1906. Before the establishment of the People's Republic of China in 1949, there were eight schools and universities offering pharmacy programs and degrees.[1] Today, there are more than 257 pharmacy schools and universities that offer the Bachelor of Science degree and higher degrees throughout China. In 2005, more than 6000 graduates received BS degrees, 800 received Master of Science (MS) degrees, and 290 received Doctor of Philosophy (PhD) degrees in pharmacy.[2] Traditionally, students receive a BS degree as an entry-level pharmacy degree. Students holding a BS degree can earn a MS degree in 3 years or a PhD degree in 5 years. Students with a MS degree can work toward a PhD with an additional 3 years of study.[3]

Pharmacy education in China focuses on the pharmaceutical sciences. Pharmacy practice curricula in these programs are centered on compounding, dispensing, pharmacy administration, and laboratory experiences, which are the traditional responsibilities of pharmacists. Additional graduate-level training is available at the MS and the PhD levels, most of which concentrate on drug discovery and drug development research.[3] After graduating, most pharmacy graduates work in hospitals and industry. Of approximately 300,000 pharmacy graduates from 1949 to 1998, 156,000 (52%) worked in hospital pharmacies, 62,000 (21%) worked in the pharmaceutical industry, and 27,000 (9%) worked in "wholesale" or community pharmacies.[4]

Licensure of Pharmacists

Pharmacists in China were not required to be licensed to practice until 1994, when the government first implemented a system of licensure for pharmacists. The Department of Human Resources in conjunction with various branches of the State Food and Drug Administration (SFDA), Peoples Republic of China, has distributed "Licensed Pharmacist Qualification System Temporary Rules" and subsequently the "Licensed Chinese Medicine Pharmacist Qualification System Temporary Rules." The SFDA is the governing body that is charged with the oversight of the licensing examination, registration of licensed pharmacists, and continuing education required for licensed pharmacists.[3]

Passing the licensure examination is not required for all areas of pharmacy practice, and the passing rate of examination is often low (12.83% in 2004, 18.18% in 2005, and 16.69% in 2006). Some fields such as pharmaceutical manufacturing, industry, and management, as well as hospital pharmacies, clinic pharmacies, and community pharmacies, require at least one licensed pharmacist. However, in these situations, the licensed pharmacist may be in a supervisory role over the unlicensed pharmacists.[3]

Clinical Pharmacy Education

In order to meet the growing demand for clinical pharmacists, the clinical pharmacy programs and additional degree offerings are being developed in China.

Clinical pharmacy education in China has developed only recently, so there is no standardization of curricula. Unlike the PharmD program in the United States, there are a variety of degrees offered from various programs. BS degrees in pharmacy or medicine, MS degrees in pharmacy or medicine, and PhD degrees in pharmacy can all have components of clinical pharmacy. From 1989 to 1999, the West China School of Pharmacy at Sichuan University offered the first 5-year clinical pharmacy BS degree. Since 2000, the Ministry of Education has allowed only pharmaceutical sciences as a first-level discipline for BS degrees. Students wishing to study clinical pharmacy at the bachelor's level may select clinical pharmacy as a second-level area of concentration under pharmaceutical sciences. As an exception, in 2008, the China Pharmaceutical University was allowed to offer a first-level, 5-year BS degree in clinical pharmacy.[3]

Peking University developed a 6-year continuous or dual degree BS/MS program in clinical pharmacy in 2001, and is the only university in China to offer such a degree. In 2007, the first 15 MS students graduated from this program at Peking University, the largest number of clinical pharmacy graduates in 1 year in China. In 2003, Peking University was permitted by the Ministry of Education to offer a 3-year postbaccalaureate MS in clinical pharmacy. Shortly thereafter, programs were approved at three other universities (Sichuan University, China Pharmaceutical University, and Shenyang Pharmaceutical University). Shandong University has another interesting degree option, the master of medicine in clinical pharmacy degree. In this program, students complete a 7-year program in medicine after graduation from high school with a concentration in clinical pharmacy.[3]

From 2005 to 2007, four universities (Peking University, Sichuan University, China Pharmaceutical University, and Shenyang Pharmaceutical University) began to recruit candidates for a PhD degree in clinical pharmacy. The first graduates from these programs appeared in late 2008. There are two possible routes for attaining/obtaining the PhD in clinical pharmacy: after graduating from a BS program, the student completes a 5-year PhD program; or after graduation from an MS program in clinical pharmacy or a related pharmacy area, the student completes a 3-year PhD program.[3]

Many large general hospitals started to differentiate a few practitioners as clinical pharmacists or hired graduates with an MS or PhD degree in clinical pharmacy. Currently, about 90% of graduates from MS in clinical pharmacy programs are working in clinical pharmacy. Additionally, some pharmacists working in hospitals and the pharmaceutical industry are electing to return to school to pursue a 3-year MS in clinical pharmacy program or a 1- to 2-year postgraduate clinical pharmacy course specifically designed for practicing pharmacists. The main venue of clinical pharmacists in China is in comprehensive medical centers and is focused on a few functions, which include patient care rounds, review medication orders, perform therapeutic drug monitoring, and provide drug information to patients and other health care practitioners during this time. However, clinical pharmacy is developing in more clinical areas and as the supply of clinical pharmacists increases, this type of practice is increasing.[3]

Pharmaceutical Care and Clinical Pharmacy

When the concept of "pharmaceutical care" came to China in the early 1990s, the emphasis in practice began to shift from medication dispensing to clinical pharmacy. In order to prepare pharmacy professionals who are able to provide pharmaceutical care, the field of clinical pharmacy has grown since 2002, when the government required all hospitals to develop clinical pharmacy programs to address drug-related problems and to promote rational drug use in hospitals, which is the core of pharmaceutical care in China.[5]

In 2002, the Ministry of Health of People's Republic of China (MHPRC), issued "Interim Provisions of Medication Management in Medical Institutions," which for the first time legally established the system of clinical pharmacists and clearly stated the role of clinical pharmacists in China. These provisions aim to address drug-related problems and to promote rational drug use in hospitals, by requiring the department of pharmacy in hospitals to establish the patient-centered model of medication therapy management (MTM).[6] The Ministry of Health established 1-year clinical pharmacy training programs for currently practicing pharmacists in January 2006. This training requires pharmacists to: (1) begin thinking of themselves as clinicians; (2) improve their knowledge base in clinical medicine, clinical pharmacy, and biology; (3) improve their knowledge of medical ethics, patient psychology, and medicine administration; (4) develop their skills in communication, computer use, and foreign language; (5) learn to participate in patient care rounds and other clinical pharmacy activities; (6) learn to employ the hospital information system (HIS) to advance the profession through activities such as establishing an adverse drug reaction database or pharmacokinetics and pharmacodynamics databases; and (7) participate in clinical professional meetings and advanced training classes.[3]

To enforce the legal provisions by MNPRC, 42 pilot hospitals were chosen as pilot hospitals to carry out pharmaceutical care services in 2008.[14] In these pilot hospitals, clinical pharmacists were required to provide pharmaceutical care services and perform their responsibilities as discussed above. The 42 hospitals were selected from 19 provinces and municipalities, which were considered as the best hospitals throughout the nation. In China, hospitals are classified into three levels: province and city level, county level, and rural and town level. Province and city level hospitals are usually considered to provide the best quality of medical services. Based on 2006 MNPRC statistics, there were 19,246 hospitals in China, and 1045 were province and city level. These pilot hospitals were all province and city level.

Due to the work at these pilot hospitals, hospital pharmacy practice is changing from "drug-centered" to "patient-centered," and the primary focus for hospital pharmacy is changing from drug supply to pharmaceutical care. Thus, the pharmacist's activities are changing from drug dispensing and compounding to rational drug use and patient care. This kind of transformation has attracted outstanding pharmacy graduates, including those with advanced degrees, to seek employment in hospitals.[3] However, there is no standard working model for clinical pharmacists currently in China because it has not been long since the establishment of the clinical pharmacist system and the pilot training of clinical pharmacists has just been completed.

Zhu et al.[7] proposed to establish a working model, a training and management system in the People's Liberation Army General Hospital (PLAGH). In 2009, PLAGH set up a clinical pharmacy department. There were six full-time unit-based clinical pharmacists in four divisions: respiratory and anti-infection, cardiovascular, endocrine, and oncology departments in the hospital. A working model was built for the clinical pharmacists in these four divisions. First, the responsibilities and working target of the clinical pharmacist were defined. After full-time unit-based clinical pharmacists were recruited, they were required to participate in daily clinical rounds and attend case discussions and clinical professional meetings; they were arranged to attend relevant advanced training programs according to their professional needs. In addition, the clinical pharmacy department held a symposium for work report and case discussion every week to stimulate clinical pharmacists' work passion. Clinical pharmacists perform the following daily clinical activities: review medication orders, give counseling for rational use of drugs and therapeutic drug monitoring to patients and other health care practitioners, provide patient education, hold lectures for the rational use of drugs, attend consultations and drug safety emergency treatment.

Second, a standard operation flow chart of medication order reviews was made. Although, clinical pharmacists treated various problems when reviewing different wards' medication orders, they faced the same issues regarding the principles of medication order reviewing and the rational use of drugs. Thus, according to the standard operation flow chart for medication reviewing, clinical pharmacists initiated medication reviews every day and focused on patients in intensive care.

Third, registration forms were standardized and the daily work for clinical pharmacists was specified. A series of registration forms was made to specify the daily work of clinical pharmacists after the completion of the standard operation flow chart for each routine work, including medication order reviews registration form, counseling registration form for the rational use of drugs, consultation registration forms and drug safety emergency treatment registration forms. By 2010, clinical pharmacists in PLAGH had communicated with physicians regarding over 200 medical orders, provided counseling for rational use of medications for more than 300 cases to the wards, attended 40 clinical pharmacy consultation cases, and dealt with 11 drug safety emergent incidents.

Fourth, clinical pharmacists in PLAGH were required to attend consultations relating to their specialty on a flexible basis. Before a consultation, a patient's clinical information such as progress notes and medical orders from the clinical pharmacy workstation was obtained. A discussion was held before a nonemergency consultation gathering all opinions on the clinical pharmacy team to improve the consultation efficiency and increase the acceptance rates of pharmacists' recommendations. A consultation registration form was to be filled in after consultations before follow-up return visits.

In addition, a clinical pharmacy service support system was established. Clinical pharmacy was added to the functions of the HIS by introducing and developing independently software for clinical pharmacy services, such as clinical pharmacy workstations, hospital medication safety monitoring and evaluation systems, and electronic medication record management systems of PLAGH. Pharmacists could provide medication-related recommendations based on comprehensive clinical information from each patient's medical record, including the medication profile, progress notes, and laboratory data, and could read dispensing data online by using clinical pharmacy workstation as well.[7]

Though pharmaceutical care and MTM services have begun to be promoted in hospital pharmacies, very little service has been provided in community pharmacies, due to the lack of clinical pharmacy professionals.

Community Pharmacy in China

Community pharmacies are retail pharmacies in China. As of December 2009, there were nearly 388,000 community pharmacies in China.[8] There is a keen shortage of pharmacists in China. In 2009, there were 380,000 pharmacists working in hospital or community pharmacies, which translate 0.29 pharmacists per 1000 population, the lowest among the Brazil, Russia, India, China (BRIC) nations (the average ratio was 0.6 in 2009).[9] To work as a community pharmacist, it is compulsory to register in a Province Pharmacists' Association. There are two professional societies, the China Licensed Pharmacist Association and CHA, representing all Chinese pharmacists in community, hospital, industry, education, scientific research, or administration.

Community pharmacists in China typically compound and dispense medications prescribed by physicians, dentists, or other authorized medical practitioners. The Fourth Chinese National Health Care Survey revealed a high prevalence rate of self-medication among the population in China, surging from 36% in 2003 to 70% in 2008.[10] The data reinforce the responsibility of community pharmacies and pharmacists in preventing patients from drug-related problems when practicing self-medication.[11] Therefore, providing pharmaceutical care as a means to solve these issues is important in community pharmacy. However, there is little information available in the literature about the extent of pharmaceutical care provision in community pharmacies in China.

In 2011, Fang et al.[11] reported their survey research, which collected information from samples of 130 pharmacists in community pharmacies in Xi'an, Shaanxi Province, northwest China in April 2008. In their survey, information on the extent of pharmaceutical care practice and the barriers to the provision of pharmaceutical care as perceived by the practicing pharmacists in community pharmacies was collected. More than 90% of the respondents reported spending some or most of their time performing prescription checks or providing patients with directions for drug administration, dosage, and precautions. In contrast, just over half the respondents reported monitoring adverse drug reaction and drug compliance among patients. They were also poor at conducting health education and promoting patients' drug safety knowledge within and outside of the community pharmacy settings.

The study also found that the lack of financial compensation was the greatest barrier in implementing pharmaceutical care with 82% of participants agreeing or strongly agreeing. In addition, insufficient communication with a physician was considered a major barrier the by respondents. It is vital to create a cooperative relationship between the pharmacist and the physician to develop an evidence-based care plan for a patient's medicine therapy and follow-up on the patient's expected health outcomes.[12]

Chinese pharmacists indicated a willingness to implement pharmaceutical care but had limited knowledge and skill of pharmaceutical care and underdeveloped pharmacy education contributed to this problem. In China, patients do not pay dispensing fees for the drugs dispensed for them. Besides, there was not an insurance program that pays pharmacists for cognitive services so far, so the lack of reimbursements discourages pharmacists' enthusiasm to offer these services.[11]

Necessity of Medication Management

The issuance of these legal provisions was due to the increased need for standards of medication management services due to several problems in China. First, there was tremendous increase in drug prices and expenditures in China from the 1990s to 2000s. According to a report from Jinshan Hospital, the Medical Center of Fudan University,[13] in the market mix of all drugs at various prices, the proportion of low-price drugs (<= 0.3 Chinese Yuan/unit) decreased from 18.76% in 1992 to 5.32% in 1999; while high-price drugs (=>10 Chinese Yuan/unit) increased from 20.11% in 1992 to 41.83% in 1999. Though there was inflation of prices between 1992 and 1994, from 1995 to 1999, national prices stayed very stable except for the rapid increase in drug price and expenditures.

Second, the increased misuse of drugs led to severe drug-related comorbidity and mortality from the late 1990s to the early 2000s. Based on the statistics of a report from the Medical and Pharmaceutical Economics Newspaper on November 29, 1999,[13] there were about 10 million people in China experiencing drug adverse reactions each year, and the associated health care costs reached 4.5 billion Chinese Yuan. It was reported that 190,200 inpatients died from adverse drug reactions; in 1990, the total number of children with hearing and speech impairment was 1.82 million, and over 1 million of these children had hearing impairment that was due to the poisoning of antibiotics.[13,14]

In order to take good control of these severe drug-related problems, the Chinese government began to promote the pharmaceutical care-based MTM services nationwide. However, the MTM services and pharmaceutical care has remained very slow in development and were poorly carried out nationwide since the issuance of Interim Provisions of Medication Management in Medical Institutions. Until the year of 2008, MTM-centered pharmaceutical care has only been practiced in pilot hospitals across the nation, specifically targeted at hospital patients. In other hospitals and community pharmacies, pharmacists' work still focuses on drug dispensing, and the patient-centered service has not yet been provided.[15]

Current Challenges of MTM Services and Recommendations

There are a number of challenges as integrated MTM services are being adopted and developed in China. These challenges are as follows:

1. The concept of patient-centered pharmaceutical care and MTM services has not been fully acknowledged and accepted. There is still a lack of

connection between the MTM theoretical framework and its application in the realistic situation in China.

2. There is a lack of skilled professionals in pharmacy practice to carry out MTM services. The social status of pharmacists in China has not been given much attention. Only since 2002, has the role of the clinical pharmacist been established. Pharmacy education in China centers on theory-based curriculum, and there is not enough teaching and practice in the clinical setting. Graduates from the pharmacy discipline have not only insufficient clinical-therapy knowledge or skills but also lack the understanding of their professional responsibilities in providing MTM services.

3. There exists a general bias that, only province and city level hospitals are qualified to carry out MTM services.

4. There is a lack of an effective theoretical framework or system to standardize and evaluate the MTM services, so health care professionals may feel confused and frustrated when providing such services.

5. There is a lack of administrative measures from government to carry out pharmaceutical care and MTM services nationwide, so there is no incentive for pharmacists to provide this patient-centered care.

Based on the barriers discussed above, the difficulty of carrying out MTM services in China mainly comes from two aspects: education and administration. As for the educational side, on one hand, there is not enough education among health care professionals about the necessity, concept, systematic framework, and specific standards of MTM; on the other hand, not enough attention has been given to pharmacists' education and social responsibilities, so pharmacists have little understanding of their value and role in their work to perform MTM services. Regarding the administrative aspect, there is no standardized evaluation system to monitor professionals' performance of MTM services, together with a lack of a payment system that gives standardized reimbursement to pharmacists or other professionals for providing MTM services, thereby giving professionals little incentive to provide MTM services to patients.

By understanding these barriers or challenges, the following suggestions are given to help improve the practice of pharmaceutical care and MTM services:

1. More education needs to be provided to health professionals, particularly pharmacists, about the theories and practical standards of MTM services not only in clinical settings but also in the university curriculum.

2. MTM practice should be promoted in community pharmacies. Pharmacists with MTM training can provide MTM services to patients who go to community pharmacies for medication information. Besides dispensing

the drug product, pharmacists can provide patient-centered care to help patients make the best decision about their medications.

3. An integrated evaluation and payment system should be established, which evaluates each itemized MTM service performed by pharmacists or other health professionals, and makes standard payments according to the services provided. For example, MTM services can be listed in health insurance coverage, providing more incentive for health professionals to perform these services.

4. Pharmacy education should be reformed to cultivate more qualified pharmacy professionals to meet the increasing demand of pharmaceutical care practice and to take more social responsibilities. More clinical practice curricular should be added to originally theory-based disciplines to strengthen pharmacy students' clinical skills. More professional opportunities and responsibilities should be provided to pharmacy graduates, which will help improve pharmacy professionals' self-perception in social role.

Conclusion

With an increasing demand for the control of drug-related problems, MTM services will become more and more popular in the health system in China, and clinical pharmacists will play an increasingly important role among health professionals providing MTM services to patients. Though there are still many challenges that need to be overcome in order to carry out MTM services nationwide from hospital pharmacies to community pharmacies, pharmacy educational reform has already been advocated and is being accomplished to provide more clinical pharmacists who are well trained and qualified to perform tasks required in MTM services. Therefore, we should be confident that pharmaceutical care-based MTM services will be developed on a broader basis in the near future in China.

REFERENCES

1. *Chinese Pharmaceutical Yearbook.* Shanghai, China: The Second Military Chinese Medical University Press; 2005:159.
2. *Chinese Pharmaceutical Yearbook.* Shanghai, China: The Second Military Medical University Press; 2006:234;247–248.
3. Ryan M, Shao H, Yang L, et al. Clinical pharmacy education in China. *Am J Pharm Educ.* 2008;72(6):129.
4. *Chinese Pharmaceutical Yearbook.* Shanghai, China: The Second Military Chinese Medical University Press; 1999:24.
5. Hu J, Cai Z, Sun H. Pharmaceutical care and integrated pharmaceutical care. *Pharm Care Res.* 2008;8(3):161–165.

6. Li A, Ping Q. The Implications of American Medication Therapy Management for China. *Med Philosophy.* 2011;1:71–73.

7. Zhu M, Guo DH, Liu GY, et al. Exploration of clinical pharmacist management system and working model in China. *Pharm World Sci.* 2010;32(4):411–415.

8. The Ministry of Commerce. *The "Twelfth Five" National Plan for Development of Pharmaceutical Distribution Industry.* 2011. Retrieved July 15, 2011 from http://www.ichainnel.com/zh-cn/read.php?id=199694_9e50f6.

9. World Health Organization. *WHO Human Resources for Health.* 2007. Retrieved July 28, 2011, from www.who.int/whosis/indicators/2007HumanResourcesForHealth/en/.

10. Ministry of Health of People's Republic of China. *The Notification of Carrying Out Pilot Clinical Pharmacy Work.* 2008. Retrieved July 29, 2011 from http://www.moh.gov.cn/publicfiles/business/htmlfiles/mohyzs/s3577/200804/18775.htm.

11. Fang Y, Yang S, Feng B, Ni Y, Zhang K. Pharmacists' perception of pharmaceutical care in community pharmacy: A questionnaire survey in northwest China. *Health Soc Care Community.* 2011;19(2):189–197.

12. Ranelli PL, Biss J. Physicians' perceptions of communication with and responsibilities of pharmacists. *J Am Pharm Assoc (Wash).* 2000;40(5):625–630.

13. Fang Z, Zeng H, Song X. Discussion on Pharmaceutical care and Calling for Good Pharmacy Practice of China. *Chinese Pharm Aff.* 2001;15(5):307–310.

14. Ministry of Health of People's Republic of China. National Health Resources Disclosure in 2006. *Chinese J Infect Control.* 2007;4:234–234.

15. The Ministry of Health People's Republic of China. *The Fourth Chinese National Health Care Survey Results.* 2009. Retrieved July 29, 2011, from www.moh.gov.cn/publicfiles/business/htmlfiles/mohbgt/s3582/200902/39201.htm.

KOREA

Eunyoung Kim, PharmD, BCPS, PhD
Assistant Professor, College of Pharmacy
Chungnam National University
Daejoeon, South Korea

Korea is located in East Asia, previously unified, but is currently divided into North Korea and South Korea. South Korea, officially the Republic of Korea, is a democratics, and free market country with memberships in the United Nations, World Trade Organization, and G-20 major economies. For this section, Korea only means the Republic of Korea.

Overview of Korean Health Care System

The population of Korea is approximately 50 million. In 2008, total expenditure on health was 6.5% of the gross national product, less than the Organization for Cooperation and Development (OECD) average of 8.9%. Drug expenditures were 23.9% of the total health care costs; it is higher than the mean of OECD at 17.1% (OECD, 2010).[1,2,3,4]

The entire Korean population is covered for the risk of medical illness, through the National Health Insurance (NHI) or the Medical Aid Program (MAP). The NHI, which has some values; mandatory coverage, payment of contributions on the basis of ability to pay, and receipt of the benefits according to need, is a social health insurance system. The MAP is a social protection program for the very poor who represent about 4% of the population, financed through general taxation before 2007. Then there was no or minimal cost sharing for MAP beneficiaries. However, since 2007, MAP beneficiaries also are required to pay cost sharing for outpatient services. The benefits are not different between NHI and MAP patients, as benefit coverage is standardized.

The predominant provider payment is fee for service. For NHI benefits fees are regulated and providers' claims reviewed. For uninsured service, fees and providers' activities are mostly unregulated. The NHI is financed through mandatory contributions. The contribution rate relates to the employee gross salary and is equally shared between the employer and the employee. Contributions for self-employed individuals are assessed by income, assets, living level, and the rate of participation in economic activities. Dependants of insures are also covered by the NHI scheme (Figure 12-3).[5]

Before 2000, both physicians and pharmacists were able to prescribe and dispense drugs. The majority of medications in Korea were dispensed and sold to patients directly by physicians during clinic visits. Pharmacists could also conduct independent evaluations of patients and dispense prescription or nonprescription drugs without a physician's prescription, based on their diagnoses. However, in recent years, public health problems, especially drug-related problems, such as drug misuse and overuse, gathered more attention. The Korean government has taken a number of steps to encourage the separation of drug prescribing from dispensing. In 1999, the Korean Medical Association, the Korean Pharmaceutical Association, and citizen's groups reached an agreement to a fundamental change in the roles of medicine and pharmacy. A new law, enacted in 2000, completely separates the professional roles of physicians and pharmacists, limiting prescribing to medicine and dispensing to pharmacy.[6]

Pharmacy Education System

There had been 20 colleges of pharmacy in Korea, but recently 15 new colleges of pharmacy have been established, for a total 35 colleges of pharmacy. Traditionally, the educational requirement was a 4-year pharmacy program. A new 6-year pharmacy educational system is being implemented starting in 2011 and requires students to take an entry test PEET (Pharmacy Education

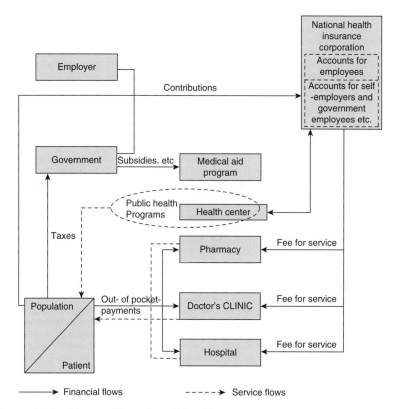

Figure 12-3 Korea: Financing of health care.
Source: OECD Secretariat, 2002, http://www.ecosante.org/oecd.htm.

Eligibility Test) (Figure 12-4). The chief reason is to provide more education in the clinical areas. Actually this 6 year pharmacy educational system (2 + 4) requires the completion of four years, including 10 months of pharmacy practice experiences, at an accredited college of pharmacy.[3]

Students applying for admission into a college of pharmacy already have either a completed undergraduate degree or they have taken 2 years of undergraduate pharmacy prerequisite classes.

The duration of this pharmacy practice experience is 40 weeks (1600 hours) for 30 credits, full-time in-service training in a community pharmacy, the pharmaceutical department of a hospital, and a pharmaceutical industry.

Pharmacies

The total number of pharmacists who are licensed to practice is 61,114 and the number of practicing pharmacists who are licensed to practice and provide direct services to clients/patients 30,000 (2010).[7]

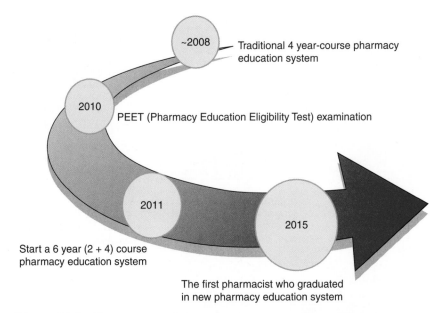

~2008 — Traditional 4 year-course pharmacy education system

2010

PEET (Pharmacy Education Eligibility Test) examination

2011

2015

Start a 6 year (2 + 4) course pharmacy education system

The first pharmacist who graduated in new pharmacy education system

Figure 12-4   Time course of new pharmacy education system.

Many pharmacists work in community pharmacies. For instance, 78% of all practicing pharmacists work in community pharmacies, while 10% work in hospitals and other health care facilities, 5% work in the industrial sector, and the remaining 7% work in other settings. The 2011 annual report of the Korea Pharmaceutical Association indicates that approximately 21,096 pharmacies serve a population of about 50 million people in Korea, which equates with 65 pharmacists per 100,000 population.[7]

The staff of a typical pharmacy includes only pharmacists. The pharmacy technician program is not implemented in Korea, so hiring pharmacy technicians is not allowed. Pharmacists are so busy dispensing prescriptions that sometimes it is disruptive to counsel patients. Hospital pharmacies focus on inpatients services, such as inpatient education, medication counseling, and multidisciplinary team approach.

Development of Clinical Pharmacy and Pharmaceutical Care

In the 1980s, a member of some Korean pharmacists in hospitals and PharmDs from the USA conducted clinical activities such as therapeutic drug monitoring consultation, participation in medical rounds, anticoagulation services, providing nutritional support services as well as other activity focused services.[8] The first hospital pharmacy residency program was implemented in 1983 at Seoul National University Hospital. It started as a 1-year course and now has become a 2-year course. Since the start of these clinical activities, the curriculum of pharmacy has changed and some clinical subjects have been added, including pharmacotherapy and pharmaceutical care.

In the 1990s, colleges of pharmacy started to engage full-time faculty who specializes in clinical pharmacy and began to teach the concept of pharmaceutical care at the universities that also stimulated care activities in practice. Pharmacy students and pharmacists became part of the health care team. Pharmacists and pharmacy residents performed patient-focused research in the hospitals. The Korean Society of Hospital Pharmacists started a clinical pharmacy program as continuing education in 1988.

Professional Activities of Pharmacists

Pharmaceutical care-related activities[9] are currently developed in two clinical settings: community pharmacies and hospital pharmacies.

Dispensing

Community pharmacies can be established by pharmacists in Korea; however, only physicians can establish hospitals. There are some chain pharmacies, but the owner of the pharmacy must be a pharmacist. The dispensing activities are done by pharmacists. Dispensing is only for physician-prescribed drugs. Nonprescription medications can be sold without a prescription but all packages of nonprescription drugs must be sealed and intact before being sold. This prevents pharmacists from mixing and packaging medications on the basis of their own decisions. Generic interchanges are allowed if there are adequate bioequivalence data recognized by the Korean Food and Drug Administration. Pharmacists are expected to evaluate the prescription before dispensing. If there are unreasonable or questionable issues, it is necessary to communicate with the physician who prescribed and verify the problem. At the beginning of the New Act in 2000, physicians did not respond to the pharmacist's questions, or refused to collaborate on a prescription. But now, they can be punished by law if they do not cooperate. Most hospitals set up automatic dispensing machines to increase effectiveness and expand their clinical roles, becoming more involved in patient care. Some hospitals implemented the unit-dose system and participate daily in clinical rounds with other health care providers.[10–16]

Patient Counseling and Drug Information

Pharmacists are requested to provide drug information to both patients and physicians. Also, pharmacists are expected to educate patients about their medications. When patients come to the pharmacy with their prescriptions, pharmacists are required to inform patients about the dispensed medicine and also counsel the patients about other medicine. A fee provided for this counseling is included in the patients' payment, though it is low (about $0.70 USD per prescription). Sometimes patients come to the pharmacy to obtain advice and information from pharmacists about diseases and the drugs they use, without a prescription, because it is free. In Korea, currently, this counseling fee is an issue. Patients complain that counseling from pharmacists is not enough or that they are not served at all. Several reasons are pointed out; one is time limitation. Most pharmacists in community pharmacies are so busy dispensing that there is not enough time to counsel. Another reason is the lack of knowledge, which may be the more important reason. The 4-year pharmacy educational system that previously existed was heavily based on the pharmaceutical sciences. Most pharmacy school graduates have started practice without adequate education or experience to carry out clinical services. They did not learn pharmacotherapy or pharmaceutical care. Many pharmacists have enrolled in continuing education programs provided by the Korean Pharmaceutical Association, Korean Society of Hospital Pharmacists, or others to overcome their deficit. To meet this request, masters degree programs in clinical pharmacy are offered in many schools these days.

Training and Education Issues

In 1990s, the clinical pharmacy Masters Program was created at a few colleges of pharmacy. The program includes four or five semesters of lectures about the diagnosis of simple ailments, pharmacotherapy, anatomy, pathophysiology, case study, communication skills, and medical statistics. Some are full-time programs, others are part-time programs for working professional pharmacists. Most of them are developing their theses and practice in community pharmacies and hospitals. Now many colleges of pharmacy have established this Masters Program. In KSHP, there are several continuing education programs, including a basic course in clinical pharmacotherapeutics. This is a 1-year course composed of disease-specific lectures and 3 days of clinical practice experience at a clinical practice site in a tertiary hospital. This program was started in 1988; and in 2009, an e-learning system was implemented to increase the effectiveness of the program. After these basic courses, specialty courses which train in one of many professional topic areas, can be taken. Usually lecturers are clinical pharmacists, physicians, and faculties in the college of pharmacy. There are also 1-year courses; specific topics such as: endocrine disorders, oncology, chronic and geriatric disorders, critical care, adverse drug monitoring, nephrotic disorders, anticoagulation services, therapeutic drug monitoring services, and nutritional services. Following the course there is a short-term clinical practice course. Special Interest Groups are also open for patient education about medicine, pharmacoeconomic evaluation, drug information, pediatric pharmacy, clinical nutrition, psychiatric pharmacy, oncologic pharmacy, clinical trials, and antibiotic therapy.[8,17]

Pharmaceutical Care

In community pharmacy, fee for patient counseling and drug information are included in the dispensing of a prescription. There are no community pharmacies where pharmaceutical care is provided. Some pharmacists record patients' basic information but it is not related to pharmaceutical care. During one continuing education program for pharmacists in community pharmacies, the Medication Therapy Management (MTM) in America was introduced and then the pharmacists were surveyed about their attitude toward medication management. Although the survey data are yet unpublished, 60% of pharmacists answered that they are interested in MTM or pharmaceutical care. But they answered they needed more clinical knowledge such as pharmacotherapy and drug information. In hospitals, pharmacists practice various kinds of clinical activities. At outpatient clinics, pharmacists practice in anticoagulation services, respiratory services, chronic renal failure services, and Parkinson's disease services. For hospitalized patients, pharmacists work with multidisciplinary teams in critical care, internal medicine, infection, pediatrics, oncology, and geriatrics. Activities of pharmaceutical care are not supported by the law and remuneration for these activities is not provided.

Future Developments

Implementation activities for pharmaceutical care in community pharmacy are necessary for the future of Korean society. The number of people aged 65 or older surpassed the 5-million mark for the first time in 2009, accounting for 10.3% of the total population. Annual taxes and fees for NHI are continuously increasing in order to support government expenditures. The role of pharmacists in achieving cost savings should be highlighted. By recommending the most appropriate medications through pharmaceutical care, pharmacists can help to lower medical expenditures.[4,18]

Pharmacists can also improve patient medication compliance through education and counseling. Now in Korea, approximately 70 pharmacists have become Board Certified Pharmacotherapy Specialist, a Board Certified Oncology Pharmacist, or a Board Certified Nutritional Supporting Pharmacist through the Board of Pharmaceutical Specialties (BPSs of the United States).[19] Within the system of health care, they are experts in the therapeutic use of medications. They provide medication therapy evaluations and recommendations about patients to other health care professionals. They provide scientifically valid information and advice regarding the safe, appropriate, and cost-effective use of medications. Most of the BPSs are working in hospitals now, but a few pharmacists are in community pharmacies. Usually pharmacists in hospitals are more familiar with pharmaceutical care. Some pharmacists who had various clinical experiences at hospitals opened a community pharmacy and tried to provide pharmaceutical care at the community pharmacy. Although it is not easy to practice pharmaceutical care in the current Korean health care system, many pharmacists recognize the need for the practice. In a few hospitals, graduate pharmacy students are supervised by university faculty. They are involved in the pharmacotherapy of individual patients and attempt to detect any problems with drug therapy during the hospital course. In addition, a few faculties in colleges of pharmacy are interested in implementing pharmaceutical care in community pharmacies. Continuing education programs for optimal pharmaceutical care, which has been developed by KSHP for hospital pharmacists, only are relatively well-organized programs and offer a good learning environment. A few continuing education programs have now been opened for the community pharmacists. This kind of collaboration among pharmacists will be helpful to work together in the same direction. An effort between pharmacists from hospital and community pharmacies, universities, and government is needed to implement pharmaceutical care.

At the beginning of New Law in 2000, most physicians were so conservative that they did not collaborate with pharmacists. Recently the relationship has improved but still pharmacists have to assure physicians that they seek to collaborate and not replace them. It is important to develop a path to share a patient's information because a patient's information is important for the work of pharmacists and other health care providers. The problems should be cautiously solved in collaboration with the other health care providers and the patients. After pharmaceutical care is implemented, a fee for providing this service should be paid. And, in order to be paid for this service, most of all, pharmacists should demonstrate the benefit of pharmaceutical care. This is yet another issue to solve.

Summary

The need for and importance of pharmaceutical care is growing quickly in Korea and is supported by laws in many countries. However, in Korea, the provision of pharmaceutical care is not supported by the laws and is not recognized by the health care department in the government. To prepare for pharmaceutical care, pharmacists must realize the importance of it and should show more concern for patients. Pharmacists' first obligation is to patients. Pharmacists help patients to receive optimal value from the medications. Collaboration with physicians and other health care professionals is essential. Recent changes in the new pharmacy educational system intensify study of pharmacotherapy, patient counseling, pharmaceutical care, and clinical practices. This will be promising for advancing pharmaceutical care. Research for development of pharmaceutical care in other countries and collaborating with pharmacists abroad will be helpful for developments in Korea. In the near future, implementation of pharmaceutical care is expected. Pharmaceutical care will be recognized by all pharmacists and supported by the patients and government in Korea.

REFERENCES

1. Health at a Glance 2009, OECD INDICATORS (ISBN 978-92-64-07555-9). http://www.oecdilibrary.org/docserver/download/fulltext/8109111e.pdf?expires=1309480458&id=id&accname=guest&checksum=2C6ED5060BEAE9F092FAA39177484FAD.
2. OECD, OECD Health Data, 2005.
3. OECD Review of Health Care systems 2003 (ISBN 92-64-29945-9).
4. World Health Report. 2010. Financial risk protection of National Health Insurance in the Republic of Korea:1995–2007.
5. *Major Statistics for Health and Welfare*. Seoul, Korea: Korean Ministry of Health and Welfare; 1999.
6. Cho HK. Challenges and opportunities posed by a new prescription law in South Korea. *Am J Health Syst Pharm*. 2002;59(18):1780–1782.
7. Annual Statistics Report, The Korea Pharmaceutical Association, 2011.
8. Choi SM, Shin HT, Choi HM, Kim JS, Ann JS, Choi KE. Development and evaluation of anticoagulation clinical pharmacy service for ambulatory patients in a community pharmacy [in Korean]. *Kor J Clin Pharm*. 1995;5(2):17–31.
9. Strand LM, Cipolle RJ, Morley PC, Frakes MJ. The impact of pharmaceutical care practice on the practitioner and the patient in the ambulatory practice setting: twenty-five years of experience. *Curr Pharm Des*. 2004;10(31):3987–4001.
10. Kim HS. *Development and Evaluation of Clinical Pharmacy practices in Hospitals*. Korean Conference on Clinical Pharmacy, practical session. 1993:79–83 (in Korean).
11. Kim CY. Financial deficits of Nation's Health Insurance and reforming the bun-up system [in Korean]. *Korean Pharm Assoc News*. 2001.
12. Kwon KH. The influence of good pharmacy practices (GPP) on Korean community pharmacies [in Korean]. *J Korean Pharm Assoc*. 1994;5(1):69–73.
13. Kim SK. Changes in health care services and prospects for the role of pharmacists [in Korean]. *J Seoul Pharm Assoc*. 1994;19(3):4–15.
14. Cho NC, Nam CH. Survey of the health-related behaviors of pharmacists working in community pharmacies and hospital pharmacies and their effect on job satisfaction [in Korean]. *J Korean Public Health Assoc*. 2000;26:116–134.
15. Epplen K, Dusing-Wiest M, Freedlund J, Harger N, Kathman S, Ivey MF. Stepwise approach to implementing ambulatory clinical pharmacy services. *Am J Health Syst Pharm*. 2007;64(9):945–951.
16. Risco AA, Foppe van Mil JW. Pharmaceutical care in community pharmacies: practice and research in Peru. *Ann Pharmacother*. 2007;41(12):2032–2037.
17. Lee EK, Lee JY. Survey of hospital pharmacy services [in Korean]. *J Korean Soc Hosp Pharm*. 1999;16:458–79.
18. World Population Ageing 2009, Economic & Social Affairs, United Nations. http://www.un.org/esa/population/publications/WPA2009/WPA2009-report.pdf.
19. http://www.bpsweb.org.

INDIA

Geeta Pradeep, MPharm
Research Scholar, School of Medical Sciences
Discipline of Pharmacy
College of Science, Engineering and Health
Royal Melbourne Institute of Technology
Victoria, Australia

Introduction

India is a confluence of cultural and ethnic diversity dating back to a 5000-year-old civilization. Her culture has evolved over time imbibing nuances from the many foreign influences that made India their home. India is the largest democracy and the second most populous country in the world today. The total population after the 2011 census program puts the population at 1.21 billion.[1] The country is geographically divided into 28 states and 7 union territories. Each region of India portrays distinct and diverse traditions, customs, religion, habits, and languages. While there are 22 "official" languages, there are over 400 mother tongues and 800 odd dialects spoken in the country.[2] English, therefore, functions as the lingua franca. In spite of a multitude of differences, India has remained the epitome of "Unity in Diversity" exemplified by its secular spirit.[1] India is a land of contrasts where one can witness opulence of society coexisting with extreme poverty and squalor in slums, scientific and technological innovations amid blind superstitions and ignorance. This societal contrast has been a decisive factor for the successes and failures of the country in various global arenas of development.

Over a span of 60 odd years after independence from the British, India has undergone an incredible political, economic, and cultural transformation that has made it a major geopolitical force of reckoning in the global affairs today.[3,4] India has one of the fastest growing economies in the developing world today with a steady growth rate of 8%.[2,5] Indeed, India is one among the very few nations which have weathered the recent global financial crisis well.[3] India has achieved global leadership in many areas such as Information Technology, business process outsourcing, telecommunications, and pharmaceutical manufacturing to name a few.[2]

The dominant presence exerted by India in various global sectors have not resulted in similar progress within the country. The health care sector, is perhaps the most neglected of public services.[3] It is true that substantial improvements have been made in population health outcomes since independence, with a doubling in life expectancy, reduction in maternal and infant mortality rates as well as reduction in the rates of infectious diseases such as polio and tuberculosis. However, by and large these improvements compare poorly with that of other developing nations with similar economies.[3] The economic boom in India has not translated into comparable tangible improvements in health determinants of the nation, probably, due to a consistent lack of political will and commitment to recognize the contribution of good health for accelerated economic growth for the country.[3] India's greatest demographic asset is its young population (650 million people younger than 30 years of age). A health system unable to cater to the needs of this demographic can undermine the economic growth trajectory of the country.[3]

Health Care Delivery in India

Health care delivery in India is provided through a public health system that consists of hospitals (both in public and private sectors), Primary Health Care Centers, and the more predominant private sector providers.[6,7] The government health expenditure is very low and often the government hospitals lack adequate supplies of essential medicines and equipment as well as well-trained staff. This situation leads to long delays and overcrowded conditions in public hospitals, forcing people to access private sector providers where every service needs to be paid for. The government hospitals which provide free health services are accessed primarily by government sector employees and the socioeconomically disadvantaged population unable to afford payments in the private sector clinics.[6] Nearly 80% of all outpatient visits and 60% of hospital admissions occur in the private sector.[6,8] As a result, nearly 82% of health expenditures occur out of pocket, giving India the dubious distinction of being the second highest spender of out-of-pocket medical expenses.[3,8] This expenditure is believed to be one of the main causes forcing 4% of the population into poverty.[3,6] Poor governance, especially corruption in public health services, also affects health outcomes of the poor. The health sector in India is the second most corrupt sector in India.[9] Bribes are expected at all hierarchies of government health services, from childbirth to postmortem services, and often it is the poorest that fall victim to these pressures.

Hence we can see a huge disparity in access to health care services primarily dependent on the ability of a person to afford the cost involved. On one hand, you have the high tech, specialist-driven care accessible to Indians in the high-economic bracket, now increasingly accessed by foreigners as part of the burgeoning medical tourism industry,[3,5] while, on the other, there is the large proportion of Indians in both rural and urban areas unable to afford even the basic medical care. Adding to this are indirect influences of inequitable economic growth, unplanned urbanization, deep rooted social caste, class and gender inequities to varying extents in different regions. This has led to an increase in chronic medical conditions, owing in part, to an increasing ageing population and more urbanized way of living, all contributory factors to the overall poor health outcomes for the nation.[3]

Medicine Use Problems

There is no doubt that medicines are the mainstay of therapy for management of acute and chronic disease conditions. India has developed a National Drug Policy as well as an Essential Medicines List, which is regularly revised. However, there still exists a significant problem of irrational medicines use. Medicines or "Drugs" as they are referred to in Indian parlance, is regulated by the Central Drugs Standard Control Organization through the Directorate General of Health Services under the Ministry of Health and Family Welfare.[8,10] A highly successful pharmaceutical industry with inadequate enforcement of existing regulations has resulted in the availability of nearly 100,000 pharmaceutical formulations in India, many of them irrational. Medicines invariably mean money, and therefore, vested commercial interests normally win out in the effort to curb irrational medications and their use in the community. Any medicine is available over the counter, without a prescription, even those legally mandated as prescription-only medicines. Prescriptions are not dated so people use the same prescriptions over and over again, at times for years, together, to self-medicate and manage their condition thereby saving the cost involved in going to a doctor.[11] Furthermore, people, tend to use medicines prescribed by alternative medicine practitioners such as ayurveda, homeopathy, sidha, or unani medicines (officially recognized alternative systems of medicine in India) along with allopathic medicines in the belief that the combinations will help dispel their symptoms faster. Some doctors also resort to prescribing medicines without appropriate indications and in inappropriate doses to appease the underlying psychological need of patients having obtained "some" treatment for "money" spent on a doctor's consultation.[12,13] Needless to say the above nonrational practices lead to preventable adverse drug reactions with the potential to cause serious morbidity and mortality. Unethical advertising, promotional gifts to prescribers to boost sales of medicines by pharmaceutical companies, the lack of awareness among medical professionals, and the general public all contribute significantly to inappropriate use of medicines.[13]

Availability of a quality health workforce is also an important determinant of a country's health status. Adequately trained and motivated health care professionals are an essential ingredient for ensuring appropriate usage of medicines and other health system resources.[14] The health care delivery in India is entirely centered on doctors.[3,6] This has in turn led to the systematic undervaluation and underutilization of other health care professionals, especially nurses and pharmacists who are sidelined in spite of having the necessary knowledge and skills to support the ever increasing workload of the doctors.[6,8]

Pharmacists form the third largest health care professional group in the world[14] and are probably the only health care professional where a patient can easily obtain health-related advice without having to wait for an appointment.[8,10] Over the recent decades there has been a paradigm shift in the practice of pharmacy. The role of a pharmacist has evolved from that of a supplier or dispenser of medicines to one of direct patient care assuming responsibility for all medication-related issues of their patients. Pharmacists in the developed world can ensure better therapeutic outcomes for patients as valued members of a collaborative practice or as independent practitioners in their own right, making them one of the most trusted professionals in the public eye.

The following section delves into the status of the profession in India and the factors that impinge upon its present situation.

Pharmacy in India

Early Beginnings

The pharmacy profession has existed in India in some form as part of the Ayurvedic and Sidha systems of traditional medicine. The advent of allopathic or modern western medicine in India can be traced back in time to the earliest Portuguese and British colonies. The modern pharmacy profession owes its early beginnings to the British colonial system. The Madras Medical College, initially instituted by the British to train both western and Indian students in the practice of allopathic medicine, started the first pharmacy class in 1860 to provide pharmaceutical instruction to students qualifying for the medical degree or diploma, apothecary grade, or hospital assistantship.[15] This later bifurcated into a diploma level chemist and druggists class to supplement the need for assistants to sell/dispense drugs as trained chemists or pharmacists under instruction from doctors in shops which came to be called "medical stores."[11,15,16] This is probably the genesis of community pharmacy practice in India that by and large, followed a pattern of development similar to Britain at the time. As there were very few qualified pharmacists on hand, the practice of both prescribing and dispensing for the vast majority of the population was carried out by doctors themselves who trained their clinic assistants to dispense medicines and help in the compounding of preparations.[11,16] A survey conducted just prior to independence puts the number of qualified pharmacists as 75 for a population of 300 million with around 27,000 compounders,[16] whose qualifications were considered beneath the level of pharmacists.

A formal pharmacy degree began much later in 1937 at Benares Hindu University toward the end of British rule in India. This 3-year pharmacy degree was probably the first of its kind in all of Asia and Africa and covered concepts of pharmaceutical chemistry, analytical chemistry, pharmaceutical economics, pharmacy, and pharmacognosy.[17–19] It geared its graduates to take on the requirements of the infant pharmaceutical industry as manufacturing and quality control specialists. At the time of independence in 1947, the system of pharmacy in the country was unorganized, poorly regulated, and without a legal foundation.[20]

Today there are 656,101 registered pharmacists as of December 31, 2010 with a ratio of 4 pharmacists per 1794 persons.[21] The world ratio stands at 1 pharmacist per 2491 persons. Data suggest that 55% are employed in community pharmacy, 20% in the hospital sector, 10% in the pharmaceutical industry and regulatory bodies, and 2% in academia.[8,22] The profession is at a crossroad today and has to take decisive steps to ensure that there is a sustainable future for pharmacists.

Let us now examine the main policies that have been instrumental in shaping the profession.

Pharmacy Regulation

The Pharmacy Act, 1948, enacted after Independence was the first step to regulate the practice and education of pharmacy in India. The Pharmacy Council of India (PCI) was formed as a statutory body to help put into effect the tenants of the Act. The practice of Pharmacy is further regulated by the Drugs and Cosmetics Act, 1940, which stipulates the manufacture, distribution, and sale of drugs.[8,20] The Pharmacy Act stipulated the minimum educational qualification of the Diploma in Pharmacy (DPharm) as the mandatory criteria for approval for a pharmacist's registration license to practice. Pharmacy education at the degree level is governed by the All India Council for Technical Education, which is responsible for planning, formulating, and ensuring quality of the higher level degree programs, namely the 4-year Bachelor of Pharmacy undergraduate degree (BPharm) and the 2-year postgraduate Master of Pharmacy (MPharmacy) in various specializations of pharmaceutics, pharmacology, medicinal chemistry, and others. A need was not perceived at the time to include any regulation for updating the skills once in practice and pharmacists once registered and initiated into their own practice did not need to undergo any professional development. This adversely affected the quality of practice in due course, as those in the retail practice were involved only in the selling of medicines and acquiring profits from the business.[8,18] This further strengthens the notion of the community pharmacist essentially being a businessman, rather than a skilled health care professional in the eyes of the public.

There are no regulations regarding the ownership of pharmacies as exists in some developed nations. Anyone who has the financial capacity to start a business can choose to start a pharmacy enterprise even if they have no qualification or experience in a pharmacy, provided the person can access a registered pharmacists's certificate which has to be in plain view in the pharmacy.[8,11] In order to achieve this, a pharmacy owned by a nonpharmacist may choose to hire the services of a registered pharmacist for a retainer fee; or more often, either manages it themselves or hands it over to someone with prior experience in a pharmacy (not necessarily qualified or registered). If the pharmacy is being managed by a non-pharmacist owner, they would hire out a registered pharmacist's certificate for a regular fee to display in the pharmacy premises. All these practices further serve to undermine the status of the pharmacist in society.

There has been no mention of pharmacy as a health care profession in any of the government's health and pharmaceutical policies.[8,10] The profession is recognized for its contribution to growth of the pharmaceutical industry but has no recognition in any other regulatory framework directly related to health care. In fact in 2002, a Parliamentary Committee Report suggested that a pharmacist was not necessary to supervise the sale of medicines in a pharmacy. This move was soon abandoned though it is strong testament to the low level of confidence in the skills of a pharmacist.

Pharmacy Education

Pharmacy education is provided as a three tier system: the diploma in pharmacy (D.Pharm), Bachelor of Pharmacy (B.Pharm), and the Master of Pharmacy (MS, MPharm, MTech) and further higher research degree programs namely Doctor of Philosophy (PhD). The DPharm program requires 2 years of didactic coursework and 3 months of workplace training to be undertaken in either a community pharmacy or hospital pharmacy.[20] The BPharm undergraduate degree is a 4-year-long course imparting mainly industry- and product-oriented instruction in basic pharmacy subjects like pharmaceutics, medicinal chemistry, pharmacology, and pharmacognosy, in addition to basic science and advanced chemistry and analytics. Neither the diploma nor the degree program had any component providing instruction in patient-centered care, the rational use of medicines, or clinical pharmacy topics, until early 1991. The postgraduate MPharm degree requires an additional 2 years after the completion of BPharm and is offered as specializations in different disciplines such as pharmacology, pharmaceutics, pharmacognosy, or medicinal chemistry. This involves 1 year of coursework and another year of a research project in the discipline of specialization. A postgraduate degree specializing in Pharmacy Practice/Clinical Pharmacy was not initiated until 1997, which will be discussed at a later stage in the chapter.

Until the early 1980s, there were only 11 universities and 26 colleges offering higher degrees in pharmacy with more government and private institutions providing the DPharm program.[20] Since then, rapid industrialization, privatization, and economic growth has led to a rapid growth in pharmacy education with over 1500 institutions, most of them in the private sector enrolling as much as 100,000 students into various pharmacy programs.[23]

Each tier of pharmacy education was designed to serve specific requirements essential for achieving national objectives for the overall development in the health sector.[8,20] The DPharm program was designed to provide the required personnel to serve as dispensing and medicines distribution specialists in the community and hospital pharmacies. Graduates from BPharm courses normally seek positions in the thriving pharmaceutical industry as marketing, manufacturing, quality control analytical, and regulatory experts. The postgraduates have options to join the industry at higher levels involved in research, formulation, and new drug development as well as clinical trials or in academia.

Growth of the Pharmaceutical Industry

Prior to independence, India primarily relied upon drug imports from Europe to satisfy its medication needs. After independence, the country, in its impoverished state, could not afford costly imports from Europe. The need of the hour was to attain self-sufficiency in the manufacture of quality yet affordable medicines to address the medicine needs of the populace. The government, therefore, concentrated its efforts toward this goal by encouraging collaborations between pharmaceutical manufacturers in India and their American and European counterparts, in both public and private sectors. This has led to a phenomenal growth of a robust pharmaceutical industry in a short span of time, catering to approximately 95% of the country's needs.[5,10] The Indian pharmaceutical industry is valued at approximately $8.0 billion.[8] Globally the industry ranks fourth in terms of volume and 13th in terms of value. In fact, 33.7% of total pharmaceutical exports from India are to developed nations. There are around 20,000 pharmaceutical firms and around 100,000 pharmaceutical products manufactured in India that has further compounded problems of irrational drug usage.

With all regulatory and educational policies concentrated toward better industrial standards and performance, there is little impetus to develop areas of patient care alongside technological advancements that culminated in a one-sided victory as far as the profession is concerned.

Patient Care initiatives: Early Developments

Clinical Pharmacy or Pharmacy Practice (the terms are often used synonymously in Indian practice) owes its birth to the slow yet persistent efforts of some clinical pharmacologists and academicians employed within the hospital pharmacy sector of major university teaching hospitals, starting in the early 1980s. These were people who had been exposed to the revolutionary changes in the role of the pharmacist that was developing in the West, especially USA. They attempted to bring in a culture of knowledge and awareness among the medical fraternity as well as the government regarding clinical pharmacy.[17] This was met with moderate success but remained within the confines of the clinical settings where they were employed.

These consistent efforts, however, helped translate into an educational regulation change in 1993–1994 when aspects of hospital and clinical pharmacy were made mandatory inclusions within the DPharm curriculum and soon after into the undergraduate BPharm curriculum as well. The movement to initiate change from a product-focused to a patient-focused profession started in earnest toward the end of the 1990s, by initiation of a postgraduate Pharmacy Practice Programme at two premier teaching hospitals in South India. The first program was the MS Programme in Clinical Pharmacy at Christian Medical College, Vellore, Tamilnadu, in 1996 followed in 1997 by the MPharm program in Pharmacy Practice at JSS College of Pharmacy In Mysore, Karnataka.[17] The MPharm was the result of a joint Indo-Australian collaboration between Repatriation General Hospital in South Australia and JSS Hospital and JSS College of Pharmacy involving the exchange of Indian pharmacists for training in clinical pharmacy services and their Australian counterparts to help setup the clinical pharmacy department in India in two hospitals across two states in South India.[12,13]

The next 5 years saw a rapid expansion of similar MPharm pharmacy practice programs in pharmacy colleges throughout the country. The curriculum involved in depth study of pathophysiology, pharmacotherapeutics, clinical pharmacokinetics, and clinical pharmacy, concentrating on direct patient care services such as patient counseling, prescription reviews, adverse reaction monitoring and reporting, therapeutic drug monitoring as well as drug information, not only in theory but also required hands-on clinical training within the hospitals. This necessitated having a hospital/clinical setting open to collaboration with the pharmacy practice faculty and students in their clinical setting. This was achieved in most cases by a symbiotic relationship between the pharmacy colleges imparting the course, investing in creating a clinical pharmacy department from where clinical pharmacy services could be provided to the hospital and the hospital in turn providing adequate space and permit the clinical training of the students.

These clinical pharmacy departments were crucial in the first initial years of the program. They spread awareness among the medical fraternity of the hospital, of the various nondispensing roles that could be taken by the pharmacist to help support the high workload of the clinicians. While it took some time to gain the support of the clinical departments in the hospital, soon the pharmacy practice interns and faculty became valued members of the health team. The faculty initiated programs to improve the use of medicines within the hospital by attempting to integrate the hospital pharmacy department into rational medicine use issues pertinent to the hospital. Until then the hospital pharmacy department, basically functioned as drug store managers within the bowels of the hospital. The MPharm course stipulated a research component in the second year of the course, which has led to increased research output and publications in national and international journals, providing a justifiable reason to argue for the sustainable role of the clinical pharmacist as the harbinger of improved and cost-effective health outcomes.

A further impetus toward the patient-centered role happened with the initiation of the professional Doctor of Pharmacy Programme (PharmD) in 2008.[20] The PharmD curriculum focused entirely on direct patient care, takes 6 years of study, with 5 years of academics and 1 year of internship or clinical residency at a practice site. Nearly 1410 students have enrolled in the PharmD course in 47 private sector colleges located mainly in the Southern states of India. There is much controversy regarding potential career options that await these graduates on completion of the course. In spite of initiating pharmacy practice programs over a decade ago, there are no viable career options for the graduate who have completed.[18] The regulatory framework has not yet recognized the need for clinical pharmacists, and therefore, there are no openings for clinical pharmacists in hospitals. This has caused clinical pharmacists to enter the pharmaceutical industry particularly in the arena of clinical research as well to migrate to developed countries that recognize their skills and offer better job prospects.

Future Directives: Challenges and Opportunities

The profession has slowly begun the paradigm shift from the product to the patient. The changes due to initiation of clinical pharmacy services have gained momentum in the past couple of years resulting in pharmaceutical care initiatives that have shown proof of value and added benefits from pharmacists involved in direct patient care services. The PCI, in collaboration with other professional and regulatory agencies, have embarked on an amendment to the Pharmacy Act to include pharmacy practice regulations and to raise the minimum qualification of registration to the level of BPharm.[8] The Government of India is planning to pilot a system of accreditation of retail pharmacies in accordance with Good Pharmacy Practice Guidelines drafted by the Indian Pharmaceutical Association.

These developments, once implemented, will serve to raise the professional credibility of pharmacy. A National Conference on Challenges and Opportunities for Pharmacy in Health care in 2007 developed a framework for policy to engage pharmacists in health system collaboration with all major stakeholders.[8] Many population-based pharmaceutical care initiatives implemented in the recent past in community pharmacies of India are slowly creating a positive feeling and growth of confidence about community pharmacy practice in India. This is happening not only among the consumers but also physicians and more importantly among community pharmacists themselves. This has improved self-esteem among pharmacists. A small proportion have started taking the lead to participate in continuing educational and professional programs and implementing patient care services in their pharmacies.[24–28] Private community pharmacies have also been actively participating in the government's TB control program (Revised National TB Control Programme), providing evidence of the positive contribution to increase the levels of awareness among the general public about TB.[29,30]

There still exists many barriers which need to be overcome before the pharmacy profession can plan toward the ideal of individualized pharmaceutical care services such as medication therapy management separate from dispensing. To make this a reality, the government needs to recognize the untapped potential of pharmacists in health care delivery and make attempts to provide better financial incentives to encourage them to elevate themselves from their current level of apathy.

At present, pharmaceutical care initiatives occur as part of research activities by academicians in pharmacy practice departments building up on the essential evidence required justifying professional pharmacy services as an integral part of health care delivery. Recently there have also been new community pharmacy initiatives by a small number of enterprising community pharmacists who have implemented innovative preventative and diagnostic services as well as counseling services within their practices as part of better business practices. It needs to be emphasized that these services normally do not mean any increase in income for the pharmacist providing them.

The profession has started to look inward, comprehend their shortcomings, and work toward raising their professional image among the general public as well as the health care fraternity. While this has started to happen, there is the need for the PCI and other pharmaceutical associations, to ensure that the new breed of pharmacy professionals has the highest levels of competence to provide patient-centered care by revising existing outdated regulations to include pharmacy practice as a legal and viable sector of patient care.

Potential Strategies to Pharmaceutical Care Practice

Regulatory Strategies

- Revision of existing regulations especially the Pharmacy Act and the Drugs and Cosmetics Act to reflect the necessary requirements of the evolving profession.
- Legally define the various professional strata for pharmacists, their credentials, and pay scales in accordance with their level of expertise and knowledge.
- Upgrade the minimum registrable qualification for a pharmacist from the existing 2-year diploma to the 4-year undergraduate BPharm degree.

- Time bound provisions to define the current diploma qualified professionals to assume the role of pharmacy technicians or assistants, working under the supervision of registered qualified graduate pharmacists.
- Design and implement professional practice standards of practice, both for individual pharmacists as well as for services provided by them in order to achieve a consistent level of practice nationwide.

Educational Strategies

- Revision of the current pharmacy undergraduate curriculum to ensure focused training in patient care services as well as clinical pharmacy topics to ensure availability of practice ready competent pharmacists qualified to enter the workforce after registration.
- Revision of the existing registration requirements to include continuing professional development as part of time-bound mandatory requirement to maintain their registration status.
- Revision of the diploma in pharmacy curriculum to include more intensive training of pharmacy assistants/technicians so that they can take up routine dispensing and compounding activities freeing the pharmacists to provide professional services.

Conclusion

India is undergoing simultaneous transformation along several fronts—urban, industrial, and economic—all of which have far reaching implications for the health sector and in particular, for pharmacy profession. Pharmacy in India can be considered to be a glass half empty or a glass half full depending on one's perceptions. The hurdles that need to be overcome are monumental. It will, doubtless, take time to effect the transition from that of an unskilled seller of medicines working invisibly in the fringes of the health care sector to that of a competent highly skilled practitioner. Pharmacists will have to demonstrate that, in addition to improving cognitive dispensing services, they are also competent to assume more direct patient care services. In time, they will find their rightful place as an integral member of the collaborative health care team, working to ensure the best possible and cost-effective treatment outcomes for patients in their care. The future holds promise for those pharmacists, bold enough to be trailblazers in the profession through their innovative services, to achieve pharmaceutical care and medication therapy management.

REFERENCES

1. *The National Portal of India.* 10 February 2011 [cited 2011 15 June]. http://india.gov.in/knowindia/profile.php.
2. *WHO Country Co-operation Strategy 2006–2011, India,* 2006, WHO.

3. Reddy KS, Patel V, Jha P, et al. Towards achievement of universal health care in India by 2020: a call to action. *Lancet.* 2011;377(9767):760–768.

4. Horton R, Das P. Indian health: the path from crisis to progress. *Lancet.* 2011;377(9761): 181–183.

5. Coopers PW, ed. *Emerging Market Report: Health in India 2007.* New York: Price Waterhouse Coopers; 2007.

6. Rao M, Rao KD, Kumar AK, Chatterjee M, Sundararaman T. Human resources for health in India. *Lancet.* 2011;377(9765):587–598.

7. Sathyanarayanan TN, Babu G. Creating a public health cadre in India: the development of a framework for interprofessional and inter-sector collaboration. *J Interprof Care.* 2011;25(4):308–310.

8. Sheth PD, Nandraj S, Nayar PCK, et al. *Challenges and Opportunities for Pharmacists in Healthcare in India,* 2007, FIP-WHO Forum of National Pharmaceutical Associations for South East Asia Region (SEARPharm Forum).

9. Sudarshan H, Prashanth NS. Good governance in health care: the Karnataka experience. *Lancet.* 2011;377(9768):790–791.

10. *Human Resources for Pharmacy Sector in India,* 2007, Advent Healthcare Group, Central Drugs Standard Control Organization, MoHFW, GOI, World Health Organisation—India Country Office: New Delhi.

11. Basak SC, Sathyanarayana D. Community pharmacy practice in India: past, present and future. *Southern Med Rev.* 2009;2(1):11–14.

12. Elliot RA. Clinical pharmacy: an evolving area of pharmacy practice in India. *Aust J Hosp Pharmacy.* 2001;31(2):147–150.

13. Nyfort-Hansen K, May FW, Clinical pharmacy a new beginning in India. *Aust J Hosp Pharmacy.* 1998;28(5):343–347.

14. *2009 FIP Global Pharmacy Workforce Report.* Wuliji T, ed. The Hague, Netherlands, International Pharmaceutical Federation; 2009.

15. Singh H. Pharmaceutical Society of India: the oldest Indian pharmaceutical organization. *Indian J History Sci.* 2000;35(1):67–76.

16. Singh H. History of modern pharmacy in India. *CRIPS.* 2006;7(3):42–44.

17. Revikumar KG, Miglani BD, eds. *A Textbook of Pharmacy Practice.* Nashik: Career Publications; 2009.

18. Basak SC, Foppe van Mil JW, Sathyanarayana D. The changing roles of pharmacists in community pharmacies: perception of reality in India. *Pharm World Sci.* 2009;31(6): 612–618.

19. Singh H. Pharmaceutical education and pharmacy practice: a historical perspective. *Pharma Times.* 2009;41(2):16–19.

20. Basak SC, Sathyanarayana D. Pharmacy education in India. *Am J Pharm Educ.* 2010; 74(4):68.

21. *National Health Profile 2010,* C.B.o.H. Intelligence, Editor 2010, Government of India: New Delhi.

22. Merlin NJ. Pharmacy careers—an overview. *Asian J Res Pharma Sci.* 2011;1(1):01–03.

23. Narayana TV. Pharmacy education in India. *Pharma Times.* 2011;43(03):35.

24. Mohanta GP, Manna PK, Valliappan K, Manavalan R. Achieving good pharmacy practice in community pharmacies in India. *Am J Health-Syst Pharm.* 2001;58(9):809–810.

25. Varma D, et al. A study on community pharmacy in Kerala. *Indian J Hosp Pharmacy.* 2000;37:49–52.

26. Ramesh A, Nagavi B, Ramanath K. A critical review of community pharmacies (drug stores) in Mysore city. *Indian J Hosp Pharmacy.* 2000;37:91–93.

27. Adepu R, Rasheed A, Nagavi B. Effect of patient counseling on quality of life in type-2 diabetes mellitus patients in two selected South Indian community pharmacies. *Indian J Pharm Sci.* 2007;69(4):519–524.

28. Carvalho S, Nagavi B. Impact of community pharmacy based patient education on the quality of life of hypertensive patients. *Indian Jo Pharm Educ Res.* 2007;41(2):164–169.

29. Rajeswari S. Balasubramanian R, Bose MS, Sekar L, Rahman F. Private pharmacies in tuberculosis control--a neglected link. *Int J Tuberc Lung Dis.* 2002;6(2):171–173.

30. Gharat M, Ambe CA, Ambe GT, Bell JS. Engaging community pharmacists as partners in tuberculosis control: a case study from Mumbai. *Res Social Adm Pharm.* 2007;3(4):464–470.

ARABIC-SPEAKING MIDDLE EAST

Nadir M. Kheir, PhD, FNZCP, MPS
Assistant Professor
Coordinator of Continuing Professional Pharmacy Development
College of Pharmacy, Qatar University
Doha, Qatar

Introduction

The impact of Arabs on medicine and pharmacy in Europe and the rest of the world cannot be overstated. Most of the earliest pharmaceutical utensils used for many years in traditional drug stores, pharmaceutical formulations prepared in pharmacies, and evidence-based pharmacotherapeutics were the products of early Arab and Muslim thinkers who pursued humanistic and scientific discourses in their search for knowledge, meaning, and values.[1] However, the development in pharmacy education and practice in Arabic-speaking Middle Eastern countries slowed down and stagnated around traditional curricula and apothecary pharmacy for decades. This recession could be attributed to multiple factors including past and current periods of conflict, occupation, social and economical pressures, and political instability.[2] As a result, the overall level of pharmaceutical services provided has been poor, particularly in the community sector but also on the public sector as well. No wonder that a common phenomenon shared by most Middle Eastern countries is that patients rarely consider community pharmacies as health care facilities. This, in turn, resulted in limited interaction (in quantity and quality) between pharmacists and patients, leading to poor public image of pharmacists in these countries.[2,3] Noteworthy is that pharmaceuticals were among the first products available to consumers in the Middle Eastern countries, and their regulation in terms of registering, licensing, and pricing dated many years back.

In more recent years, herbal medicines were subjected to comprehensive regulation in most countries in the region, and as an example, in 1990s, the Office of Complementary and Alternative Medicine was established at the United Arab Emirates (UAE) Ministry of Health to regulate herbal medicines and license pharmacists and pharmacy technicians practicing in this area.[4] However, pharmacy regulations governing the sale, classification, prescribing, and dispensing of medications (and ultimately the public's access to medications) are still inadequate. In most of these countries, only antibiotics, male sex hormones, narcotics, psychotropic medicines, hypnotics, tranquilizers, and other agents that can cause dependence require a prescription at community pharmacies. A wider range of medicines, which otherwise in other countries are considered prescription-medicines, are sold over-the-counter in Middle Eastern countries. These medicines include, but not limited to, non-steroidal anti-inflammatory drugs, drugs for wide range of gastrointestinal problems, asthma inhalers, insulin and other antidiabetics, cholesterol-lowering and antihypertensive medications, to mention a few. Such a situation has the potential for presenting a plethora of drug-related adverse consequences. More importantly, this situation places (or should place) an additional burden of responsibility on the pharmacist.

The emergence of the philosophy and practice of pharmaceutical care worldwide has challenged pharmacists everywhere to change their old ways and embrace a new paradigm that focuses on outcomes of care rather than on products or tasks. In a time of globalization, this move must have had an effect on how pharmacy is practiced in the Middle East region as it did elsewhere. Apart from few studies that attempted to provide some idea about the status of pharmacy practice in a few of the Middle Eastern countries, no work was done to assess the extent this new evolving practice had in this region or the challenges it faces. Our aim in this section is to provide a snapshot of the status of pharmaceutical care (and more specifically medication therapy management as defined elsewhere in this book) in the Middle East.

We selected nine countries in the Arabic-speaking Middle Eastern region for this synopsis and those were Egypt, Jordan, Kuwait, Lebanon, Oman, Qatar, Saudi Arabia, Sudan, and the UAE. Of these countries, five (Kuwait, Oman, Saudi Arabia, Qatar, UAE) constitute most of the countries that form the Gulf Cooperation Council (GCC), and they are in close geographical and cultural proximity to each other.[2] Two countries (Egypt and Sudan) are situated in the neighboring continent of Africa, and both countries lie in the Eastern Mediterranean region (http://www.who.int/about/regions/en/index.html published literature).

First, we searched the literature using key words (and Boolean search where needed) and phrases including medication therapy management, pharmaceutical care, and pharmacy, in conjunction with each of the listed countries. Relevant publications were located and retrieved. Second, we identified, through personal contact and through the websites of Universities and other relevant pharmacy organizations in the countries listed, individuals who at the time of information collection were working for at least 5 years in the respective country either in pharmacy academia and/or practice, and/or who we know have good understanding of the pharmacy environment in the respective country, and we targeted those who had scholarly contributions in the area of the pharmacy profession (publications, teaching, or policy). These individuals were considered to be *key informants* in our endeavor to collect credible information on medication therapy management in this part of the world. The use of key informants has origins in the fields of anthropology, sociology, and psychology, and is now being applied on other branches of research that evaluates health services. A key informant is an expert source of information, who is deemed familiar with the particular area in which the researcher is interested.[5] The individuals selected were invited by email to contribute information in response to a set of standardized questions relating to medication therapy management, pharmacy education, and pharmacy practice. For data validation purposes, we adopted methodology that had been used in previous studies.[2] Data and input received or collected were entered in a spreadsheet that was updated regularly with information received from the respective country representatives, and whenever possible, more than one key informant per country was included to maximize data accuracy.

General Information

The majority of pharmacy graduates from Universities in the countries examined hold baccalaureate in pharmacy, and most graduates from Egypt, Lebanon, Sudan, and Jordan joined the community pharmacy practice or drug companies, followed by the hospital sector. The situation is the reverse in respect to site of employment in the GCC countries, where the hospital sector presents the most attractive employment opportunity for the national graduates, while expatriate pharmacists may be employed in both the public and community practice positions, which traditionally pay less salary. Some countries (e.g., Lebanon, Jordan, Egypt, Sudan) only permit nationals to practice pharmacy within their borders.[2] So far, only a few Universities award the PharmD instead of baccalaureate (e.g., the Lebanese American University in Lebanon, King Faisal University in Kingdom of Saudi Arabia (KSA), and Jordan University of Science and Technology in Jordan).

Egypt

With a population of over 82 million, Egypt is the most populous of the countries identified. The College of Pharmacy at Cairo University is considered the oldest pharmacy program among all other programs in the Middle East (opened in 1824 AD).

In recent years, some of Egypt's pharmacy programs started to offer undergraduate clinical pharmacy courses, which is a significant development considering the slow pace at which the practice of pharmacy was moving.[6,7]

Total annual admissions to Egypt's universities are estimated to be in the range of 11,000 to 13,000 students.[2] With this rate, Egypt is considered a major exporter of graduates to GCC countries. There is an estimated 138,000 pharmacists and 60,000 community pharmacies in Egypt.[8]

Egypt's health care system has been criticized for not doing enough to move the pharmacy profession forward. Lack of funding as a consequence of the unhealthy economy is a major issue confronting Egypt's health care in general and pharmacy in particular. As a result, contemporary pharmacy practices, like medication therapy management, are not currently widely applied in Egypt.[7] However, pharmacists in two hospitals (the National Cancer Institute and the Children's Cancer Hospital) are making concerted efforts toward applying the concepts of medication therapy management on the individual patient's level, and separate from the routine dispensing process. This being said, these could be considered personal rather than structured and planned organizational efforts. Oncology care in Egypt is currently an area with some potential, but overall the primary task of pharmacists remains to be dispensing. The same level of sporadic efforts could be seen in several other hospitals in Egypt. These individual attempts to practice medication therapy management are made by a small number of U.S-trained pharmacists as well as a few pharmacists who were able to seek U.S board certification.[9] To date, no formal training is offered to equip pharmacists with the right skills for providing pharmaceutical care in the country, and experiential training is not well organized yet.[9,10]

Historically, the modest awareness of the concept of pharmaceutical care and subsequently its inconsistent application as medication therapy management services was preceded by a slow introduction of clinical pharmacy in what had been pharmacy curricula totally dominated by traditional, chemistry-based courses. The first attempt for the introduction of "some" therapeutics and clinical pharmacy courses was made by the then-Dean of the Faculty of Pharmacy in Tanta University who visited the University of Tennessee in Memphis in the early 1980s and returned to introduce clinical pharmacy to the curriculum in Tanta University. This University then provided scholarships to four of its graduates to pursue PharmD/PhD in the United States (University of Tennessee, University of the Pacific in California, and University of Minnesota). Only two of the four returned to Egypt and are later seconded to colleges of pharmacy in Saudi Arabia and Kuwait. Later on the concepts of clinical pharmacy, pharmacy practice and pharmaceutical care propagates to other colleges of pharmacy specially in private universities.[9]

On a governmental level, there was resistance to create a larger role for pharmacists in health care settings, although there were some attempts to establish hospital and clinical pharmacy departments at the Egyptian Drug Authority and the Ministry of Health to set the grounds for such practice. Lately, there are voices calling for redefining pharmacy practice from a legislative point of view in Egypt. Some pharmacy practitioners argued that current legislation does not offer a clear, detailed, and workable scope of practice, which includes professional and legal requirements for the provision of such services like medication therapy management. Indeed, the professional arena now lacks a clear scope of practice with respect to the clinical pharmacy practice too, which is still perceived by some health care professionals outside the pharmacy field as intrusion in their professional pitch. Presently, a good proportion of pharmacists resists practicing any form of clinical pharmacy and medication therapy management as a "compulsory service" before the development of clear legislation, terms of reference, and scope of practice.[7]

It has been suggested that research is an area that will grow exponentially in the next few years in Egypt.[10] Again, budget and manpower allocation should allow for greater opportunities and potential for research in Egypt. There are, however, signs that research in pharmacy-related topics is going the right direction, and there are expectations that it addresses the impact and application of pharmaceutical care on health outcomes when the environment is conducive enough for such practices.[10]

Jordan

Jordan has a population of about 6.5 million, of which 41% are under the age of 20, and only 3% are over the age of 65.[11] It has more than 8800 registered pharmacists and over 1600 community pharmacies.[12]

Pharmacy education is provided by two public and six private faculties of pharmacy graduating about 1000 pharmacists per year.[12] This places Jordan in a comfortable status with respect to the ratio of faculty to population, especially when compared to more populous countries like Saudi Arabia and Egypt. The Bachelor of Science (BSc) degree in pharmacy is still the only undergraduate pharmacy degree offered by the private universities in Jordan. Two public schools offer a PharmD or similar degree. The first faculty to adopt the PharmD program in Jordan was the faculty of pharmacy at Jordan University of Science and Technology in 2000, followed by The University of Jordan in 2005.[12] Jordan is the third country in the Middle East after Lebanon and KSA to run a PharmD program.[3]

Pharmaceutical care and medication therapy management services are still new concepts in Jordan; therefore, their implementation is limited to some governmental and private hospitals, and fewer community pharmacy outlets. The main hospitals that host the service are King Abdulla University Hospital, University of Jordan Hospital, Royal medical services, King Hussein

Cancer Center, and few private hospitals. Most providers of the service are holders of PharmD or Master of clinical pharmacy degrees. Only a few have ASHP-accredited residencies and fellowships. Those involved in the provision of medication therapy management cover from third to half of the hospital beds in the hospitals they work in. Clinical pharmacists who provide the service are mostly paid some financial incentive. It is likely that application of the medication therapy management service involves providing a standard of care that ensures each patient's medications are individually assessed to determine that they are appropriate for the patient, effective for the medical condition, safe, and that the patient is willing to take or administer them as intended. However, whether the standard of service provided includes the development of an individualized care plan and commits to scheduled follow-up to monitor patient-specific outcomes remains to be seen, and was not clearly identified as one of the service deliverables.

In respect to the level of acceptance of the service, patients in Jordan who experience this patient-centered and caring professional interaction with the pharmacist appreciate it and are likely to demand it.[13] However, many pharmacists are still not ready to include it in their daily practice because they feel they are not yet equipped with the required attributes that would allow them to provide the full service. Others (usually new graduates) are enthusiastic and want to be involved. Tahaineh suggests that older pharmacists are much more resistant than younger pharmacists to the application of medication therapy management.[13] In terms of physician acceptance to these new roles of the pharmacist, Tahaineh, Wazaify, and colleagues found out that physicians in hospitals in Jordan were more likely to accept or recognize traditional pharmacy services than new services. They suggested that there is need for more education and interaction with members of the health care team if this perception is to change.[13]

In community pharmacy, the practice is still dominated by dispensing and selling products. The concept of medication therapy management and pharmaceutical care is rarely put into practice. However, one chain community pharmacy presents a quite different model. This community pharmacy provides medication therapy management to a wide population of patients in Amman (Jordan's capital city) and other major cities in the country, in addition to branches in the United States (Miami), KSA, and several other Middle Eastern countries.

Jordan's pharmacy profession is privileged with many dedicated researchers in the pharmacy practice field. Their publications helped to draw a clear picture of the country's professional scene and helped to identify different areas of strengths, weakness, and priorities. The future of medication therapy management in the country will in no doubt be helped by the work of these and other dedicated individuals.

Kuwait

Kuwait, with a population of 2.5 million, has one public pharmacy school. This nationally accredited public program at the University of Kuwait offers a 5-year baccalaureate degree.[2] More than half of the pharmacists in Kuwait work in the public hospital sector. Clinical pharmacy services are limited, but efforts are being made to increase direct patient responsibilities of the hospital pharmacists.[2] Community pharmacies are not being fully utilized as sources for quality health care provision, and as such provide product-centered services dominated by selling drug products with little counseling and little patient-centered care.

Medication therapy management is not yet widely available. However, some junior pharmacists with bachelor degree in pharmacy (BPharm) in addition to some graduates from the United Kingdom with a Master in Clinical Pharmacy and a few U.S. graduates with the PharmD have started the implementation of inconsistent patient-centered services since the last 4 years.[14]

There are sporadic continuing professional development (CPD) and continuing education activities that aim at providing training to pharmacy practitioners in the country. These are held as monthly presentations by pharmacists on different diseases and their management or different drug groups related to the pharmacists' field of work and interest. The Faculty of Pharmacy at Kuwait University and the Kuwait Pharmaceutical Association organize some of these introductory CPD workshops on the pharmaceutical care of chronic diseases.[14]

Like the case in Jordan and Egypt, junior pharmacists are taking the lead in trialing these new services, while most of the "older" pharmacists find their safety zone in the traditional roles of compounding and dispensing medications.[14] This attitude could be the result of a lack of confidence in their technical skills and their outdated knowledge. However, provided with the necessary training, pharmacists in Kuwait may be more willing and able to embark on providing more patient-centered medication therapy management. Consequently, this could help in changing the public's view of what pharmacists can do, and allow other health care practitioners to accept the pharmacist into the health care team. Currently, physicians vary in their acceptance level; some are more comfortable than others with the pharmacist taking a more clinical role.[14]

The setting where the practice comes closest to medication therapy management is usually in the inpatient pharmacy when preparing medications for patients. This is when pharmacists have access to the patients' notes and laboratory results so they are able to make clinical decisions in respect to the patient's drug therapy. In some instances, although very few pharmacists go up on the ward and deliver "partial" medication therapy management to selected patients.[14]

In the undergraduate pharmacy education front, the concept of pharmaceutical care is widely introduced in the curriculum of the Faculty of Pharmacy in Kuwait University. In the 3rd year of the faculty of pharmacy, the students apply their communication skills and therapeutics knowledge in conducting simple medication reviews, dispensing medications, and provide patient counseling. Students also are trained on how to respond to symptoms through assessment of patients and to decide the need for referral. In the 4th year, the students acquire knowledge and skills required for identification of drug therapy–related problems and the development of an individualized care plan that achieves the intended goals of therapy with appropriate follow-up to determine actual patient outcomes through a variety of simulated case studies to reinforce the practice of pharmacy. In addition, the students are involved in clinical placements to expose them to real-life situations in polyclinic pharmacies. In the final undergraduate year, the pharmacy students spend more time in clinical placements at pharmacy departments and medical wards in hospital settings. Concepts of clinical pharmacy and pharmaceutical care are integrated in deciding drug treatment plans for patients. Through various courses in pharmacy practice, the student is able to acquire the skills needed for a competent pharmaceutical care practitioner to handle real-life patients' drug therapy problems.[14] However, after graduating, the new graduate is disillusioned by the reality of the practice, the absence of regulations that support the pharmacists in their new roles, and a practice that is still focused on the traditional role of pharmacists as being dispensers for drugs. On the bright side, the Faculty of Pharmacy in Kuwait University was granted approval from Kuwait University and the Ministry of Health for the Post-Baccalaureate PharmD degree program, which is expected to start in 2012. The PharmD degree program will enable the graduates to become leaders in pharmacy not only as clinicians and patient care providers but also as educators and clinical researchers.

Finally, the Kuwaiti Ministry of Health is planning to establish clinical pharmacy services in Kuwait in the near future. Pharmacists in Kuwait aspire to provide more structured medication therapy management on the individual patient level through their clinical pharmacy roles in hospitals. Considering all the circumstances and activities happening at this time, the future of medication management services in Kuwait looks promising, with an estimated time frame of 2 to 5 years to take shape in small and specialized setting, and to spread more widely in around 8 years.[14] So far, no reimbursement is currently provided for pharmacists for providing patient-centered services.

Lebanon

Lebanon lies on the eastern shore of the Mediterranean Sea, and has a population of over 4 million people. Currently, five universities offer pharmacy programs in Lebanon. Two of the five universities, the Saint-Joseph University and the Lebanese University, follow the French system in which students graduate with a 5-year license degree (equivalent to a bachelor's degree) or a 6-year degree, "*Doctorat d'exercice en pharmacie.*" The Beirut Arab University and Lebanese International University offer a 5-year bachelor's degree program, taught in both Arabic and English.[15] The School of Pharmacy at the Lebanese American University (LAU), which was opened in 1995, and its program is consistent with the American pharmacy educational system.[15] In 2002, the PharmD degree program offered by LAU secured accreditation from the Accreditation Council for Pharmacy Education (ACPE), making it the first and only PharmD degree program outside of the United States to have ACPE accreditation. Graduates of LAU are now eligible to take the North American Pharmacy Licensure Examination and can be licensed to practice in the United States.[2] There are approximately 1800 community pharmacies and 148 hospitals in Lebanon, and a growing number of graduates are expected to compete to work in the limited available jobs. An ongoing economic crisis in the country is further impacting the job satisfaction of Lebanese pharmacists.[16] and prevents the government from supporting or delivering any reimbursement scheme for additional patient care activities provided by the pharmacists.

In 1950, the Lebanese Order of Pharmacists (LOP) was established and it subsequently issued a structured scope of practices, which is considered the foundation of pharmacy laws and regulations in Lebanon.[15] However, the LOP plays very limited role in terms of advancing the profession pharmacy in Lebanon.

Medication therapy management is still in its infancy in Lebanon. Only recently, after graduating PharmD students from LAU, was clinical pharmacy more widely accepted in hospital settings in the country. The practice of pharmacy in Lebanon, especially in the community, is still circling around dispensing and the selling of medications, a phenomenon shared by several neighboring countries. While some universities like LAU and LIU (Lebanese International University) are actively preparing their students to provide pharmaceutical care by delivering pharmacy courses that mirror the U.S. undergraduate and PharmD courses, many of their graduates are either leaving the country to seek job overseas (especially in the rich Gulf country region or in north America) or are working as medical representatives with pharmaceutical companies, mainly focusing in detailing and selling limited medicinal products to private clinics and community pharmacies.

United Arab Emirates

The UAE is an oil-rich federation situated in the southeast of the Arabian Peninsula in Southwest Asia on the Persian Gulf, and is divided into seven emirates. The UAE's population is over 5.6 million people, of which less than 20% are UAE nationals or Emiratis.[17] Abu Dhabi is the most populated Emirate with 38% of the UAE population.

Pharmacy education is offered by seven pharmacy schools in UAE.[18] The Gulf Medical University is the only university that offers a PharmD program in UAE. Like in other neighboring Gulf countries, pharmacy practice in the UAE is in a state of evolution, though still dominated by traditional pharmacy and inconsistent service provision.[19]

Modern pharmacy courses, including pharmaceutical care, were included in most pharmacy college curricula; however, the provision of medication therapy management services has not been a reality, especially in the community sector, due to several factors. The most important of these are workload, shortage of qualified staff, level of acceptance by patients and physicians, and lack of remuneration scale.[19] Furthermore, the health regulatory agencies in the UAE did not pass legislation that organizes or empower pharmacists from a professional point of view. Because there is still no detailed legislation to organize the practice of pharmacy, no specific level of competency is needed to provide cognitive services, and all that pharmacists need is to obtain a license from the Ministry of Health to practice pharmacy. There is now, however, a requirement to obtain a set number of CE units for renewal of licensure. In some private hospitals in the UAE, medication therapy management can be provided only by licensed pharmacist with *evidence of clinical training*. However, the picture in the hospital setting is somewhat different. Several hospitals in the UAE now recruit holders of PharmD and advanced degrees from the United Kingdom and the United States, and these hospitals are introducing, or had introduced, advanced clinical pharmacy services to their patient populations.[20]

In respect of acceptance level of the provision of medication therapy management, a professional hierarchy still places the physician at the top of other "allied" health professionals, and this still dominates the health care scene not only in Kuwait but also in other neighboring countries. Pharmacists are still widely perceived as medication dispensers, and patients' expectations do not go beyond that except at those instances when patients experience individualized pharmacy services provided during their stay in one of the hospitals that provide medication therapy management. These still remain the minority, however, and much remains to be done to change that state of affairs.

The future of medication therapy management in the UAE will probably be determined by the quality of the undergraduate pharmacy education, and the introduction of more PharmD programs in the country. Currently, pharmacy colleges are helping to draft standards of practice and they are taking an active role in advancing the practice in the country. Key to the success of these services is the development of more advanced, workable, and detailed pharmacy legislations in the UAE.[19]

Qatar

The State of Qatar (Qatar), an Arab Emirate that lies on the northeasterly coast of the Arabian Peninsula, has a population of approximately 1.7 million people, of which approximately 80% are expatriates.[21] Gas and oil produced and exported from this small country make it one of the countries with the highest gross domestic product per capita in the world. Qatar is also known as one of the two least-taxed sovereign states in the world.[22]

To date, there is no autonomous professional pharmacy association or society that regulates the practice of pharmacy and represent or promote the profession of pharmacy in Qatar.[23] These roles fall under the jurisdiction of the Supreme Counsel of Health.

Qatar's only national pharmacy program was opened in 2007 in Qatar University, making it the newest public College of Pharmacy in the Gulf region at the time this section was being written. Admission to the program requires completion of U.S-based pharmacy college admission test as a component of the application process.[2] Admission also requires attending a structured interview, in addition to providing a personal statement and references. The College had secured provisional international accreditation from the Canadian Council on Accreditation of Pharmacy Programs (CCAPP) in 2008, making it the first and only accredited pharmacy program by the CCAPP outside Canada. The College had its plans for PharmD degree approved in early 2007, and its first candidate will start their degree in September 2011. The PharmD degree program was designed to meet western accreditation standards and to provide advanced professional training opportunities for students wishing to pursue specialized clinical careers.

Pharmaceutical care features prominently in this college, where its Mission states: [*to prepare students to provide optimal pharmaceutical care, to promote research and scholarly activity and to serve as a pharmacy resource for Qatar and the Middle East region*].* Pharmaceutical care is therefore introduced early in the course of study, and continues as a thread in the following years. Course integration and teaching strategy introduces disease-based teaching and management strategies that use pharmaceutical care approaches. Medication therapy management is introduced as the clinical application of pharmaceutical care at different semesters, and students are given assignments to write proposals for the implementation of medication therapy management services in Qatar or to write research proposals that focus on assessing the impact of medication therapy management in managing health conditions.

The College of Pharmacy in Qatar University adopts a strategy of involvement with health care policy and practice in the country through linking with multiple practice sites and multiple local Stakeholders Group meetings

---

*http://www.qu.edu.qa/pharmacy/mission_vision.php

involving hospital, community, and other pharmacy practitioners, as well as supporting organizations.[24]

A new pharmacy technician program has also recently opened in Qatar. This program is operated by the Qatar branch of the College of North Atlantic (Canada), and its graduates are trained to support local pharmacists in the delivery of competent health care.[2]

So far, most pharmacists practicing in Qatar are expatriates and the majority of pharmacists received their degrees in Egypt, India, or Jordan.[2] Practice opportunities resemble those in other regional countries and are primarily in private community pharmacies, publicly funded hospitals, and public health and private clinics.

There is good awareness of pharmaceutical care in Qatar, though the term is often used interchangeably with clinical pharmacy. However, like in other Middle Eastern countries, medication therapy management is not a commonly used term. From that perspective, there are recognizable pockets of medication therapy management in most government hospitals, but there is a shortage of people with training in basic clinical skills, and liberating pharmacists from the dispensary is one of the main challenges facing the development of medication therapy management in Qatar.[25] No structured medication management services exist in the non-Government sector in Qatar apart from a few individual initiatives by pharmacists who completed online, distant-learning courses with the Peters Institute of Pharmaceutical in the College of Pharmacy at the University of Minnesota (United States) (http://www.pharmacy.umn.edu/centers/peters/about/home.html). These pharmacists started using their new skills in their daily practice in non-Government and semi-Government health care institutions. In 2006, a cohort of pharmacists including several Qatari nationals completed an in-house foundation program in clinical pharmacy, and over half of these are still working as clinical pharmacists. Several government hospitals have also motivated pharmacists to obtain advanced pharmacy degrees and attend clinical ward rounds to make real contribution to inpatient care. In 2010, the first Qatari national graduated with a PharmD.[25]

To date, at least five public hospitals offer some sort of clinical pharmacy service. However, one of these hospitals (specialized in cancer therapy) adopts full clinical pharmacy services provided by two experienced clinical pharmacists (covering a total of 50 beds), and the department of pharmacy of this hospital has plans for adoption of pharmaceutical care and medication therapy management in its strategic future programs.[26] The only published research that looked at physicians' acceptance of cognitive services provided by pharmacists in public hospitals showed that physicians were comfortable with the pharmacists role in patient care but that there were many unmet expectations.[27]

The first baccalaureate and PharmD graduates from Qatar's College of Pharmacy will enter the workforce in 2011 and 2012, respectively. It is anticipated that these graduates will mark the beginning of qualitative improvements in how pharmacy is practiced in this country and may lead to fast track the introduction of medication therapy management practices in several pharmacy outlets in Qatar. As per the strategic planning of the pharmacy services at the main government provider (Hamad Medical Corporation), pharmacy technicians will start to provide most of the preparative and dispensing services, and most pharmacists will be deployed to provide clinical pharmacy services using the pharmaceutical care approach outside of the pharmacy units.[25]

The visibility of pharmacy academics, their deliberate engaging strategies with stakeholders, coupled with an active Continuing Professional Pharmacy Development (CPPD) program and an organized Structured Practical Experience Program that allows students to spend training time in community and hospital pharmacies during their undergraduate course are all important factors that maximize the chances of advancing pharmacy practice in Qatar.

Qatar's National Health Strategy of 2011–2016, which articulates its goal of developing a comprehensive world-class health care system, describes the introduction of disease management, health insurance, and greater integration between government and the private sector. The document also advocated "a community pharmacy network supported by appropriate policy and process, decreasing the reliance on hospitals for filling drug prescriptions, leading to increased efficiency and enhanced access."[28] These policies and plans exemplify the politics that will be necessary to provide the impetus for an improved pharmacy practice complete with effective patient-centered services like medication therapy management and disease management programs run by Qatar pharmacists in a few years time.

Saudi Arabia

The oil-rich KSA is the third largest Arab country and has a population of about 28 million people, of which over 5.5 millions are noncitizens. KSA has at least five public and four private pharmacy programs.[2] Formal education of pharmacy in KSA started in 1952 with the establishment of the College of Pharmacy at King Saud University (KSU) as a 4-year pharmacy program.[29] As in other countries in the region, basic and foundation sciences (pharmaceutics, pharmacology, pharmacognosy and pharmaceutical chemistry) dominated the curriculum during all the earlier years, and students graduated with Bachelor of Pharmacy and Medicinal Chemistry.[30] In 1964, a 5-year program that awarded Bachelor of Pharmaceutical Science (BScPharm) replaced the 4-year program. As a result, new courses were introduced (industrial pharmacy, biostatistics, biological standardization, and applied pharmacognosy). From 1970 onward, the College of Pharmacy at KSU and subsequently other colleges of pharmacy started and maintained links with some U.S. universities for the purpose of curriculum improvement.[29] These strategies led to two landmark results, introducing clinical pharmacy courses, and years later (in 2008) the initiating of the first PharmD degree program in Saudi Arabia.

Like the case in several other countries in the region, KSA suffers from a shortage of qualified pharmacy practitioners and academics, and it has been estimated that at least 17,000 pharmacists are needed by 2026 in KSA.[2,31] Most pharmacy graduates in this country join the hospital sector where services are progressive and clinical pharmacists are well paid.[3] Saudi has an active professional pharmacy society (The Saudi Pharmaceutical Society), which has an established pharmacy continuous education program and publishes pharmacy-related periodicals and a peer-reviewed journal (Saudi Pharmaceutical Journal).

Pharmaceutical care is taught as a 3-credit hour course in the 4th and 5th year on the BSc.Pharm and PharmD programs, respectively. However, like in other countries in the region, clinical pharmacy services dominate the practice and grab the interest of pharmacists. Indeed, clinical pharmacy is well established in many large Saudi hospitals (like the National Guard Hospital, King Khalid University Hospital, and Security Forces Hospital), and some practicing pharmacists integrate clinical pharmacy with the provision of pharmaceutical care and medication therapy management to their patients. However, while the pharmaceutical care idea is widely recognized especially by fresh graduates, it is clear that so far a full process of medication therapy management that utilizes the pharmaceutical care concept does not exist and will require years to be a recognized practice.[32]

Sudan

Up to the time of writing this chapter, Sudan, which has a population of 39 million people, is the largest country in Africa and the Arab world, and 10th largest in the world by area.[33] It is bordered by Egypt to the north, the Red Sea to the North East, Eritrea and Ethiopia to the east, Kenya and Uganda to the southeast, the Democratic Republic of the Congo and the Central African Republic to the southwest, Chad to the west, and Libya to the northwest. The world's longest river, the Nile, divides the country between east and west sides.

There are around 9300 registered pharmacists in Sudan, graduated from 12 public and 3 private colleges of pharmacy and from overseas universities as well.[34] Like Egypt, Sudan is one of the major sources of pharmacists working in oil-rich Gulf Countries, which has recognizable impact on the pharmacy work force at the national level. The concept of pharmaceutical care was introduced in Sudan very late, possibly in 2004, and now only about 40% of the existing colleges of pharmacy include aspects of pharmaceutical care in their curricula.[34] While some of these colleges have reasonably well-established pharmacy practice departments, only a few have qualified faculty members to deliver courses with pharmaceutical care or medication therapy management as their main focus. An international meeting about pharmaceutical care was held in 2010 in Khartoum (Capital city of Sudan) in an attempt to raise awareness about pharmaceutical care among pharmacy academicians. As a result of this and other such initiatives, several pharmacy programs started to target recruiting faculty with expertise in pharmaceutical care teaching or course development.[34]

A Sudanese Union of Pharmacists (a self-appointed group established in 1989) is responsible for the social and cultural activities of the pharmacists, in addition to organizing regional conferences and delivering continuous pharmacy education. It established the CPD Centre in 2005 to "oversee the provision of continuing education and continuing professional development opportunities for all pharmacists in Sudan."[35] However, the Sudan Medical Council (SMC) is the main body that manages the legal and administrative aspects of pharmacists in Sudan (registration, ethical, and professional issues). The SMC is governed by directives and laws approved by the Council of Ministers. The Sudanese Ministry of Health has recently appointed a committee to look into the future of pharmacy in Sudan. This committee is entrusted to carry out situation analysis, find the gaps, and propose solutions in the form of a road map for Pharmacy in 2021.

There is currently a realization among many Sudanese pharmacy graduates that they were not adequately prepared during their undergraduate years for provision of pharmaceutical care. A number of CPD workshops and training courses on diverse bundles of skills and competencies are offered by the General Directorate of Pharmacy of Khartoum State, which has started to advocate and support clinical pharmacy practices in hospitals, including pharmaceutical care services of some sort, in the hospital setting. Some Sudanese pharmacists who have advanced degrees and who live and work outside Sudan had started organizing continuous education workshops on pharmaceutical care and other pharmacy practice subjects in coordination with non-Governmental health care Sudanese groups and organizations. These are usually well attended, but do not provide recognized qualifications.[36]

Only a handful of community pharmacists started their own pharmaceutical care practice (that is separate from the dispensing process) through personal initiatives.[37] The health problems mostly targeted are diabetes, dermatology, asthma, and hypertension. Patients may or may not pay for these services, and when payment is made, it is a nominal charge. The community pharmacists that provide these services all have separate patient counseling rooms that ensure confidentiality. The qualifications of pharmacists providing these cognitive services in the hospital setting are usually Masters in Clinical Pharmacy, but no specific training, formal certification, or postgraduate qualification is required to provide medication therapy management or pharmaceutical care.[35]

Education is only slowly changing due to the scarcity of qualified faculty, lack of motivation, and barriers facing the application of medication therapy management. Leaders of the profession in Sudan plan to continue setting up more scientific meetings, seminars, and workshop to increase the awareness of pharmacists, policy makers, and educators to adopt a new approach that is hoped to improve the health delivery system by introducing pharmaceutical care and medication therapy management as a means of achieving good outcomes for the patients.

Conclusion

As a term, medication therapy management is still largely unknown in the Middle East region. Pharmacists in this region are more used to pharmaceutical care, which had been introduced relatively recently. Both terms, however, are still confused with clinical pharmacy, which remains a priority in several countries in the region. Pharmacy education is witnessing rapid change in many of the countries in the Middle East, and several pharmacy programs either have introduced or are planning to introduce the PharmD degree program to replace the traditional Baccalaureate degree. These changes are hoped to reflect a wider recognition and application of medication therapy management in the hospital and community settings. However, there is still a vague and poorly defined role for professional pharmacy associations in the Middle East, which slows down progress in the practice of pharmacy.

At the time this Section was written, the Middle East was passing through a tsunami of political and social change led by an aspiring generation of young Arabs. It will not be surprising that these changes also bring about changes in pharmacy education and practice in the Middle East. The challenge facing the wider application of pharmaceutical care and medication therapy management in this region remains to be not if they happen, but when they happen. It is a matter of time.

REFERENCES

1. Hadzovic S. Pharmacy and the great contribution of Arab-Islamic science to its development. *Med Arch.* 1997;51(1–2):47–50.
2. Kheir N, Zaidan M, Younes H, El Hajj M, Wilbur K, Jewesson P. Pharmacy education and practice in 13 middle Eastern countries. *Am J Pharm Educ.* 2009; 72(6):1–13.
3. Al-Wazaify M, Matowe L, Albsoul-Younes A, Al-Omran Oa. Pharmacy education in Jordan, Saudi Arabia, and Kuwait. *Am J Pharm Educ.* 2006;70(1):18.
4. Hasan S. Continuing education needs assessment of pharmacists in the United Arab Emirates. *Pharm World Sci.* 2009;31(6):670–676.
5. Marshall MN. The key informant technique. *Fam Pract.* 1996;13(1):92–97.
6. Khalifa S. Medication therapy management in Egypt. (Personal Communication) 2011. March 24, 2011.

7. Sabri N. Medication therapy management in Egypt. (Personal Communication) 2011.
8. Ministry Of Health. Statistics, Ministry of Health and Population of Egypt, Cairo, Egypt. 2011
9. Khalifa S. Email Communication. 2011. March 24, 2011.
10. Elmahdawi M. Medication therapy management in Eygpt. 2011.
11. Encyclopedia of the Nations—Asia and the Pacific: Jordan. 2011.
12. Albsoul-Younes A, Wazaify M, Alkofahi A. Pharmaceutical care education and practice in Jordan in the new millennium. *Jor J Pharm Sci.* 2008;1(1):83–89.
13. Tahaineh Lm, Wazaify M, Albsoul-Younes A, Khader Y, Zaidan M. Perceptions, experiences, and expectations of physicians in hospital settings in Jordan regarding the role of the pharmacist. *Res Social Adm Pharm.* 2009;5(1):63–70.
14. Awad A, Al-Ebrahim S, Abahussain E. Pharmaceutical care services in hospitals of Kuwait. *J Pharm Pharm Sci.* 2006;9(2):149–157.
15. Dib JG, Saade S, Merhi F. Pharmacy practice in Lebanon. *Am J Health Syst Pharm.* 2004;61(8):794–795.
16. Antoun RB, Salameh P. Satisfaction of pharmacists in Lebanon and the prospect for clinical pharmacy. *East Mediterr Health J.* 2009;15(6):1553–1563.
17. United Arab Emirates. Wikipedia the free encyclopedia. 2011. September 4, 2011.
18. Ladygin SI. Pharmacy in the United Arab Republic. *Farmatsiia.* 1967;16(6):74–76.
19. Abduelkarem A. Medication therapy management in the United Arab Emirates. 2011.
20. Dajani S. Gold, golf, and pharmacy in the Gulf. *Pj.* 2011;273:930–931.
21. Qatar Information Exchange. Population. http://www.Qix.Gov.Qa/Portal/Page/Portal/Qix/Subject_Area?Subject_Area=176, 2011.
22. Maps of the World.Com. Qatar Gdp. http://www.Mapsofworld.Com/Qatar/Economy/Gdp Html, 2011.
23. Wilbur K. Continuing professional pharmacy development needs assessment of Qatar pharmacists. *Int J Pharm Pract.* 2010;18(4):236–241.
24. Jewesson P. Qatar University pharmacy program targets for the academic year 2007–2008. 2008.
25. Fahey M. Medication therapy management in Qatar. (Personal Communication) 2011. June 6, 2011.
26. Zaidan M. Pharmaceutical care and medication therapy management in Al Amal and the cardiology hopsitals in Qatar. 2011.
27. Zaidan M, Singh R, Wazaify M, Tahaineh L. Physicians' perceptions, expectations, and experience with pharmacists at Hamad Medical Corporation in Qatar. *J Multidiscip Healthc.* 2011;4:85–90.
28. Executive Committee Shc. Qatar National Health Strategy 2011–2016. 2011
29. Asiri Y. Emerging frontiers of pharmacy education in Saudi Arabia: the metamorphosis in the last 50 years. *Saudi Pharm J.* 2011;19:1–8.
30. Al-Wazaify M, Matowe L, Albsoul-Younes A, Al-Omran Oa. Pharmacy education in Jordan, Saudi Arabia, and Kuwait. *Am J Pharm Educ.* 2006;70(1):18.
31. King Saud University College of Pharmacy website. 2011.
32. Al-Draimly M. Medication therapy management in Saudi Arabia. 2011. March 5, 2011.
33. Sudan.Net. Republic of the Sudan. 2011. June 6, 2011.
34. Elkhawad A. Medication therapy management in Sudan. (Personal Communication) 2011.
35. Sudan pharmacists continuing professional development center. 2011. July 6, 2011.
36. Hamed A. Medication therapy management in Sudan. (Personal Communication) 2011. June 4, 2011.
37. Eltaeb M. Medication therapy management in the community pharmacy sector in Sudan. 2011. April 4, 2011.

GERMANY

Jochen Pfeifer, PharmD, MRPharmS
Clinical Assistant Professor, Professional Education
University of Minnesota, College of Pharmacy
Owner and Head Pharmacist
Adler Apotheke Velbert, Germany

Andreas Niclas Föerster, PharmD
Clinical Assistant Professor, Professional Education
University of Minnesota, College of Pharmacy
Senior Pharmacist
Adler Apotheke Velbert, Germany

Introduction

This section will analyze the development and structure of pharmaceutical care practice in Germany with particular regard to community pharmacies.

In 2010, there were 21,441 community pharmacies in Germany and 48,695 licensed pharmacists. Approximately 4 million people out of approximately 80 million inhabitants visit German community pharmacies every day.[1]

In contrast to other countries, the owner of a community pharmacy in Germany has to be a pharmacist. A pharmacist may own one main pharmacy and up to three subsidiaries. Under German law, three requirements apply to the establishment of subsidiaries. First, the pharmacist personally manages the main pharmacy. Second, the owner employs a responsible pharmacist in each of the subsidiaries. Third, all subsidiaries must be located within the same or a neighboring district—which can still stretch over a very large area in certain German states.[1]

In 2009, the European Court of Justice confirmed that each member state of the European Union might take its own measures to guarantee a high level of consumer protection in health care. In this context, Germany's ownership requirement was ruled to be in line with European law and even considered an effective measure of consumer protection.[2]

Therefore, German pharmacists are either independent professionals who own their pharmacy or are employed in a community pharmacy, fulfilling the daily tasks.[3] They commonly depend upon themselves to complete the traditional activities of the dispensing pharmacists (Figure 12-5).

But German pharmacy is currently under economic pressure and facing changes in demand from consumers and government to provide some limited cognitive pharmaceutical services.[3,4,5]

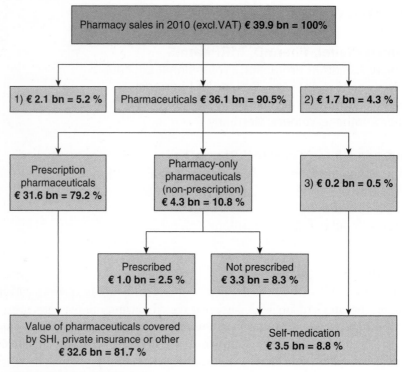

1) Supplementary assortment
2) Patient care products
3) Unrestricted OTC pharmaceuticals*

Figure 12-5 Structure of pharmacy sales in 2010 (in €).[1]
*Pharmaceuticals, which may be sold outside pharmacies (e.g., by chemists)

Strand has defined pharmaceutical care as a "practice in which the practitioner takes responsibility for a patient's drug-related needs, and is held accountable for this commitment."[6] Therefore, the pharmacist who provides pharmaceutical care services in Germany is providing a professional practice, like those of medicine or dentistry because the pharmacist will be responsible for satisfying unique health care needs of a patient.[7]

In Germany, the term "pharmazeutische Betreuung" (pharmaceutical care) is commonly used in a different way.[8]

There are tendencies to establish the notion that any kind of services by pharmacists to a patient, which go beyond the dispensing only, should be considered as *pharmaceutical care* per se. Also the definition of pharmaceutical care as care of the pharmacist around pharmaceuticals for the benefit of the patient is too simple and of questionable value.[9] The term *cognitive services*, which is often used to describe certain aspects of pharmaceutical care, adds to the confusion about a correct definition.[10]

Eickhoff and Schulz[11] divide community pharmacy services in Germany into the following activities:

- dispensing of drugs
- provision of appropriate drug information and advice
- optimization of drug therapies and solution of drug-related problems (DRPs) as well as cooperation with physicians
- preventive care services
- contribution to health promotion
- "provision of pharmaceutical care, the responsible and continuous provision of drug therapy for the purpose of achieving definite outcomes that improve a patient's health-related quality of life, including medication management"[11]

This chapter will focus on the level of systematic pharmaceutical care as it has been implemented or suggested thus far and will conduct a review on what level of the provision of pharmaceutical care that improve a patient's health-related quality of life in Germany has been achieved.

Historical Development in Germany

The evolution of the service has been a slow and unsteady process.

Implementing pharmaceutical care practice in Germany has been discussed in Germany by the Federal Union of German Associations of Pharmacists (Arbeitsgemeinschaft Deutscher Apothekerverbände [ABDA]) since the early 1990s.

ABDA issued a concept paper in 1993.[12] According to the ABDA "this was the official starting point of the change that led to community pharmacists moving from the image of a person primarily dispensing medicines toward a highly qualified advisor taking responsibility for patients' drug-related needs."[11]

Several studies[8,11] show that pharmaceutical care and other pharmaceutical services are feasible in German community pharmacy practice, and that patients could benefit from these services.

Starting also in 1990, the Federal Chamber of Pharmacists (Bundesapothekerkammer [BAK]) has issued a growing number of guidelines pertaining to the correct implementation of structured pharmaceutical processes into German community pharmacy.[13] The BAK is the federal cooperation of the regional boards of pharmacy. As their mission is to define professional behavior, the BAK issues guidelines, which are not legally binding but as a whole, describe the standard of practice in Germany.

Those guidelines aim to assist pharmacists and pharmaceutical personnel by way of recommending standard procedures for specific pharmaceutical processes or the workflow during for instance the dispensing of over-the-counter (OTC) or Rx medications also encompassing some specific indications. They include recommendations on how to provide pharmaceutical advice and information. Providing pharmaceutical advice and information is legally required by Article 20 of the Ordinance of the Operation of Pharmacies (Apothekenbetriebsordnung).[14] They do not, however, reflect a pharmaceutical care practice as laid out in this book.

Present State of Comprehensive Medication Management Services in Germany And Differences in Terminology

The situation of the German community pharmacy, relatively stable and successful over the years, has changed dramatically with the emergence of new competitors such as mail-order pharmacies, new legal restrictions such as rebate limits with wholesalers, new forms of access to prescription drugs for patients, and the focus on extreme price sensitivity in the OTC sector–unlike regulated reimbursements for Rx medication, German pharmacists can decide freely on OTC prices. The issue is how German pharmacists adjust to the increasingly competitive situation.

The risk of paying for pharmaceutical services exclusively through the sales price of a product–as practiced in the current system in Germany–fosters the minimization of pharmacist's services to logistics.[15]

The tendency of many German pharmacists to perceive their Unique Selling Proposition, their main distinction from competing pharmacies, and therefore, the patient's reason to choose this pharmacy solely in the discount pricing of an OTC drug is a critical development.[15]

A great number of pharmacists' marketing efforts do not focus on their pharmaceutical quality but rather on discount pricing. Examples for this development are the introduction of "Happy Hours" with 15% or higher rebate on all OTC products during specific times, for example on Saturdays, to attract customers to purchase OTC products and additionally fill their prescriptions in that specific pharmacy.[15]

Within the traditional dispensing role of pharmacy in Germany, the pharmacist is mainly responsible for allocating the "right product to the right patient."[16]

Even though the pharmacist is obliged to deliver state-of-the-art services, as defined by the BAK guidelines for example, the enforcement of changing standards lacks persuasiveness and thus slows the development.

More emphasis should be shifted in German pharmacy toward understanding that pharmaceutical care practice is not about a specific physical site such as the independently owned and operated community pharmacy. Pharmaceutical care does not occur only in the hospital, and is not about the pharmacist but the patient.[17]

Per definition pharmaceutical care practice can happen wherever there are patients, such as at home, in the community pharmacy, or at senior citizens' homes.[7] The realization of this fact is crucial, when defining the role of the pharmacist within the system. There has not yet been made a distinction between this service and the logistical role of the dispensing community pharmacy in this country with different levels of care being offered by German pharmacists.

Therefore, it is essential to differentiate between "pharmaceutical advice" and "pharmaceutical care".

Pharmaceutical **Advice** (Level 1)	Provision of appropriate drug information and advice for patients and other health professionals
	Use of Information Systems for pharmacists like the ABDA-databank
Pharmaceutical **Advice** (Level 2)	Pharmacist's involvement and interaction with the patient to detect and prevent DRPs
Pharmaceutical **Advice** (Level 3)	Intervention by pharmacists to solve DRPs, for example by communication with prescribing physician
	Preventive care projects in community pharmacies
Pharmaceutical **Care** (Level 1)	Review of a patient's drug regimen conducted by the pharmacist through cooperation with the patient's physician
	Examples: Medication Therapy Management, Home Medication Review
Pharmaceutical **Care** (Level 2)	Monitoring for Adherence and Drug Therapy Outcomes as part of a Medical Home in cooperation with physicians
	Implementation of Evidence Based Medicine
	Pharmacotherapy Counselling for Physicians

(Continued)

Pharmaceutical **Care** (Level 3)	Pharmacist being actively involved in patient's therapy decision in consultation with physicians, prior to a prescription being written.
	The role of the pharmacist is in the vast majority of cases reactive by responding to physician's decisions without having the possibility to intervene actively. Therefore, the specialist knowledge of the pharmacist is not utilized at the time when it is most useful: at the time of prescribing[18,19]

Data from Germany reference 19.

Levels 1-3 of the "Pharmaceutical Advice" class can be considered to be a part of traditional pharmaceutical services but not pharmaceutical care practice as defined in this book.

German community pharmacists perform these three pharmaceutical advice levels very successfully. In 2010, the Voluntary Report Service for suspected cases of medication risks to the Drug Commission of the German Medical Association received reports of 8300 cases. Main complaints referred to unwanted medication effects and reports of misuse (31%), errors in packaging (30%) as well as galenic deficiency (18%).[1]

In 2009, Schulz et al. analyzed nature and frequency of DRPs in daily community pharmacy practice in Germany.[20]

Findings of this study were:

- Almost every fifth patient request for self-medication pharmaceuticals was associated with one or more DRP,
- 72% of DRP occurred in conjunction with the four most common indications such as pain, respiratory, gastrointestinal, and skin disorders,
- 75% of DRP were inappropriate self-medication, inappropriate product request, wrong dosage, and the duration of drug use (including abuse) was too long,
- Significantly more cases of wrong dosage and drug-drug interactions could be identified when the patient had a medication record in that particular community pharmacy
- 90% of DRP could be resolved in community pharmacies.

A recent study on pharmaceutical care in German community pharmacies[21] established that pharmacists routinely screened patient records, verified patient understanding, and validated filled prescriptions, but pharmacists infrequently documented activities related to patient care, evaluated patients' perceived status, engaged in implementing therapeutic objectives and monitoring plans, evaluated patient satisfaction, or self-evaluated their performance in providing pharmaceutical care on regular basis.

This European study[21] investigated the provision of pharmaceutical care by community pharmacists across Europe and examined the various factors that could affect its implementation.

With regard to Germany, the findings of this study suggest that the provision of pharmaceutical care in community pharmacy is still limited. There was a response rate of less than 10% to the provided questionnaires from the contacted community pharmacies. Of those who responded, indicated that pharmacists were routinely engaged in general activities such as patient-record screening but were infrequently involved in patient-centered professional activities such as the implementation of therapeutical objectives and monitoring patient plans or in self-evaluation of performance of the patients.

The long-lasting success of the traditional dispensing and advisory services appears to make the realization difficult for German pharmacy that the addition of a pharmaceutical care practice adds a new set of responsibilities and objectives to the working system of the community pharmacy. This change, however, urgently mandated by the healthcare system would be achieved easiest, if implemented through a shift in the training of new pharmacists.[6,22,23]

At the same time, the patient may be confused in his perception of the pharmacist, if the traditional role of the dispensing German community pharmacist cannot be clearly demarcated from his practice of pharmaceutical care.

A feasible option for the German community pharmacist who does not want to separate those two kinds of services would be to physically separate them from each other within the same building as demonstrated by the authors in a community pharmacy in Velbert in 2009.[24]

Since 2009, the authors are cooperating with the College of Pharmacy of the University of Minnesota in offering an international Advanced Pharmacy Practice Experience in a German community pharmacy according to U.S. rules and regulations in order to implement international best practice elements into each country's health care and pharmacy systems.[25]

As a result of this cooperation the following overview on the implementation of optimized practice components to offer comprehensive medication management by pharmacists in German community pharmacies has been developed.[26]

Practice component:	Specific examples:	Optimal practice	Implementation in Germany
Medication reconciliation	Computerized drug-interaction software	Implementation of a computerized drug-interaction software system with well-designed training programs	Basic software already available New modules to be developed and applied
	Pharmacist clinical review	Utilization of Medication Therapy Management services and implementation of a pharmacist clinically reviewing medications	Not yet implemented in Germany
	Drug-utilization review	Implementation of a utilization review	Not yet implemented in Germany
Patient dispensing safety	Authenticity	Utilization of Good Manufacturing Practices (GMPs) and regulations as primary source of product verification	Discussion in German on developing new safety measures against drug forgeries
	Electronic prescribing	Implementation of an electronic prescribing system	Essential for implementing better pharmaceutical care modules in Germany but at this time politically not yet accepted by pharmacists
	Labeling medication	Labeling medication with patient-specific information including directions for use	Not yet mandatory in Germany but needs to become mandatory in order to guarantee drug safety and compliance
	Quantity dispensed	Dispensing amount of medication tailored for the patient needs	Not yet implemented. In Germany, drugs are only dispensed in so-called normed sizes "N1, N2 and N3"

Patient education	Education by pharmacist, when no clinical decisions need to be made	In many community pharmacists
	Implementation of mandatory patient education on all new prescriptions	This U.S. regulation should be implemented in Germany to enhance patient care
Education of personnel — Pharmacist education	Education with a clinical pharmacy focus and requiring continuous education	Mandatory continuous education for pharmacists has to be implemented in Germany. For political reasons at the moment (December 2011) unlikely
Quality measurement — Patient-satisfaction surveys	Measuring correct quality parameters	Not yet implemented in Germany
Documentation systems — Computer documentation	Implementation of computer-documentation systems	Not yet fully implemented in all German pharmacies
Documentation of compounding	Implementation of mandatory documentation of various parameters when compounding	Has to become mandatory in Germany, even though the current pharmacy law does not require it yet
Documenting patient education	Implementation of a clinically based patient education documentation system	This U.S. model should be implemented in German community pharmacy

While the introduction of the pharmaceutical care practice might pose a challenge, the German pharmacist would be well advised to also work on his profile as an equal partner in the patient's health service team. When it comes to the medication of the patients, it is the pharmaceutical care practitioner who must understand the patient's medication experience because it is the duty of the pharmacist who provides pharmaceutical care to optimize the patient's medication experience.[7]

Payment for Services

As mentioned in the beginning, the reimbursement structure for Rx medications that links the pharmaceutical service to the dispensing of the product cultivates a focus on the product and the sale thereof.

Article 78 Arzneimittelgesetz (German Drugs Act)[27] and Section 3 Arzneimittelpreisverordnung (Ordinance on the Operation of Pharmacies)[14] as well as agreements between the German pharmacists associations and the Association of German Social Health Insurances regulate the payment structure for community pharmacists in Germany.[28] In January 2004, the German government changed the law of reimbursement of pharmacists by introducing dispensing fees for each prescription-only drug.[28] There is basically no additional remuneration for medication management services and until this day, there are only regulations regarding dispensing fees for community pharmacists, which cover all legally required services by community pharmacists.

Such a context does not advance the implementation of services for the patient-focused outcome improvement.

In order to incentivize the implementation of pharmaceutical care practice into German pharmacy, the payment structure should be modified by redefining the pharmacists' input from only dispensing inventory, which includes pharmaceutical advice to additional reimbursement schemes for the numbers of patients for whom they identify, solve, and prevent DRPs.[16]

This would mean the introduction of a "pay for performance" structure for pharmacists in Germany.

Qualification of Practitioners in Germany

In order for German pharmacists to work as clinicians in the described setting, they would have to adopt a conceptual framework that would contain all the questions, organization of patient-specific data, and encompasses the clinical decisions inherent in the pharmaceutical care process.

In the profession, education also evolves slowly toward clinical topics. Because of its grown, traditional structure, education is dominated by the traditional subjects of chemistry, compounding, pharmaceutical technology, and biology. In 2001, changes were implemented to include a limited exposure to courses in clinical pharmacy.[11]

In addition, although pharmacists are obliged by law to engage in continuous education programs when their original training is completed, there has been no control over their commitment or requirement for pharmacists to substantiate the successful participation in those programs.[11]

The following minimum requirements for education programs for German community pharmacists would enable them to perform comprehensive medication management services.

Clinical Pharmacy	Advanced knowledge of pharmacology, clinical pharmacy, and pathophysiology
	Work on patient cases
	Monitoring
	The practice of pharmaceutical care
Interdisciplinary Communication	Communication with doctors, patients
	Communication technology
	Negotiation skills
Ethical requirements	Privacy policy
	Pharmacist as a consultant to the doctor; therapy sovereignty remains with the doctor
	The patient's medication-related needs as the center of the pharmacist's activity
	Commitment to continuous education
Practice Management	Documentation, preferably electronically
	Consultation areas
	Structured counseling program for patients
	Structured counseling program for interdisciplinary communication
Quality Management	Certification according to DIN EN ISO 9001/2008
	Continuous improvement
	Commitment to the evaluation of achievements

Selective Pharmaceutical Care Projects in Germany

I.   Funding Project "Pharmaceutical Care" of ABDA

To promote pharmaceutical care research and implementation in Germany, ABDA has introduced a funding project with the following goals:[29]

- Assistance in developing the scientific foundations and practical implementation of pharmaceutical care
- Promotion of pilot projects
- Promotion of studies on the effectiveness of pharmaceutical care
- Raising public awareness of the pharmaceutical care

In November 2011, an Internet data base was established for members of this project, which gives an overview on all pharmaceutical care projects in Germany.[30]

II. Geriatric Pharmacy

The ABDA passed a resolution on implementing continuous education programs for a specialization in geriatric pharmacy on November 25, 2009.[31]

Only a few of 17 state pharmacy boards in Germany have implemented this additional level of qualification.

Specialists for geriatric pharmacy collect, analyze, prevent, and solve DRPs, and improve pharmaceutical care for geriatric patients with regard to effectiveness, safety, and rationality. They work closely with doctors, nurses, and relatives of the patients and offer their services in the community, hospital, and nursing homes.

There are certain requirements for pharmacists to participate in this new geriatric pharmacy project:

- Participation in at least 100 hours of seminars with small groups of maximum 25 participants each
- Proof of a completed training of nursing staff in hospitals or nursing homes
- Proof of a 3-day placement: either at least 2 days in a nursing home, with the optional third day in a hospital setting or 3 days at a geriatric hospital
- Examinations

Learning objectives for geriatric pharmacists:

- identification, resolution, and prevention of drug risks through monitoring and structured advice on DRPs,

- quality assurance and optimization of pharmaceutical care processes including identification, resolution, and prevention of typical medication errors,
- medical, pharmaceutical, social, and economic importance of acute and chronic diseases in old age,
- patient-centered care,
- cooperation with physicians, nurses, relatives, and senior citizens groups
- clinical pharmacy practice,
- collection, management, and evaluation of drug information for geriatric patients
- planning and implementation of education and training for nursing staff, caregivers, and patients.

As a consequence, some areas in Germany have a limited number of these specialized pharmacists. Unfortunately until now (December 2011) there is no additional reiumbursement for the provision of these services. Therefore, there is limited incentive for pharmacy owners to either undergo the training themselves or have their staff be trained with those skills.

The introduction of geriatric pharmacy into Germany is a very promising step for implementing new patient services. It is unfortunate that the participation is purely voluntary for pharmacists who supply nursing homes.

III. Pharmacist-led Intervention to Improve Inhalation Technique in Asthma and Chronic Obstructive Pulmonary Disease Patients

For the first time, pharmacists are now involved systematically in the asthma care process in Germany supporting assurance of a correct inhalation technique in close collaboration with the prescribing doctors.[32,33]

The significance of this project lies in the fact that this is the first time that pharmacists are mentioned alongside the medical doctor in a guideline or scope of practice and that it was issued by a national expert panel of physicians. Unfortunately, the utilization of the community pharmacist is limited to ensuring patient understanding of the device[33] (Figure 12-6).

IV. ABDA-KBV Project 2011

Doctors and pharmacists have developed a promising new approach of collaboration in Germany to reduce medication risks, increase patient compliance, and to improve the quality of the supply and reduction of health care costs.

Developed jointly on a federal level by the Federal Associations of Statutory Health Insurance Physicians (KBV) and ABDA this new concept is the first joint approach to medication safety. It is built around the central element of medication management,[34] with the utilization of a medication catalog

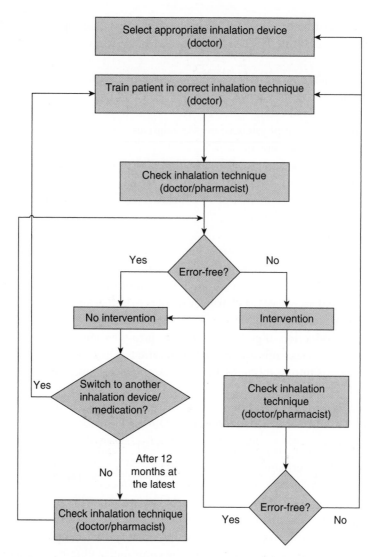

Figure 12-6 Intervention to improve inhalation technique. (Reproduced with permission from Hämmerlein A, Müller U, Schulz M. Pharmacist-led intervention study to improve inhalation technique in asthma and COPD patients. *J Eval Clin Pract.* 2011;17(1):61–70.)

and the prescription of the medication by the International Nonproprietary Names only.

This requires knowledge both of all prescribed drugs and the self-medication of patients with OTC products and, therefore, an extensive exchange of information between doctors and pharmacists and patients.

Medication management is designed for chronically ill patients who take at least five drugs permanently. With the patient's consent and this person's choice of one specific doctor and one specific pharmacist, the patient will be followed continuously for 1 year. The total medication including self-medication will be checked for potential adverse drug effects and will lead to comprehensive consultations with the goal to resolve DRPs, increase compliance, and to coordinate and optimize the medication prescribed by several physicians.

A medication catalog names certain drugs of choice for specific diseases and reserve agents. The physician's right to deviate from this catalog remains. This will be a nationwide uniform approach, which will be SHI-comprehensive and guidelines-oriented to ensure quality and compliance.

This systematical interdisciplinary cooperation of pharmacists and physicians could, if fully implemented, significantly enhance the quality of patient care in Germany.

Future of Pharmaceutical Care Practice in Germany

Germany has to find its own way to implement new patient-centered services such as comprehensive medication management in the existing system. It is not possible to just adapt U.S. or Australian models into German pharmacy without taking the specific German differences in pharmacy practice and the health care system into consideration. Although the practice itself is universal, the profession has to appeal to people with different cultural background and expectations from their pharmacists.

Pharmacists should also take the recommendations of the Advisory Council on the Assessment of Developments in the Health Care System 2009 for the German Ministry of Health to their hearts.[35] The Advisory Council supports the idea of the individual practice focusing on the patient's needs and the results of therapy in an integrated approach.

Its recommendations read as follows:

In a future health care system that will be cross-sectoral, community-based care, community pharmacies must position themselves as institutions that bear more responsibility than now for the quality and efficiency of the choice of medication being involved in an integrated care network.

We also believe that community pharmacies should organize future care units both regionally and supra-regionally in which cases associations of pharmacies that agree on communicable and verifiable quality standards could be a sensible solution.

"Cooperation with doctors within the context of community-based care makes special professional qualifications appear essential (e.g. in clinical pharmacy). The resultant differentiation between pharmacies and the liberalisation of the 'collective contract' that has been in existence to date (framework contract according to Article

129 Social Code, Book V)[36] *for the pharmacies involved in SHI care, as well as competition for contract models in drug provision, will lead to more integration and cooperation in medical treatment processes, as in primary and secondary medical care.*"[35]

Germany has one major advantage for implementing new medication management services—unused until now. Unlike the United States, German pharmacy technicians are fully trained professionals with a 2.5-year professional training.[37] They are considered "pharmaceutical personnel," may dispense medication and perform certain forms of counseling (pharmaceutical advice stages 1 to 3 of the above scheme) under the supervision of a pharmacist. Therefore, the utilization of pharmacy technicians should become more intense than it is today.

This step would yield open time for pharmacists to spend more time in the newly developed pharmaceutical care practice.

Implementation of comprehensive medication management into Germany will strengthen the position of the pharmacist and improve the cooperation between the medical professions to improve patient care.

REFERENCES

1. German Pharmacies; Bundesvereinigung Deutscher Apothekerverbände ABDA. Available at http://www.abda.de/983.html. Accessed December 01, 2011. German population figures provided by http://www.statistik-portal.de/Statistik-Portal/de_zs01_bund.asp. (Accessed December 1, 2011).
2. Urteil des EuGH vom 19. Mai 2009, verb. Rs. C-171/07 und C-172/07–Apothekerkammer des Saarlands u.a./Saarland.
3. Glaeske G. Von der Zunft in die Zukunft—Mehr Qualitätswettbewerb im Apothekenmarkt. TOP Jahreskongress 2009. Published by Zentrum für Sozialpolitik, Universität Bremen. Available at http://www.zes.unibremen.de/homepages/glaeske/downloads/081205_ Apotheke 2009.pdf. (Accessed June 29, 2011).
4. Benrimoj SI, Feletto E, Gastelurrutia M, Martinez Martinez F, Faus M. A holistic and integrated approach to implementing cognitive pharmaceutical services. *Ars Pharm.* 2010;51(2):69–88.
5. Hoffmann F, Glaeske G, Pfannkuche MS. The Effect of introducing rebate contracts to promote generic drug substitution, on doctors' prescribing practices. *Dtsch Arztebl Int.* 2009;106(48):783–788.
6. Strand L. Re-visioning the profession. *J Am Pharm Assoc (Wash).* 1997;37(4):474–478.
7. Cipolle R, Strand L, Morley P. *Pharmaceutical Care Practice: The Clinician's Guide.* New York, 2004.
8. Schaefer M, Schulz M. Manuale zur Pharmazeutischen Betreuung, Band 1: Grundlagen der Pharmazeutischen Betreuung, Eschborn; 2000.
9. Foppe van Mil JW, Schulz M. A review of pharmaceutical care in community pharmacy in Europe. *Harvard Health Policy Review.* 2006;7(1):155–168.

10. Roberts A, Benrimoj SI, Chen T, et al. Understanding practice change in community pharmacy: a qualitative research instrument based on organisational theory. *Pharm World Sci.* 2003;25(5):227–234.

11. Eickhoff C, Schulz M. Pharmaceutical care in community pharmacies: practice and research in Germany. *Ann Pharmacother.* 2006;40(4):729–735.

12. Schulz M, Morck H, Braun R. Neues Apothekenprofil: good pharmacy practice und pharmaceutical care. *Pharm Ztg.* 1993;138(41):3191–3197.

13. Bundesapothekerkammer: Leitlinien, http://www.abda.de/leitlinien0.html (Accessed June 19, 2011).

14. Ordinance on the Operation of Pharmacies (*Apothekenbetriebsordnung—ApBetrO*), last amended pursuant to Art. 2 of the Ordinance amending the Ordinance on Prescription-only drugs and the Ordinance on the Operation of Pharmacies dated December 2, 2008 [Federal Law Gazette I p. 2338]. This consolidated version was developed as a working aid by ABDA (Federal Union of German Associations of Pharmacists). Only the texts published in the Federal Law Gazette are legally binding.

15. Pfeifer J. Medication Therapy Management, Profilierungschance gegenüber Versandapotheken, dm und Co. PZ online 2008. http://www.pharmazeutische-zeitung.de/index.php?id=5690 (Accessed June 19, 2011).

16. Sakthong P. Comparative analysis of pharmaceutical care and traditional dispensing role of pharmacy. *Thai J Pharm Sci.* 2007;31:100–104.

17. Cipolle C, Cipolle R, Strand L. Consistent standards in medication use: The need to care for patients from research to practice. *J Am Pharm Assoc (2003).* 2006;46(2):205–212.

18. Leape L, Cullen D, Clapp M, et al. Pharmacist participation on physician rounds and adverse drug events in the intensive care unit. *JAMA.* 1999;282(3):267–270.

19. Benrimoj SI, Roberts AS. Providing patient care in community pharmacies in Australia. *Ann Pharmacother.* 2005;39(11):1911–1917.

20. Eickhoff C, Griese N, Hämmerlein A, Schulz M: ABP in der Selbstmedikation. Chance und Auftrag für die Apotheke. Pharm, Ztg, 2009; 154(39): 3606–3615.

21. Hughes C, Schaefer M. et al. Provision of pharmaceutical care by community pharmacists: a comparison across Europe. *Pharm. World Sci.* 2010;32(4):472–487.

22. Strand LM, Cipolle RJ, Morley PC, Perrier DG. Levels of pharmaceutical care: A needs-based approach. *Am J Hosp Pharm.* 1991;48(3):547–550.

23. Strand LM, Cipolle RJ, Morley PC, Frakes MJ. The impact of pharmaceutical care practice on the practitioner and the patient in the ambulatory practice setting: twenty-five years of experience. *Curr Pharm Design.* 2004;10(31):3987–4001.

24. "Excellence Award Apotheke 2009: Spitzenleistungen ausgezeichnet", PZ online 2009 http://www.pharmazeutische-zeitung.de/index.php?id=31618 (Accessed June 19, 2011).

25. Pfeifer J, Förster A. Die pharmazeutische Kompetenz besser nutzen. *Dtsch Apoth Ztg.* 2009;149(34):3810–3816.

26. Modified and adapted from Vierkant MJ, Isetts B. December 4, 2009, University of Minnesota, (Personal Communication).

27. Medicinal Product Act of the Federal Republic of Germany (Arzneimittelgesetz) Last amended pursuant to Article 1 of the Ordinance of September 28, 2009 (Federal Law Gazette I p. 3172), which entered into force on October 3, 2009.

28. Denda R. Steuerungsinstrumente im Arzneimittelbereich. PZ online 2010, http://www.pharmazeutische-zeitung.de/index.php?id=33331 (Accessed June 16, 2011).

29. Förderinititiave Pharmazeutische Betreuung. http://www.abda.de/fi.html (Accessed December 1, 2011).

30. http://www.foerderinitiative.de (Accessed December 1, 2011)

31. ABDA (Federal Union of German Associations of Pharmacists): Geriatrische Pharmazie. http://www.abda.de/1042.html (Accessed June 19, 2011).
32. Hämmerlein A, Müller U, Schulz M. NVL Asthma, Apotheker sind miteingebunden, PZ online 2010. http://www.pharmazeutische-zeitung.de/index.php?id=32759 (Accessed June 19, 2011).
33. Hämmerlein A, Müller U, Schulz M. Pharmacist-led intervention study to improve inhalation technique in asthma and COPD patients. *J Eval Clin Pract.* 2011;17(1):61–70.
34. Zukunftskonzept Arzneimittelversorgung: Gemeinsames Eckpunktepapier von KBV und ABDA. http://www.kbv.de//ais/38730.html (Accessed June 19, 2011).
35. Advisory Council on the Assessment of Developments in the Health Care System Coordination and Integration-Health Care in an Ageing Society, Special Report 2009 (abridged). http://www.svr-gesundheit.de/Startseite/Startseite.htm (Accessed June 19, 2011).
36. Sozialgesetzbuch V, http://www.gesetze-im-internet.de/sgb_5 (Accessed June 19, 2011).
37. Apothekerkammer Nordrhein: Pharmazeutische Technische Assistentin (PTA), http://www.aknr.de/fortbildung/berufe/pta.php (Accessed June 19, 2011).

THE NETHERLANDS

Johan J. de Gier, PharmD, PhD
Professor, Department of Pharmacotherapy and Pharmaceutical Care
Faculty of Mathematics and Natural Sciences
University of Groningen
Groningen, The Netherlands

Introduction

This Chapter describes medication management services in primary care settings in the Netherlands and explains the development and evolution of patient-centered pharmaceutical care practices. It will explain how those services were developed from existing medication surveillance activities and patient information practices. Furthermore, it describes the practices based on the philosophy of pharmaceutical care, which have been evaluated and serve the purpose of defining future directions in developing the medication management services in the Netherlands.

In 2010, there were 1976 community pharmacies in the Netherlands, 32% of these owned by chains. An average community pharmacy has 1.45 (fte, full-time equivalent) pharmacist and 5.67 fte pharmacist assistants as professional staff. With a total population of about 15 million inhabitants, an average number of 7800 patients are served by each pharmacy. An average fee per prescription is €7.91, but pharmacists and health insurers have the possibility of making additional written agreements regarding fees for quality processes, including those in medication therapy management.[1]

In 65 hospital pharmacies, about 400 hospital pharmacists are providing clinical pharmacy services.

Van Mil[2] clearly described the development of patient information, clinical pharmacy, and medication surveillance (checking prescriptions to avoid drug–drug interactions, double medications, contraindications, compliance, and dosing problems) in the Netherlands. The role of the patient in the Dutch pharmacy practice setting was founded on the vision presented in the late seventies by the professional organization of pharmacists that "the patient is a human being for whom we care, and for whom we feel the same responsibility as the physician." Controversies with physicians (e.g., about exchange of clinical data such as diagnoses and laboratory values) during those years resulted in a slow development of an active role of pharmacists in the provision of drug information to patients, which showed significant developments in the late 1980s.

Clinical pharmacy in the Netherlands was first described in the early 1970s, focusing on hospital pharmacists' needs to develop pharmacokinetic-oriented services to improve outcomes of pharmacotherapy. It was like looking at the patient through the glasses of a medicine. However, not much attention was given to the development of more patient-centered services. A major change was observed by the development of computer software for keeping patient drug history files and medication surveillance based on those patient data in the late 1970s. This development was primarily influenced by community pharmacists who played a significant role in setting standards. In the late 1980s, counseling practices and medication surveillance started to become integrated activities and patient-centered information services focused at patients starting to use (chronic) treatments. In those years, individualized patient leaflets written in lay language were introduced with the name of the patient and individualized instructions and warnings for use integrated in the text. In addition, more individualization was achieved according to the patient's characteristics (e.g., age, gender, contraindications). However, community pharmacists presented themselves as drug specialists, responsible for checking prescriptions by performing medication surveillance and drug information counseling services to patients.

During the 1980s, emphasis on cost containment was dictated by health policy developments at that time and rational pharmacotherapy was linked to activities in which pharmacists tried to position themselves as drug specialists who complied to the health policy agenda and at the same time showed interest in providing patient-centered services. But this focus was hard to observe and in the eyes of the public community pharmacists were seen as distributors of medicines, advising patients how to use these. Other professional roles, such as medication surveillance and advising physicians, were not at all acknowledged.

The First Approaches to Develop Pharmaceutical Care

The switch to delivering comprehensive patient care did not start until the early 1990s. During various World Pharmacy Congresses, the philosophy of pharmaceutical care practice as advocated by Hepler and Strand was introduced.[3] Many Dutch community pharmacists were inspired by these developments and started to create the right circumstances for software developers to invest in new patient-centered modules. A clear example was the introduction of an electronic dossier for documenting the assessment of drug-related needs and problems, its evaluations, and subsequent interventions during patient counseling in the Pharmacom system, a software package used by the majority of Dutch community pharmacists.[4]

At the same time, the first research efforts were performed to establish the effects of pharmaceutical care activities in community pharmacy. Two studies were conducted by Van Mil.[2] Both studies were designed as controlled (cohort) studies with internal and external reference groups. A first study (carried out in 18 pharmacies) was focused on the effects of pharmaceutical care in asthma patients applying the therapeutic outcomes monitoring and self-assessment approach as developed by Grainger-Rousseau et al.,[5] aiming at better control of the disease, better coping behavior, and, as a result, improved health-related quality of life (according to the SF36). A second study by the same research team was conducted in 21 pharmacies to investigate the effects of pharmaceutical care in the elderly over 65 years, using four or more different drugs and living independently.[2] The focus in this study was on rationality of treatment and better control over side effects by interventions of the community pharmacist, and health-related quality of life as one of the outcomes. For both studies, carried out between 1995 and 1997, a 2-year study design was decided to allow for the process and outcomes to be as complete as possible. In both studies, only pharmacists (not pharmacy assistants) provided the full scope of pharmaceutical care, including an intake, frequent pharmacist–patient contact (every time a prescription is dispensed), a consultation with the pharmacist every 6 months (focus on medication-related problems and analyses of the drug use profile), and interventions whenever needed, discussed with the patient before contacting the general practitioner. Additional care in the asthma patients study was described as follows: installation of a self-management program in co-operation with the general practitioner and regular inhaler instruction and evaluation of the Peak Expiratory Flow measurement results, at least every 6 months, provided by the pharmacists. Additionally, in the elderly polypharmacy patients, home visits were conducted, whenever a patient was unable to visit the pharmacy for the 6-monthly consultations or whenever necessary, as well as an effort to decrease the use of benzodiazepines. All pharmacists in both studies were provided four half-day training sessions before the start of the studies. During the study, a half-day training was provided every 6 months on drug-use evaluation and medication analysis, relationship and communication, disease state management, and some comprehensive care issues (such as documenting drug-related problems (DRPs), patients needs, and interventions).

The results of the asthma patients' study show that more patients receiving care in the intervention group of pharmacies started to use peak-flow meters and became more involved in self-management than patients who were offered usual care by the reference group pharmacists. Better asthma control was shown by a decrease in the amount of reliever and rescue medication, and knowledge about illnesses related to asthma improved. Intervention group patients indicated improved health-related quality of life. However, asthma patients might not appreciate a 2-year long study, since a high dropout rate of 63% was observed in the intervention group. A high dropout rate (50%) was also observed in the elderly polypharmacy patients using four or more different medicines. The pharmaceutical care provided by the intervention group pharmacists led to a high degree of satisfaction among patients. No major influence was observed on knowledge or quality of life. No clear conclusions were drawn from the data on compliance with the use of diuretics, and no influence on the use of benzodiazepines could be reported, probably due to the low number of patients at the end of the study and the short prestudy period of available drug data. Although pharmacists reported a decreasing number of DRPs (mainly dealing with side effects) while providing pharmaceutical care, patients could not report a difference based on experiencing those DRPs.

Both studies are important examples of early "real-life" studies in the evaluation of pharmaceutical care practice in the Netherlands and show some impact on patient outcomes. But these studies also illustrate that most pharmacists at that time were not used to changing their organizational and practice models for the provision of pharmaceutical care and to modify prescriptions in collaboration with physicians, other than in checking drug–drug interactions, double medications, and contraindications. After publication and discussion of both studies, not very much change in the development of pharmaceutical care was observed. Most pharmacists felt a need to change their practices but incentives were not provided and work load was given as major barrier for taking new initiatives.

Expanding Patient-Centered Activities

Most of the activities in the late 1990s were dedicated to expanding the patient-centered activities in community pharmacies, specifically the implementation of the pharmaceutical dossier for documenting patient consultations. The professional organizations "The Royal Dutch Society for the Advancement of Pharmacy (KNMP)" and an organization for the development of professional content to be used in Pharmacom-pharmacy software systems, "Health Base Foundation (HBF)," developed protocols and guidelines and focused on developing new professional norms and standards for pharmacy care. However, the definition of pharmaceutical care as originally formulated by Hepler and Strand (1990) was modified and described by the KNMP as the care provided by the pharmacy team (including assistants) in the field of pharmacotherapy, and aimed at the patient's improving quality of life. No standards were developed to explain the process of assessing patient needs and concerns, how to perform structured medication review, and how to develop the pharmaceutical care plan and the process follow-up evaluations, and its documentations. HBF's developments in the field of pharmaceutical care were guided by the more practice-oriented definition: pharmaceutical care is a practice in which the practitioner takes responsibility for a patient's drug-related needs, and is held accountable for this commitment.[6] A group of about 80 to 100 early adopters of the philosophy of pharmaceutical care at that time, who started to use a documentation system for patient needs, assessment of DRPs, and evaluation of interventions, such as described above,[4] was able to make a difference in providing comprehensive care.

After the 1990s, cost containment strategies by the Dutch government developed further, and most of the community pharmacists became frustrated knowing that their time and efforts could not be reimbursed within the system that was installed as a fee for prescription system. They felt that innovations in pharmaceutical care were not recognized by health insurers and policy makers. If these were discussed the question asked always pointed at the value of those innovations for insurers (lower costs and better quality) and society (better patient outcomes), expected approval by prescribers if community pharmacists proposed recommendations to change medication for patients, and if the new role of the community pharmacist was a sustainable one.

A study in which one of the health insurers and community pharmacists collaborated in investigating whether a community pharmacist-led intervention reduces the number of potential DRPs in the elderly, was performed in 2002 by Vinks et al.[7] A pharmacy-based controlled trial was conducted from June 2002 until June 2003 in 16 community pharmacies. Elderly patients aged > 65 years using six or more drugs concomitantly were included. Patients were randomly selected from the pharmacy prescription database, as well as the matched control patients (for age and gender), and patients whose GPs were unable or willing to provide relevant diagnostic data concerning all medications used were excluded. Patients were not consulted about their concerns, needs and actual use of medicines. Potential DRPs were determined and grouped into three categories: (i) patient-related potential DRPs (noncompliance); (ii) prescriber-related potential DRPs (expired indication, double medication, over- and underdosage, undertreatment, off-label use, inconvenience of use); (iii) drug-related potential DRPs (contraindications, drug–drug interactions, drug treatment of adverse drug reactions). The primary outcome was the change in the number of potential DRPs; the secondary outcome was related to the change in number of medicines used between the intervention group (n = 87) and the control group (n = 87), at baseline and 4 months after the start of the study. A significant reduction in mean number of DRPs per patient was observed (mean difference 16.3%; 95% CI –24.3, –8.3); the mean number of drugs per patient was not significantly reduced (mean difference –4.7%; 95% CI –9.6, 0.2). Although the authors conclude that the results could show a positive influence of the community pharmacist in reducing potential DRPs in the elderly, they also concluded that focus on actual outcomes, including quality of life, morbidity, and mortality, should be given in future research. It was interesting to observe that this study was developed with the support of pharmacists who were actively collaborating with each other in a regional pharmacy practice research network. The collaboration with a major health insurer was a starting point for future developments where groups of 15 to 30 pharmacies started to make written agreements to provide cognitive services. Those regional activities included in total about 200 pharmacies at the national level.

Appropriateness of prescribing among elderly patients in a Dutch residential home was investigated in an observational study of outcomes after a pharmacist-led medication review by Stuijt et al.[8] in a 12-month period in the years 2003–2004. A health care professional team consisting of a GP, care home staff, and a pharmacist included all 54 residents of one residential nursing home in a rural area in the Netherlands. This study was also financially supported by a local insurance company (only for compensating participating GPs). For all kinds of good reasons, 24 patients could not be included, resulting in an evaluation of 30 patients, mean age 85.8 (SD 6.7) years. Patients were assessed using the Medication Appropriateness Index (MAI) by a group of 13 independent clinical pharmacists recruited as assessors from five hospitals in the Netherlands and all having experience in providing pharmaceutical care for elderly in nursing homes. Each patient was assessed twice on April 1, 2003 (before the intervention) and April 1, 2004 (after intervention) by a fix pair of independent reviewers, using the patient medication profile and the patient's medical record. The intervention consisted of a pharmacist-led medication review and the development of a pharmaceutical care plan, which described clinical outcomes or therapeutic objectives to be obtained in the future, and was also meant to incorporate adherence to professional guidelines. After the development of the care plan in collaboration with the team members, a consultation with the patient could be conducted by the GP, the pharmacist, or nursing staff. The pharmacist identified 115 DRPs, ranging from 1 to 11 with a mean (SD) of 3.1 (1.9). The total number of accepted recommendations was 78 (67.8%). High frequency of prescribed medicines without a documented or current medical condition resulted in the highest number of DRPs. There was a statistical significant difference between overall pre- and postintervention summed MAI scores ($P = 0.013$). This study underlines the importance of looking at the quality of prescribing, and supports the formal integration of a clinical pharmacist (not being a community pharmacy-based pharmacist) into the health care team. At that time hospital pharmacists were primary focusing on the pharmacotherapy of the individual patient by checking alerts on abnormal dosages, duplicate medication, drug–drug interactions, and nonformulary medication at the end of the day by screening lists. The pharmaceutical care evaluation was, however, developing slowly by using a model to evaluate the choice of the medical therapy, dosing regimen, side-effects, therapeutic duplication, and so on while participating in physician rounds.[9]

Another example of research efforts to determine the effects of treatment reviews conducted by community pharmacists was conducted in 2004 by Denneboom et al.[10] The investigators determined which procedure for treatment review (case conferences with physicians versus written feedback) resulted in more medication changes in a randomized, controlled trial, with randomization at the level of the community pharmacy. Treatment reviews were performed by 28 pharmacists and 77 GPs including 738 elderly patients (>75 years) on polypharmacy (more than five medicines), and costs and savings related to the type of intervention were determined as secondary aim of the study. In the case-conference group, significantly more medication changes were initiated (42 versus 22, $P = 0.02$); this difference was also present 6 months after the treatment reviews (36 versus 19, $P = 0.02$). Nine months after the reviews, the difference was no longer significant (33 versus 19, $P = 0.07$). Additional costs in the case-conference group were covered by the slightly greater savings in this group.

Measuring health status and clinical outcomes were not done by the authors because they felt it was noticed from trials published at that time that no statistical differences were found. It was suggested that studies including large populations of older people should be performed to measure clinical consequences, health status, hospital admissions, health-related patient satisfaction, and mortality.

The recommendation of the authors to integrate performing treatment reviews for older people in the routine collaboration between GPs and pharmacists was very well chosen because at that time, the interest from physicians' and pharmacists' organizations to discuss the medication review activities in primary care started to become an issue that attracted most attention. This discussion resulted in a clear and accepted definition of a clinical medication review: a structured assessment of issues relating to the patient's use of medicines in the context of their clinical condition performed by the patient, his/her GP, and pharmacist, as well as access to patient's notes and prescription medicines.

The development of a pharmaceutical care plan was not included yet, which illustrated the need for more emphasis to be focused on the developments of more advanced patient-centered services.

By accepting the definition of clinical medication review at a national level, and reviewing all practice research between 2000 and 2005, the need for a comprehensive assessment of patient needs and DRP for polypharmacy patients were established in health care practice. About 15% of all community pharmacies could provide comprehensive care, and GPs were supporting the development based on local networks.

Hospital Admissions Related to Medication Caused an Impact

A major change in thinking about the need to develop more patient-centered practices was caused by the publication of the HARM-study (Hospital Admissions Related to Medication), a prospective multicenter study conducted in 2005–2006 to determine the frequency and patient outcomes of medication hospital-related hospital admissions.[11] A case–control design, including 21 hospitals, was chosen to assess risk factors for potentially preventable hospital admissions. During 40 days, all unplanned admissions were assessed, controls were patients admitted for elective surgery. The frequency of medication-related hospital admissions, potential preventability and outcomes were determined and for preventable medication-related admissions, risk factors were identified. In total, 714 (5.6%) of almost 13,000 unplanned admissions were found to be medication-related, and half of these (46.5%) were potentially preventable. Data from 332 cases were matched with 332 control patients. The most important determinant of preventable medication-related hospital admission was impaired cognition (OR 11.9; 95% CI 3.9–36.3), followed by four or more comorbidities (OR 8.1; 95% CI 3.1–21.7), dependent living situation (OR 3.0; 95% CI 1.4–6.5), impaired renal function (OR 2.6; 95% CI 1.6–4.2), nonadherence to medication (OR 2.3; 95% CI 1.4–3.8), and polypharmacy (OR 2.7; 95% CI 1.6–4.4). Based on these results, many organizations involved in developing pharmacy-related activities focused on these outcomes. Discussions on the identified risk factors provided a starting point for further development of research efforts for increasing knowledge, and information technology to address the issues of preventing DRPs. Pharmacy responded by developing national strategies how to involve a larger proportion of community pharmacy in a transition mode, for example, by offering postgraduate education programs for training pharmacists in developing pharmaceutical care services. At the university level, developing pharmaceutical care plans after assessing patient needs and DRPs was addressed substantially in the pharmacy curriculum, for example, during internships, whereas more practice research projects were initiated.

A follow-up on the outcomes of the HARM-study was the pHARM-study (Preventing Hospital Admissions by Reviewing Medication), conducted in 2008–2009 by Leendertse et al.[12] This study was designed as an open, controlled, multicenter study in an integrated primary care setting. Patients with a high risk on a medication-related hospital admission were included in the study. The intervention consisted of a patient-centered, structured, pharmaceutical care process, consisting of the following steps: a pharmaceutical anamnesis, review of the patient's pharmacotherapy, the development and execution of a pharmaceutical care plan combined with the monitoring of follow-up evaluations. The patient's own GP and community pharmacist carried out the intervention. The control group was included by another GP than the intervention GP and received usual care. The primary outcome of the study was the frequency of hospital admissions related to medication within the study period of 12 months of each patient. As secondary outcomes survival, quality of life, adverse drug events, and severe adverse events were determined. In 42 primary health care settings of at least one pharmacist and at least two GPs, 364 intervention and 310 control patients were included. In the control group, more medication-related hospital admissions were found than in the intervention group, respectively 10 and 6 admissions. No statistically significant differences were found between the intervention and control group in the secondary outcomes survival, adverse drug events, and quality of life.[13]

The pHARM-study demonstrated that the patient's own pharmacists together with its own GP and the patient as codevelopers of a pharmaceutical care plan may prevent hospital admissions with a medication-related cause. This was quiet a breakthrough in thinking of how the process of pharmaceutical care could be developed with the primary care health care providers and the patient together. The principles and processes of pharmaceutical care, although accepted by those who were involved in research and education, were shown to become real in practice settings and were accepted by many others after the completion of this study. Not only health care professionals but also health insurance companies, policy makers, and developers of software packages for pharmaceutical care acknowledged the support for the development of pharmacy practice in order to address the needs of patients with DRPs.

Community Pharmacist Recognized as Health Care Provider

During those years, the discussion on the role and position of the community pharmacist in the health care team was becoming a political issue again—

this time with favorable outcomes for community pharmacy. By law, it was recognized as of the July 1, 2007 that community pharmacists are health care providers, with their own therapeutic relationships with their patients. The new law was meant to protect the patient in treatment settings. In other words, no longer was the GP found responsible for the outcomes of treatment, but the pharmacist who did not ensure that the patient could make the best use of his or her medicine could be held accountable for that as well. It was a stimulation for the development of more pharmaceutical care–related projects in pharmacy practice research and started discussions on new developments in the reimbursement system (see below). The number of practices in which comprehensive care could be provided increased to about 300, whereas about 900 to 1000 community pharmacies could use an integrated system for documenting patient consultations. The development of a pharmaceutical care plan for an individual patient still needed a time-consuming process of data entry in nonintegrated software packages and was hampering this development. At the same time, the Ministry of Health and politicians addressed more issues in preventive health care and called upon health care professionals to become more health care team players. An initiative by the Dutch Government to establish a national electronic patient dossier available to all health care providers in the Netherlands was not approved by the Senate in 2011, due to privacy-related issues. However, many initiatives at the local level already exist and can ensure patient data to be exchanged between health care providers, if needed, for the benefit of the patient who has to visit different health care providers in primary care settings. For ensuring medication data exchange during hospital admission, a similar technology exists, although staffing at hospitals is not always adequate to take care of medication checks during this transfer.

More interesting developments for further recognition of community pharmacy to become reimbursed for their pharmaceutical care activities were accomplished in November 2010. The Dutch Health Authority proposed a guideline with several performance descriptions allowing pharmacists to make a contract with health insurers for delivering pharmaceutical care services to patients. The list of proposed contracted activities related to pharmaceutical care is presented in Table 12-4.

In case health insurers want to negotiate the pharmaceutical care services with community pharmacists, contracted prices are free to determine. Examples in practice settings where pharmaceutical care services are already reimbursed show that payments of time spent by the pharmacist vary from 45 minutes (pharmacist only) to 3 hours (shared between GP and pharmacist). As of the 1st of January 2012, the new reimbursement rules will be contracted if pharmacists can show their documented activities in terms that are in concordance with the rules. Based on these proposed rules,

Table 12-4 Proposed contracted activities for reimbursement of pharmaceutical care services

Pharmaceutical care–related performance rule	Description
Clinical medication review for patients with chronic treatment	If there will be an indication for the review, the following activities have to be conducted: • Documenting the objective of the medication review • Structured critical evaluation of medical, pharmaceutical, and medication use data, in concordance with accepted treatment guidelines and evidence based medicine • Assessment of the individual needs of the patient and care givers • Sharing outcomes of the clinical medication review among involved patient and health care providers • Execute the interventions, if needed • Follow-up evaluation of outcomes (versus objectives of treatment) • Documentation of the clinical medication review and its evaluation in an electronic patient dossier
Critical medication review after discharge from hospital	If the patient is in need of (repeat) medication after discharge from hospital the following checks are needed: • Structured critical evaluation of medical, pharmaceutical, and medication use data, in concordance with recent patient records and medication files of the community pharmacy • Assessment of the individual needs of the patient and care givers • Execute interventions, if needed • Follow-up evaluation of outcomes • Documentation of the critical evaluation of the new medication regimen and its evaluation in a electronic patient dossier
Home visits for clinical medication review in all situations as mentioned above	If needed, the above rules comply but with additional reimbursement for home visits

the establishment of pharmaceutical care services will increase involvement of community pharmacists in defining the role of their profession in the new health care contracts that will be developed in the coming years. Opportunities exist to negotiate more activities than listed in Table 12-4, if they are needed and agreed between health insurers and community pharmacists. At this moment, small-scale projects for contracting 100 clinical medication reviews for polypharmacy patients with chronic treatment per year per pharmacy are most frequently observed. Reimbursement varies between € 200 and € 300 per review.

New Perspectives for Pharmaceutical Care in the Netherlands

Present research projects in the Netherlands focus on more extensive pharmaceutical care developments, including home medication review and the application of web-based pharmaceutical care plans. Home medication review in the Netherlands is derived from the Australian model (the Home Medicines Review), where clinical medication review was introduced by including patient interviews held during home visits by a pharmacist.[14] Based on this approach, an intervention study was carried out by Kwint et al.[15] For each patient, medication records (including drug-dispensing records) and information on comorbidity and/or drug intolerances, relevant patient notes, were collected by the community pharmacist. The patient's GP was asked to provide clinical records including diagnoses, disease burden, and laboratory data. The patient's community pharmacist visited the patient at home for a face-to-face interview with the patient about the medicines and to identify possible DRPs. During the home visit, the community pharmacist captured data on all the patient's medications (including discontinued prescription medicines, use of over-the-counter medicines, complementary and alternative medicines). Patients were asked to identify dosage regimens of all known medication. All DRPs were registered for discussion with the GP.

A clinical medication review was performed by the community pharmacist using the data from sources as mentioned above. Community pharmacists used both implicit and explicit criteria to identify potential DRPs. Explicit criteria consisted of a list of prescription indicator tools based on Dutch treatment and prescription guidelines. Implicit criteria for identifying DRPs were based on a structural assessment by Cipolle et al.[16] in the rational order of indication, effectiveness, safety and practical issues (including compliance), also applied by Leendertse et al.[12] DRPs were prioritized based on the patient's perspective, focusing on those that cause the most concern. Results of this study are not yet known because the writing of the scientific article is still in progress.

Another interesting development is the implementation of the web-based pharmaceutical care plan in a research project, as well as in routine community practice settings. The project carried out by Geurts et al.[17] focuses on integrated pharmaceutical care with an emphasis on the development of the pharmaceutical care plan by patients and their community pharmacist and GP. The web-based application can be used independent of existing software packages for community pharmacy and GP practices. It can be accessed by the pharmacist and GP using the Internet in a secured network and (relevant), medical and pharmaceutical data are made available from the original source. After an upload of those data (with patient consent) in an automatic process, the following sections of the pharmaceutical care plan are presented for review and follow-up:

A. General patient information (name, address)
B. Reason for assessment pharmacotherapy (problem/question by whom)
C. Medical situation (diagnoses)—uploaded automatically
D. Pharmaceutical situation (medicines)—uploaded automatically
E. Lifestyle (smoking, alcohol use, diet)
F. Lab results—uploaded automatically
G. Assessment pharmacotherapy (patients' perspective)
H. Care plan with follow-up.

A clinical medication review follows the structures as provided in A–G; the pharmaceutical care plan with evaluation and follow-up activities are structured according to H. It is expected that preparation of a clinical medication review and development of a care plan will require less time than if prepared in a paper-based manner. A patient-friendly printable version of the care plan has been made available to patients included in the project. The aim of the ongoing project involving eight practice sites is to solve complex medication problems among poly-pharmacy patients ($\geq$60 years with $\geq$5 medications) with cardiovascular disorders using a web-based pharmaceutical care plan. Randomization in intervention and control group is at the patent level, where the intervention group will be provided the clinical medication review and care plan, whereas the control group will receive care as usual. Follow-up activities will be reviewed for 1 year. Outcomes will consist of DRPs (according to the classification by Cipolle et al.,[6] patient questionnaires (Beliefs About Medicines Questionnaire-general and EQ-5D), adherence to therapy (according to prescription refill rates), clinical values and lab results, and data from interviews with pharmacists. Community pharmacists and GPs will receive a total of €210 (equivalent of 3 hours work) per intervention-group patient, which is paid for by a health insurance company who showed interest in patient outcomes, time invested by pharmacist and GP, and the ultimate business case.

Concluding Remarks

Pharmaceutical care in the Netherlands has become a major practice for community pharmacy in developing the profession and the foundation for new reimbursement strategies supported by the Dutch Government, professional organizations and health insurance companies.

The implementation of comprehensive care in community pharmacy is still limited to around about 300 community pharmacies (out of 2000). Early and late adopters are involved in research projects and contract negotiations with insurers and will present best practices in the coming years. But the majority of pharmacists is still waiting for "more reimbursement options" and have not organized their practice model accordingly. A challenge will be to change the business and practice models from prescription-driven to patient care–driven. Without substantial support from the national association of pharmacists in developing strategies for developing local networks with GPs and health insurers, learning opportunities in practice (postgraduate courses, internships for master students), the highly motivated practitioners who have adjusted their practices already will not grow substantial in numbers.

Another challenge for the future will be how to change the organizational model of community pharmacy, in order to be able to process patient consultations instead of prescriptions as a routine activity. There is still a lack of knowledge and expertise in the field of organizational management in pharmacy. The discussion on whether or not to separate dispensing from providing comprehensive care is starting up on a very limited scale. But there is growing interest, and with all the recent changes in mind, pharmacy practice is expected to change in the near future.

Finally, for hospital pharmacy, the challenge will be to decide whether their focus will be on developing health systems to prevent medication errors and to act as health systems pharmacists, or to become more patient-centered and develop services based on patient needs, particularly at moments of patient's admission to and discharge from hospital with an open eye for collaboration with community pharmacy.

REFERENCES

1. SFK (Foundation for Pharmaceutical Statistics (Stichting Farmaceutische Kengetallen) February 2011, The Hague, the Netherlands.
2. Van Mil (2000). Pharmaceutical care: the future of pharmacy. PhD Thesis, University of Groningen, January 2000.
3. Hepler CD, Strand LM. Opportunities and responsibilities in pharmaceutical care. *Am J Hosp Pharm.* 1990;47:533–543.
4. de Gier JJ. The Electronic Pharmaceutical Dossier: an effective aid in documenting pharmaceutical care data. *Pharm World Sci.* 1996;18(6):241–243.

5. Grainger-Rousseau TJ, Miralles MA, Hepler CD, Segal R, Doty RE, Ben-Joseph R. Therapeutic outcomes monitoring: application of pharmaceutical care guidelines to community pharmacy. *J AM Pharm Assoc (Wash)*. 1997;NS37(6):647–661.

6. Cipolle RJ, Strand LM, Morley PC. *Pharmaceutical Care Practice*. 1st ed. The McGraw-Hill Companies Inc., 1998.

7. Vinks ThHAM, Egberts ACG, de Lange AM, De Koning GHP. Pharmacist-based medication review reduces potential drug-related problems in the elderly: the SMOG controlled trial. *Drugs Aging*. 2009;26(2):123–133.

8. Stuijt CCM, Franssen EJF, Egberts ACG, Hudson SA. Appropriateness of prescribing among elderly patients in a Dutch residential home: observational study after a pharmacist-led medication review. *Drugs Aging*. 2008; 25(1):947–954.

9. Bosma A, Jansman FGA, Franken AM, Harting JW, Van den Bemt PMLA. Evaluation of pharmacist clinical interventions in a Dutch hospital setting. *Pharm World Sci*. 2008;30:31–38.

10. Denneboom W, Dautzenberg MG, Grol R, De Smet PA. Treatment reviews of older people on polypharmacy in primary care: cluster controlled trial comparing two approaches. *Br J Gen Pract*. 2007;57(542):723–731.

11. Leendertse AJ, Egberts AC, Stoker LJ, van den Bemt PM. Frequency of and risk factors for preventable medication-related hospital admissions in the Netherlands. *Arch Intern Med*. 2008;168(17):1890–1896.

12. Leendertse AJ, De Koning FH, Goudswaard AN, et al. Preventing hospital admissions by reviewing medication (PHARM) in primary care: design of the cluster randomisation, controlled, Multi-centre PHARM-study. *BMC Health Serv Res*. 2011;11:4.

13. Leendertse AJ. *Hospital Admissions Related to Medication: Prevention, Provocation, and Prevention*. PhD Thesis, University of Utrecht, September 2010.

14. Sorensen L, Stokes JA, Purdie DM, Woodward M, Elliott R, Roberts MS. Medication review in the Community: results of a randomised, controlled effectiveness trial. *Br J Clin Pharmacol*. 2004;58(6):649–664.

15. Kwint HF (2011). Personal communication.

16. Cipolle RJ, Strand LM, Morley PC. *Pharmaceutical Care Practice: The Clinician's Guide*. 2nd ed. The McGraw-Hill Companies Inc., 2004.

17. Geurts MME (2011). Personal communication.

SPAIN

Manuel J. Machuca, PhD, PharmD
Community Pharmacist
Clinical Pharmacist at a Unit for Drug-Therapy Optimization
Seville, Spain

Introduction: A Health Care Picture of Spain
Spanish health care system control is a responsibility of the 17 autonomous states in which the country is divided. Health services are offered by the different autonomous states, with their own laws and portfolio. Only medication regulation is reserved to the central government.

Acknowledgements: to Debbie Pestka, for the revision of this manuscript.

Public health care is universal and obligatory for Spanish citizens and foreigners working in Spain. Just 10% of population has additional private services. Every service, except medication, is free and financed as part of the salary and income taxes. Workers must pay 40% of the price of medication that they need, with the exception of chronic diseases, in which the patient only pays 10% or up to € 2.64 per box of medication. Those that are retired receiver their medications for free. The price of medications is fixed by the central government, and patients staying at hospital do not have to pay for the medication they need.

The public health system includes general practitioners (family doctors), nurses, and specialists. Family doctors work at health centers with nurses, while specialists work at other primary care centers and in hospitals. Community pharmacists work outside of the public health system, but they have an agreement with the public health system to provide prescription and nonprescription drugs. There are hospital pharmacists, included in the public health system as other health professionals, to provide medication needed for their patients. There are also primary care pharmacists, included in the public health system. They work to preserve the rational use of drugs, but they do not have any activity related to comprehensive medication services. They supervise the rational use of drugs prescribed by family doctors but mainly from the evidence-based medicine proposals. They have no clinical responsibilities, but rather are focused on helping physicians acquire good prescribing practices. More than 10 years ago, there were experiences in Galicia (North-West of Spain) with pharmacists' consultation offices into the health centers. But they only took responsibilities for drug compliance, and reinforcing educational tasks. Nowadays they are focused on the practice described above.

In Spain, every patient who needs public health assistance must make an appointment with his or her family doctor, who decides to treat or to refer the patient to a specialist.

Andalusia (South of Spain) has been the first autonomous state to develop electronic prescribing in primary care. Family doctors can prescribe medicines for a maximum duration of 1 year. The purpose of this is to provide better care to the patients who need real assistance, rather than patients only interested in refill their prescriptions. It is possible for community pharmacists to assume responsibilities for medication management, but neither pharmacists nor health authorities have tried to face this opportunity.

The Present State of Comprehensive Medication Management Services in Spain

Comprehensive medication management services are not being widely delivered in Spain. Although some projects have been developed to provide these services since 2000, there are very few practitioners, none of which are being reimbursed. There are some differences in the terminology used in Spain to describe the practice. For example, comprehensive medication management services are known as drug therapy follow-up. The term used to define drug therapy problems is negative medication outcomes,[1] and the limited number of practitioners that practice pharmaceutical care use a three-item classification (necessity, effectiveness, and safety); compliance is not included. The care plan is defined as an action plan, and the process of developing a care plan is also defined differently. Although this system is based on what Cipolle et al. described in 1998,[2] it is less developed, and the medication experience is only considered as the patient's concerns and expectations and does not include components such as cultural and religious influences. The most important challenge is how to classify drug therapy problems, instead of discussing how to achieve goals of therapy, or the level of responsibilities to be assumed by patients or practitioners in this new practice.

Historical Development of Medication Management Services in Spain

Spanish pharmacists began discussing Pharmaceutical Care in the mid 90s. The development of pharmaceutical care in Spain started at the first Consensus of Granada.[3] The principle topic of discussion was drug-related problems, which has remained the main topic of discussion throughout this historical process. Following discussion of this topic, a Spanish school was created based on pharmaceutical care and adopted the theories and concepts of Cipolle et al.[2] from the discussion that we were having in Spain. From this moment on, a new concept of drug therapy problems was created along with a new classification system. This new system consisted of six classification categories, as opposed to seven developed by Cipolle et al. The majority of the members of this Consensus were community pharmacists who saw this as an opportunity to give a more professional feel to what they were doing. On the other hand, hospital pharmacists did not include themselves in this discussion because they felt that pharmaceutical care was not needed for their line of practice and that it was a problem basically dealing with community pharmacists. In 1999, a group of Spanish pharmacists attended a Pharmaceutical Care course at the University of Minnesota and, upon their return to Spain, decided to create the Dader Program on pharmaceutical care. The name was later changed to Dader Program on drug therapy follow-up as a result of changing the term "pharmaceutical care" to "drug therapy follow-up."[4]

From that time on, the Dader Program has been the main tool to practice pharmaceutical care. A practical guide was created, based on the work that was done at the University of Minnesota, which produced an intense teaching tool to incorporate pharmacists into the practice of drug therapy follow-up. The principle characteristic of this teaching model was providing classes based on the theory of pharmaceutical care with practical examples about how to implement this practice. The participants of these courses learned the theory of pharmaceutical care, and later had to present their own in-practice cases with patients and send them to a database where they incorporate the identified and resolved drug therapy problems. Thanks to this program, more than 500 pharmacists joined the practice of pharmaceutical care. However, due to various reasons, they began abandoning the practice. The extra work, the increased responsibility that comes with the practice, and the time that is spent and not compensated for have been the main reasons for abandoning this new practice.

Continuing with this historical process, there was a time when the term Pharmaceutical Care, defined as the standard of care to ensure that each patient's medications are appropriate, effective, safe, and convenient, changed to drug therapy follow-up. It was in the following Consensus that the Spanish Consensus on Pharmaceutical Care was formed.[5] In this Consensus, they accepted the term Pharmaceutical Care to define every practice performed by a pharmacist in relation to the patient including dispensing services, compounding services, drug prescription to treat minor symptoms, Pharmacovigilance and drug therapy follow-up.

Later, in 2002, another Consensus on drug-therapy problems took place in Granada.[6] The main difference was to adapt the correlative number of drug-safety problems to the classification set forth by Cipolle et al., and to rewrite the different problems to highlight the concept as a health problem because there were too many pharmacists classifying drug-therapy problems without a real goal of therapy.

While this Consensus took place, and during the following years, the Dader Program continued on course, incorporating new pharmacists into the program, while other pharmacists were abandoning it too. There was a flow of pharmacists in both directions, and continuance was difficult because it was difficult to coexist with dispensing services. Also during these years, the Dader Program was exported to other countries, mainly Argentina and Brazil, but in other Latin American countries as well.

The desire to find a way to classify comprehensive drug therapy problems was carried out in 2005 by Fernández-Llimós et al.[1] They published a letter in the *American Journal of Health-System Pharmacy*, suggesting the term of negative clinical outcomes be used to substitute drug-related problems. As they argued, it was difficult to separate causes from problems with the existing classifications. From this point of view, they proposed to abandon the term "drug related problems" and use "negative clinical outcomes" instead because it was more precise.

This led to the publication of the Third Consensus of Granada in 2007[7] using the term negative outcomes associated with medications, instead of drug therapy problems, and using drug-related problems to all that could lead to a negative outcome.

In 2008, a new document was published called *Foro de Atención Farmacéutica* (Pharmaceutical Care Forum) in which diverse scientific organizations and professionals had worked since 2004 with the intention of developing the concept of pharmaceutical care. This was proposed in 2001 for the Minister of Health,[5] and is the last effort made.[8] Despite all of this, medication therapy management services do not formally exist in Spain, and there are very few practitioners that dedicate their time to this practice.

Delivering the Services in Spain

Although there is a lack of practitioners in Spain, a lot of work has been done to establish the concept of pharmaceutical care. Today, only a few practitioners are delivering these services. There are no data to support how many practitioners are involved in this practice. Currently, these services are being delivered by some community pharmacists, while hospital pharmacists are still not involved. Nevertheless, much research has been done in Spain to demonstrate that drug therapy problems cause important injuries to patients.[9–13] These investigations have created a picture of the problem: about 33% of patients admissions in an emergency room are caused by drug therapy problems, and 75% of them can be avoided with medication management services.

There are also several investigations with interventions to reduce the impact of drug therapy problems, in hospital[14–15] and community settings,[16–17] but implementation of comprehensive medication services is still a great challenge.

The community pharmacists that are practicing pharmaceutical care are not being reimbursed for this practice. Despite this, there are many pharmacists, especially in hospitals, that claim that they are performing this type of practice, although in reality what they are doing is counseling about the prescribed medication and how to improve adherence. Patients are not individually assessed to determine that each medication is appropriate for him or her, effective for the medical condition, safe given the medical conditions and other medications being taken, and able to be taken as intended.

Practitioner's Qualifications to Provide
Medication Management Services

There are no qualification programs to deliver these services. In Spain, since 1997, it has been required that community pharmacists provide information and follow-up on patient's medications.[18] It is difficult to understand how legislation anticipated this law before this practice was implemented in the real word. It is impossible to understand if you do not understand Spaniards obsession to have laws, as the first step to infringe upon them.

The only necessary qualification is to have gone through the pharmacy course work. In the Colleges of Pharmacy, there is no traditional course work related to pharmaceutical care, nor is there a course on medication therapy management. There is no patient contact, except during the final 6-month clerkship, which can be done in community pharmacies or hospital pharmacies, but neither one has regulations about the activities within these establishments, and it is possible there will be no work dealing with patient care. These clerkships last 6 months, but they are not rotations. At the most, a student can go to two different locations, 3 months in each. As a result, Spanish pharmacists have the legal capacity to provide medication therapy management services without any practice or experience within this area. Consequently, legislation and education together are putting patients at risk rather than caring for them.

There are masters programs in pharmaceutical care, but they are not mandatory for any specific clinical practice. They are only necessary in order to obtain a PhD degree but nothing more. Only some of the programs focus on the practice of pharmaceutical care. The intention of the rest of the programs is to bring pharmacologic acknowledgement more up to date. But the philosophy of comprehensive medication services has not been adopted as the core of the program.

Recently, another master program will be implemented, at the University of San Jorge, as an on-line program but with a real focus on comprehensive medication services. Nevertheless, all the practice required to obtain this degree must be done by the student alone, without the help of experienced practitioners.

There is also no specialization or residency program for practitioners. The only residency program for pharmacists is for hospital pharmacists. It is a 4-year program in which the fourth year is dedicated to going through the different medical services, but there is no integration of evaluating all of the patient's drug-related needs.

Formal and Informal Training to Prepare Practitioners

There is no formal training to implement comprehensive medication services and to prepare practitioners. There is a week-long course, certified by the Health Quality Agency, to implement comprehensive medication services. Students directly watch how a practitioner provides comprehensive medication services during the first 3 days of the course. The next 2 days students provide care to volunteer patients, and the practitioner watches and discusses the patient care process provided by the students.

Students must develop a care plan for these patients and design a business plan to develop these services. However, this is considered informal training because there is no obligation to do it before delivering medication management services. It is remarkable to know that several laws expect medication management services to be provided by pharmacists, but there is no formal learning to implement them. Therefore, pharmacists can legally become practitioners with no formal training.

The Current Status of Medication Management Services in Spain

Medication management services do not formerly exist in Spain. The number of practitioners delivering medication management services is insignificant, although a great number of pharmacists has intended to implement them and many pharmacists state they are practicing pharmaceutical care on a daily basis. Several factors can describe this situation. First of all, although there is legislation concerning this practice, it does not well define which kinds of services must be provided.[18,19] There is an uncertain mix of prescription-focused and patient-centered approaches.[8] Moreover, practitioner's responsibilities are not defined, and no certification programs guarantee practitioners' training to assume these responsibilities. Furthermore, reimbursing is not recognized. Taking into account that patients who can benefit from these services usually have chronic and important diseases, it is easy to assume why medication management services are still not widely implemented in Spain. Medication management services have not been considered as a general practice, which can be implemented in every setting. It has been considered a practice closely connected to a place, instead of to a philosophy of practice. It is mandatory in Spain to put the practice before the pharmacy or the pharmacists.

The Level of Acceptance by Pharmacists, Patients, Physicians, and Patient Care Providers

In the early years, medication management services were enthusiastically accepted by community pharmacists because they considered these services as a means to save them the profession. But later, they have recognized that many changes must occur to assume the new practice; these changes are still unrealized.

Patients who have experienced these services accept them, but it is difficult for them to perceive them as a different practice because there is a lack of practitioners providing medication management services. Many of them consider his or her practitioner as a competent pharmacist, but it is difficult to realize that this is a new practice because there are few practitioners.

What is being described for patients can be said about physicians. There are no practitioners working in a comprehensive and rational approach, in the same setting as physicians. So, these practitioners are considered as pharmacists with a high level of commitment, and many of them think of this practice as a way to their own practice, instead of perceiving it as a new clinical approach. It is necessary to separate this practice from other different practices or business.

But from the point of view of professional associations and councils, comprehensive medication services are not widely known and Pharmaceutical Care was seen by physicians as professional interference.[20–23] It is very difficult to separate professional prejudices from a new and still unknown practice.

The main patient care provider in Spain is the government, through several regional health agencies. These agencies do not consider medication management services as a part of their portfolio. They are not promoting any legislative development to implement them. Although they have supported some projects to research these services, no decisions have been made about the practice.

Private patient care providers do not reimburse medication management services either. These companies do not offer any support concerning medication. The Spanish health system is universal for everyone who lives in Spain, and everyone must be included, by means of deduction from their salary. Moreover, there are several companies providing private insurance, but it must be additional because people cannot choose between public or private insurance.

The Role of Colleges of Pharmacy
In the last few years, some changes have been made in Europe. The Bologna Process aimed to create a European Higher Education by 2010. Colleges of Pharmacy have changed their curricula to accommodate subjects related to pharmacy services. But once again, these changes are not directed at medication management but to prescription-focused services. They are not based on a philosophy of practice but to the different services provided by community pharmacies.

Before the Bologna Process, medication management services were not in the curricula. This is true today, but colleges of pharmacy believe they have really changed.

The Future of Medication Management Services in Spain
Nowadays, the future of medication management services is uncertain. Many barriers are still in the way, before these services will become a reality.

It is mandatory to create a pilot project to deliver these services, and to demonstrate their benefits to pharmacists, patients, physicians and patient care providers. Medication management services are embedded in a vicious circle: no practice, no practice improvement, no philosophy acceptance, no discussion about practitioner's responsibilities, unspecific teaching, unspecific learning, unspecific laws, no reimbursing, and so on.

Professors, politicians, and pharmacists still blame one another, but up until now, medication management services have been a failure. A lot of work has been done but in the wrong direction.

There is no future for medication management services in Spain, if we force community pharmacists to develop these services alone, without formal teaching, training, and reimbursement. We must accept that medication management services do not have to be provided just in community pharmacies; we have to conceptualise a real practice because a practice is not a setting. There will be a future for medication management services if we face the real challenge to deliver a real practice, focused on patient's drug-related needs. No profession will survive if its focus is outside of the needs of the population. It is obvious that comprehensive medication services are needed in our society. If pharmacists do not assume this challenge, another profession, new or old, will. The experience provided by other countries, in ambulatory clinic practices, with a high level of satisfaction by patients, physicians, and other caregivers and providers, demonstrates that it is possible to achieve a real and profitable practice. As in other countries, comprehensive medication services will be possible.

It is necessary to pursue medication management services, by means of a research center to know the economic, clinical, and quality of life benefits of this practice. As soon as this practice is better known, teaching will be realized in a logical manner, and patient care providers will pay for and support it.

The current state only benefits those who talk about these services but are just interested to talk, not to act; to those who put first their own self-interest before patients needs and suffering. There will not be any logical practice, teaching, reimbursing, or legislation if Spanish pharmacists do not begin to develop a model, which leads to a real practice, and to enrich the future, focused on patient's drug-related needs.

If we want to implement medication management services in Spain, we have to think beyond pharmacies; even beyond actual pharmacists. We have to create a real practice, focused on a real philosophy of practice. When we will be able to deliver a high level of practice to our patients, we will be able to demonstrate to patients, to physicians, and to providers the real value of this practice. Then, we will be able too to discuss how this professional must be qualified, and we will decide if he or she will be a pharmacist. But in Spain, nowadays, we have too many questions, which are paralyzing us, and it is impossible for us to respond to them now. When we will achieve a high level of practice, all these questions will have been forgotten.

REFERENCES

1. Fernández-Llimós F, Faus MJ. From "drug- related problems to "negative clinical outcomes". *Am J Health Syst Pharm.* 2005;62(22):2348–2349.
2. Cipolle R, Strand LM, Morley PC. *Pharmaceutical Care Practice.* New York: McGraw-Hill; 1998.
3. Consensus panel ad hoc. Consensus of Granada on Drug-related Problems. *Pharm Care Esp.* 1999;1:107–112.
4. Sabater D, Silva-Castro MM, Faus MJ. Método Dáder. *Guia de seguimiento farmacoterapéutico* (3ª Ed). Granada: GIAF-UGR; 2007.
5. Consensus on Pharmaceutical Care. Madrid: MSyC; 2001.
6. Second Consensus of Granada on Drug Therapy Problems. *Ars Pharm.* 2002;43(3–4): 175–184.
7. Consensus Committee. Third Consensus of Granada on Drug Related Problems (DRP) and Negative Outcomes Associated with Medication (NOM). *Ars Pharm.* 2007;48(1):5–17.
8. Consensus Forum. Foro de Atención Farmacéutica. Documento de Consenso (Pharmaceutical Care Forum. Consensus Document). Madrid: CGCOF; 2008.
9. Tuneu L, García-Peláez M, López Sánchez S, et al. Drug related problems in patients who visit an emergency room. *Pharm Care Esp.* 2000;2:177–192.
10. Otero MJ, Bajo A, Maderuelo JA, Domínguez GA. Evitabilidad de los problemas relacionados con medicamentos en un servicio de urgencias. *Rev Clin Esp.* 2000;199:796–805.
11. Martín MT, Codina C, Tuset M, et al. Problemas relacionados con medicamentos como causa de ingreso hospitalario. *Aten Farm.* 2001;3:9–22.
12. Tuneu L, García PM, López S, Serrá G, Alba G, Irala C. Problemas relacionados com los medicamentos em usuarios que visitan um servicio de urgencias. *Pharm Care Esp.* 2002;2:177–192.
13. Baena MI, Faus MJ, Martín R, Zarzuelo A, Jiménez-Martín J. Problemas de salud relacionados con los medicamentos en un servicio de urgencias hospitalario. *Med Clin (Barc).* 2005;124:250–255.
14. Silva-Castro MM, Calleja MA, Tuneu L, Fuentes B, Gutiérrez-Sáinz J, Faus MJ. Seguimiento del tratamiento farmacológico en pacientes ingresados en un servicio de cirugía. *Farm Hosp.* 2004;28(3):154–169.
15. Campos-Vieira N, Bicas-Rocha K, Calleja MA, Faus MJ. Seguimiento farmacoterapéutico em pacientes ingresados em el Servicio de Medicina Interna del Hospital Infanta Margarita. *Farm Hosp.* 2004;28(4):251–257.
16. Fornos JA, et al. Evaluación de un programa de seguimiento farmacoterapéutico a diabéticos tipo 2. *Aten Primaria.* 2004;34:48–54.
17. Gastelurrutia MA, Faus MJ, Fernández- Llimós F. Providing patient care in community pharmacies in Spain. *Ann Pharmacother.* 2005;39(12):2105–2109.
18. Cortes Españolas. Ley 16/1997, de 25 de abril, de regulación de los servicios de las oficinas de farmacia. BOE 1997; (100 de 26 de abril):13450–13452.
19. Cortes Españolas. Ley 29/2006, de 26 de julio, de garantías y uso racional de los medicamentos y productos sanitarios. BOE 2006; 178:28122–28165.
20. Costas Lombardía E. Análisis crítico de la atención farmacéutica. *Med General.* 2000;25:591–596.
21. Costas Lombardía E. La amenaza de la atención farmacéutica. El País 2001, 9nov. Page 39.
22. Anonymus. El 73% de los médicos considera que la farmacia debería limitarse a dispensar. El Global. El Global 2004; 13 a 19 de diciembre.
23. Anonymus. La OMC rechaza el papel que el Plan de Sanidad da a la atención farmacéutica. El Global 2005; 28 de febrero al 6 de marzo. Page 8.

ICELAND AND SCANDINAVIA

Anna Birna Almarsdóttir, PhD
Professor, Faculty of Pharmaceutical Sciences
University of Iceland
Reykjavik, Iceland

Preamble

I am native Icelandic but have spent considerable time in Denmark and Sweden both studying and working. I communicate well in the Scandinavian languages, although my native language differs from these. I am currently not involved in any pharmaceutical care project in the other Nordic countries. This chapter is not a comprehensive review of activities in the Nordic countries but a perspective of a person who has worked within academia relating to pharmaceutical care for about 20 years. I wish to thank my informants for their valuable input by pointing me toward reports and articles of interest in this section. It is also important to note before reading the section that many documents pertaining to pharmaceutical care have not been published in English and many are only to be found in the gray literature.

Introduction

Scandinavia consists of Norway, Sweden, and Denmark. The term Nordic countries include in addition the sovereign states of Finland and Iceland. The Nordic countries are a political entity and outsiders often see them as a unified whole. There are strong cultural ties between the countries and they have governmental cooperation—the Nordic Council of Ministers. In spite of this, neither Scandinavia nor the Nordic countries can be viewed as a block of homogenous countries, although there is substantial collaboration across borders.

In the health care arena, Vallgårda[1] identified many similarities between Denmark, Norway, and Sweden in their approach to dealing with health problems in the population; for example, all three countries were informed by welfare state and social democratic values. However, she also found significant differences in the explanations for and solutions to these problems. The pharmacy sector is no exception. Holmberg et al.[2] found major differences in how distribution is organized, service level offered, division of labor between the various actors, and how legislation/regulations are formed.

The organization of community pharmacy in the countries has developed in very different directions in recent decades. Denmark historically has had a system of granting community pharmacy privileges to licensed pharmacists by the government.[3,4] Iceland having been Denmark's colony and later commonwealth country until 1944 adopted Danish legislation in the field of pharmaceuticals. This Danish-looking system was changed in 1996[5] when pharmacists lost monopoly on the right to ownership. Norway followed Iceland in 2001, and the ownership of community pharmacies quickly changed from all being privately owned by Norwegian pharmacists to the great majority belonging to European wholesaler conglomerates.

In Sweden, all community and hospital pharmacies in Sweden were state-owned from 1971 to 2009, meaning that all Swedish pharmacies were organized into one single, government-owned chain, Apoteket AB.[6] On July 1 2009, new legislation was implemented, deregulating pharmacy ownership in Sweden.[7] Community pharmacies are being sold out of Apoteket AB and thus opening the market to new forms of ownership.

The primary health care systems also differ between the Scandinavian countries. Sweden emphasizes top-down management on a regional level, whereas Denmark and Norway have had a more professional initiative in the primary sector with privately run GP clinics and offices. Iceland adopted the Swedish approach in the 1970s.[8]

Description of Pharmaceutical Care Services in the Area

Understanding of Concept and Operationalization

It is safe to say at this point that comprehensive medication management services is hardly known as a concept, but the concept of pharmaceutical care has been embraced by pharmacist associations in these countries. Rarely is the term *Practice* added when the concept is being discussed, that is, pharmaceutical care practice. I have therefore chosen to focus the discussion on the concept of pharmaceutical care.

We first need to look at which definitions of pharmaceutical care have been used to better understand how this concept has been interpreted and operationalized in these countries. The definition in the article by Hepler and Strand[9] is commonly used to introduce the concept in documents describing pharmaceutical care–related work. However, the definitions from two books of Cipolle et al.[10,11] are seldom used in published papers or the gray literature.

The concept appears in both the work of community as well as hospital-based (clinical) pharmacy. However, when looking at published work and the gray literature in the area, the term is usually omitted from the titles, and other concepts used to identify the activities relating to pharmaceutical care practice. The concepts that are promoted currently are *Medication Review* (mostly in Norway and Denmark), *Booked counseling with follow-up* (earlier called *Patient Medication Records*, Sweden), and the hospital-focused Lund Integrated Medicines Management Model (LIMM) (mostly in Sweden). The term *clinical pharmacy* is also used often implicitly to describe pharmaceutical care practice in hospital pharmacy.

The classification of drug-related problems or drug therapy problems is one of the cornerstones of pharmaceutical care practice.[11] It is notable that the same classification is not in use across Scandinavia and Iceland. Many leaders in community pharmacy belong to Pharmaceutical Care Network Europe (PCNE), which has devised its own classification. The PCNE classification, which is based on the work of Westerlund et al.,[12] is therefore used widely, although sometimes modified as in the case of Norway.[13,14] In other cases, Norwegian researchers use a modified version of Cipolle et al.'s classification,[15] and the Icelandic hospital pharmacists have adopted a modified version of the classification by Viktil et al.[15]

Health care professionals in the Nordic countries are obliged to keep medical records of all care provided to patients. The same is not required for the care provided by pharmacists—especially not when the service is provided in community pharmacies. Most electronic medical record systems do not accommodate pharmacists' needs for record keeping for patient care with the notable exception of Apoteket AB's service.

Promoters/Key Actors

It is important to note who the main promoters of pharmaceutical care are in the countries in order to understand the political and practical framework for the services.

In Iceland, pharmaceutical care has been solely in the realm of hospital pharmacy and promoted by a couple of clinical pharmacists who have focused on specific wards within Landspitali—The National University Hospital of Iceland (LSH). LSH is the only place that can be said to provide services related to comprehensive medication management services. Pharmaceutical care practice as defined and operationalized by Cipolle et al.[10,11] has been used, although the standard of care stressed there has not yet permeated the practice in the hospital.

Denmark has one large player Pharmakon, which has been instrumental in promoting pharmaceutical care within community pharmacy. Pharmakon is owned by the community pharmacy owners' association (*Apotekerforeningen*). This body has long and strong ties to the government[3,4] and has managed to maintain the monopoly on pharmacy ownership in the hands of pharmacists in spite of a number of attempts to change this. Pharmakon is therefore a development institute for the pharmacies and the view of the owners of what constitutes services is apparent in its projects.

There is a tendency at Pharmakon to segment pharmacists' interventions into studies of medicines use/compliance, clinical pharmacy, patient safety, medication reviews, and dose-dispensing activities. The activity termed medication review may come closest to the concept of pharmaceutical care. A number of local projects relating to medication reviews have also been carried out in Denmark.[16] Regions within Denmark manage their own health care budgets and have in their service pharmacists who work on promoting rational medication use.[17]

With resources from the Norwegian owners' association, the institute called *Apoforsk* was founded in 2002 to conduct independent research and development in cooperation with other professional actors, increasing the use of pharmacists' and pharmacies' competencies for individuals and society and helping to increase rational use of medicines. Their mandate was to study among other topics pharmaceutical interventions and drug-related problems in the elderly. The institute was closed in 2009 after the board of directors changed course from an independent research-based model to a highly dependent service development model. Some of the activities of Apoforsk were related to pharmaceutical care. One medication review project was carried out on patients with type 2 diabetes[14,18] and another on elderly living in nursing homes.[13]

Until recently, Sweden had one large player in the field of pharmaceutical care, namely the state owned Apoteket AB. It had a research and development unit, which worked with the pharmacies in the country. After deregulation in 2009, this unit was dismantled. Apoteket AB started a counseling service in 2002. The service was called *Bokad rådgivning med uppföljning* (*Booked counseling with follow-up*).[6]

Another important player within Sweden is the University of Lund where the university hospital's clinical pharmacists in collaboration with other health care professionals constructed and implemented the so-called LIMM model (Lund Integrated Medicines Management model).

Medication Reviews

The concept of medication reviews (Danish: *lægemiddelgennemgang*, Norwegian: *legemiddelgjennomganger*) seems to be of choice in the Scandinavian countries currently. The concept is not unified, and the understanding of it varies.

A study of medication review models by the Danish Pharmakon's specialists underscores how diffuse the concept is Thomsen LA et al.[16] The results show that there are four basic models in use in primary care: (1) Opportunistic *ad hoc* review of medication orders which focuses on the drug and administrative issues in drug distribution; (2) Technical review of the patient's medication profile to assure rational use of medicines but more focused on the individual patient than model 1; (3) Review of patient's medical treatment with the goal of optimizing drug therapy with a focus on the patient's total therapy and the outcomes; (4) Patient-centered medication review which in addition to what is stated in model 3 focuses on how the patient uses the medication.

Model 4 is probably the one that comes closest to pharmaceutical care practice. These models are used in community pharmacies, medical clinics, nursing homes, home health services, health care centers, or homes of the handicapped. Most often they focus on the frail and polypharmacy patients. The practitioners carrying this out can vary from a physician alone to an active cooperation between the physician, pharmacist, nursing staff, health education staff, and the patient. The practice is usually based on a protocol of some kind and is most often documented systematically.

In 2005, the government of Norway presented a white paper for the use of pharmaceuticals.[19] The white paper emphasized medication reviews. On the background of this report, the Ministry of Health and Care Services decided to start pilot projects in four main areas: (1) in hospitals in relation to patient information; (2) in nursing homes; (3) for users of home nursing care; and (4) for certain patient groups in community pharmacies in cooperation with their physicians. The Norwegian Directorate of Health issued a report in 2011 on proposed measures for elderly patients in nursing home and home care.[20]

On the basis of these official reports, it is important to understand what the key concept *medication reviews* means in the Norwegian context. From the 2011 report, it is clear that this means that a health care practitioner evaluates each medication that the patient receives with respect to appropriateness for his/her therapy. It stresses that medication review should be done in a cross-disciplinary team of physician, pharmacist, and nurse. The review consists of considering indications, safety issues, contraindications, interactions, dosing, and minimizing polypharmacy. Medication reviews can result in changes in the patient's therapy and it may be necessary or useful to discuss this with the patient and/or a caregiver if they ask for it. It is therefore clear that in Norway, the patients' active participation is not emphasized.

Projects focusing on medication reviews are ongoing based on the Norwegian government's whitepaper. At present, a few projects focus on developing a standard pharmaceutical care plan document. One such project is ongoing in the Western Health Region to facilitate a systematic approach to assessing and resolving drug-related problems. This tool is meant to be helpful to pharmacists who are not experienced in medication reviews but are starting to offer them as part of their services. Such a document has not been developed nationally.

Booked Counseling with Follow-up

This counseling service, resting on the principles of pharmaceutical care (as described by Cipolle et al.),[10,11] was developed and implemented in 2002 by Apoteket AB (The National Corporation of Swedish Pharmacies). The service, initially called *Läkemedelsprofiler* (*Patient medication records, PMR*), was introduced on a trial basis in 11 community pharmacies and evaluated by researchers at Uppsala University.[21] Representatives from doctors' professional associations were involved in reference groups and local GPs at the project locations were informed personally.

The overall aim of this service was to support patients with pharmaceutical interventions and advice in order to achieve optimal effect from drug therapy. The outline of the service included a booked initial consultation (approximately 30 minutes) in a separate or semiseparate area of the pharmacy and shorter follow-up evaluations.

The service was provided by pharmacists and prescriptionists who were specifically trained in the theories and practice of pharmaceutical care, communication skills, and reflective practice (7 days of effective training in total). Prior to entering the training program, practitioners were required to pass a test on their pharmacological knowledge. There were one or two practitioners per pharmacy.

The service was documented: the medications used, DRPs identified (classification system based on Westerlund et al.),[12] issues discussed, and advice given. The service was not targeted at specific patient groups. Pharmacies did not receive any third-party payments for this service, which was voluntary and free of charge to the patient. Financing was through Apoteket AB's overall profit margin, as a public service. This service had become a permanent part of pharmacy practice in about 260 out of 900 community pharmacies before the change was made in ownership and some pharmacies sold to private owners.

A doctoral dissertation defended at Uppsala University in 2009[6] was initiated by Apoteket AB (The National Corporation of Swedish Pharmacies) in 2002 to evaluate the service in collaboration with Uppsala University. The main findings in this thesis were that the practitioners' level of patient-centeredness varied. Focus on the computer during consultations limited PC practitioners' abilities to practice patient-centered care. Follow-up evaluations were carried out for about half of the patients signing up for the service. The number of patients enrolled in the service per pharmacy predicted whether follow-up evaluations took place more than patient characteristics. Patients who received the service were characterized by old age and use of multiple medications.[6]

Hospital-based Models

The hospital-based models relating to pharmaceutical care are most prominent in Sweden with the LIMM model. Two concepts seem to be central to the LIMM model. First, *Medication reconciliation*, which is a process that involves comparing the medications a patient is receiving to what he or she actually should be receiving, and then resolving the discrepancies.[22] Second, LIMM includes *medication reviews*, although again this is not a well-defined concept.

LIMM was built on the concept of *integrated medicines management*, which was developed in Northern Ireland.[23] *Medicines management* is a concept used in British health care, especially the National Health Service.[24] Medicines management as a concept is closely tied to a managerial way of thinking, although the professional and patient angle is becoming more important as the concept is developed.[25] Central to the LIMM model are a number of systematic and validated instruments for use in clinical pharmacy services during the patient's hospital stay and beyond, but the service is carried out by hospital staff.[26] The Mid-Norway Health Region has recently started to build medicines management based on the Swedish LIMM model.

Another important development in Sweden is at the Uppsala University Hospitals where a randomized clinical trial of patients 80 years and older showed important effect of pharmacist and health care team collaboration on outcomes.[27] It was important to note that physicians proclaimed at a national meeting where this study was presented that they "do not want medication review, they want a pharmacist by their side."[28]

Efforts are underway in Iceland to work directly from Cipolle et al.'s practice guidance, and parts of Norway are starting to use the Swedish *LIMM* model. In Denmark, hospital pharmacy mainly uses the term *clinical pharmacy*. However, it seems that *medication reviews* are central to patient-related activities in Danish hospitals (Unpublished Discussion notes April 5, 2011. Obtained from Ellen Westh-Sorensen).

Professionals Involved and their Qualifications

It is of interest to describe who works in community and hospital pharmacies. Although pharmacists are most often the instrumental workers in outpatient pharmaceutical care–related activates, the practice or projects almost always includes physicians, nurses, nurses' aides, and sometimes even social workers. The hospital setting has an even tighter cooperation in multiprofessional teams consisting of physicians, nurses, and pharmacists among others.[16,23]

Professionals in Pharmacy

The Nordic countries have three kinds of professionals working in community pharmacies. About 60% of pharmacy personnel in Denmark and Norway are pharmacy technicians. In Norway, the other 40% is mostly made up of pharmacists, with a 5-year master's degree or a 3-year bachelor's degree. In Denmark, the remaining 40% divided into other personnel (24.8%) and pharmacists with a master's degree (13.7%). Iceland stands out in this comparison, having more than half of all pharmacy personnel unskilled, the other half composed of pharmacists (ca.30%) and pharmacy technicians (ca.20%).[29] Approximately, 40% to 60% of the pharmacy staff in Sweden have university pharmacy education.[6]

Sweden and Norway have official bachelor degree programs for pharmacy; in Sweden, these professionals are called prescriptionists (*receptarier*), and in Norway, bachelor pharmacists (*reseptarfarmasøyter*). Denmark and Iceland do not have these job categories, but Denmark educates their technicians (called *farmakonom*) for 3 years to a level closer to the bachelor level pharmacist compared with other countries and have granted them commensurate rights such as managing pharmacies.

A similar picture can be drawn of the workforce situation in hospitals, although in many cases master-level pharmacists have further formally qualified in clinical pharmacy. Formal education in this area is currently available in the Scandinavian countries (not in Iceland) and a few have been trained in the United Kingdom or the United States.

Formal Training to Prepare Practitioners

Formal training in the practice of pharmaceutical care consists of the basic degree programs to become a pharmacist or pharmacy technician, although there are some continuing education options available in each of the countries.

The formal training as a basic qualification in pharmacy has traditionally been chemistry- and biology-focused with social and clinical pharmacy playing a minor role within the programs. The share of these disciplines has gradually been increasing in the past two decades, although many pharmacists involved in patient care have found this to be too slow. This impatience has now resulted in a new Masters Degree Program in clinical pharmacy being established at the University of Southern Denmark, thus abolishing the former monopoly of the University of Copenhagen on pharmacist education in Denmark. In addition, a new 2-year masters degree in clinical pharmacy is starting at the University of Oslo, Norway, and a 5-year program is starting up at the University of Lund in Sweden in 2012.

European Union rules stipulate that in order to be registered as a pharmacist in the union countries, the pharmacy student who has finished the 5-year university program has to have completed a 6-month internship in a community or hospital pharmacy. The university programs in Denmark, Norway, and Sweden are in charge of these 6-month internship periods and use this time to a varying degree to train students in patient care.

The University of Copenhagen's internship program started in 2008 a practice research project in which the internship students were involved in patient care as well as data collection. This project called *Medisam* had as objective to develop, implement, and evaluate a model of cooperation for medication review and reconciliation involving patients, pharmacists, and general practitioners in a multiprofessional dialogue aimed at solving drug-related problems by involving patients in decision making around their medication. The project was supported by funds from the Danish Ministry of Health and Prevention in 2008–2011 (DKK 1.2 million). The regions in Denmark have gone another route and have trained GPs to do medication review.[30]

Continuing Education in Pharmaceutical Care

In general, it can be stated that continuing education is conducted through two avenues, as part of large pharmaceutical care implementation projects or by one of the promoters of pharmaceutical care on a more continual basis. In Denmark, Pharmakon offers a number of continuing education courses and in addition to the Danish regions, trains all personnel involved in certain projects. Norway had a special institute for continuing education (*VETT*) operating within the University of Oslo. It has now been dismantled, and there is currently a need to find new ways to keep continuing education going in the country. Sweden has a professional society called *Apotekarsocieteten* (http://www.lakemedelsakademin.se/), which has offered a few courses through the years. Most continuing education in pharmaceutical care has been within the hospital projects and Apoteket AB. Iceland has only had very few *ad hoc* continuing education activities related to specific projects.

Acceptance of Pharmaceutical Care

Acceptance by Pharmacists

Research carried out in Iceland in the late 1990s showed that community pharmacists were thinking in a drug-focused paradigm, which was evident when they talked about missing the role of compounding.[31] Sweden has until recently been looked upon by the neighboring countries' pharmacists as having the most opportunity to promote pharmaceutical care due to its ownership and close ties to research and development. Certainly, Apoteket AB acted on this with their service *Booked counseling with follow-up*. With changes in the system, this may be disappearing. According to Montgomery's evaluation of the Apoteket AB's service, pharmacists and prescriptionists who provided this service experienced a positive influence on their daily work and made more use of their pharmaceutical knowledge.[6]

There is growing interest in specializing in clinical pharmacy in the Nordic countries, which may indicate that pharmacists are increasingly interested in patient care.

Acceptance by Patients

Icelandic research in the late nineties involving focus groups with pharmacy customers showed that when the term quality of pharmacy services is mentioned, they immediately started to discuss the quality of prescribing by physicians. They generally did not know what pharmacists do and were not aware that the pharmacy can provide "care", i.e., they had low expectations.[32] Similar results can be seen in an unpublished Danish study of pharmacy customers (Traulsen JM. Do Patients' views and expectations of pharmacists match those of the profession? FIP invited speaker 2010. Pharmacy as a profession: today and tomorrow monday 30th of August 2010. Organized by the FIP Board of Pharmaceutical Practice) and a new study from Sweden.[33]

The dissertation from 2009 showed that patients receiving the Swedish Apoteket AB's service reported that they felt a genuine interest from the pharmacist, received important information, and felt better prepared for doctor visits to a greater extent than did patients receiving standard service.[6]

Acceptance by Health Care Professionals

A new unpublished study from the LSH hospital in Iceland indicates that nurses and younger physicians are well aware of the patient care provided by pharmacists in wards and consider them very important members of the care team. Older and more specialized physicians, however, are not aware of this pharmaceutical care activity and do not share the opinions of their younger colleagues and nurses.[34]

In Sweden, Södergaard et al.[35] described how a satellite pharmacy at a HIV clinic increased the satisfaction and health care personnels' acceptance of pharmacists working more closely with HIV patients. Although the term pharmaceutical care was used to describe the work of the pharmacist, there was no indication that he provided direct patient care but mostly had the task to provide drugs. The Apoteket AB's evaluation study showed that some physicians were positive toward the service due to a perceived increased safety of drug treatment but some were disturbed by pharmacists' attention to nonclinically relevant therapy problems.[6]

The health care personnel's (nurses and physician) attitudes toward the LIMM model was studied by Bergkvist et al.[23] using a questionnaire. The health care personnel estimated the clinical pharmacy service in general, specific clinical pharmacy activities, and the pharmacist in the health care team to be of great benefit. Evaluation projects are underway in Norway after the government granted special funds for medication review activities, but no reports are out on the subject yet (Anne Gerd Granas email communication May 5, 2011).

Curricula in Colleges of Pharmacy

Substantial differences exist between the education of pharmacists in the Nordic countries as compared to U.S. colleges of pharmacy. When scanning program evaluation reports and curricula, it is evident that the focus of most pharmacy programs at the masters level is on producing pharmacists with wide array of skills within the natural sciences and in technology. The graduates of the programs go upon graduation to a much larger extent to industry than is known in the United States, although this varies by the country's pharmaceutical industry presence.

This view on pharmacists' competencies and job prospects certainly impacts the way subdisciplines such as pharmacy practice and clinical pharmacy are viewed within the profession of pharmacy. They are considered valuable, but since not all students will need them, whereas they are viewed to generally need the more natural science oriented subdisciplines, not much room is given to patient-oriented disciplines and the integration of pharmaceutical knowledge into patient care.

A further hurdle is the fact that clinical pharmacy and pharmacy practice (social pharmacy) faculty members are often separated organizationally within colleges of pharmacy. This weakens the opportunity to collaborate and give a holistic picture of how the budding pharmacists can use their skills in patient care from a theoretical and practical standpoint. The 6-month internship stipulated by European Union is used to a varying degree to train students for the patient care role, and it is apparent that they in these 6 months are mainly under the supervision of one pharmacist most often in isolation from the health care system and other health care professionals. The university departments in charge of the course (usually social pharmacy) forge ties with practice in this way, but it is uncertain whether they can impact practice to a large extent through internship programs.

Government/Payer Recognition and Reimbursement for Services

Government (national, regional or local) is usually the payer for health care services (including hospital care) in the Nordic countries. This implies that the government usually pays directly or indirectly the salary of hospital personnel involved in pharmaceutical care practice. Many hospital pharmacists who are involved also have other obligations than direct patient care, such as distribution to wards.

No examples of payment of patient care services for outpatients can be shown, although the government has in the case of Denmark and Norway put funds into pilot projects in medication review.[36] In Denmark, one community pharmacy service, which cannot be labeled pharmaceutical care, is currently reimbursed, Inhaler Technique Assessment Service (*Tjek på inhalationen*).[37,38]

In April 2011, 42 Danish stakeholders (patient organization reprehensive, policy makers, and researchers) met to discuss medication review as part of health care (Unpublished Discussion notes April 5, 2011. Obtained from Ellen Westh-Sorensen). Among the projects presented were *Medisam* (the university-pharmacy project) and clinical pharmacy in Danish hospital pharmacy. The symposium concluded that there should be a national effort put into medication reviews with national clinical guidelines. In addition, that specific patient groups should be targeted such as polypharmacy patients.

The Future of Medication Management
Services in Scandinavia and Iceland

This chapter started by stating that it is difficult to view even the Scandinavian countries as a unified whole. However, there are important commonalities to be seen in how pharmaceutical care is being seen and practiced in these countries.

First, there is a tendency to focus attention on certain types of patients, either relating to disease categories, age groups (the elderly), or the number of medicines used. The reasons for this could be pharmacists' fear that taking on a general population may be too difficult to master from a pharmacotherapeutic point of view. Another probable reason is that in order to sell the idea to policy makers, pharmacists need to show study results on seriously ill populations whose morbidity has been studied more extensively with the implicit expectation on all parts that this will be where pharmaceutical care will have the greatest impact.

Second, there is a general confusion about what the concepts mean within pharmaceutical care practice. The findings of Pharmakon[16] are very telling about how medication review can be anything from a very technical exercise without patient involvement to something that could probably be called comprehensive medication management. It seems that it is easy to sell the concept of medication review to politicians and policy makers rather than the concept of care. Medication reviews seem to be something tangible and imply more specific tasks than pharmaceutical care.

The term pharmaceutical care has been used freely to describe activities that are almost solely related to drug distribution and information provision as seen in a study of HIV patient clinic.[39] This lack of clarity and loose use of terms lead to a lack of standards of care preventing the understanding and adoption of pharmaceutical care practice. Researchers (not excluding the author) are also to blame for the lack of unified definitions.[40] They have been willing partners in designing protocols for studies on pharmaceutical care and carrying out research in cooperation with practitioners without rigorous attention to a common understanding of practice.

Third, within community pharmacy, the brunt of work within this field has been research and evaluation projects, which have not led to permanent changes in practice. Only Apoteket AB's efforts seemed to promise a permanent change, but the change in ownership threatens to close down this service. It is more promising to see developments within inpatient care where the practice change has been seen as permanent from the start and focused on health care professions working together centering on the patient's therapy. Denmark has forged ahead with making the GP the central actor in medication review. This has taken many pharmacists by surprise. It looked as if pharmacists outside hospitals do not understand yet that physicians view themselves and are viewed by patients as the central actor in patient care (pharmaceutical or otherwise).

It will be interesting to see the results from the large Norwegian effort, but as previously mentioned, many issues have not been taken into account there such as philosophy, clarity, and permanence of practice. The Swedish community pharmacy model—long thought to be the most likely to succeed due to its size and support systems—is being dismantled. The Danish community pharmacy system is yet again under siege. It is evident from all the four countries that when public debate turns to community pharmacy, politicians and the public do not see health care in pharmacies but immediately start discussing prices of drugs.

The brightest prospect for comprehensive medication management services in the near future lies within the hospitals in Scandinavia and Iceland. Clinical pharmacists there are often researchers and teachers in addition to being practitioners. They therefore document their services and teach their students the philosophy of practice. The traditional pharmacy education institutions focus on a broad pharmacy education—a "one size fits all" ranging from community pharmacy to drug development. They do not realize that the pharmaceutical industry does not require a registered health care professional and that they as a result may lose their reason for existence if community pharmacy disappears as a profession. The deprofessionalization within community pharmacy started when compounding disappeared. The opening up of ownership to nonpharmacists in the last two decades has further escalated this trend. On the bright side, new clinical pharmacy education programs are being started, which provides hope that comprehensive medication management services will be a reality in a few years within both primary and tertiary care.

REFERENCES

1. Vallgårda S. Public health policies: a Scandinavian model? *Scand J Public Health.* 2007;35(2):205–211.
2. Holmberg C, Kjellberg H, Axelsson B. *Läkemedelsdistribution i Norden—en komparativ studie av aktörer, resurser och aktiviteter. [In Swedish. Drug distribution in the Nordic countries—a comparative study of actors, resources and activities.] SEE/EFI Working paper series in business administration (vol.10).* Center for Marketing, Distribution and Industry Dynamics: Stockholm no. 2003.
3. Larsen JB, Mount J, Kruse PR, Vrangbæk K. Dynamics of Pharmacy Regulation in Denmark, 1932–1994: a study of profession-state relations. *Pharm Hist.* 2004;46(2):43–61.

4. Larsen JB, Mount J, Kruse PR, Vrangbæk K. Dynamics of Pharmacy Regulation in Denmark, 1546–1932: a study of profession-state relations. *Pharm Hist.* 2004;46(1):3–25.

5. Morgall JM, Almarsdóttir AB. No struggle, no strength: how pharmacists lost their monopoly. *Soc Sci Med.* 1999;48:1247–1258.

6. Montgomery A. Counseling in Swedish Community Pharmacies. Understanding the Process of a Pharmaceutical Care Service. Acta Universitatis Upsaliensis. Digital Comprehensive Summaries of Uppsala Dissertations from the Faculty of Pharmacy 107. 71 pp. Uppsala. ISPN 978-91-554-7622-9.

7. Swedish Law. Lag om handel med läkemedel [Statute on drug retailing] SFS 2009:366.

8. Johnsen JR. *Health Systems in Transition: Norway.* Copenhagen, WHO Regional Office for Europe on behalf of the European Observatory on Health Systems and Policies; 2006.

9. Hepler CD, Strand LM. Opportunities and responsibilities in pharmaceutical care. *Am J Hosp Pharm.* 1990;47:533–543.

10. Cipolle RJ, Strand LM, Morley PC. *Pharmaceutical Care Practice.* New York: McGraw-Hill Companies Inc; 1998.

11. Cipolle RJ, Strand LM, Morley PC. *Pharmaceutical Care Practice: The Clinician's Guide.* 2nd ed. New York: McGraw-Hill Companies Inc; 2004.

12. Westerlund LT, Almarsdottir AB, Melander A. Drug-related problems and pharmacy interventions in community pharmacy. *Int J Pharm Pract.* 1999;7:40–50.

13. Halvorsen KH, Ruths S, Granas AG, Viktil KK. Multidisciplinary intervention to identify and resolve drug-related problems in Norwegian nursing homes. *Scand J Primary Health Care.* 2010;28:82–88.

14. Granas AG, Berg C, Hjellvik V, et al. Evaluating categorisation and clinical relevance of drug-related problems in medication reviews. *Pharm World Sci.* 2009;32:394–403.

15. Viktil KK, Blix HS, Reikvam A, et al. Comparison of drug-related problems in different patient groups. *Ann Pharmacother* 2004;38(6):942–948.

16. Thomsen LA, Herborg H, Rossing C. Pharmakon. Models for medication reviews in the Danish primary health care sector [in Danish: Modeller for medicingennemgang i den danske primære sundhedssektor] Version 1.1 (5. april 2011). 2011. ISBN 978-87-91598-47-0.

17. IRF. County-based medicinal advisers of medicinal products and the Danish regions' treatment guidelines [in Danish: Regionale lægemiddelkonsulenter og regionernes behandlingsvejledninger. Accessed August 16, 2011 from http://www.irf.dk/dk/om_irf/alke.htm

18. Haukereid C, Horn AM, Berg C, Granas AG. Medication reviews for patients with type 2 diabetes. [in Norwegian: Legemiddelgjennomganger for pasienter med type 2-diabetes]. *Norsk farmaceutisk tidsskrift* 2008;7–8:18–22.

19. Helse- og Omsorgsdepartementet. In Norwegian: Stortingsmelding nr. 18 (2004–2005). Rett kurs mot riktigere legemiddelbruk. 2005. Accessed April 24, 2011 from http://www.regjeringen.no/nb/dep/hod/dok/regpubl/stmeld/20042005/Stmeld-nr-18-2004-2005-.html?id=406517.

20. Helsedirektoratet. In Norwegian: Riktig legemiddelbruk til eldre pasienter/beboere på sykehjem og i hjemmesykepleien. Forslag til tiltak. [homepage on the Internet]. 2011 cited 2011 April 24]. 2011. Available from: http://www.helsedirektoratet.no/vp/multimedia/archive/00330/IS-1887_Tiltak_for__330569a.pdf.

21. Kettis Lindblad Å, Ring L. *Internal Report 2: Customer evaluations* [in Swedish: Kundutvärdering Projekt Läkemedelsprofiler, delrapport 2]. Apoteket AB; 2003.

22. Institute for HealthCare Improvement. Prevent Adverse Drug Events with Medication Reconciliation. Accessed April 24, 2011 from: http://www.ihi.org/explore/adesmedication-reconciliation/Pages/default.aspx.

23. Bergkvist Christensen A. A systematic approach to improving pharmacotherapy in the elderly. Lund University, Faculty of Medicine Doctoral Dissertation Series 2010:123, 61 pp. Lund. ISBN 978-91-86671-39-6.
24. Audit Commission. *A Spoonful of Sugar—Medicines Management in NHS Hospitals.* London: The Audit Commission. 2001. http://www.audit-commission.gov.uk/national studies/health/other/Pages/aspoonfulofsugar.aspx.
25. Barber N. Pharmaceutical care and medicines management—is there a difference? *Pharm World Sci.* 2001;23(6):210–11.
26. Scullin C, Scott MG, Hogg A, McElnay JC. An innovative approach to integrated medicines management. *J Eval Clin Pract.* 2007;13(5):781–788.
27. Gillespie U, Alassaad A, Henrohn D, et al. A comprehensive pharmacist intervention to reduce morbidity in patients 80 years or older a randomized controlled trial. *Arch Intern Med.* 2009;169(9):894–900.
28. Bergqvist K. In Swedish: Bort med läkemedelsgenomgångar, in med apotekare i vården. Läkartidningen 2008-11-28 (48). 2008. Accessed June 29, 2011 from http://www. lakartidningen.se/engine.php?articleId=10912#comment
29. Jónsdóttir, HÞ. Deregulating outpatient pharmacies in Denmark, Iceland and Norway— a comparison of key parameters [in Icelandic]. MS thesis. Reykjavik: University of Iceland.
30. Glintborg D. Medication reviews in general practice [in Danish: Medicingennemgang i almen praksis]. Månedsskrift for Praktisk Lægegerning. January 2011.
31. Almarsdóttir AB, Morgall JM. Technicians or Patient Advocates?—still a valid question. (Results of Focus Group Discussions with Pharmacists). *Pharm World Sci.* 1999;21(3):127–131.
32. Morgall Traulsen J, Almarsdóttir AB and I Björnsdóttir. The lay user perspective on the quality of pharmaceuticals, drug therapy, and pharmacy services. *Pharm World Sci.* 2002;24(5):196–200.
33. Renberg T, Wichman Törnqvist K, Kälvemark Sporrong S, Kettis Lindblad Å, Tully MP (in press). *Pharmacy Users' Expectations of Pharmacy Encounters: A Q-methodological Study.* Health Expectations 2011, Vol. 14 Issue 4, p361–373.
34. Jósteinsdóttir OA (2011) Clinical work of pharmacists at LSH—the impact of interventions and the attitudes of other health care professionals [in Icelandic]. MS thesis. Reykjavik: University of Iceland.
35. Södergaard B, Barretta K, Tully MP, Kettis Lindblad A. A qualitative study of health care personnel's experience of a satellite pharmacy at a HIV clinic. *Pharm World Sci.* 2005;27(2):208–115.
36. Bernsten C, Andersson K, Gariepy Y, Simoens S. A comparative analysis of remuneration models for pharmaceutical professional services. *Health Policy.* 2010;95(1):1–9.
37. Herborg H, Sorensen EW, Frokjaer B. Pharmaceutical care in community pharmacies: practice and research in Denmark. *Ann Pharmacother.* 2007;41:681–689.
38. Kaae S. Analysis of the local organizational situation's impact on a permanent implementation of the first officially reimbursed pharmacy service "Inhaler Technique Assessment Service". [PhD thesis. In Danish: Analyse af lokale organisatoriske forholds betydning for varig implementering af de forste offentligt betalte apoteksydelse "Tjek på inhalationen"]. Copenhagen: University of Copenhagen; 2009.
39. Södergaard B. *Adherence and readiness to antiretroviral treatment.* Acta Universitatis Upsaliensis. Digital Comprehensive Summaries of Uppsala Dissertations from the Faculty of Pharmacy 43. 2006; 82 pp. Uppsala. ISBN 91-554-6719-9.
40. Björkman IK, Sanner MA, Bernsten CB. Comparing 4 classification systems for drug-related problems: processes and functions. *Res Social Adm Pharm.* 2008;4:320–331.

UNITED KINGDOM

Dr. Paul F. Grassby, BSc, PhD, MRPharmS
Deputy Head of Pharmacy, School of Pharmacy
University of East Anglia, Norwich
Norfolk, United Kingdom

"A great and novel undertaking."

Aneurin Bevan

In order to fully understand the current state and issues with respect to the development of comprehensive medication management services in the United Kingdom it is necessary to briefly outline the history and structure of the National Health Service. On the 5th July 1948 the Minister for Health, Aneurin Bevan launched the National Health Service for the United Kingdom. It was, and continues to be, based on three key principles:

1. That it will meet the needs of everyone.
2. That it will be free at the point of delivery.
3. That it will be based on clinical need, not the ability to pay.

The National Health Service brought together hospitals, general practitioners, pharmacists, dentists and others under one umbrella. It still remains essentially free at the point of care and is financed from general taxation—thus the rich pay more in absolute terms for comparative benefits. Outside the old Soviet bloc, few countries have used this model—most relying on insurance schemes. Consequently, in terms of medicines, the majority of patients obtain all their regular medicines via a free prescription from their general practitioner, even for quite minor self-limiting conditions. The National Health Service remains one of the country's most cherished institutions—belonging to and for the people. Because of this fact, it was and remains almost impossible for politicians to make dramatic changes to the service, and/or its underlying principles. However with the aging population it is argued that productivity within the service must increase if the founding principles are to remain intact, but attempts to introduce competition into the service have and continue to prove extremely difficult.

The National Health Service employs 1.7m people making it the world's fourth largest employer—only the Chinese People's Liberation Army, the Wal-Mart supermarket chain and the Indian Railways directly employ more people. The National Health Service is divided into primary and secondary care structures, but it is the primary care trusts that control 80% of the health care budget and commission secondary care as well as managing primary care in their areas. There are 151 individual primary care trusts in England.[1]

Health care is devolved to Scotland, Wales and Northern Ireland. In Scotland there are 12 Health Boards under the control of the Scottish Government and similar arrangements are in place in Wales and Northern Ireland under their respective elected assemblies.

It is extremely difficult to measure the efficiency of the National Health Service in a consistent and systematic way, and patients themselves are very reluctant to criticize or sue the National Health Service for negligence. Patients will always support "their" local hospital (even if it is killing them!), and independent members of parliament have been elected on the back of threatened local hospital closures. A significant number are even embarrassed to raise the question of sub-standard care. Dr. Keith Brent of the British Medical Association says *"What they want is an explanation. It's not really money that they want. It's an explanation, an apology. And perhaps some kind of assurance that, hopefully, if something has gone wrong that shouldn't have gone wrong, that won't happen again to other people."*[2] In addition recent opinion polls show that 92% of patients continue to trust their doctors (compared with only 71% for clergymen!).[3]

An understanding of these facts is important in appreciating some of the challenges that have faced pharmacists in attempting to extend their roles and develop other patient care services beyond a simple supply function. Prior to the National Health Service, dispensing accounted for less than 10% of a pharmacists' income—after the creation of the National Health Service this increased overnight to 94%, and is little changed today. The National Health Service has created and strengthened the patients' perception that it is doctors who are solely responsible for the management of their treatment in terms of appropriateness, effectiveness, safety and compliance. The pharmacist (or chemist) is still largely regarded as having mainly a supply function in terms of dispensing and sales of over the counter medicines. This is confirmed by a number of studies that have highlighted that patients regard the general practitioner as the first choice for all health advice, and that there is even concern expressed by patients about pharmacists extending their role—in particular concerns with access to patient records and their escalating workloads.[4]

Medication Reviews: "All Things to All People"

The term *"medication review"* is commonly used by many National Health Service organizations and has been defined as *"a structured, critical examination of a patient's medicines with the objective of reaching an agreement with the patient about treatment, optimising the impact of medicines, minimising the number of medication-related problems and reducing waste."*[5] Taken at face value, this would appear to fulfill some requirements of *"comprehensive medication management"* that is the focus of this discussion. In practice the term *"medication review"* has referred to all and any activities that involve a review of medicines! The term has been applied across different settings and across different contractual frameworks. These are quite diverse and will be discussed below. Four levels of medication review were first described in 2002 in a report entitled "Room for Review" which was produced by a taskforce of many stakeholders by the National Prescribing Centre[5] which has been used by many organizations to inform service development:

Level 0: *Ad hoc:* unstructured opportunistic review.
Level 1: Prescription review: a technical review of a list of a patient's medicines (paper-based).
Level 2: Treatment review: a review of medicines with the patients full notes (not necessarily with the patient present).
Level 3: Clinical medication review: face-to-face review of medicines and condition with the patient.

The National Health Service National Service Framework for Older People has suggested that: "All people >75 should have a medication review every 12 months OR if they are prescribed four or more regular items the review should be carried out every 6 months."[6]

Medication Reviews by General Practitioners

The General Medical Services (GMS) contract for general practitioners contains a Quality and Outcomes Framework,[7] for which general practitioners are paid for meeting certain targets. This framework covers 134 indicators and a total of 1000 points can be achieved. In relation to medication reviews it is expected that *"A medication review is recorded in the notes (by way of recording a specific payment code) in the preceding 15 months for all patients being prescribed four or more repeat medicines (7 points), or for patients on any repeat medications (8 points)"*. The guidance includes the statement that *"it is expected that at least a level 2 medication review will occur"* so the minimum standard does not even require the patient to be present.

The most recent analysis of the Quality and Outcomes Framework achievement, based on the code recorded in patient's notes is 97%. As each point is worth approximately $200 per general practitioner, this equates to $3000. Just including patients over 65 years on their list who are taking four or more medications for review this equates to 8% or 144 patients for a typical general practitioner, or just $20 per medication review. Although there is guidance on the underlying principles of a medication review—that it must be carried out in a systematic way, the reviews are not recorded in enough detail to be assessed for quality in terms of structure, time spent or outcomes. One can only speculate on the time spent and the quality of these reviews and recent research has suggested that general practitioners miss 85% of pharmaceutical care issues.[8]

Medication Reviews by Primary Care Pharmacists

Some pharmacists are employed directly by the primary care organizations, called Primary Care Trusts which manage the National Health Service budget within their locality and commission health services. These pharmacists may have a lead role for all issues relating to medicines management within their Primary Care Trust. This may include promoting evidence based prescribing, developing and managing local formularies, financial management of prescribing budgets and interfacing with local hospitals. They also play a role in education and training and some are employed to work for general practitioners' practices. Their roles include conducting clinical medication reviews within the surgery, in nursing and residential homes, or by paying home visits. There are some excellent examples of good practice in terms of structures and outcomes in the literature;[9,10,11] however other studies have reported poor outcomes, including one showing a significant increase in hospital admissions.[12] Primary care pharmacists are employed either by the Primary Care Trusts, or directly by general practitioners or other organizations that provide a range of medicines management services to general practice. This group of pharmacists actually carry out a similar number of clinical medication reviews as general practitioners at all levels. However it is proposed by the new government that Primary Care Trusts should be disbanded and that general practitioners should now take responsibility for the primary care budget and will be responsible for commissioning services. Currently this is having a significant impact on the morale and number of primary care pharmacists employed by these organizations.

Medication Reviews by Hospital Pharmacists

Hospital pharmacists are engaged in a range of activities including traditional procurement, supply and manufacturing services, developing and auditing guidelines, education and training and clinical pharmacy services with direct patient contact. In December 2001 the Audit commission published "A Spoonful of Sugar"[13] a national report on medicines management in hospitals. The report stressed that pharmacists have a central role in ensuring the optimal use of medicines, and should be regarded as a core clinical service. Recently the commission reported findings from the "Acute Hospital Portfolio"[14] a collection of audits for use within hospitals, one of which was medicines management. The report suggested the results should drive the establishment of standards for good practice. It was observed that in some hospitals pharmacists spend more than twice as much time on clinical activities compared with others, and this ranged from 20% to 80%. However in many hospitals the pharmacist spent just 10 minutes per patient.

There is no clear definition of what a medication review is in the acute setting. One standard states that an accurate drug history should be taken within 24 hours of admission. This is not always achieved. The Health Care Commissions report "The Best Medicine—the management of medicines in acute and specialist trusts"[15] recognizes that the term "review" is more than that and reported that the number of patients undergoing a "comprehensive medication review" was on average only 54%, and 81% of these did not involve the patient. The review also established that if a patient was taking more than five medicines, a change was normally required. The commission went on to state that more clarity was needed on what was meant by a "medication review", and that it was not simply a pharmacists' review of drug charts. The reviews should involve a full drug history (including failed drugs and side effects) and considering wider clinical information. Of course it was recognized that patients may only be in hospital for a short time, and that changes to medication should be made explicit to general practitioners and that some changes should be initiated by general practitioners and monitored for effectiveness. It is also stated that more work is needed to define the range of functions that relate to a medication review.

Medication Reviews by Community Pharmacists in England and Wales

All community pharmacies have a contract with the National Health Service, which is negotiated at a national level, to provide a range of services. These pharmacists may be independent pharmacists or more usually part of large multi-national organizations, which now make up the bulk of community pharmacies in the United Kingdom.

The current (2005) pharmacy contract[16] for England and Wales is made up of three levels of service:

- **Essential services**: provided by all contractors that include dispensing, public health initiatives, signposting and support for self-care.
- **Advanced Services:** provided once accreditation requirements are met which include Medicines Use Review and Prescription intervention service and a New Medicines Service.
- **Enhanced Services:** commissioned by local Primary Care Trusts which include a diverse range of services including free emergency contraception, vascular health checks, minor ailment services, pharmacist prescribing and full clinical medication reviews.

The Medicines Use Review was introduced in the new pharmacy contract in 2005 as an advanced service for community pharmacists. Currently each pharmacy can perform up to 400 Medicines Use Reviews in one year on any patients taking multiple medicines, particularly with long-term conditions. The new contract reforms were supported by pharmacists as they were intended to make better use of pharmacists' knowledge and skills, and promote feelings of competence and autonomy.

The underlying purpose of the Medicines Use Review is to improve adherence by improving the patients knowledge and use of drugs by establishing the patients' actual usage; their understanding and experience of taking drugs; identifying, discussing and resolving poor or ineffective use of drugs; identifying side effects and drug interactions that may affect the patients compliance and improving the cost-effectiveness of drugs prescribed to patient's thereby reducing the wastage of such drugs. Thus, it was not intended to be a clinical medication review, but an *"adherence centered review."*

In order to perform a Medicines Use Review a pharmacist must obtain independent accreditation (typically a free on-line or face to face training and examination), and there must be a consultation area within the pharmacy. The service is free to patients, and the pharmacists are paid a fee of $40 per consultation, which is paid for by the Primary Care Trust.

This service does not fit into the previous defined levels of a medication review as it is a concordance review with the patient (level 3), but with no access to the patient's notes (level 2). For this reason three levels of medication review are now proposed as:[10]

Type 1: Prescription review
Type 2: Concordance and compliance review
Type 3: Clinical Medication review

The MUR falls within a level 2 review. The uptake of Medicine Use Reviews by community pharmacists has steadily increased to 1.7 million in 2009–10. In 2008 59% of community pharmacists were providing Medicine Use Reviews with an average of 65 per pharmacy. Uptake varies significantly according to ownership category (i.e., independent or multiple), as more than twice as many Medicine Use Reviews were performed by multiple pharmacy chains.[17,18]

The experience and opinions of pharmacists working with the new contract shines some light on the value of Medicine Use Reviews. While some pharmacists reported that MUR's were worthwhile and fulfilling, others reported that they were bordering on fraudulent.[17] This has been seized on and highlighted by medical publications for general practitioners, with headlines such as *"Pharmacists' medicines-use reviews 'bordering on fraud'."*

In addition others reported that due to targets being imposed by employers they had become a source of pressure rather than fulfillment and tensions developed between pharmacists and patients. Many patients felt no need for a review by a pharmacist (as it was done by the doctor), pharmacists found it difficult to be pro-active in recruiting patients, and appreciating that the latter may want to exercise a degree of strategic noncompliance and choice with prescribed medication regimes to enable them to achieve a balance in their lives and to attain a sense of well-being and control.[17]

Pharmacists also reported frustrations with respect to general practitioners' opinions of the service and a target driven tick box culture. Although the initial Medicines Use Review discussions and documentation had many similarities with "comprehensive medication management", and resembled the pharmaceutical care pharmacotherapy work-up, the final versions removed sections on medical history, allergies, adverse drug reactions and previous drug history becoming little more than a list of drugs with tick boxes for: directions followed; knowledge of medicine; appropriate formulation and side effects. The only actions available for pharmacists are providing general information to the patient about their medicines and referral to the general practitioner.

Some have argued that the current Medicines Use Review, while providing and opportunity for pharmacists to extend their role and responsibilities is having the opposite effect, and in terms of pharmaceutical care is trying to address compliance with medicines, without taking into account appropriate indication, efficacy and safety. In terms of their quality, there is anecdotal evidence that there is considerable variation.[19]

In a recent report on the role of community pharmacy in the modern National Health Service[20] Senior Liberal Democrat Norman Lamb Member of Parliament and Chief Parliamentary and Political Advisor to the Deputy Minister Nick Clegg has been reported as saying: "The role of pharmacists does have to be effectively coordinated. I was shocked when recently visiting a general practitioners' practice to be told that they have great piles of forms with the results of Medicine Use Reviews which pile up and are never really used in any meaningful way—this looks dangerously like spending a lot of money heating the atmosphere to no real benefit. The principle of the Medicine Use Review is very good, but the results must be utilized to improve patient care"[20] The report goes on to recommend that MURs should be fully integrated into care pathways and strong communicative relationships must be made with general practitioners.

On 15th March 2011 the National Health Service employers announced that in the future it will be important to demonstrate the benefits of the Medicines Use Review service and provide assurance that it is a high quality, value for money, service of benefit to patients, and agreed to a number of changes. It has been agreed that 70% of Medicines Use Reviews should be carried out on target groups (high risk medicines, recently discharged from hospital, and in specific therapeutic areas such as respiratory disease) and that outcome measures be developed and agreed to prior to implementation.

Clinical Medication Reviews are one of a number of enhanced services within the community pharmacy contract. Enhanced services are currently responsible for only about 1% of a pharmacists' income.[14]

The service is described as "A structured, critical examination of a patient's medicines with the objective of reaching an agreement with the patient about the continued appropriateness and effectiveness of the treatment, optimizing the impact of medicines, minimizing the number of medication-related problems and reducing waste". It is described as a "Level 3 medication review" requiring access to a patient's medical notes and in particular, supporting those with complex medicine regimens.

The outcomes are described as follows:

1. To ensure patients are on optimum therapy by reviewing and making recommendations to improve therapy to the prescriber:

   - effectiveness of treatment;
   - appropriateness of treatment based on latest evidence;
   - adverse drug effects;
   - test results, interpreting them and acting on them where required; and whether the recommendations of previous reviews have been acted upon;
   - recommend new treatments, for example, aspirin or statins in patients with coronary heart disease; and
   - if the pharmacist is a prescriber they would be able to make changes to the patient's treatment as agreed with the doctor.

2. To improve patient compliance with therapy by:

   - providing an opportunity for the patient to discuss concerns and ask questions about their medicines;
   - improving the patient's understanding of their medicines;
   - simplifying the medication regimen and drug ordering process where appropriate;
   - identifying practical problems in medicine taking and referring the patient for assessment of support required if necessary;
   - providing advice and support to the patient and carer, including referral to specialist centers or other health and social care professionals where appropriate; and
   - ensuring that there is active participation of the patient, with shared decision making and agreement about any changes.

In contrast to Medicines Use Reviews, this is a full clinical medication review that meets many of the requirements of comprehensive medication management, and is one of a range of 15 enhanced services, which need to be commissioned by a local Primary Care Trust. As such the actual enhanced services which are commissioned vary considerably from one Primary Care Trust to another. Although many Primary Care Trusts offer popular enhanced services, such as free emergency contraception, free smoking cessation clinics and free cardiovascular risk checks through community pharmacies. The exact specifications of the services and payment vary considerably from region to region.

Community pharmacy contractors in England in 2009–10 provided 29,526 local enhanced services.[14] The most frequent services provided in 2009–2010 have remained unchanged since 2006–2007. These were stop smoking support, supervised administration of methadone, minor ailment schemes and free medicines supply via Patient Group Directions. The number of individual pharmacies reported as being contracted to provide a "medication review service" was reported as 2357 or 8% of the total. Because these are locally commissioned services, and there are no agreed national definitions of many enhanced services, "medication review services" can vary widely, and while many may indeed be comprehensive medication reviews, they also include services such as targeted medicines management services to care homes, disease-specific services and also include extended or targeted MUR services, for example, in a patients' home, or targeted at a particular patient group.[21]

New legislation has placed a statutory duty on all local primary care trusts to carry out and publish a Pharmaceutical Needs Assessment which is defined by the National Health Service as *"a key tool for identifying what is needed at local level to support the commissioning intentions for pharmaceutical services and other services that could be delivered by community pharmacies and other providers"*. The regulations are intended to be permissive and allow primary care trusts to interpret how any of the enhanced services should be commissioned (which include clinical medication reviews), its scope and method of delivery. As there are 151 primary care trusts, each carrying out an individual Pharmaceutical Needs Assessments, one will be discussed as typical.

Norfolk primary care trust[22] have identified a need to develop pharmacy services that amongst other things support long term conditions and ensure that medicines are used safely and effectively. It concludes that their existing medicines review service, which is an enhanced service, should remain a necessary service. This service involves an assessor conducting a medication review on vulnerable patients in their own homes and making recommendations for improved compliance. There are no recommendations for a more comprehensive medication management service, although a recent publication suggests that medication reviews should have a high priority in terms of a pharmaceutical needs assessment in primary care.[23]

In terms of improving and addressing concerns regarding the quality assurance and accountability of this range of services, which vary considerably throughout the country, the "Healthy Living Pharmacy" concept has emerged from a 2008 government White Paper—"Pharmacy in England: Building on Strengths, Delivering the Future."[24]

Launched initially in the city of Portsmouth, and about to be launched at a number of pathfinder sites in England, this model outlines a more structured and tiered approach addressing a number of health needs: including smoking, obesity, alcohol, physical activity, sexual health, men's health, substance misuse, minor ailments and long term conditions.[25] Associated with these are four levels of pharmacies: core, level 1 (promotion), level 2 (prevention) and level 3 (protection). Clinical medication review being a level 3 service, requiring advanced clinical skills. It is intended that this framework will inform the commissioning of pharmacy services, and pharmacies will receive a Healthy Living Pharmacy quality mark.

Medication Reviews by Community Pharmacists in Scotland

The management of health services is devolved to the Scottish Parliament, and community pharmacists in Scotland supply pharmaceutical services to National Health Service Scotland. A recent document entitled "Right Medicine – A Strategy for Pharmaceutical Care in Scotland"[26] outlined the commitment to make better use of pharmacists' skills and expertise to improve patient care. The Chronic Medication Service[27,28] is a core service, to which all 1223 community pharmacies have signed up. The first stage of its implementation commenced in April 2010 and by the end of November 2010 19,000 patients had been registered by 1100 pharmacies.

The Chronic Medication Service requires voluntary patient opt-in prior to participation and has three stages:

Stage 1: Registration of patients
Stage 2: Pharmaceutical Care Planning and Patient Profiling
Stage 3: Shared care with the patient's GP establishing a serial prescription for either 24 or 48 weeks and support for the patient using disease-specific protocols.

It is stated that the key intervention within the chronic medication service is the pharmaceutical care planning (stage 2) process with the following key steps:

Step 1: Identifying Pharmaceutical Care Needs and Issues
Step 2: Formulating the Pharmaceutical Care Plan, and documenting the issues, outcomes and actions.

Documentation of the pharmaceutical care plan and patient profile will be done using a web-based pharmacy care record.[29] This will allow the pharmacist to create and maintain pharmaceutical care plans. The care plan will form the basis of ongoing monitoring and review of the patient to ensure the issues identified are actioned.

Step 3: Implementing, monitoring and reviewing the pharmaceutical care plan. This step includes monitoring progress towards each of the outcomes identified and review.

Pharmacists will be expected to monitor and review the care plan on an ongoing basis. Implementation might be counseling the patient, ensuring they have their medication monitored appropriately or referring to the GP due to a loss of symptom control if required. It states explicitly that pharmaceutical care planning is a dynamic process and it is important that regular review of the care plan is undertaken.

The Chronic Medication Services is in its early days and is currently in the process of implementation. The current implementation payments consist of a monthly fixed fee and banded payments if the pharmacists meets targets in relation to their dispensing volume.

The Education and Training of Pharmacists

To register as a pharmacist within the United Kingdom you are required to complete a 4-year MPharm degree from an accredited School of Pharmacy, followed by 52 weeks preregistration training, within which students have to meet a set of performance standards, and pass a national registration examination. The General Pharmaceutical Council (GPhC) which is the regulator for pharmacists in England, Scotland and Wales has recently published "Future Pharmacists – Guidance on Standards for the initial education and training of pharmacists,"[30] which specifies learning outcomes for the "novice professional, which includes disease and chronic medicines management, medicines use review and care planning.

Although many pharmacy students do not undertake a specific course in comprehensive medicines management, they are increasingly devoting more time in developing their communication and clinical skills, which will underpin their new clinical roles including clinical medication reviews. Within my own locality at the School of Pharmacy at the University of East Anglia, Norwich, students prepare a range of individualized pharmaceutical care plans, and have some (albeit limited) opportunity to practice with patients. In addition as part of a research project final year students in 2011–12 will be trained in the necessary skills to conduct comprehensive medication reviews and identify pharmaceutical care issues using patients within local

GP practices. Finally the Government is currently in the process of examining a proposal for a 5 year integrated pharmacy qualification to enable pharmacists to deliver a wider range of clinical services.[31]

With regards to medical education, 75% of new doctors believe they have had too little pharmacology, therapeutics and prescribing training, and only 20% believed they had been adequately assessed in these areas.[32] In response to such concerns a national prescribing skills assessment is being developed in conjunction with the British Pharmacological Society for all new doctors.

However many community pharmacists will not have had any opportunity at university to develop these clinical skills. To support the Medicines Use Review implementation in England and Wales, pharmacists require accreditation by way of a short "on-line" course.[33] To support the Chronic Medication Service National Health Service Scotland provided full funding for community pharmacists to undertake 50 hour short course over six months to prepare themselves[34] with on-line support.[35] In addition there are opportunities for community pharmacists to participate in a range of postgraduate courses, such as the Diploma in General Pharmacy Practice (Joint Programmes Board), which includes pharmaceutical care planning and medication review within the curriculum.[36]

A Tale of Two Nations

There are many excellent examples of individual pharmacists providing excellent pharmaceutical care throughout the United Kingdom, but it appears to be sporadic with little consistency and little documentation or follow up. In common with the rest of the world the need for comprehensive medication management services is paramount and will undoubtedly increase as the population ages and resources become scarcer. In terms of improving the efficiency of the health service the care of the elderly and patients with long-term conditions is now high on the political agenda.

It has always been joked about that if a sportsman from Scotland loses, he is Scottish, but if he wins he is British! To that end we should claim that the Scottish Chronic Medication Service (CMS) is an excellent British example of an emerging comprehensive medication management service! This service involves the development of individualized care plans with appropriate follow up and documentation. It is also built within a collaborative national contractual framework with GP's and patients.

In contrast the Medicines Use Review in England is a poor relation, which has few of the required attributes of comprehensive medication management. It is essentially an adherence review with no care planning or follow-up. However on the positive side it could provide an excellent platform for the service to be developed in the future, and there are already some excellent examples of some pharmacists providing more comprehensive medication reviews as part of an enhanced service.

The new coalition government in the UK is currently in the process of attempting to change the National Health Service structure in England. In contrast to Scotland the purchasing or commissioning of services is to be devolved to consortia of general practitioners at a local level supported by others. This is intended to put the health care budget for England in the hands of local GP's who will decide on priorities. It has been argued that this change will encourage a degree of competition and increase the accountability of individual GP's– and is a way of politicians absolving themselves of hard decisions with respect to the allocation of resources. It is an attempt to remove the politics from health care, and give the power to the general practitioners at the coal face. Paradoxically because a coalition government is in place in the United Kingdom it has actually become an immense political issue particularly with any reference to competition and the changes are being considerably watered down as I write, with the new mantra of integrated care. However given the high degree of drug-related morbidity and mortality it is without saying that local commissioning must include comprehensive medication management services in order to make better use of our existing medicines and improve the productivity of the health system. It is now imperative that pharmacists in England and Wales acquire the knowledge, skills, enthusiasm, tools and commitment to invest in and develop patient-centered medication management services and effectively market these services to local commissioners. How this is managed is questionable. Perhaps pharmacists should wait for their negotiating body, the Pharmaceutical Services Negotiating Committee to follow the Scottish example and enshrine medication management services within a national arrangement. Perhaps England is more suited to a bottom up local approach, due to the local nature of health care commissioning. The impetus for this change must therefore come from individual pharmacists who understand the need for change, and the need to develop their services beyond a supply function in a unique way that meets a societal need. This will require investment by individuals in terms of education and time to develop medication management services that can meet a societal need and subsequently marketed to commissioners of health care.

REFERENCES

1. About the NHS (NHS Choices). http://www.nhs.uk/NHSEngland/thenhs/about/Pages/overview.aspx. Accessed June 15, 2011.
2. British reluctant to sue health system. Marketplace (American Public Media). http://marketplace.publicradio.org/display/web/2010/01/06/pm-nhs-docs-sued/. Accessed June 15, 2011.

3. Ipsos MORI Doctors remain the most trusted profession. http://www.ipsos-mori.com/researchpublications/researcharchive/2478/Doctors-Remain-Most-Trusted-Profession.aspx. Accessed June 15, 2011.

4. Iversen L, Mollison J, MacLeod TNN. Attitudes of the general public top the expanding roles of community pharmacists: a pilot study. *Fam Pract.* 2001;18:534–536.

5. Room for Review. Taskforce on Medicines Partnership and the National Collaborative Medicine management Services Programme at the National Prescribing Centre. 2002. http://www.keele.ac.uk/schools/pharm/npcplus/medicinespartnership/room for review.htm. Accessed June 15, 2011.

6. The National Service Framework for Older People. Department of Health. 2007. http://www.dh.gov.uk/en/Publicationsandstatistics/Publications/PublicationsPolicyAndGuidance/Browsable/DH_4096710. Accessed June 15, 2011.

7. NHS employers Quality Outcomes Framework. http://www.nhsemployers.org/PayAndContracts/GeneralMedicalServicesContract/QOF/Pages/QualityOutcomesFramework.aspx. Accessed June 15, 2011.

8. Krska J, Ross SM and Watts M. Medication reviews provided by general medical practitioners (GP's) and nurses: an evaluation of their quality. *Int J Pharm Pract.* 2005;13:77–84.

9. Zermansky AG, Alldred DP, Petty DR, Raynor DK, Frteemantle N, Eastaugh J and Bowie P. Clinical medication review by a pharmacist of elderly people living in care homes –randomised controlled trial. *Age and Ageing.* 2006;35:586–591.

10. A Guide to Medication Review. National Prescribing Centre. 2008. http://www.npc.nhs.uk/review_medicines/intro/resources/agtmr_web1.pdf. Accessed June 15, 2011.

11. Lowe CJ, Pettey DR, Zermansky AG and Raynor DK. Development of a method for clinical medication review by a pharmacist in general practice. *Pharm World Sci.* 2000;22(4):121–126.

12. Holland R, Lenaghan E, Harvey I, et al. Does home based medication review keep older people out of hospital? The HOMER randomised controlled trial *BMJ,* doi:10.1136/bmj.38338.674583.AE (published 24 January 2005).

13. Audit Commission. A spoonful of Sugar Medicines Management in NHS Hospitals. Audit Commission 2002. http://www.audit-commission.gov.uk/health/nationalstudies/other/Pages/aspoonfulofsugar_copy.aspx. Accessed June 15, 2011.

14. Audit Commission. Medicines Management. Review of National Findings (2002). http://www.audit-commission.gov.uk/health/nationalstudies/other/Pages/medicinesmanagement_copy.aspx. Accessed June 15, 2011.

15. The Best Medicine—The Management of Medicines in Acute and Specialist Trusts. Commission for Healthcare Audit and Inspection. 2007 http://www.cqc.org.uk/_db/_documents/The_Best_Medicine_acute_trust_tagged.pdf. Accessed June 15, 2011.

16. The Pharmacy Contract. http://www.psnc.org.uk/pages/introduction.html. Accessed June 15, 2011.

17. The impact of incentives on the behavior and performance of primary care professionals. A Report for the National Institute for HealthResearch Service Delivery and Organisation programme. Queen's Printer and Controller of HMSO 2010 http://www.sdo.nihr.ac.uk/files/project/158-final-report.pdf. Accessed June 15, 2011.

18. NHS Information Centre. http://www.ic.nhs.uk/statistics-and-data-collections/primary-care/pharmacies/general-pharmaceutical-services-in-england-2000-01-to-2009-10. Accessed June 15, 2011.

19. James DH, Hatten S, Roberts D and John D Identifying criteria for assessing the quality of medicines use review referral documentation by community pharmacists. *Int J Pharm Practice.* 2008;16:365–374.

20. Delivering enhanced pharmacy services in a modern NHS: Improving outcomes in health and long term conditions. The Bow Group. www.bowgroup.org. Accessed June 15, 2011.

21. PSNC Services database http://www.psnc.org.uk/services_db.php Accessed June 15, 2011.

22. NHS Norfolk Pharmaceutical Needs Assessment. 2011. http://www.norfolk.nhs.uk/sites/default/files/Pharmaceutical%20Needs%20Assessment%20(PNA).pdf.

23. Williams SE, Bond CM, Menzies C. A pharmaceutical needs assessment in a primary care setting. *Br J Gen Pract.* 2000;50:95–99.

24. Pharmacy in England: building on strengths—delivering the future. Department of Health. 2008. http://www.dh.gov.uk/en/Publicationsandstatistics/Publications/PublicationsPolicyAndGuidance/DH_083815. Accessed June 15, 2011.

25. Healthy Living Pharmacy. NHS Portsmouth. http://www.portsmouth.nhs.uk/Services/Guide-to-services/Healthy-Living-Pharmacy.htm. Accessed June 15, 2011.

26. The Right Medicine: A Strategy For Pharmaceutical Care In Scotland. The Scottish Government. 2002. http://www.scotland.gov.uk/Publications/2002/02/10633/File-1. Accessed June 15, 2011.

27. Chronic Medication Service. The Scottish Government. http://www.scotland.gov.uk/News/Releases/2010/08/30095953/. Accessed June 15, 2011.

28. Chronic Medication Service. Community Pharmacy Scotland. http://www.communitypharmacyscotland.org.uk/nhs_care_services/chronic_medication_service/what_is_the_chronic_medication_service.asp. Accessed June 15, 2011.

29. Pharmacy care record user guide. NHS Education for Scotland. 2010. http://www.communitypharmacy.scot.nhs.uk/documents/PCR_user_guide.pdf. Accessed June 15, 2011.

30. Future Pharmacists. Guidance on standards for the initial education and training of pharmacists. 2010. (http://www.pharmacyregulation.org/pdfs/consultations/gphcdraftstandardsfortheinitialeducationandtrainingofpharmacists.pdf. Accessed June 15, 2011.

31. Modernising Pharmacy Careers Programme Board. Medical Education England. http://www.mee.nhs.uk/programme_boards/modernising_pharmacy_careers_p.aspx. Accessed June 15, 2011.

32. Heaton A, Webb DJ and Maxwell SRJ Undergraduate preparation for prescribing: the views of 2413 UK medical students and recent graduates *Br J Clin Pharmacol.* 2008;66(1): 128–134.

33. MUR Online http://www.medicines-use-review.co.uk/murtools.asp. Accessed June 15, 2011.

34. Clinical Skills for Chronic Disease Management. Robert Gordon University. http://www4.rgu.ac.uk/pharmacy_life/courses/page.cfm?pge=80807. Accessed June 15, 2011.

35. Supporting the Pharmacy Contract. NHS Education Scotland http://www.nes.scot.nhs.uk/disciplines/pharmacy/supporting-the-pharmacy-contract-/chronic-medication-service-(cms)/cms-general-info. Accessed June 15, 2011.

36. Joint Programmes Board. Diploma in general Pharmacy Practice. http://www.jpbsoutheast.org/ Accessed June 15, 2011.

BRAZIL

Djenane Ramalho de Oliveira, BSc, RPh, MSc, PhD
Professor, Social Pharmacy Department
College of Pharmacy, Universidade
Federal de Minas Gerais, Belo Horizonte, Brazil

Researcher and MTM Pharmacist Specialist, Medication Therapy
Management Department, Fairview Pharmacy Services
Minneapolis, Minnesota

Adjunct Faculty, Department of Pharmaceutical Care & Health
Systems
College of Pharmacy, University of Minnesota
Minneapolis, Minnesota

> *"I have not been formally prepared to do this [pharmaceutical care]. Nobody ever taught me how to take care of patients in the college of pharmacy. But, I have had some good teachers in the last years... My teachers have been patients who take medications every day. I keep learning a lot with them."*
>
> *Sofia*

The opening quotation is an account of one of the 28 pharmacists who responded to an online questionnaire that inquired about pharmaceutical care practices in Brazil in May 2011. The questionnaire was sent by this author to 85 individuals who are publicly known to be involved with pharmaceutical care by teaching it, researching it or supervising/providing the service in Brazil. The questionnaire had 11 questions that accounted for the following topics: pharmacist training, practice setting, practice model, patient recruitment, flow of service, collaboration with other health care professionals, documentation, outcomes of the service, quality assurance and perspectives on how pharmaceutical care can be better implemented and advanced in Brazil.

A Peek at Brazil

Brazil is a federative republic that covers 47% of South America with an estimated population of 190,732,694 in 2010.[1] It is the world's fifth most populous country with a multiethnic population. Brazil was a Portuguese colony until 1822 and it became a republic in 1889. Its political system is composed of several political parties and three levels of autonomous government–federal government, 26 states and a federal district, and 5563 municipalities.[2] Health sector reform in Brazil was motivated by civil society rather than by the government. The Brazilian health reform that started in the 1970s and culminated with the creation of the Unified Health System (Sistema Único de Saúde [SUS]) regarded health as a social and a political issue to be addressed by the public instead of a solely biological issue to be resolved by medical services.[3] SUS was instituted in Brazil by the constitution of 1988 and is based on the principle of health as a citizen's right and the state's duty. Subsequently, SUS was organized with principles of universality, integral care, health promotion, and community participation.[2] The principle of health as a constitutional right means that all Brazilian citizens have the right to preventive care, medical care, and pharmaceuticals. It should be noted that Brazil also has a private health care system, which is overseen by the government.

Regarding medication use, as most medical interventions in Brazil involve the prescription of medications, it is imperative that the government establish ways to guarantee not only the broad access but also the appropriate and safe use of medicines. Pharmacy services in the public health care system, known in Brazil as "Assistência Farmacêutica," includes research, development, and production of pharmaceuticals as well as their acquisition, distribution, dispensing, and the follow-up of their utilization in order to guarantee not only the quality of the product but also their impact in patients' lives in terms of effectiveness, safety, and quality of life.[4] However, pharmaceutical care, as a comprehensive assessment and follow-up of all of a patient's medications, is not a service commonly offered in the Brazilian public health care system.

In 2010, there were 142,841 licensed pharmacists in Brazil, 82,204 private pharmacies, 8379 public pharmacies, 7351 compounding pharmacies, 5631 hospital pharmacists, and 1053 homeopathic pharmacies.[5] In 2008, there were 321 schools of pharmacy in Brazil: 255 private and 66 public schools.[6] It is worth mentioning that the number of both private and public pharmacy schools continues increasing in Brazil.

Pharmacists, Pharmacy, and Pharmaceutical Care Practice

From the 28 pharmacists who responded to the questionnaire, 20 are providing pharmaceutical care in ambulatory clinics associated with universities and serving as a rotation site for pharmacy students; six deliver pharmaceutical care in ambulatory clinics at the public health care system and two in community pharmacies (one commercial community pharmacy and one teaching community pharmacy attached to a pharmacy school). It is interesting to highlight that 70% of these practices are not connected with dispensing, 60% of the practices are in primary care clinics and 40% in specialty clinics (hepatitis C, HIV, Hansen, Tuberculosis, Hematology, Oncology, Chronic Kidney Disease, Anticoagulation, and Transplant). Furthermore, 80% of the respondents referred to the "Pharmacotherapy Workup" and the philosophy of pharmaceutical care, as proposed by Strand, Cipolle, and Morley,[7,8] as their practice framework.

Currently, it is not known how many pharmacists provide pharmaceutical care in Brazil. Sofia (a fictitious name), one of the questionnaire respondents, graduated from a pharmacy program in 2004 and has been providing pharmaceutical care services since 2007 in an ambulatory clinic attached to a public hospital of a major city in Brazil. As the majority of pharmacists in Brazil, Sofia has not received formal training in the practice of pharmaceutical care or medication therapy management services in her pharmacy school. Nonetheless, she learned by scanning the literature and through apprenticeship with more clinically experienced pharmacists. Sofia has a very good understanding of what pharmaceutical care entails and the importance of having high-quality standards of practice. She assesses all medications her patients are taking to identify drug therapy problems, develops a care plan for each of the patient's medical conditions, and follows up with patients to measure the actual outcomes of their drug therapy. The care provided and the actual outcomes are documented in forms designed specifically for the practice. She works closely with physicians, a nutritionist, a psychologist, and a social worker in a geriatric clinic, and sees herself as a key part of the team.

Sofia's experience is a very common one in Brazil as most colleges of pharmacy do not prepare pharmacists for clinical practice. Silva,[9] in his compelling PhD thesis, carried out an in-depth critique of the education of pharmacists in Brazil highlighting the incongruence between the needs of the health care system, the reality of pharmacy practice, and what is taught in colleges of pharmacy. In his work, he discusses how pharmacists in Brazil are more often than not prepared to comprehend pharmacy as a set of skills and techniques instead of a professional practice. For the most part, the person, or the patient, is not presented as the spotlight of the curriculum and it is not obvious what the responsibilities of the pharmacist are in the health care interdisciplinary team. It is common to encounter pharmacy students in their last year of pharmacy school who cannot elaborate on what their responsibility is in the health care system. As recently underscored by Ramalho de Oliveira,[10] a detrimental assumption in the profession of pharmacy, which is particularly true in Brazil, is one that surmises that the more "activities" pharmacists are able to perform the more social legitimation they will achieve. Regarding this issue, the author emphasized:

"Actually, the expansion in the number of pharmacists' activities complicates the positioning of the pharmacist in the health care team since the understanding of his or her responsibilities becomes even more obscure. Again, the pharmacist is perceived as one who does many things but does them superficially. At this point in time, it is not possible to negate that pharmacy as a profession needs to better define itself and elucidate the unique contribution the pharmacist is going to grant to the health care team."[10] (p. 288)

In 2002, the Ministry of Education established new curriculum standards for the preparation of a generalist pharmacist in Brazil.[11] I concur that this curriculum might present a larger focus on the patient, is more tailored to the Brazilian Public Health Care System, and creates more space for the teaching of pharmaceutical care than the previous one.[12] However, as previously discussed,[9,10,12] this curriculum does not introduce standards of practice that define and clarify the professional responsibility of the pharmacist as a health professional in the care team. Once again it lists numerous activities pharmacists should be taught to augment their professional's scope of practice. I believe that this is a significant oversight the profession is sustaining over the years and it is hurting the pharmacist's professional identity. The fact is that most pharmacy schools in Brazil are NOT preparing pharmacists with the capability to apply a unique body of knowledge for the benefit of patients.

As Sofia, Mario, a pharmacist who works with primary care at the municipal level of the public health care system, was not prepared as a clinician in his college of pharmacy, but he had the opportunity to participate in theoretical training offered by the board of pharmacy of his state. He states:

"My school of pharmacy never made patient care a priority. To be honest, I didn't even know what pharmaceutical care really meant… So I took the introduction to pharmaceutical care course offered by the board and I fell in love with it. So, even though we did not have to take care of real patients during that course, I got my first patient just after that. And I haven't stopped since then."

Mario

For all respondents of the questionnaire, education is the rate-limiting step in making pharmaceutical care a reality in Brazil. It should be emphasized that the clinical pharmacy movement that happened in the United States of America in the 1960s did not occur in Brazil until the 1980s.[13] Also, this was a very small and isolated movement that took place only in a few Brazilian public universities. In Brazil, with the expansion of the pharmaceutical industry and the loss of control over the production of medicines, in the 1970s and the 1980s pharmacists moved away from the pharmacy and migrated to areas such as food technology, laboratory analysis, toxicology, and basic science research.[9,10] Moreover, new professions with a clearer definition of their professional responsibilities are emerging in Brazil (e.g., biomedicine), and these new professionals are quickly occupying a larger space in the market as compared to pharmacists. This might be due to the lack of clarity in the mission of pharmacy as a profession as well as to its crowded and superficial "generalist curriculum." Thus, differently from the USA, pharmacy education in Brazil did not shift toward clinical practice. In general, the curricula of colleges of pharmacy in Brazil do not focus on pharmacy practice nor have a clinical orientation. Pereira and Freitas,[14] in their article on the evolution of pharmaceutical care in Brazil, advocate for a more robust training of pharmacists on therapeutics, physiopathology, and problem-based learning as a meaningful means to encourage the development of the practice. In a chapter about the need to prepare a new pharmacist in Brazil, Ramalho de Oliveira[10] stresses the need to rethink the pedagogical project of a college of pharmacy whose mission is to prepare a practitioner who is capable to assist the health care team with managing patients' medications. The curriculum must provide the necessary experiences and nurture a culture that enables the preparation of pharmacists to assume responsibility for the outcomes of drug therapy.

It also should be mentioned that most colleges of pharmacy, especially the long-established ones in public universities, do not have clinical faculty members. Most professors are trained in basic sciences and perceive pharmacy education as a path to move students into graduate school rather than into clinical practice. However, it should be noted that new colleges of pharmacy are moving faster than the traditional ones in the direction of preparing a health care professional able to competently insert herself as a dynamic player into the health care system. Also, in the last decade clinical faculty members are becoming a little more prevalent in the new schools. But, it is worth emphasizing that a larger change in focus, or I would dare to say "an educational revolution," is crucial if a clinical pharmacist is to be prepared in Brazil.

Mario also mentions that currently his most significant challenge is the lack of support from pharmacy administration, which expects him to build a pharmaceutical care practice but still do dispensing and run the pharmacovigilance program. The bureaucratic and logistic aspects of drug distribution are still his major responsibility in the primary care clinic. He utters:

> *"I cannot do it all. I will get crazy! How can I get better in what I do and expand my practice if I cannot increase the number of patients I see every day? I need management to understand what it really takes to build a practice."*
>
> *Mario*

For this reason, Mario can only dedicate two half-days a week to his clinical practice and often he has to share his time between inventory control, dispensing, and medication management. He recognizes that accumulating all these responsibilities has not been working well because building a practice requires dedication, time, and a completely different set of skills than doing dispensing or administrative types of work. It is well discussed in the literature that pharmaceutical care and dispensing are different types of business that require different management systems and knowledge so that they should be separated.[7,8,10,15–18] But, for Mario's supervisor, all these activities are part of what she understands as "Atenção Farmacêutica" or pharmaceutical care.

A proposal of a national consensus in pharmaceutical care was published in Brazil in 2002, and according to the consensus dispensing, counseling, health education, and pharmacotherapeutic monitoring are all components of pharmaceutical care.[19] As pointed out by Freitas et al.,[20] defining pharmaceutical care as an umbrella that encompasses several pharmacy activities can be seen as problematic in the sense that it looks like we are giving new names to old activities instead of elucidating or even redefining the pharmacist's responsibility in direct patient care. However, it should be underscored that this consensus represented an important step toward a broader national debate about the role of the pharmacist in the health care system and an invitation to the pharmacy profession to envision new possibilities in creating a pharmacist practitioner. Since then several pharmaceutical care seminars and conferences have taken place in the country, organized both by professional organizations and the different levels of government. Also, the federal government has provided financial resources specifically for research in the area of pharmaceutical care.[12,21,22] Funchal-Witzel[23] conducted a descriptive study of the articles published by Brazilian authors between 1990 and 2007. She identified 324 peer-reviewed publications and a significant increase in the number of publications since 2006. Therefore, since the publication of the Brazilian consensus in pharmaceutical care in 2002, it is apparent that there is an increased interest and discussion about pharmaceutical care as well as an explicit effort to implement new practices and conduct research projects in diverse settings in Brazil.

Another pharmacist, Elena, is a professor at a college of pharmacy in Brazil and has been studying, teaching, and providing pharmaceutical care since 2005. With the objective to make pharmaceutical care a reality for her students, Elena partnered with the city government to supervise pharmacy and master students in a primary care ambulatory clinic. Thus, the practice is run by her and pharmacy students under her supervision. She states:

> *The primary care clinic is the perfect scenario for pharmaceutical care. In the Family Health Strategy we have health care teams taking care of a population and we can help the team to better manage their patients' medications by providing pharmaceutical care. It is unquestionably the best fit for a pharmacist practitioner."*
>
> *Elena*

The Family Health Strategy (*Estratégia Saúde da Família* or ESF) is the government's strategy launched in 1994 for restructuring municipal health systems in the SUS. This strategy emphasizes the reorganization of primary clinics to focus on families and communities to integrate medical care with health promotion and public health actions.[24] ESF is organized through family health care teams that are composed of one doctor, one nurse, one auxiliary nurse, and four to six community health works. These family health teams are assigned to specific geographical areas and defined populations of 600 to 1000 families.[2] The teams are focused on the social and physical environment of the family allowing for a broader perspective on the processes and experiences of health and illness. One of the assumptions of the ESF is to promote teamwork, which requires respect among all members of the team and the perception that the preparation of other professionals is not subordinate to medical training. It is expected that teamwork requires the establishment of new routines by all professionals[11,25,26] and new ways of teaching health care professionals.[27] In one of its official documents about the ESF, the Ministry of Health emphasizes the importance of a different and innovative approach to teamwork:

> "It proposes a new conception of work, a new form of relationship between members of the team, unlike the traditional biomedical model, allowing greater diversity of actions and continuous search for consensus. This relationship, based on interdisciplinarity, and no more associated with multidisciplinarity, connected with the nonacceptance of the refuge in the biological positivism, requires an approach that questions professionals' certainties and encourages ongoing horizontal communication between the components of a team. Thus, meaningful changes are necessary in professional approaches to individuals, families and communities, in order to occur, in fact, the effective implementation of a new model of health care."[25]

Even though the pharmacist was not included as an integral part of these teams, in 2008, the government introduced a bill to incorporate other health care providers (pharmacist, psychologist, physical therapist, physical educator, etc.) as supporting personnel to the ESF teams—Núcleo de Apoio a Saúde da Família or NASF.[28] Each supporting professional is expected to assist several health care teams. Pharmacists have been playing diverse roles in the ESF, which goes from inventory control to patient education to the delivery of medication management services.[29–31] A study conducted from May 2006 to January 2008 in Belo Horizonte (Minas Gerais) describes the process of implementation of pharmaceutical care services in a public primary care clinic and the introduction of the pharmacist as a team member in the ESF.[31–35] This study sheds light on the perspectives and experiences of patients, pharmacists, and other health professionals with the new service and unearths the challenges and benefits of adding a pharmacist in the care of patients in primary care. The work of Soler et al.[30] uses diverse ways to utilize pharmacists in the care of a population assigned to the ESF. This study depicts pharmacists doing group visits with patients living with specific chronic conditions (e.g., asthma, diabetes, and tuberculosis), participating in case management of high-risk patients, providing individual patient education, among other preventive actions. It should be emphasized that because of the focus on public health and population health by all spheres of government in Brazil, pharmacists are frequently involved in the design of policies and programs associated with health promotion and medication use. As discussed by Vieira,[36] besides being an actor in the strategies of health promotion in the area of population health, pharmacists should be more effectively incorporated into the health care team as a crucial effort to improve the use of medicines in the Brazilian health system. As pointed out numerous times in this text, what is missing in Brazil, as in other parts of the world, is the profession's definition of a standard of practice that unmistakably defines the clinical role of the pharmacist independently of the setting in which she or he works. As any other professional in health care, pharmacists need a patient care process that can be used with any patient in any kind of setting, and this is what pharmaceutical care practice offers to the profession of pharmacy. This does not mean that the pharmacist would not be able to be utilized in other ways to influence the health of a population, as they are presently utilized in Brazil. As one pharmacist observed:

"It is great that we are involved in health promotion and in making sure patients have access to medicines! But, we still need only one practice so that we can communicate to each other, to other professionals and to our patients."

The Family Health Strategy most likely represents the best opportunity for Brazilian pharmacists to demonstrate their value to the health care team,[10,28,30,31] and therefore, many pharmacists, such as Elena, perceive this as their possibility to implement and advance the practice of pharmaceutical care.

However, Elena emphasizes that the pharmacists who are part of the NASF are being more often than not utilized for inventory control and other administrative tasks. Furthermore, she is concerned that the pharmaceutical care practice she supervises is completely dependent on her students to function. For this reason, she is currently negotiating with the city government so that they can make a pharmacist available specifically to provide pharmaceutical care.

One concern several Brazilian pharmacists have, including myself, is the fact that several pharmaceutical care practices around the country are implemented for the sake of research. Master and Doctoral students implement a practice so that they can answer their specific research questions. Nonetheless, these practices tend to fade away as soon as the student has collected the necessary data for the completion of his or her work. This is an important problem that needs to be jointly addressed and resolved by the health care system and the academy.

In the other end of the continuum, there are Brazilian pharmacists building their practices in hospital settings and in community pharmacies with various degrees of success. For instance, a couple of respondent pharmacists have been providing pharmaceutical care in community pharmacies for over 8 years and they have reached significant clinical results and patient satisfaction.

As in other parts of the world, in Brazil pharmaceutical care can mean different things to different people. Pharmaceutical care might stand for the pharmacist's caring attitude toward the patient, or the act of sitting with a patient in a semiprivate room to educate him on a medical condition, or to assess and follow-up a patient using a specific medication, usually a very expensive one. In their questionnaire responses, several pharmacists describe their pharmaceutical care practices as the care they provide to patients using high-cost medications. In these cases, they do not refer to a holistic approach to the patient, which would mean to assess all of the patient's medical conditions and medications, but an approach that follows the treatment protocol for certain conditions such as hepatitis C, transplant, Hansen, tuberculosis, several types of cancer or HIV. Of course this is a very important approach for the Brazilian health care system, which is spending large sums of money to make these treatments available to the population. However, as previously discussed,[10] this is an old problem of the profession of pharmacy in that it endeavors to create a specialized practice before clearly defining and implementing a generalist one. Pharmacy needs a clear understanding of its mission in the health care system and a good way to start is by defining itself as a generalist practice with specific standards of practice that can be provided to the population as a whole, independently of the medication or the medical condition. Contrary to what is understood by most pharmacy organizations and colleges of pharmacy in Brazil, a generalist pharmacist is not someone who is able to engage superficially in many different activities, but one who is capable of providing a consistent service to any patient to prevent and resolve specific problems in the health care system.

What Might Lie Ahead?

Considering the current health care environment and established programs in Brazil (e.g., Family Health Strategy), this could be an exciting time for pharmacy and for pharmacists. The health care system has an interdisciplinary team that calls for pharmacists' expertise and a culture that values a holistic approach to patient care. It is the perfect time for pharmacists to stand up and become a key partner in the care of patients. In order for that to happen, colleges of pharmacy and the health care system need to align their interests and efforts to prepare the desired pharmacist, one who is truly capable of assuring the effective, safe, and convenient use of medications in Brazilian society. Nevertheless, some pharmacy faculty members like Maria do not foresee pharmacy education going through such a dramatic change. She states:

> "I am afraid pharmacy will never take this responsibility... if we consider the rigid structure of the more traditional colleges of pharmacy with faculty members without any clinical experience nor an understanding of what pharmaceutical care really is... Even in the newer colleges of pharmacy, where there are some clinical faculty, most of the financial resources go to basic research and the majority of teachers are interested in laboratory-based work. I have a pessimist vision towards the profession of pharmacy as I don't see that this profession will take responsibility for direct patient care, for the drug therapy of patients... We would have to create a new profession with a new mission."
>
> Maria

In view of the reality of the practice and the education of pharmacists in Brazil, in order for pharmaceutical care to prevail major changes and innovations must occur. First, the preparation of pharmacists has to be dramatically transformed. Colleges of pharmacy have to understand what a clinical practice really means in the health care system so that a specific and well-understood professional practice can be accepted by all faculty members and taught to all students. Furthermore, it is crucial that curricula create opportunities for students to acquire a great deal of experience with patients, with other members of the health care team and with the reality of the health care system. Interdisciplinary education is urgently needed in Brazil in order to create a culture of teamwork that might be later on transferred to the health care system.

It should be mentioned that in 2008 a new university reform was launched in Brazil. Among other measures, a massive investment plan called REUNI is doubling the federal university network in size, allowing for the implementation of interdisciplinary undergraduate courses.[37] For education of the health workforce, the SUS is provoking a strong political demand to replace the reductionist, disease-oriented, hospital-centered, specialization-driven pattern of professional education by one that is more humanistic, health-oriented, focused on primary health care, and socially committed.

In this context, the State, pushed by social movements, created initiatives such as REUNI and, particularly, the Pró-Saúde—a SUS-based program to reform higher education for the health workforce.[21] This should be seen as the biggest opportunity to include the pharmacist as an active member of the health care team in the public Brazilian health care system in the last decade or so.

Secondly, there must be more congruence between what is taught at colleges of pharmacy and what the health care system needs in terms of more cost-effective and safer use of medications in the Brazilian society. Perhaps, the federal government should find ways to encourage and reward universities to prepare pharmaceutical care practitioners who are capable of working collaboratively with other health professionals in the Family Health Strategy.

Thirdly, the federal government should build and introduce a pharmaceutical care policy that offers standards of practice and guidance on the process of building pharmaceutical care practices in the health care system. This would expound the right language and a consistent patient care process to be utilized by all professionals (e.g., pharmacists, nurses, physicians) who will be providing the service. For instance, the primary care department ("Departamento de Atenção Básica") at the federal level of SUS could define the standards of care, introduce, and monitor the outcomes of pharmaceutical care practices in the country. The "Departamento de Atenção Básica" operationalizes the Family Health Strategy's policy within the federal management, develops mechanisms of control and evaluation, and provides technical cooperation to municipalities and states in the implementation and organization of the Family Health Strategy. Thus, the same type of processes could be used to operationalize the implementation of pharmaceutical care at the primary care level in Brazil.

Therefore, for the profession of pharmacy to take charge of pharmaceutical care in Brazil, major changes have to occur in the education of future pharmacists. Moreover, the government can have a significant role in defining a practice that is consistent and follows specific quality standards across the country. This would guarantee that patients receive the same quality of service, independently of where she or he receives health care.

In Brazil there is an understanding that all the activities and services related to medicines—"Assistência Farmacêutica"—have to be perfectly organized before pharmacists can become involved in the provision of direct patient care. I believe this is a fallacy, and I would go further to state that it might be an excuse for not changing what pharmacists do. It is essential to guarantee access to medicines, but it is not enough! Especially in a time when Brazil is taking off as possibly the fifth largest economy in the world, there must be a way to guarantee that Brazilian patients will also benefit and not get harmed from the medicines they have access to. Even though it is not clear if pharmacy will be the profession to take the responsibility for the provision of pharmaceutical care in Brazil, it is apparent that patients have the right to receive a service that assures the best possible results from their drug therapy. Accordingly, pharmaceutical care must move from the everyday rhetoric and theorization of pharmacists to a reality in the lives of Brazilian patients, or another professional will have to step in and take this charge. Despite all the challenges the profession of pharmacy in all likelihood has to reinvent itself as a clinical profession. We must recognize that we have a professional practice—pharmaceutical care—that is well described and recognized and that if it is properly implemented and delivered to patients it can grant us the designation of a true health care provider. The Brazilian pharmacists cannot miss the ride!

REFERENCES

1. IBGE—Instituto Brasileiro de Geografia e Estatística. *Séries estatísticas & séries históricas.* Rio de Janeiro: O Instituto; 2010. http://seriesestatisticas.ibge.gov.br/lista_tema.aspx?op=0&no=10. Accessed June 15, 2011.
2. Paim J, Travassos C, Almeida C, et al. The Brazilian health system: history, advances, and challenges. *Lancet.* 2011;37:1778–1797.
3. Pego RA, Almeida CM. Teoria y práctica de las reformas de los sistemas de salud: los casos de Brasil y Mexico. [Theory and practice from health care reforms: the cases of Brazil and Mexico]. *Cad Saúde Pública.* 2002;4:971–989.
4. Conselho Federal de Farmácia. A assistência farmacêutica no SUS/Conselho Federal de Farmácia, Conselho Regional de Farmácia do Paraná; organização Comissão de Saúde Pública do Conselho Federal de Farmácia, Comissão de Assistência Farmacêutica do Serviço Público do CRF-PR. Brasília: Conselho Federal de Farmácia; 2010:60 p.
5. CFF—Conselho Federal de Farmácia. Estatísticas. 2010. Available at http://www.cff.org.br/pagina.phr?id=16&menu=16&titulo=estat%c3%adsticas. Accessed July 11, 2011.
6. Anuário das Graduações em Saúde 1995–2008. 2008. Observa RH—Estação de Trabalho IMS/UERJ. Available at http://www.obsnetims.org.br/atlas/farmacia.pdf. Accessed July 14th 2011.
7. Cipolle RJ, Strand LM, Morley PC. *Pharmaceutical Care Practice.* New York: McGraw-Hill; 1998.
8. Cipolle RJ, Strand LM, Morley PC. *Pharmaceutical Care Practice: The Clinician's Guide.* 2nd ed. New York: McGraw-Hill; 2004.
9. Silva WB. *A emergência da atenção farmacêutica: um olhar epistemológico e contribuições para o seu ensino* [The emergence of pharmaceutical care: an epistemological glimpse and the contributions for teaching]. 2009:305 p. Thesis (Doctorate in Scientific and Technological Education). Centro de Ciências da Educação, Universidade Federal de Santa Catarina, Florianópolis.
10. Ramalho de Oliveira D. *Atenção farmacêutica: da filosofia o gerenciamento da terapia medicamentosa* [*Pharmaceutical Care: From Its Philosophy to Medication Therapy Management*]. São Paulo: RCN Editora; 2011:328 p.

11. Brasil. Ministério da Educação. Resolução no. CNE/CES 2, de 19 de fevereiro de 2002. Institui as diretrizes curriculares Nacionais do Curso de Graduação em Farmácia. Diário Oficial da União, Mar 04, 2002.

12. Castro MS, Correr CJ. Pharmaceutical care in community pharmacies: practice and research in Brazil. *Ann Pharmacother.* 2007;41:1486–1493.

13. Funchal-Witzel MDR. *Aspectos conceituais e filosóficos da Assistência Farmacêutica, Farmácia Clínica e Atenção farmacêutica* [Conceptual and philosophical aspects of pharmaceutical assistance, clinical pharmacy and pharmaceutical care] In: Storpirtis S, et al. *Ciências Farmacêuticas: farmácia clínica e atenção farmacêutica.* Rio de Janeiro: Editora Guanabara Koogan; 2008.

14. Pereira LRL, Freitas O. A evolução da Atenção Farmacêutica e a perspectiva para o Brasil [The evolution of pharmaceutical care and the perspective for Brazil]. *Braz J Pharm Sci.* 2008;44(4):601–612.

15. Pereira ML, Ramalho de Oliveira D, Mendonça SM, et al. *Atenção Farmacêutica: implantação passo-a-passo* [*Pharmaceutical Care: Implementation Step by Step*]. Belo Horizonte: Faculdade de Farmácia, Universidade Federal de Minas Gerais; 2005.

16. Pereira ML, Ramalho de Oliveira D, Tirado MGA, Frade JCQP. Da Teoria à Prática: Relatos da Experiência de Implantação da Clínica de Atenção Farmacêutica em Minas Gerais, Brasil [*From theory to practice: experiences of implementation of pharmaceutical care in Minas Gerais, Brazil*]. *Latin Am J Pharm.* 2009;28(6):869–875. Available at http://www.latamjpharm.org/trabajos/28/6/LAJOP_28_6_1_10_8A8907011I.pdf. Accessed May 12th 2011.

17. Ramalho de Oliveira D, Brummel AR, Miller DB. Medication therapy management: 10 years of experience in a large integrated health care system. *J Manag Care Pharm.* 2010;16:185–195. http://www.amcp.org/data/jmcp/185-195.pdf. Accessed May 2011.

18. Ramalho de Oliveira, D. *The Reality of Pharmaceutical Care-based Medication Therapy Management: Patients', Pharmacists' and Students' Perspectives.* Koln: Lambert Academic Publishing; 2010:382 p.

19. OPAS—Organização Pan-americana da Saúde. *Consenso Brasileiro de Atenção Farmacêutica: proposta* [*Brazilian Consensus on Pharmaceutical Care: A Proposal*]. Brasília: Organização Pan-Americana da Saúde; 2002. http://bvsms.saude.gov.br/bvs/publicacoes/PropostaConsensoAtenfar.pdf. Accessed May 11, 2011.

20. Freitas EL, Ramalho de Oliveira D, Perini E. Atenção farmacêutica-teoria e prática: um dialogo possível? [Pharmaceutical Care—Theory and Practice: A Possible Dialogue?] *Acta Farm. Bonaerense.* 2006;25(3):447–453.

21. Ministério da Saúde, Ministério da Educação. National program for reorientation of professional preparation in health. 2007. http://prosaude.org/rel/pro_saude1.pdf. Accessed August 10, 2011 (in Portuguese).

22. Ministério da Saúde, Secretaria de Ciência, Tecnologia e Insumos Estratégicos, Departamento de Assistência Farmacêutica e Insumos Estratégicos. *O ensino e as pesquisas da atenção farmacêutica no âmbito do SUS* [*Education and Research in Pharmaceutical Care in the Unified Health System*]. Brasília: Ministério da Saúde; 2007:74–78.

23. Funchal-Witzel MDR. *Produção científica brasileira na área de atenção farmacêutica entre 1990 e 2007* [*Scientific Brazilian Production in the Area Of Pharmaceutical Care Between 1990 And 2007*]. 2009:94 p. Thesis (Master in Public Health). Programa de Pós-Graduação em Saúde Pública da Faculdade de Saúde Pública da Universidade de São Paulo, São Paulo.

24. Ministério da Saúde. *Saúde da Família: uma estratégia para reorientação do modelo assistencial.* [Family Health: a strategy to reorient the patient care model] 1997. http://bvsms.saude.gov.br/bvs/publicacoes/cd09_16.pdf. Accessed May 3, 2011.

25. Brasil. Ministério da Saúde. Cadernos de Atenção Básica: Programa de Saúde da Família. *A implantação da unidade de saúde da família. Caderno 1.* Brasília: Ministério da Saúde; 2000.

26. Brasil. Ministério da Saúde. Apostila: O Programa Saúde da Família e a atenção básica no Brasil, Brasília; 2002.

27. Santos MAM, Cutolo LRA. A interdisciplinaridade e o trabalho em equipe no Programa de Saúde da Família [The interdisciplinarity and teamwork in the Health Family Program]. *Arquivos Catarinenses de Medicina.* 2003;32(4):31–40. http://www.acm.org.br/revista/pdf/artigos/182.pdf. Acessed June 23, 2011.

28. Ministério da Saúde, Secretaria Atenção à Saúde. Portaria 154 de 18 de março de 2008. http://dab.saude.gov.br/nasf.php. Acessed June 23, 2011.

29. Severino P, Zanchetta B, Cavallini ME, Leme ALSA. A inserção do profissional farmacêutico no Programa de Saúde da Família [The insertion of the pharmacist in the Health Family Program]. *Rev Bras Farm.* 2008;89(1):56–58.

30. Soler O, Rosa MB, Fonseca AL, et al. Assistência farmacêutica clínica na atenção primária à saúde por meio do Programa Saúde da Família [Clinical Pharmacist assistance in primary care services offered through the family health program]. *Rev Bras Farm.* 2010;91(1): 37–45.

31. Ramalho de Oliveira D, Furtado BT, Mendonça SAM, Freitas EL. *Atenção Farmacêutica e a Estrategia Saúde da Família: Processo de implantacao e as experiencias dos profissionais envolvidos* [Pharmaceutical care and the Family Health Strategy: the implementation process and the experiences of the health professionals involved]. In review by Brazilian Journal of Pharmaceutical Sciences. Submitted December, 2011.

32. Ramalho de Oliveira D, Mendonça SAM, Furtado BT, Freitas EL. Programa Saúde da Família e Atenção Farmacêutica: Construindo uma nova realidade [Family Health Program and Pharmaceutical care: constructing a new reality]. [Abstract] In: I Seminário Internacional para Implementação da Atenção Farmacêutica no SUS, 2006, Brasília. *Anais do I Seminário Internacional para Implementação da Atenção Farmacêutica no SUS.* 2006;1: 1–121.

33. Ramalho de Oliveira D, Mendonça SAM, Furtado BT, Freitas EL. Atenção Farmacêutica no Programa Saúde da Família [Pharmaceutical care in the Family Health Program]. [Abstract] In: 2° Seminário de Atenção Básica do SUS BH, 2007, Belo Horizonte. *Livro de Resumos do 2° Seminário de Atenção Básica do SUS BH.* 2007;1:1–246.

34. Ramalho de Oliveira D, Mendonça SAM, Furtado BT, Freitas EL, Silva L. A Estratégia Saúde da Família e a prática da atenção farmacêutica [The Strategy of Family Health and pharmaceutical care practice]. [Abstract] In: I Congresso Nacional de Saúde da Faculdade de Medicina da UFMG, 2008, Belo Horizonte. *Rev Méd Minas Gerais.* Belo Horizonte: Coopmed; 2008;18:40–40.

35. Ramalho de Oliveira D, Mendonça SAM, Furtado BT, Freitas EL, Silva L. "Yo no sabía que había farmacêutico": La integración de la atención farmacêutica en los equipos de salud, en Belo Horizonte, Brasil ["I didn't know there was a pharmacist": the integration of pharmaceutical care in the health care team, Belo Horizonte, Brazil]. [Abstract] In: VI Congreso Nacional de Atención Farmacéutica, 2009, Sevilla. *Rev Pharm Care Esp.* Barcelona: Ediciones Mayo. 2009;11:32–33.

36. Vieira FS. Possibilidades de contribuição do farmacêutico para a promoção da saúde [How pharmacists can contribute to health promotion]. *Ciência e Saúde Coletiva.* 2007;12(1):213–220.

37. Almeida-Filho N. Higher education and health care in Brazil. *Lancet.* 2011;377: 1898–1900.

CANADA

Barbara Gobis Ogle, BSc(Pharm), ACPR, MScPhm

Pharmacist Consultant
North Vancouver, British Columbia, Canada

Health Care in Canada

A Publicly Funded System

Canada's 34 million citizens receive most of their health care through a publicly funded health care system as outlined in federal legislation known as the Canada Health Act.[1] The federal government establishes criteria and conditions for insured health services and extended health care services, and provides funding to the provinces and territories to administer health care at the local level. The goal is to ensure that all eligible residents of Canada have reasonable access to insured health services on a prepaid basis, without direct charges at the point of care.[2]

Payment for Drugs and Pharmacist Services

Drug therapies are not covered within the Canada Health Act except in a hospital setting. Provincial and territorial governments offer drug programs to help people with their drug costs, with drug coverage typically being determined by need (presence of disease), and ability to pay. Of the $21 billion spent on prescribed drugs in Canada in 2006, 46% was financed by the public sector, and 36% was funded by private insurers. The remaining $3.9 billion was paid directly out-of-pocket by Canadian households.[3]

As the largest payers for drug therapies, the provincial and territorial governments make decisions on which products and services are paid for, what prices are paid, and the drug coverage policies within their own jurisdictions. The pharmacist services covered under public drug programs have traditionally been related to dispensing events. In recent years, public payers have become increasingly interested in exploring different ways to pay pharmacists for patient care–related services independent of dispensing the prescription. For example, both Ontario and British Columbia (BC) pay pharmacists fees for providing medication review–type services and preparing current medication lists for patients.[4,5] BC also pays pharmacists fees for adapting prescriptions and administering publicly funded vaccines to eligible residents.[6,7]

Pharmacists in Canada

Regulation

Pharmacy is a self-governing profession in Canada. Pharmacists must meet legal requirements, be registered, and maintain a license in good standing with the appropriate provincial or territorial regulatory authority in order to practice.

As of January 1, 2010, Canada had 32,586 licensed pharmacists and 8718 accredited, licensed pharmacies (of note—Northwest Territories, Yukon, Nunavut, and Quebec do not license pharmacies, only pharmacists)[8] (Table 12-5).

Education and Training

Ten Canadian universities offer educational programs leading to an undergraduate (Bachelor of Science) degree in pharmacy. Most undergraduate pharmacy programs are 4 years in length and require the completion of at least 1 year of additional undergraduate study prior to entering the pharmacy program.[9] Bridging programs are also available to assist foreign-trained pharmacists in getting licensed to practice in Canada.[10]

The University of British Columbia and University of Toronto (Ontario) both offer a 2-year postbaccalaureate Doctor of Pharmacy Degree (PharmD) and produce 6 to 21 graduates per year.[11,12] This postgraduate degree is different than the entry-level Pharm D in that it prepares the student to be an advanced practitioner over and above the entry-to-practice requirements. The Canadian Pharmacists Association and the Association of Faculties of Pharmacy of Canada support the transition of all entry-level pharmacist education programs in Canada to the entry-level Doctor of Pharmacy program.[13,14]

Two universities now offer the PharmD as the first professional degree, without the prerequisite Bachelor of Science of Pharmacy degree. The

Table 12-5 Pharmacists and Pharmacies in Canada: National Statistics[64]

National pharmacists/pharmacies statistics	2010
Total licensed pharmacists	32,586
Pharmacies*:	
Community pharmacies	8,428
In-patient hospital pharmacies, if licensed by regulatory authority	290
Total licensed pharmacies	8718

* Northwest Territories, Yukon, Nunavut, and Québec *do not* license pharmacies; figures are for information purposes only.

University of Montreal (Quebec) enrolled its first entry-level PharmD class in September 2007 and the University of Laval (Quebec) enrolled its first class in 2010.[15,16] Most other Canadian universities are exploring program changes to offer the PharmD as the first professional degree.[17]

Pharmacy educational programs in Canada continue to evolve to provide graduates with the knowledge, skills, and values needed to

- carry out their primary practice responsibility of direct patient care,
- with the goal of decreasing drug-related morbidity and mortality, promoting health, and preventing disease,
- through the provision of pharmaceutical care.[18]

Pharmacists must maintain a high level of competence throughout their careers to maintain their license to practice pharmacy in Canada as outlined in the National Association of Pharmacy Regulatory Authorities (NAPRA), National Model Continuing Competence Program for Canadian Pharmacists.[19] Competency assessment programs are administered provincially and can include pharmacists collecting a minimum number of continuing education credits, pharmacists completing written knowledge assessment exams, or pharmacists preparing a portfolio of documentation for their clinical practice.[20]

Where Pharmacists Practice

The majority (over 70%) of licensed pharmacists in Canada work in community pharmacies, whereas 15% work in hospitals.[21] Pharmacists also work in the pharmaceutical industry, governments, colleges and universities, and associations.

Individual pharmacists usually do not have billing numbers or other means to bill third-party payers directly for services they provide to patients. Within the community setting, public and private third-party payers typically have agreements with pharmacy owners/managers for service delivery and payment. Consequently, most pharmacists work as employees. Only a select few work as consultants or independent clinical practitioners.

Pharmacists working in hospitals, clinics, and other clinic-type settings are usually salaried, unionized employees of the local, publicly funded health authority. Community-based pharmacists are usually salaried employees working for private, for-profit drugstore chains or individual small business owners. Some provinces maintain a requirement that a pharmacy owner must be a pharmacist, but most are not and the Canadian drugstore sector tends to be driven by the retail business agenda.

Most practicing pharmacists in Canada have the entry-level BSc pharmacy degree. The small number of graduate-trained pharmacists (PharmD or

MSc) in Canada usually work in management, hospital, or atypical advanced practice settings.

Pharmacist Practice Change in Canada

Canada's health care system is facing significant pressure due to increased demand, finite budgets, and limited capacity to meet this demand. Payers continue to seek ways to maximize efficiency in health care delivery and maximize value for the health care dollar.

Within every challenge lies opportunity, and Canadian pharmacy leaders have been actively working with health care payers and decision makers to expand the focus of pharmacist practice from primarily a product-based (dispending) model to a broader, patient care–based model.

In 2007, a Task Force was formed to undertake a consultation process with a broad range of pharmacy stakeholders across Canada, and define a vision and clear action plan for the future of pharmacy.[22] The result was a "Blueprint for Pharmacy" with a vision for pharmacy of, "optimal drug therapy outcomes for Canadians through patient-centered care."[23] This Blueprint includes key strategic actions for pharmacy human resources; education and continuing professional development; information and communication technology, financial viability, and sustainability; and legislation, regulation, and liability.[24]

Within each province and territory, regulatory changes are either in development or in place to expand the pharmacist's scope of practice to include administration of injections and immunizations, authority to adapt (renew and change) prescriptions, and initial prescribing of drug therapy in specific clinical situations.[25]

Government Initiatives

Around the same time as the pharmacy Task Force was formed, provincial governments started making changes to the traditional compensation models for community pharmacies.[26] Public (government) payers have used a variety of strategies to introduce policies that "drive down" drug prices and increase transparency in drug prices. In return for their cooperation, government payers are re-investing some of the savings from drug prices into community pharmacies in the form of funding for pharmacist practice change initiatives.[27]

Although the end goal is for Canadian pharmacists in all patient-care settings to provide comprehensive medication management, pharmacist practice change has been occurring at different rates and in different ways in two general streams in Canada:

- within the hospital and health authority environment,
- within the community pharmacy environment.

Medication Management in Canada

Hospital-based Practice

Pharmacists have been providing pharmaceutical care to patients in hospital settings since the early 1990s.[28] The challenge of implementing a comprehensive medication management service with limited staff resources triggered a study comparing the drug-related problems identified and resolved using pharmaceutical care versus traditional clinical drug monitoring at a 350-bed community hospital in BC.[29] Data collection was carried out prospectively over two 8-week periods on two general medicine wards. In the first phase, pharmacists provided drug monitoring of target patients receiving specific drugs. After receiving 4 months of training to learn and practice providing pharmaceutical care, the same pharmacists returned to the wards and provided care to patients using a pharmaceutical care approach. The researchers concluded that focusing clinical services on selected patients and providing comprehensive pharmaceutical care to these patients resulted in the identification and resolution of significantly more drug-related problems than using equivalent staff to carry out drug-specific or problem-specific monitoring for a larger number of patients.

The Clinical Pharmacy Services Study (CPSS) provided further evidence of the value of having pharmacists spend more time providing comprehensive services to patients and less time on drug distribution and drug-specific monitoring.[30,31] In the CPSS, 15 Ontario hospitals provided data from pharmacists providing three different levels of care to hospitalized patients: Drug Order Review (the regular screening of drug orders for general accuracy), Basic Pharmacotherapy Monitoring (synonymous with clinical drug monitoring where a patient's care is reviewed for the purposes of evaluating specific drug therapy), and Concurrent Pharmacotherapy Monitoring (synonymous with comprehensive medication management and ongoing monitoring of patients, their drug therapies and response to therapy).

In terms of return on investment, the median "recommendations per hour of total pharmacist time" was 0.67 (Drug Order Review), 0.98 (Basic Pharmacotherapy Monitoring), and 1.22 (Concurrent Pharmacotherapy Monitoring). Extrapolating these results to a hypothetical 37-bed medical ward, the number of pharmacist recommendations expected per day would be 1 (when only Drug Order Review services are provided), 3 (when Basic Pharmacotherapy Monitoring services are provided), and 11 (when Concurrent Pharmacotherapy Monitoring services are provided). These figures raise the question, "what are the consequences of unresolved drug-related problems in hospitals with less pharmacist monitoring available?"

Concurrent Pharmacotherapy Management services were shown to provide greater benefit to patients and also require an investment in resources (staff and technology), education and training of pharmacists, reorganization of workload to maximize pharmacists' time for patient care and organization of service delivery so pharmacists have unlimited access to patients.[32]

In spite of fiscal pressures, hospital pharmacists have had success pressing for the necessary changes so pharmacists can focus their time on providing comprehensive medication management to patients.[33,34] One example is the regulation of pharmacy technicians in several Canadian jurisdictions.[35,36]

IMPACT Project and Pharmacists on Family Health Care Teams in Ontario

IMPACT was a demonstration project supported by the Ontario Primary Health Care Transition Fund from 2004 to 2006.[37] The goal of IMPACT was to improve drug therapy using a collaborative care model that integrates pharmacists into the primary health care team. The pharmacists' main role in the team was conducting individual patient assessments to identify, prevent, or resolve drug-related problems. The Primary Health Care Transition Fund was a large-scale federal initiative where the Government of Canada provided $800 million in funding to the provinces and territories to support their efforts to reform the primary health care system.[38] IMPACT received project funding specifically from the Ontario funding envelope.

The IMPACT demonstration project involved multiple sites, seven pharmacists (two with PharmD degrees and the rest with BSc degrees), approximately 70 physicians and care to approximately 150,000 patients. Family physicians from a range of practice models (Ontario Family Health Networks, Primary Care Networks (PCNs), and other types of family physician group practices) participated. Within each practice site, a pharmacist was paid a salary through the project to work 2.5 days per week for 1 year, and coordinate a multifaceted intervention, including patient assessments to identify and resolve medication problems, to optimize drug therapy and improve patient outcomes.[39] IMPACT pharmacists received project-specific training and underwent a major transformation in how they thought, practiced and related with other health care professionals during the project.[40]

The IMPACT project itself has provided a wealth of information and learning about the process of integrating pharmacists with primary health care teams and the impact of the comprehensive medication management services on patients.[41] For example, pharmacists learned the importance of, and how to, document their patient assessments. A specific identity and role for pharmacists also developed within the health care team. The researchers developed tools to assess pharmacist contributions to patient care within a team, and pharmacists learned practical primary care skills (such as interviewing a patient, conducting an assessment, taking a blood pressure measurement, and prioritizing multiple drug-related problems).

The efforts of IMPACT, in conjunction with other local initiatives and policy changes, have paved the way for longer-term change in health care delivery in Ontario.[42] The use of multidisciplinary care teams has evolved into interdisciplinary practice groups called Family Health Teams (FHTs). Since April 2005, 170 FHTs have been created across the province. It is expected that the 170 teams will improve access to health care for more than 2.7 million Ontarians. In August 2010, the government announced 30 more teams bringing the total number of FHTs in Ontario to 200.[43]

All the practice locations involved in the IMPACT project became FHTs and have elected to include a pharmacist position within their staffing compliment. As of 2008, 67 full-time equivalents (FTEs) for pharmacist services had been approved and funded for FHTs across Ontario.[44] References and tools from the IMPACT project continue to be available to any pharmacist wanting to enhance their practice within a family health care team.[45] Examples of available tools include resources for the clinic manager (pharmacist job descriptions, orientation for staff, and how to identify patients who might benefit from consultation with a pharmacist), resources for the practicing physicians (orientation for pharmacy services, sample pharmacist consult letters, and examples of practice innovations), and support for the pharmacist (sample consults, support materials, and educational resources).

The Ontario Ministry of Health and Long-Term Care has made extensive resources available on-line to assist practitioners in setting up FHTs in Ontario communities.[46] Guidelines for hiring and compensating nonphysician interdisciplinary health care providers are also available. The salary range for a full-time (1 FTE) pharmacist is $61,685 CAN to $88,869 CAN plus an additional 20% for benefits. This salary does not include overhead compensation and is based on a 40-hour work week. Part-time and sessional rates are derived from the salary ranges provided.[47]

Other Regionally Funded Pharmacist Positions: Saskatchewan and Alberta

Other Canadian provinces are at various stages of piloting, evaluating, implementing, and funding pharmacist positions within health teams in local health authorities. Two such initiatives are in Alberta and Saskatchewan.

In 2003, Alberta Health and Wellness, the Alberta Medical Association and Alberta's Regional Health Authorities (now Alberta Health Services) established the Primary Care Initiative (PCI) to improve patient access to family physicians and other frontline health care providers in Alberta. The purpose of the PCI was to develop PCNs and support them in meeting the objectives of the program.[48] The "Integrating Pharmacists into Primary Care Networks" pilot project was started in April 2006 to improve medication therapy and patient outcomes. Four million dollars in funding was committed to support implementation and evaluation of 30 pharmacists working part time in PCNs.[49] In the project, pharmacists engaged by PCNs worked collaboratively with patients, physicians and other allied health professionals offering "structured medication reviews" to identify, prevent, and resolve drug-related problems in challenging, complex and chronic care patients. Results of the evaluation have not been widely released and, in the meantime, pharmacists continue their PCN work.

Saskatchewan Health currently funds 23 primary health care (PHC) pharmacists practicing part-time in Primary Care Sites across the province. These PHC pharmacists report directly to the PHC Director and/or the Director of Pharmacy within each Region and are physically co-located with other members of the PHC teams. Minimum requirements for PHC pharmacists include a bachelor's degree in pharmacy and experience practicing Pharmaceutical Care, including activities such as conducting patient interviews and medication reviews; developing, implementing, and monitoring patient care plans; and communicating or collaborating with the interdisciplinary care team as required.[50,51] Another 20 to 30 (part-time) pharmacists receive ongoing funding through local health authorities to provide selected specialty services in urban specialty practice sites.

Community-based Initiatives

Canadian pharmacists in community settings have been slower at integrating patient-focused comprehensive medication management into their practices.[52] Pharmacy owners generally agree that new models for pharmacist services and compensation are needed. They are calling for strategies to manage the transition to a funding model based on pharmacist services in collaboration with public payers, rather than proceed directly to comprehensive medication management.[53]

The governments of Alberta and BC have taken the biggest steps to support the development of comprehensive medication management as the standard patient care service provided by community pharmacy-based pharmacists.

Demonstration Project: The Alberta Pharmacy Practice Models Initiative

In 2008, Alberta Health and Wellness provided funding to the Alberta Pharmacists Association to

- build an innovative service model that utilizes the full scope of pharmacist's knowledge, skills, and competencies to achieve optimal drug utilization in the community setting,
- run a demonstration project to show the impact of services on patient outcomes,

- provide decision makers with useful information to help create new remuneration models for patient care services.[54]

The service model chosen for the Alberta Pharmacy Practice Models Initiative (PPMI) was based on the pharmaceutical care philosophy and combined a standard comprehensive medication management care process with the unique scope of pharmacist practice in Alberta and the Alberta Standard of Pharmacist Practice.[55] Other elements of the Alberta PPMI service model were

- provided independent of dispensing,
- suitable for appointments,
- pharmacist training and support,
- documentation of care,
- integrated quality management,
- remuneration using a resource-based relative value model,
- on-line billing procedures.

Figure 12-7 provides an overview of the patient care process used in the Alberta PPMI.

The remuneration model used for the PPMI was a bundled fee per service episode. Fees were calculated in two parts

- a baseline fee for the patient assessment, care plan, and evaluation,
- a premium for specific interventions that required the pharmacist to accept additional, direct responsibility for patient care (e.g., adapting a prescription, prescribing in an emergency, advanced prescribing authorization, administering an injection, or diabetes education for self-management).

The baseline fee was determined using a Resource-Based Relative Value Scale (RBRVS) to reflect the variable intensity and duration of service as

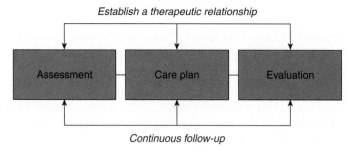

Figure 12-7 Alberta Pharmacy Practice Models Initiative: steps in the patient care process.[65]

Table 12-6   Drug therapy problem summary for 18,623 patients with 33,993 encounters in the Alberta PPMI[65]

Drug therapy problem type		Number of drug therapy problems
Indication	Unnecessary drug therapy	832 (2%)
	Needs additional drug therapy	21,575 (55%)
Effectiveness	Ineffective drug	1235 (3%)
	Dosage too low	6811 (17%)
Safety	Adverse drug reaction	2170 (5%)
	Dosage too high	1717 (4%)
Compliance	Noncompliance	5177 (13%)
Total		39,517

determined by patient complexity and need. Baseline fees also included extra funding to cover project-related costs, and ranged from $54 to $126 for a new contact and from $36 to $108 for a follow-up contact depending on patient complexity. Patient complexity was determined by the number of medications (Rx, OTC, or natural health product), medical conditions and drug therapy problems present.[56]

Between March 1, 2009 and June 30, 2010, 186 pharmacist participants working at 107 pharmacy sites engaged a total of 18,623 patients in 33,993 encounters, resulting in the resolution of 39,517 drug therapy problems. The total amount billed by pharmacies during the project was $2,133,263.40, with an average of $114.22 per patient and $62.36 per encounter. A total of 39,517 drug therapy problems were identified and resolved among the 18,623 patients. Table 12-6 provides a detailed summary of the types of drug therapy problems identified and resolved.[57]

The pharmacists with the greatest success in the PPMI were those who effectively delegated technical and administrative tasks to others, had buy-in and ongoing support of pharmacy management, and had collaborative relationships with local physicians and other health care providers.

Although the Alberta government intended to develop a payment model for ongoing medication management services based on the PPMI, the results were insufficient to meet decision-making needs. As of May 2011, the future of medication management service provision by community-based pharmacists in Alberta remains on hold as the government takes more time to work with pharmacy representatives and other health care professionals to define a service and payment model that pharmacists can successfully implement within their current work environments.[58]

Demonstration Project: The British Columbia Medication Management Project   In BC, the Pharmaceutical Services Division (PSD) of the BC Ministry of Health and the BC Pharmacy Association entered into an agreement in 2008 whereby government would re-invest some savings from drug policy changes in the design, development, and future implementation of demonstration projects for medication management and review.[59]

The result is the BC Medication Management Project (BCMMP), which got underway in the fall of 2010 with 291 pharmacists from 118 community pharmacies located across the province.[60] The project's purpose is to support pharmacists in providing a standardized medication management service to patients in the community, thereby improving patient care, drug therapy outcomes, and the sustainability of the health care system.[61]

The BCMMP involves a comprehensive medication management service where the pharmacist develops a relationship and works together with the patient to optimize safe and effective medication use and improve health outcomes. The service includes

- preparing and reviewing a detailed medication history,
- identifying any medication management issues (drug-related problems),
- setting patient-focused goals,
- implementing solutions to address issues and meet goals,
- monitoring effects and modifying solutions according to changing patient need,
- documenting care,
- communicating and collaborating with the patient's health care team.[62]

Data collection in the project will continue until January 31, 2012, and an evaluation of the results will be used to inform decision making about future services provided by community pharmacists and associated remuneration models. Interim results are not yet available.

Although some aspects of BCMMP are similar to the Alberta PPMI, a few significant differences exist. The BC service model is based on comprehensive medication management without the region-specific modifications added in Alberta. Pharmacists in BC can provide comprehensive medication management without the requirement for any additional scope of practice. Both projects use an RBRVS in the remuneration model, but in BC the service fees payable are based on the services rendered, with separate allowance payments built into the project to support the extra work and expense associated with IT set-up, pharmacist training and data collection. The Alberta PPMI used bundled service fees that combined remuneration for service and project support together.

The biggest difference to date is that, in BC, the Ministry of Health entered into a subsequent agreement with the BC Pharmacy Association and Canadian Association of Chain Drugstores whereby a commitment was made to fund transitional clinical pharmacy services, such a medication reviews, for all community-based pharmacists in addition to project funding. These clinical pharmacy services allow pharmacists outside the project to prepare themselves for the transition to comprehensive medication management in the future.[63] In Alberta, only a subset of pharmacists participated in the PPMI and service provision stopped once the project (and funding) stopped in 2010. Negotiations continue on how to define, fund and integrate comprehensive medication management services into existing and emerging health care delivery models.

Challenges and Opportunities

The future of comprehensive medication management in Canada will ultimately depend on the ability of pharmacists to maintain their focus on patient care services in the face of ongoing economic, political, and retail pressures.

Public and Private Funding Models

Third-party (mainly government) payers are working with pharmacy leaders to establish workable payment models and policies to support pharmacist practice change. The system, however, does not have new money to pay for these new services. Payers expect new services to be funded by savings generated from efficiencies, reduced costs and reduced utilization of existing health resources, and produce improved patient outcomes. These conversations are challenging, especially since they are happening at the same time as other sectors of health care including hospitals and medical physicians are asking for more funding.

Private payers in Canada traditionally position themselves as the second payer with public payers as the first payer. Private payers are therefore expected to wait until the public payers have defined the specific payment levels, deliverables, and eligibility criteria for comprehensive medication management before developing programs to cover pharmacist patient care services. Moreover, private payers will respond when their customers (the employers) start asking for these kinds of services to be covered. Pharmacists need to demonstrate the value of comprehensive medication management services to decision makers on the front line.

Pharmacist–physician Relationships

Relationships between pharmacists and physicians have evolved in recent years but still have a long way to go. Individual physicians working with individual pharmacists in the care of mutual patients generally have a positive view of pharmacists if the working relationships are also positive. Some pharmacists just do not understand the importance of this working relationship and, in these situations, physician opinions of pharmacists tend to be less favorable.

Physicians at the political and advocacy levels generally view pharmacists as competition for limited health care dollars and as threats to physician control of patient care. The typical issues raised by physician groups are

- pharmacists should not be trying to "practice medicine,"
- pharmacist reports and phone calls increase physician workload,
- pharmacist efforts increase fragmentation of patient care,
- pharmacist efforts can erode the sacred patient–physician relationship.

Pharmacists need to be aware of the importance of relationships with other health care professionals and persevere in a respectful and collaborative manner and eventually physician issues will go away.

Innovative Practice Settings
Perhaps the greatest challenge pharmacists face in their practice change efforts relates to the complex, interdependent relationship pharmacists have with community pharmacy owners. Some pharmacists are becoming increasingly frustrated with the challenge of being a professional within a retail environment. This frustration is driving more pharmacists to seek innovative practice settings such as employment contracts with regional health authorities, participation in demonstration projects and even seeking out nontraditional employers like home care agencies. A small number of pharmacists are exploring ways to become licensed as nondispensing, clinical pharmacies so they can sign agreements and submit claims to public payers using existing pharmacy payment mechanisms.

Pharmacists will need to be increasingly creative in community practice settings. Pharmacy technicians are becoming regulated and licensed to take over technical dispensing functions, and the cost of dispensing technologies is coming down. The net result will be a reduced need for pharmacists to do traditional dispensing work in Canadian retail community pharmacies.

At all levels, the key for pharmacists is to maintain a clear vision for their role within the Canadian health care system and not let political, market-share, or retail agendas distract them from providing comprehensive medication management services for patients.

No matter what barriers exist or arise, pharmacists must not waver from their focus of taking care of patients. Patients who do receive comprehensive medication management services from a pharmacist are generally very satisfied with the care and health benefits they receive. Ultimately, the benefits to patients are all that really matter. Individual pharmacists who are determined to provide comprehensive medication management to patients, decision makers, and relatives of decision makers will lead the way and eventually they will reach the tipping point whereby comprehensive medication management becomes the generally accepted standard for all pharmacists in Canada.

REFERENCES

1. Statistics Canada. *Population Estimates and Projections.* http://www40.statcan.ca/l01/cst01/demo23b-eng.htm. Accessed April 23, 2011.
2. Health Canada. *Health Care System. Canada Health Act.* http://www.hc-sc.gc.ca/hcs-sss/medi-assur/cha-lcs/index-eng.php. Accessed April 23, 2011.
3. Canadian Institute for Health Information. *Pharmaceutical Care and Utilization.* http://www.cihi.ca/CIHI-ext-portal/internet/en/Document/types+of+care/pharmaceutical/FAQ_PCU_DID_YOU_KNOW. Accessed April 23, 2011.
4. Ontario Ministry of Health and Long-Term Care. *Public Information: About MedsCheck.* http://health.gov.on.ca/en/public/programs/drugs/medscheck/. Accessed April 23, 2011.
5. Medication Review Services Guidelines for Pharmacists. *BC PharmaCare.* April 1, 2011. http://www.health.gov.bc.ca/pharmacare/pdf/medrevguide.pdf. Accessed July 13, 2011.
6. BC PharmaCare Newsletter. March 25, 2011 Edition 11–004. http://www.health.gov.bc.ca/pharmacare/newsletter/news11-004.pdf. Accessed July 13, 2011.
7. Resource Guide for Pharmacists and Publicly Funded Vaccine. October 2010. http://www.health.gov.bc.ca/pharmacare/pdf/ResourceGuideforPharmacistsandPubliclyFunded-Vaccine-FINAL.pdf. Accessed July 13, 2011.
8. National Association of Pharmacy Regulatory Authorities. *Pharmacy Practice and Regulatory Resources.* National Statistics. http://napra.ca/pages/Practice_Resources/National_Statistics.aspx. Accessed April 23, 2011.
9. Canadian Pharmacists Association. Directory. *Canadian Faculties and Schools of Pharmacy.* http://www.pharmacists.ca/content/about_cpha/about_pharmacy_in_can/directory/associations.cfm?main_heading=Canadian$Faculties$and$Schools$of$Pharmacy.Accessed April 23, 2011.
10. University of Toronto. Lesley Dan Faculty of Pharmacy. International Pharmacy Graduate Program. http://www.ipgcanada.ca/. Accessed April 24, 2011.
11. University of British Columbia. Faculty of Pharmaceutical Sciences. Doctor of Pharmacy Program Overview. http://www.pharmacy.ubc.ca/programs/degree-programs/PharmD. Accessed April 23, 2011.
12. University of Toronto. Lesley Dan Faculty of Pharmacy. Doctor of Pharmacy. http://pharmacy.utoronto.ca/programs/pharmd.htm. Accessed April 23, 2011.
13. *CPhA Position Statement on a Doctor of Pharmacy Degree as an Entry-Level to Practice.* Canadian Pharmacists Association. 2009. http://www.pharmacists.ca/content/about_cpha/who_we_are/policy_position/pdf/PharmD%20Entry%20Level.pdf. Accessed April 23, 2011.
14. *Educational Outcomes for First Professional Degree Programs in Pharmacy (Entry-to-Practice Pharmacy Programs) in Canada.* Association of Faculties of Pharmacy of Canada. Annual General meeting, Vancouver BC, June 3, 2010. http://afpc.info/downloads/1/AFPC_Education_Outcomes_AGM_June_2010.pdf. Accessed April 23, 2011.

15. Universite de Montreal. Faculte de pharmacie. Doctorat en pharmacie. http://www.pharm. umontreal.ca/etudes_cycle1/pharmd.html Accessed April 23, 2011.

16. Universite Laval. Faculte de pharmacie. Admission au doctorat de premier cycle (Pharm D). http://translate.google.com/translate?hl=en&sl=fr&u=http://www.pha.ulaval. ca/&ei=OjCzTby-PIKosQOt08ThCw&sa=X&oi=translate&ct=result&resnum=6&ve d=0CEMQ7gEwBQ&prev=/search%3Fq%3DU%2Bof%2Blaval%2BPharm%2BD% 26hl%3Den%26safe%3Doff%26client%3Dfirefox-a%26hs%3DMuj%26rls%3Dorg. mozilla:en-US:official%26prmd%3Divns. Accessed April 23, 2011.

17. Koleba T, Marin JG, Jewesson PJ. Entry-level PharmD degree programs in Canada: some facts and stakeholder opinions. *Can Pharm J.* 2006;139(6):42–50. http://www. pharmacists.ca/content/cpjpdfs/nov_dec06/EntryLevelPharmD_Koleba.pdf. Accessed April 25, 2011.

18. AFPC Mission Statement for Pharmacy Education in Canada. Association of Faculties of Pharmacy of Canada. http://www.afpc.info/content.php?SectionID=2&Language=en. Accessed April 23, 2011.

19. National Model Continuing Competence Program for Canadian Pharmacists. National Association of Pharmacy Regulatory Authorities. 2002. http://napra.ca/pages/Practice_ Resources/contiuning_competence.aspx?id=2091. Accessed July 13, 2011.

20. College of Pharmacists of BC. Professional Development and Assessment Program. http:// www.bcpharmacists.org/professional_development/professional_development/index.php. Accessed April 23, 2011.

21. Canadian Pharmacists Association. *About Pharmacy in Canada.* http://www.pharmacists. ca/content/about_cpha/about_pharmacy_in_can/index.cfm. Accessed April 24, 2011.

22. Task Force on a Blueprint for Pharmacy. *Blueprint for Pharmacy: The Vision for Pharmacy.* Ottawa (ON): Canadian Pharmacists Association; 2008. http://www.pharmacists. ca/content/about_cpha/whats_happening/cpha_in_action/pdf/BlueprintVision.pdf. Accessed April 24, 2011.

23. *Blueprint for Pharmacy: The Vision for Pharmacy. About the Vision.* http://blueprintforpharmacy.ca/home. Accessed April 24, 2011.

24. Task Force on a Blueprint for Pharmacy. *Blueprint for Pharmacy: The Vision for Pharmacy.* Ottawa (ON): Canadian Pharmacists Association; 2008. http://www.pharmacists.ca/ content/about_cpha/whats_happening/cpha_in_action/pdf/BlueprintVision.pdf. Accessed April 24, 2011.

25. *Blueprint for Pharmacy: The Vision for Pharmacy. Policy Changes by Region.* http://blueprint-forpharmacy.ca/policy-changes-by-region Accessed April 24, 2011.

26. Turning Point for Pharmacy. *2010 CACDS Report.* Canadian Association of Chain Drug Stores; 2010:4–14. http://www.cacds.com/supplement/index.html. Accessed April 24, 2011.

27. *Blueprint for Pharmacy: The Vision for Pharmacy. Policy Changes by Region.* http://blueprint-forpharmacy.ca/policy-changes-by-region. Accessed April 24, 2011.

28. *Pharmaceutical Care: Information Paper on the Evolution of Patient Pharmacotherapy Monitoring to Pharmaceutical Care.* Canadian Society of Hospital Pharmacists; 1994.

29. Shalansky S, Nakagawa B, Wee A. Drug-related problems identified and resolved using pharmaceutical care versus traditional clinical monitoring. *Can J Hosp Pharm.* 1996;49(6):282–288.

30. Ogle BG, McLean WM, Poston JW. The Clinical Pharmacy Services Study: a study of clinical services provided by pharmacists in Ontario hospitals. *Can J Hosp Pharm.* 1996;49(1):S1–S25.

31. Brown G. The Clinical Pharmacy Services Study: rocket fuel. *Can J Hosp Pharm.* 1996;49(1):1–2.

32. Ogle BG, McLean WM, Poston JW. The Clinical Pharmacy Services Study: a study of clinical services provided by pharmacists in Ontario hospitals. *Can J Hosp Pharma.* 1996;49(1):S1–S25.

33. *Pharmaceutical Care: Guidelines on Optimizing the Use of Limited Resources to Provide Pharmaceutical Care.* Canadian Society of Hospital Pharmacists; 2001.

34. *Hospital Pharmacists: Information Paper on Direct Patient Care and Beyond.* Canadian Society of Hospital Pharmacists; 2010.

35. Pharmacy Technician Regulation. College of Pharmacists of British Columbia. http://www.bcpharmacists.org/about_us/key_initiatives/index/articles27.php. Accessed April 24, 2011.

36. The Regulation of Pharmacy Technicians. Ontario College of Pharmacists. http://www.ocpinfo.com/client/ocp/OCPHome.nsf/web/Tech_Overview. Accessed April 24, 2011.

37. *IMPACT: Integrating Family Medicine and Pharmacy to Advance Primary Care Therapeutics.* A Primary Health Care Transition Fund Demonstration Project (G03–02671). http://www.impactteam.info/impactProject.php. Accessed April 24, 2011.

38. Primary Health Care Transition Fund. *Health Canada.* http://www.hc-sc.gc.ca/hcs-sss/prim/phctf-fassp/index-eng.php. Accessed April 24, 2011.

39. Dolovich L, Pottie K, Kaczorowski J, et al. *IMPACT: Project Summary.* http://www.impactteam.info/impactProject.php. Accessed April 24, 2011.

40. Pottie K, Haydt S, Farrell B, et al. Pharmacist's identity development within multidisciplinary primary health care teams in Ontario; qualitative results from the IMPACT project. *Res Soc Adm Pharma.* 2009;5:319–26. http://www.impactteam.info/documents/Pottieetal2009.pdf. Accessed April 24, 2011.

41. IMPACT. Results and News: Publications. http://www.impactteam.info/publications.php. Accessed April 24, 2011.

42. Farrell B, Pottie K, Haydt S, et al. Integrating into family practice: the experiences of pharmacists in Ontario, Canada. *Int J Pharma Pract.* 2008;16:309–315. http://www.impactteam.info/documents/Narrativereportpaper1stfourmonthsIMPACT.pdf. Accessed April 24, 2011.

43. Ontario Ministry of Health and Long-Term Care. *Family Health Care Teams: Public Information.* http://www.health.gov.on.ca/transformation/fht/fht_mn.html. Accessed April 24, 2011.

44. IMPACT Resources for Pharmacists. *Practice Enhancements.* http://www.impactteam.info/practiceEnhancements.php. Accessed April 24, 2011.

45. IMPACT Resources for Pharmacists. *Practice Enhancements.* http://www.impactteam.info/practiceEnhancements.php. Accessed April 24, 2011.

46. Ontario Ministry of Health and Long-Term Care. *Family Health Teams: Information for Family Health Teams.* http://www.health.gov.on.ca/transformation/fht/fht_guides.html. Accessed April 24, 2011.

47. Ontario Ministry of Health and Long-Term Care. *Family Health Teams: Advancing Family Health Care. Guide to Interdisciplinary Provider Compensation (Version 3.2, Updated May 2010). Appendix A: Salary Benchmarks for Interdisciplinary Health Care Providers.* http://www.health.gov.on.ca/transformation/fht/guides/fht_inter_provider.pdf. Accessed April 24, 2011.

48. Alberta Primary Care Initiative (PCI). *About the PCI.* http://www.albertapci.ca/AboutPCI/Pages/default.aspx. Accessed April 24, 2011.

49. Alberta Primary Care Initiative (PCI). *Pharmacy Pilot Project.* http://www.albertapci.ca/AboutPCI/RelatedPrograms/Pages/Pharmacy.aspx. Accessed April 24, 2011.

50. Government of Saskatchewan. *Primary Health care in Saskatchewan.* http://www.health.gov.sk.ca/primary-health-care-in-saskatchewan. Accessed April 24, 2011.

51. Pharmacy Association of Saskatchewan. *Media Release: Pharmacist Awareness Week Celebrates 100 Years of Provincial Pharmacist Regulation in Saskatchewan. March 7, 2011.* http://www.skpharmacists.ca/media/34952/prescriptive%20authority%20media%20release%20-march%207,2011.pdf. Accessed April 24, 2011.

52. Ramaswamy-Krishnarajan J, Hill, DS. Pharmaceutical care in Canada: an exploratory study of 81 community pharmacies. *Can Pharm J.* 2005;138(4):p46–p50.

53. Value of Pharmacy: Building on a Firm Foundation. *CACDS Report.* Canadian Association of Chain Drug Stores; 2010:27–29. http://www.cacds.com/supplement/index.html. Accessed April 24, 2011.

54. Tachuk M. Alberta Pharmacy Practice Models Initiative. Presentation at the Canadian Pharmacists Association Annual Conference. June 2009. http://www.pharmacists.ca/content/about_cpha/whats_happening/cpha_in_action/pdf/Matt%20Tachuk_Blueprint_CPhA_2009.pdf. Accessed April 24, 2011.

55. Alberta College of Pharmacists. *Health Professions Act: Standards for Pharmacist Practice.* April 1, 2007. https://pharmacists.ab.ca/Content_Files/Files/HPA_Standards_FINAL.pdf. Accessed April 24, 2011.

56. *Alberta Pharmacy Practice Models Initiative: Evaluation Report.* Alberta Pharmacists Association. March 28, 2010. http://www.rxa.ca/Content_Files/Files/PPMIEvaluationReport.pdf. Accessed April 24, 2011.

57. *Alberta Pharmacy Practice Models Initiative: Final Data Summary.* Alberta Pharmacists Association. September 20, 2010. http://www.rxa.ca/Content_Files/Files/PPMIExtension-Report.pdf. Accessed April 24, 2011.

58. Letter from the Alberta Minister of Health and Wellness to Alberta Pharmacists and Pharmacy Owners. June 29, 2010. http://www.rxa.ca/Content_Files/Files/Zwozdesky_Jun292010.pdf. Accessed April 24, 2011.

59. Interim Agreement between the Ministry of Health Services and the BC Pharmacy Association. December 12, 2008. http://www.health.gov.bc.ca/pharmacare/suppliers/ia.pdf. Accessed April 24, 2011.

60. De Jong I. *How Medication Management is Changing Pharmacy Practice.* The Tablet: Official Publication of the BC Pharmacy Association; 2011:10–12.

61. Studies and Reviews. *Information for Pharmacists and Other Medical Suppliers.* PharmaCare Program. BC Ministry of Health. http://www.health.gov.bc.ca/pharmacare/suppliers.html. Accessed April 24, 2011.

62. De Jong I. *How Medication Management Is Changing Pharmacy Practice.* The Tablet: Official Publication of the BC Pharmacy Association; 2011:10–12.

63. Pharmacy Services Agreement. *Between the BC Ministry of Health, BC Pharmacy Association and Canadian Association of Chain Drug Stores.* July 7, 2010. http://www.health.gov.bc.ca/pharmacare/suppliers/psa.pdf. Accessed April 24, 2011.

64. National Association of Pharmacy Regulatory Authorities. *Pharmacy Practice and Regulatory Resources.* National Statistics. http://napra.ca/pages/Practice_Resources/National_Statistics.aspx. Accessed April 23, 2011.

65. *Alberta Pharmacy Practice Models Initiative: Final Data Summary.* Alberta Pharmacists Association. September 20, 2010. http://www.rxa.ca/Content_Files/Files/PPMIExtension Report.pdf. Accessed April 24, 2011.

UNITED STATES

Brian J. Isetts, PhD, BCPS
Professor, Department of Pharmaceutical Care & Health Systems
University of Minnesota College of Pharmacy
Minneapolis, Minnesota

Introduction

A dialogue about comprehensive medication management in the United States often commences with reflections from the 1990 "wake-up call" issued by Hepler and Strand in their landmark article focusing on opportunities and responsibilities in pharmaceutical care.[1] Acknowledging the need for a practitioner to do more than simply ensure the accuracy of medications dispensed to patients nearly gave rise to a renaissance period in the profession of pharmacy. Use of the words pharmaceutical care became fashionable for a number of years, until it became apparent that building a practice to take responsibility for all of a patient's drug-related needs was much different than the business of dispensing medications. An important lesson learned in the Minnesota Pharmaceutical Care Demonstration Project of 1993–1997 was that attempting to provide comprehensive medication management commingled with daily dispensing activities soon culminates with the colloquial definition of multitasking, "doing two or more jobs poorly at the same time." Also, critical to successful implementation is understanding the relationship of medication therapy management services to the practice of pharmaceutical care.

Background

The purpose of this chapter is to summarize the history and present state of comprehensive medication management services in the United States, including key developments, emerging opportunities, and future challenges to ensuring that each patient's medications are assessed to determine the appropriate indication for use, effectiveness, safety, and ability to be taken by the patient as intended. Important historical aspects of building a comprehensive medication management infrastructure in the United States starts with articulating the need for a redesigned medication use system, describing a consistent and systematic patient care process, conducting research necessary to establish evidence supporting the delivery of services that address the need represented by drug-related morbidity and mortality, attaining recognition in official health reporting nomenclature, obtaining compensation, and establishing the capacity for widespread availability.

Historical Perspectives

"Those who don't know history are destined to repeat it."

Edmund Burke (1729–1797)
British Statesman and Philosopher

The purpose of reviewing historical developments is to frame the context of serving as a health professional providing consistent and systematic care in a manner recognized by society to fulfill a specific social need that includes a philosophy of care, a standard patient care process, and a practice management system. It is important to present key historical developments to provide a perspective on the journey pharmacists have taken to arrive at the current state of affairs, and to learn from previous successes and challenges. The context for this historical review is the social need generated as a result of drug-related morbidity and mortality associated with medication use.

Drug-related Morbidity and Mortality: 1780 to Present

Drug-related morbidity and mortality, defined as the incidence and prevalence of disease, illness, harm, and death associated with drug therapy, is the primary social need that has facilitated the evolution of pharmacists' patient care contributions for many decades. Apothecaries in colonial America made house calls to treat patients, accurately measured and compounded safe and effective substances to meet the needs of individual patients, and counseled patients on health.

However, the post–World War II growth of commercial drug manufacturers, combined with the 1951 Durham-Humphrey Food and Drug Law Amendments introducing physician-only prescription status, led to the development of the modern day pharmacist as a dispenser of premanufactured drugs. In addition, there was an important decision made by pharmacy leaders in the 1950s affecting the status of pharmacists as health professionals for more than half a century. It was decided that payment for pharmacists' professional services should be included in the dispensing fee for medications. At the time, it was determined that a "parts and labor" billing system would have placed pharmacists in the light of a trade association similar to plumbers and home construction contractors. Pharmacy owners did fairly well economically for many years due to a sizable markup on the cost of prescriptions. However, an understanding of what pharmacists actually did to justify the "professional services component" of dispensing fees remained a mystery for many decades.

Nevertheless, drug-related morbidity and mortality persisted throughout this period of time and contributed to the emergence of clinical pharmacists functioning in hospitals. The growing complexity of medications necessitated the need for a health professional with extensive expertise in the pharmacokinetics and pharmacodynamics of medications administered to acutely ill patients. Another response to drug-related morbidity and mortality occurred with the implementation of a 1974 law mandating that a consultant pharmacist review the records of each skilled nursing facility resident to assess the appropriate use of medications. Initiatives such as the Minnesota Pharmaceutical Care Demonstration Project and legislation to implement medication therapy management services represents responses to drug-related morbidity and mortality in ambulatory patients.

It is important to recognize that drug-related morbidity and mortality is much more than adverse drug events and drug interactions. It also relates to the ineffective and unanticipated consequences of medication use. For instance, resolving a drug therapy problem based on a patient's lack of knowledge of how a medication will help him means that a barrier to appropriate use has been removed. Eliminating a barrier to appropriate use means that the patient need not suffer from access to a medication that has an intended use, that the medication can be effective and safe for the patient to take. In other words, a patient who is not achieving his intended goals of therapy is experiencing a problem because he is not benefiting from the use of an effective and safe medication.

The relationship of drug therapy problems to patient safety was recently highlighted by colleagues reporting on results from a Medicaid health information technology demonstration project in Connecticut. The classification of medication safety using the National Coordinating Council—Medication Error and Reporting Prevention algorithm was expanded to encompass not only the dangerous effects of drugs, but also the ineffective and unanticipated consequences of medication use, and 75.9% of drug therapy problems resolved by pharmacists providing medication therapy management services were classified as preventable medication errors.[2]

Drug-related morbidity and mortality represents a significant challenge by imposing a $200 billion annual burden on the U.S. health care system,[3,4] and improper medication use by patients has been estimated to cost the health system up to $290 billion a year.[5] In addition, prescription drug expenditures comprise 10% ($249 billion) of total U.S. health expenditures representing the third most costly component of the nation's health spending behind hospital care (31%) and physician and clinical services (21%).[6] This nearly 1:1 ratio of drug expenditures to spending for undesirable medication effects is cause for concern supporting the call for medication management interventions and efforts to address appropriate medication use and nonadherence.[5,7]

Replicating the Science of Clinical Drug Trials at the Patient's Bedside

Although the etiology of drug-related morbidity and mortality is multifactorial, the lack of a consistent postmarketing scientific process similar to the science of clinical drug trials is an important consideration.[8] A systematic patient care process applied to the manner in which patients use medications has been designed to help patients achieve desired drug therapy treatment goals and resolve drug therapy problems impeding progress toward goals.[9] This approach, recognized in official health reporting nomenclature as medication therapy management services,[10,11] has the potential for increasing the quality of care and reducing health expenditures with a positive return on investment.[12,13]

Replicating the science of clinical drug trials at the patient's bedside will require a reexamination of health care from a "systems" perspective. The noted Harvard scholar, former Medicare Administrator, and health reform proponent Dr. Donald Berwick has often commented that, "Every system is designed perfectly to produce the results it gets."[14] W. Edward Deming advocated for the widespread application of a systems approach to improve nearly all aspects of the human condition. Dr. Deming's systems approach methods call for continuous process analysis for improvement. The use of medications can also be viewed from this process improvement perspective. Unfortunately, it can be argued that there are no systems and processes in place to guide the use of medications in the homes of patients across America.

A rational medication use system is one that focuses on helping patients to achieve their intended goals of therapy and resolving drug therapy problems impeding progress toward achieving those goals. A rational medication use system includes a consistent and systematic patient care process that is applied to the care of patients across all practice settings. It is recognized that implementing this vision will take time, and there will need to be coordinated efforts to connect successful programs and initiatives currently in place. Suggestions for accelerating efforts to build a rational medication use system are presented in the conclusion of this section.

Recognition of the Service and the Provider

Although pharmacists might have done all sorts of nice things for patients and engaged in a variety of clinical activities prior to 2005, they did not have a recognized service in official U.S. health reporting nomenclature, and they did not have standard national provider identification (NPI) numbers. Without official recognition of a reportable health service and provider identification it follows that pharmacists were not considered to be health professionals. During the early portion of this journey to create a rational medication use system, circa 2000, I recall pharmacists bemoaning the fact that, "if we only had billing codes and provider identification numbers we could really do a lot to take care of patients." Well, be careful what you ask for, you might just get it.

Current Procedural Terminology (CPT), created in 1966, is a means for systematically classifying and reporting health procedures and services.[15] A consistent health reporting nomenclature was needed to standardize health procedures and services across the United States. The primary purpose of CPT as official health reporting nomenclature is often overshadowed by one its secondary administrative functions, namely health care billing and reimbursement. Another important administrative function of CPT is in the development of performance benchmark measurements. Performance benchmark measurements are becoming a central component of a new and evolving health care financing system referred to as "value-based health care."[16] The role of medication management in value-based health financing is discussed briefly in the chapter conclusion.

The journey toward recognition of medication management as a health service and acknowledgment of pharmacists as providers of medication management services in official health reporting nomenclature can be traced to the efforts of many pioneers and stakeholders. However, a little known clause contained in regulations associated with the Health Insurance Portability and Accountability Act of 1996 (HIPAA) opened a door for the profession of pharmacy to petition the CPT Editorial Panel for inclusion in official health reporting nomenclature. In August 2000, the U.S. Department of Health and Human Services released the final rule for implementation of HIPAA, which sought to simplify administrative aspects of the health care claims system and enable a more efficient electronic transmission of certain health information. Of relevance to the profession of pharmacy is that the final rule dictated use of electronic data interchange transaction standards for professional services claims from all health professionals, including pharmacists. This regulation to include pharmacists' professional services in electronic transaction standards for the health care reporting system created an opportunity to petition for inclusion in CPT coding.

The American Medical Association (AMA) oversees proceedings of the CPT Editorial Panel and services as publisher of *Current Procedural Terminology*. In 2002, a coalition of eight national pharmacy organizations was created to work with the American Medical Association and the CPT Editorial Panel to begin the process for submitting a formal medication therapy management (MTM) services code proposal. The coalition, know today as the Pharmacist Services Technical Advisory Coalition (PSTAC), was recognized as the official "medical specialty society" of pharmacy in matters related to CPT, and Daniel Buffington was approved by the AMA as pharmacy's representative on the Health Care Professionals Advisory Committee of the CPT Editorial Panel.

The original CPT code proposal submitted by PSTAC in 2004 requested a permanent Category I MTM coding system based on patient complexity using a resource-based relative value scale similar to that used by the medical profession for evaluation and management service codes (e.g., 99201–99205). Evidence of the effectiveness and safety of MTM contained in the original CPT code proposal was derived from the literature on the practice of pharmaceutical care. Relationships between pharmaceutical care (first described in 1975) and MTM (a procedure or service provided in the practice of pharmaceutical care) were included in this body of evidence.[10]

The description of MTM services contained in the PSTAC CPT code proposal was derived from the literature on pharmaceutical care practices. Fundamental components of the MTM service description included pharmacists performing a face-to-face comprehensive medication review and assessment to identify, resolve, and prevent drug therapy problems; formulating a medication treatment plan to achieve patients' goals of therapy; and monitoring and evaluating patient outcomes of therapy. The CPT Editorial Panel approved the following description of MTM services: "Medication Therapy Management Service(s) (MTMS) describe face-to-face patient assessment and intervention as appropriate, by a pharmacist. MTMS is provided to optimize the response to medications or to manage treatment-related medication interactions or complications."[10,11,17]

The CPT codes for MTM services provided by pharmacists were assigned Category III (temporary) CPT code status. Category III CPT codes are used for reporting new or emerging procedures and services and can be used for up to 5 years while evidence is gathered to petition for migration to Category I (permanent) CPT codes.[15] Shortly after the CPT Editorial Panel assigned temporary Category III status, colleagues in the PSTAC coalition got to work to obtain evidence on the availability of MTMS nationwide. A provider survey was developed and disseminated to gather information on the number of pharmacists providing MTMS as defined in *CPT 2006*. A nine-item survey instrument was developed by the PSTAC in consultation with CPT Editorial Panel members, advisors, and staff. The electronic survey instrument was distributed using a variety of invitation methods to several groups of pharmacists who were known or believed to be engaged in the provision of MTM services. A total of 240 practice sites responded to the provider survey. Practices offering MTM services were identified in all 50 states, the District of Columbia, and Puerto Rico. The vast majority of responses (86%) originated from ambulatory care practice sites, including community pharmacies, clinic and physician office practices, outpatient pharmacies, employer work sites, and home and hospice care locations. Results of this survey revealed that there were a total of nearly 2.8 million MTM encounters over the prior 2-year study period (2005, 2006). Based on the results of this survey, a code-change proposal was submitted by PSTAC to the CPT Editorial Panel and MTMS CPT codes were assigned permanent Category I status in 2007.[10]

Current State of Medication Management in the United States

Relationship of Medication Therapy Management Services to the Practice of Pharmaceutical Care

It's important to not only understand the origins of medication therapy management, but also its relationship to the practice of pharmaceutical care. One of the most important aspects of this chapter is to understand that all health services must have a practice to support the delivery of those services. Otherwise, the health service is nothing more than an uncoordinated activity destined to fail. All dental procedures are supported by the practice of dentistry, all surgical procedures are supported by the practice of surgery, and all clinic visits are supported by the practice of medicine. A practice is defined as, "the creative application of knowledge, guided by a common philosophy and patient care process, to the resolution of specific problems in a manner and at a standard accepted by society."[9] In other words, MTMS is provided in the context of a practice philosophy (e.g., meeting a social obligation to reduce drug-related morbidity and mortality and assume responsibility for patients' drug therapy outcomes), a patient care process (e.g., the systematic assessment, care plan, and follow-up evaluation of all of a patient's drug-related needs), and a practice management system (e.g., workload management, performance appraisal, documentation, appointment scheduling, billing and revenue generation).

Origins of the term medication therapy management services are shrouded in a bit of mystery and intrigue. Even the popular but dubious on-line reference *Wikipedia* tells a story about the origins of MTMS that are inaccurate, although almost believable. In the mid-1990s legislation introduced in Congress intended to reimburse pharmacists for pharmaceutical care services utilized medication management, drug management, and collaborative drug therapy management in an attempt to capture the essence of pharmaceutical care services.

In 2002, the Medicare Payment Advisory Commission (MedPAC) prepared a report for Congress on Medicare payment of nonphysician providers. This report recognized drug-related morbidity and mortality generally, and the inappropriate use of medications among the elderly specifically. Drug management was described as, "an evolving approach to care in which drug therapy decisions are coordinated collaboratively by physicians, pharmacists, and other health professionals together with the patient," with a specific recommendation that the Secretary of the U.S. Department of

Health and Human Services should, "assess models for collaborative drug therapy management services in outpatient settings."[18] This Report also addressed the need to optimize the drug therapy of Medicare beneficiaries with complex drug regimens. These observations about the inappropriate use of medications in the elderly also set the stage for initiating a Medicare drug benefit with medication management services as described in the following section.

The Medicare Part D Drug Benefit

In 1965, Congress enacted Medicare as part of the vision for the Great Society. The roots of this vision can be traced to the work of Presidents Franklin Delano Roosevelt, Harry S. Truman and others as America struggled to emerge from the Great Depression of the 1930s. When Medicare was enacted it included coverage for hospitalizations and physician office visits in elderly patients. Medicare Part A represents hospital coverage and Medicare Part B includes coverage for physician office visits. However, coverage of prescription medications was not included in the Medicare legislation. Popular legend has it that the average cost of a typical prescription in 1965 was less than the administrative cost of submitting an insurance claim for prescriptions. However, competing priorities related to the potentially devastating hospitalization costs of individual retirees coupled with an aggressive attack on Medicare legislation as "socialized medicine," precluded inclusion of a prescription drug benefit at that time.[19]

In the 40 years since Medicare was enacted the average cost of pharmaceuticals increased substantially. The burden of prescription drugs on the pocketbooks of elderly Americans became a significant concern, although financing of a Medicare prescription drug benefit was a matter of intense debate. Although it was recognized that the Medicare program desperately needed a drug benefit, the MedPAC report on payment of nonphysician providers highlighted the concept of including medication management so that we were not just throwing drugs at the elderly and leading them down a path of certain drug-related morbidity and mortality. The MedPAC report noted that, "as part of multi-faceted program reforms, the Congress could consider drug management services together with comprehensive care coordination for Medicare beneficiaries." And the report went on to specifically state that, "as the Congress contemplates creating a Medicare drug benefit, including a drug management benefit may provide a mechanism to optimize drug therapy for a subset of Medicare beneficiaries who have complex drug regimens."[18]

The Medicare Modernization Act of 2003 (MMA) under title 42 CFR Part 423, Subpart D, established a Medicare Part D prescription drug benefit, as well as requirements that Part D plans and sponsors must meet with regard to cost control and quality improvement including requirements for medication therapy management programs (MTMPs). The Medicare Part D prescription drug benefit provided 25 million Medicare beneficiaries with guaranteed access to a drug benefit in 2008. Interestingly, actual drug expenditures were nearly 40% lower than originally projected budget estimates, due in part to the use of competition among prescription drug plans and pharmacies.[20]

The MMA set forth broad goals for medication therapy management as programs to optimize therapeutic outcomes for targeted beneficiaries by improving medication use and reducing adverse events. The initial CMS regulations for MTMPs established a general framework that allowed sponsors' flexibility to promote best practices, as each Part D sponsor is required to incorporate a MTM program into their Plan's benefit structure.[21] Furthermore, funding for the Medicare Part D MTM program has been designed as a component of the administrative fees paid to Part D plans and sponsors, as compared to payments for most other health services, which are paid to health providers or health care organizations.

In an ideal world, it would have been nice to construct and fund the Medicare MTM Program similar to other health services. This situation is remarkably similar to that of incorporating MTM into official health reporting nomenclature in that the initial temporary, time-based CPT reporting and billing codes represented an exception to standard procedures and protocols. Credit this state of affairs to pharmacists serving predominantly as purveyors of a commodity they put into a bottle—and a decision made nearly 60 years ago to eschew a "parts and labor" business model as unprofessional. However, as described below, there is a silver lining and a growing body of evidence and support for pharmacists serving as full-fledged health team members in patient-centered health homes.

From the "glass is half full perspective," pharmacists have made fairly significant progress over the previous 6 to 7 years in terms of meaningful contributions to addressing drug-related morbidity and mortality and constructing a rational medication use system. The Medicare Part D MTM Program is an excellent example of how stakeholders can work together to strengthen a program that was originally designed with very few clearly defined guidelines, standards of practice, or service level expectations. Colleagues in the Medicare Drug Benefit and Parts C & D Data Group have been working to monitor progress, track results, educate beneficiaries, validate and publicly report outcomes, promote best practices, and improve the quality of services provided to Medicare beneficiaries. The 2011 *Medicare Part D MTM Fact Sheet* provides a nice overview of the progress made to date, as well as providing a road map for future service level expectations and research directions using a process referred to as "signaling" in the Summary section of the Fact Sheet.[21]

The centerpiece of all Medicare MTM Programs is the "Comprehensive Medication Review" or CMR. A CMR is, "a review of a beneficiary's medications, including prescription, over-the-counter (OTC) medications, herbal therapies and dietary supplements, that is intended to aid in assessing medication therapy and optimizing patient outcomes."[21] The CMR must be completed at least annually through an interactive person-to-person consultation with eligible beneficiaries, and the assessment may be either face-to-face or through other interactive methods such as the telephone. In 2011, every MTM Program offers the interactive, person-to-person CMR consultation via the phone, and roughly one-fourth (27.0%) of programs also offer face-to-face consultations (up slightly from 25.8% in 2010).[21] Due to the fact that Medicare Part D MTM Program beneficiary-level data are being validated, it will be possible to measure quality and outcomes in the future.

Measuring the Quality of Therapeutic Decisions made by Medication Management Practitioners

The quality of medical care delivered in the hospital and ambulatory care settings has been evaluated using a variety of measurement tools and methods.[22] The quality of therapeutic decisions made by pharmacists providing comprehensive medication therapy management services has also been evaluated using structured implicit review, a methodology applied to the evaluation of medical care.[23]

The quality of therapeutic determinations made by pharmacists within a collaborative practice of pharmaceutical care was studied by a 12-member panel of physicians and pharmacists who used randomly selected patient records. This was a quality improvement and care process validation component of a study evaluating the effects of drug therapy management in patients receiving prepaid medical assistance. Peer review by physicians and pharmacists was performed to evaluate interventions of pharmaceutical care practitioners intending to identify and resolve drug therapy problems and achieve the therapeutic goals of patients in an ambulatory health care setting.[23] The results of this study suggest that decisions made by pharmaceutical care practitioners working in collaboration with physicians and other caregivers to provide medication management are clinically credible. It is anticipated that this same methodology could be used to evaluate the quality of care provided in the Medicare Part D MTM Program. In addition, the Pharmacy Quality Alliance or PQA (a stakeholder organization created to develop performance measures applicable to the Medicare Part D Program) has been developing consensus on prospective measures of the quality of CMRs in the Medicare Part D MTM Program.[24]

The Role of Pharmaceutical Care Demonstration Projects

There have been a number of pilot studies and demonstration projects that have contributed to the knowledge base for medication management in the United States. The Minnesota Pharmaceutical Care Demonstration Project described previously, as well as the Asheville Project and the American Pharmacists Association-Foundation Project ImPACT studies are a few examples of important initiatives contributing to the knowledge base of medication management.[9,25-27]

Many of the lessons learned from these and other studies have been incorporated into a dynamic profession-wide consensus effort to establish essential service level expectations for medication management in the United States.[28,29]

A variety of Medicaid programs administered by the States have had in important influence in these efforts. In 1998, Mississippi became one of the first states to pay pharmacists to provide pharmaceutical care services for Medicaid patients as a result of a waiver granted from the Health Care Financing Administration (now known as the Centers for Medicare & Medicaid Services). Under the Mississippi plan, appropriately credentialed pharmacists were reimbursed for managing the drug-related needs of patients with asthma, diabetes mellitus, hyperlipidemia, or coagulation disorders.[30] The Wisconsin Medicaid Program Incentive-Based Pharmacy Payment System used a slightly different approach, electing to have pharmacies bill for pharmaceutical care services using an enhanced fee reimbursement system in which the dispensing fee was waived.[31] Medicaid programs in Iowa and North Carolina have also been documented in the literature.[32,33] In addition, at least 18 states have had some recent medication management initiatives in place as reported by the National Conference of State Legislatures.[34]

Case Study: The Minnesota Medicaid MTM Care Law

The Minnesota Medicaid Medication Therapy Management Care Law provides an example of how one state utilized lessons learned from other states' Medicaid programs, the CPT Editorial Panel, and previous demonstration projects to carefully construct a medication management program based on best practices and other program successes. Enactment of the Minnesota Medication Therapy Management Care Law (Minnesota Statute §256B.0625, subd. 13h., 2005) was a 12-year effort characterized by extensive collaboration among legislators, payers, and stakeholder organizations. Key components of the Minnesota Law include defining the medication therapy management component of pharmaceutical care services, recognition of qualified pharmacists as providers, authorization for program evaluation, initial stewardship of program implementation through a Department of Human Services (DHS) Medication Therapy Management Advisory Committee, a resource-based relative value scale reimbursement system cross-walked to the MTM CPT codes, a resource-rich Web site, and recipient awareness and education.[35]

The legislatively mandated program evaluation conducted after the first 10 months of the program used data from the first 259 Minnesota Medicaid recipients to receive services under the MTM Care Law. In this evaluation, pharmacists identified and resolved 789 drug therapy problems in these 259 recipients (3.1 drug therapy problems per recipient), with inadequate therapy (e.g., dose too low for effectiveness, needs additional therapy, and noncompliance) representing 73% of resolved drug therapy problems. Based on the number of drug therapy problems resolved, the number of medical indications (6 indications/recipient), and the number of drugs (14 drugs/recipient), demonstrates that State of Minnesota medical assistance and general assistance medical care recipients with complex medical and drug-related needs were served in the initial stages of the program.[36]

Experiences of the Minnesota Medicaid MTM Care Program are serving as an incentive, and as a model, for other state legislative initiatives. In addition, it is noted that the MTM Grant Program provisions of the Affordable Care Act to implement medication management services in treatment of chronic diseases (Public Law 111–148, companion Reconciliation Act P.L. 111–152, Title III, Subtitle A, Sec. 3503, and Public Health Services Act, 42 U.S.C. 201, 2010 Amendments to the P.H.S. Act, Sec. 935) contains all of the service level expectations articulated in the Minnesota MTM Care Law.[37]

Future Directions

The purpose of this section is to provide an educated estimate of future directions and important decisions that will need to be made to create a rational medication use system for every American that extends from cradle to grave. As noted previously, America does not currently have a rational medication use system in place. The disjointed, uncoordinated, and fragmented nature of medical care in general has not been conducive to addressing medication use in a systematic manner. Fortunately, there are scientific principles applied to the approval of new drugs that is helping to serve as a model for assessing medications to ensure intended medical use, effectiveness, safety, and convenience of use postmarketing. The three main areas of discussion in this section are the projected capacity of medication management for every American, characteristics of the medication management provider workforce, and curricular implications for medication management. In addition, the expanding capacity of health information technology and the exchange of health information will be addressed.

Projected Capacity of Medication Management for Every American

As noted previously, it is anticipated that not every pharmacist in America today will be willing or able to assume responsibility for all of a patient's drug therapy outcomes. An analysis of the psychological profiles of individuals electing to enter the profession of pharmacy over the past 50 years is beyond the scope of this presentation. Suffice to say that many pharmacists have become very comfortable, even complacent, serving as purveyors of a drug product commodity with an occasional discussion of how the patient should take their drugs. This is not an indictment so much on the values of pharmacists in general, as it is acknowledging realities of the drug product dispensing enterprise. Nevertheless, there are many examples of pharmacists who have overcome the entrepreneurial "inertia" of dispensing to build medication management practices complementing their drug distribution businesses.

Estimates for the number of medication management providers that will be needed to assume responsibility for the drug therapy outcomes of every American are drawn from a number of sources. These information sources include data from early demonstration projects such as the Minnesota Pharmaceutical Care Demonstration Project, experiences from health systems that have integrated medication management in care model redesign, and findings from a patient-centered medical home program implemented in 2005 in Ontario. It is noted that these projections are based on the need for generalist practitioners to serve the entire U.S. population. Credible projections for specialists in medication management are difficult to construct without first having a full complement of generalist practitioners in place. In addition, the term medication management provider will be used to describe those individuals who will assume responsibility for all of a patient's drug therapy outcomes. Pharmacists have the training and expertise to serve society in this capacity; however, a medication management provider may also include other health providers who learn the patient care process, develop the expertise and step forward to fulfill the demand.

One of the first key assumptions of note from the Minnesota Project is that a single pharmacist can reasonably assume responsibility for 750 to 1000 patients at any point in time. This is a "steady state" estimate in which the majority of patients are established patients with medication management care plans in place, while the remainder of patients is new to the practice. Steady state refers to the fact that established patients will exit any given care system to be replaced by patients new to care.[9]

The second assumption is derived from practices that have integrated pharmacists in patient-centered, team-based care model redesign. As patient-centered health homes and accountable care organizations shift from volume-based to value-based reimbursement in which compensation is based on performance benchmarks, care is being managed by smaller "teamlets" of health providers within clinics.[38] For example, a modest sized clinic of 3000 patients may have three teamlets of providers. In one Minneapolis-based health clinic of 3000 patients the services of one full-time equivalent (FTE) pharmacist are being analyzed. This is to say that, of the 3000 patients in the clinic approximately one-third of patients have complex drug-related needs requiring comprehensive medication management services of the pharmacist necessary to complement work of the teamlets.

The third assumption is drawn from findings of Ontario's Family Health Team Model, which includes funding by the Ministry of Health of one pharmacist for every 10,000 lives.[39,40] This estimate includes patients who frequent the medical care system, as well as individuals who are generally in good health and may not necessarily need to visit a primary care clinic or be under the care of a primary care provider.

Therefore, from these estimates and assumptions a projected range of the number of medication management generalist practitioners can be calculated based on an estimated 300 million inhabitants of the United States. If one were to use the estimate of one medication management provider for every 3000 individuals, then there will need to be about 100,000 providers. If the estimate of one medication management provider for every 10,000 individuals is used, then there will need to be 30,000 providers. The two key variables in these estimates are the impact of health insurance reform in which over 92% of individuals in America will have health insurance, and the impact of health information technology and the exchange of health information. If America can move from its current burden of illness health system to a prevention of illness model, and there is free exchange of health information with appropriate electronic safeguards, then these estimates may vary. Although the range of 30,000 to 100,000 generalist medication management practitioners may be fairly wide, it is interesting to note that this nation could re-deploy the more than 200,000 licensed pharmacists to build a rational medication use system and still have over 100,000 pharmacists remaining for specialist roles in medication management and to oversee medication distribution.

Characteristics of the Medication Management Provider Workforce

As described in this and other pharmaceutical care textbooks and medication management resources, the practitioner must have a core set of values with a patient-centered philosophy of care, a consistent and systematic patient care process, and a practice management system. As reiterated almost *ad nauseam* throughout this chapter, the medication management practitioner must have an inner drive to assume responsibility for all of a patient's drug therapy outcomes and to be held accountable for this commitment. For those individuals who have never held the life of a patient in their hands, this can be a little scary. There are complementary attributes related to the art of developing a therapeutic relationship with the patient, and technical competence in the actions, reactions, pharmacokinetics, and pharmacodynamics of medications.

One of the lessons learned in the Minnesota Project is that a pharmacist is never too old to become a medication management provider. Careful attention to the patient's medication experience and dedication to developing a therapeutic alliance can serve as a springboard for gathering the technical knowledge necessary to establish competence. Patients do not expect you to "know everything," which is why we teach students and practitioners to tell the patient that they will look it up or do research on their behalf to address drug therapy problems. However, it is acknowledged that a medication management provider who is integrated into the patient's health or medical home will be recognized by other health care providers as a true peer with unique contributions. Similar to other health professions, there will need to be some type of provider recognition so that society can differentiate medication management providers from other providers. Therefore, provider credentialing for licensure and reimbursement will be important to the future of medication management providers in the United States.

Curricular Implications for Medication Management

Nearly 20 years ago the American Association of Colleges of Pharmacy accepted pharmaceutical care as the mission of pharmacy practice and as the mission of pharmacy education. However, there is little consistency across schools and colleges of pharmacy in the tenets of providing medication management services within the practice of pharmaceutical care. Some schools attempt to integrate the consistent and systematic patient care process of medication therapy management throughout the curriculum from day one of pharmacy school. Others teach about medication management as a module at the end of the student's third year of school. In addition, there is growing dissention among the profession related to whether or not we are graduating too few or too many pharmacy students. Unfortunately the answer is both! We're graduating too many students for careers in medication distribution and too few students for careers in medication management.

Any college of pharmacy that has attempted to reconstruct their curriculum will tell you that this is no small undertaking. There certainly are a number of challenges that need to be overcome. One suggestion for a first step in this direction may be to gain consensus on the core competencies to be taught in all schools and colleges of pharmacy. A recent thoughtful PhD dissertation combined an exhaustive literature review with ethnographic observation and interviews of established pharmaceutical care practitioners to build the case for seven fundamental core competencies.[41] These competencies need to become the starting point for curricular revision around the world.

Summary

In summary, there have been a number of significant developments over the past 15 to 20 years supporting the development of a rational medication use system in the United States. Data and information on the outcomes of medication management services provided within the practice of pharmaceutical care have been useful in establishing official health reporting and billing codes for medication therapy management. Medication management services cannot stand alone as an uncoordinated health service, and therefore are directly related to, and supported by, the practice of pharmaceutical care. The Medicare Part D MTM Program was launched without clear service level expectations, but has grown so that it is now possible to validate the outcomes and measure the quality of a comprehensive medication review. Patient awareness of medication management may not be strong, although stories of drug-related morbidity and mortality are far too common. Developing the business case for medication management may be challenging, although outcome studies to date provide useful patient-centered outcomes research and comparative effectiveness studies. The fundamental question before America today is whether or not the $200 billion annual cost of drug-related morbidity and mortality is an acceptable cost of doing business?

REFERENCES

1. Hepler CD, Strand LM. Opportunities and responsibilities in pharmaceutical care. *Am J Hosp Pharm.* 1990;47:533–543.
2. Smith MA, Giuliano MR, Starkowski MP. Connecticut: improving patient medication management in primary care. *Health Affairs.* 2011;30:646–654.
3. Johnson JA, Bootman JL. Drug-related morbidity and mortality: a cost-of-illness model. *Arch Intern Med.* 1995;155:1949–1956.
4. Ernst FR, Grizzle AJ. Drug-related morbidity and mortality: updating the cost-of-illness model. *J Am Pharm Assoc.* 2001;41:192–199.
5. Engleberg Center for Health Reform at Brookings and the Dartmouth Institute for Health Policy and Clinical Practice. *Brookings-Dartmouth Accountable Care Organization Toolkit.* Washington DC: The Brookings Institution; 2011:119. Available at https://xteam.brookings.edu/bdacoln/Documents/ACO%20Toolkit%20January%202011.pdf. Accessed July 19, 2011.

6. Martin A, Lassman D, Whittle L, Catlin A, National Health Expenditure Accounts Team. Recession contributes to slowest annual rate of increase in health spending in five decades. *Health Aff (Millwood).* 2011;30(1):11–22.

7. Aspen P, Wolcott JA, Bootman JL, eds. *Preventing Medication Errors.* Institute of Medicine. Washington: National Academy Press; 2007.

8. Cipolle CL, Cipolle RJ, Strand LM. Consistent standards in medication use: the need to care for patients from research to practice. *J Am Pharm Assoc.* 2006;46:205–212.

9. Cipolle RJ, Strand LM, Morley PC. *Pharmaceutical Care Practice: The Clinician's Guide.* New York: McGraw-Hill; 2004.

10. Isetts BJ, Buffington DE. CPT code-change proposal: national data on pharmacists' medication therapy management services. *J Am Pharm Assoc.* 2007;47:491–495.

11. American Medical Association. *CPT Changes 2006: An Insider's View.* Chicago: American Medical Association; 2005:309–312.

12. Smith MA, Bates DW, Bodenheimer TS, Cleary PD. Why pharmacists belong in the medical home. *Health Aff (Millwood).* 2010:29(5);906–913.

13. Patient-Centered Primary Care Collaborative. *The patient-centered medical home: Integrating comprehensive medication management to optimize patient outcomes.* 2010. Available at http://www.pcpcc.net/content/medication-management. Accessed July 19, 2011.

14. Carr S. *A quotation with a life of its own.* Quotation often attributed to Donald Berwick, W. Edward Deming, and Paul Batalden as a guiding principle for quality improvement. *Patient Safety Quality Healthcare E-Newsletter,* July/August 2008. Accessed July 19, 2011. http://www.psqh.com/julaug08/editor.html.

15. American Medical Association. *About CPT®.* Accessed July 19, 2011. http://www.ama-assn.org/ama/pub/physician-resources/solutions-managing-your-practice/coding-billing-insurance/cpt/about-cpt.page?

16. Porter ME, Teisberg EO. *Redefining Health Care: Creating Value-based Competition on Results.* Boston: Harvard Business School Press; 2006.

17. Pharmacist Services Technical Advisory Coalition. *Medication Therapy Management Service Codes.* Accessed July 19, 2011. http://www.pstac.org/services/mtms-codes.html.

18. Medicare Payment Advisory Commission, Hackbarth GM (Chair). *Report to the Congress: Medicare Coverage of Nonphysician Practitioners.* Washington DC, June 2002; 21–26. Accessed July 19, 2011. http://www.medpac.gov/documents/jun02_NonPhysCoverage.pdf.

19. Oliver TR, Lee PR, Lipton HL. A political history of Medicare and prescription drug coverage. *The Milbank Quarterly,* 2004;82(2):283–354. Available through The Henry J. Kaiser Family Foundation (2004 Milbank Memorial Fund, Blackwell Publishing). http://www.kff.org/medicare/upload/A-Political-History-of-Medicare-and-Prescription-Drug-Coverage.pdf.

20. Benner JS, Kocut SL. Medicare Part D: good for patients and an opportunity for pharmacists. *J Manag Care Pharm.* 2009;15:66–70.

21. Centers for Medicare and Medicaid Services. *Medicare Part D Medication Therapy Management (MTM) Programs 2011 Fact Sheet,* updated June 30, 2011. Accessed July 15, 2011. https://www.cms.gov/PrescriptionDrugCovContra/Downloads/MTMFactSheet2011.pdf.

22. Goldman RL. The reliability of peer assessments: a meta-analysis. *Eval Health Prof.* 1994;17:3–21.

23. Isetts BJ, Brown LM, Schondelmeyer SW, Lenarz LA. Quality assessment of a collaborative approach for decreasing drug-related morbidity and achieving therapeutic goals. *Arch Intern Med.* 2003;163:1813–1820.

24. Pharmacy Quality Alliance, Medication Therapy Management Work Group. Accessed July 1, 2011 at http://www.pqaalliance.org/MTMCare.htm.

25. Cranor CW, Bunting BA, Christensen DB. The Asheville project: long-term clinical and economic outcomes of a community pharmacy diabetes care program. *J Am Pharm Assoc.* 2003;43:173–190.

26. Bluml BM, McKenney JM, Cziraky MJ. Pharmaceutical care services and results in Project ImPACT: Hyperlipidemia. *J Am Pharm Assoc.* 2000;40:157–165.

27. Goode JV, Swiger K, Bluml BM. Regional osteoporosis screening, referral, and monitoring program in community pharmacies: findings from Project ImPACT: Osteoporosis. *J Am Pharm Assoc.* 2004;44:152–160.

28. Bluml B. Definition of medication therapy management: development of profession-wide consensus. *J Am Pharm Assoc.* 2005;45:566–572.

29. American Pharmacists Association, National Association of Chain Drug Stores Foundation, et al. Medication therapy management in pharmacy practice: core elements of an MTM service model (version 2.0). *J Am Pharm Assoc.* 2008;48:341–353.

30. Medicaid to pay Mississippi pharmacists for disease management. *Am J Health Syst Pharm.* 1998;55:1238–1239.

31. HMOs adopt Wisconsin Medicaid pilot project for commercial enrollees. *Payment Strat Pharmaceut Care.* 1998;3:1,2,5–8.

32. Chrischilles EA, Carter BL, Lund BC, et al. Evaluation of the Iowa Medicaid pharmaceutical case management program. *J Am Pharm Assoc.* 2004;44:337–349.

33. Michaels NM, Jenkins GF, Pruss DL, Heidrick JE, Ferreri SP. Retrospective analysis of community pharmacists' recommendations in the North Carolina Medicaid medication therapy management program. *J Am Pharm Assoc.* 2010; 50:347–353.

34. National Conference of State Legislatures. *Medication Therapy Management: Pharmaceutical Safety and Savings.* Updated June 2011. Accessed July 19, 2011 at http://www.ncsl.org/default.aspx?tabid=19064.

35. State of Minnesota Medicaid Medication Therapy Care Program documents and information available at: http://www.dhs.state.mn.us/ Advanced Keyword Search: medication therapy management. Accessed July 1, 2011.

36. Isetts BJ. *Evaluating Effectiveness of the Minnesota Medicaid Medication Therapy Management Care Program—Report to the Legislature.* State Contract Number B00749, Posted December 14, 2007. Accessed July 19, 2011 at http://www.dhs.state.mn.us/main/groups/business_partners/documents/pub/dhs16_140283.pdf.

37. Affordable Care Act, 2010: *Medication Management Services in Treatment of Chronic Diseases, Grants or Contracts to Implement Medication Management Services in Treatment of Chronic Diseases.* Public Law 111–148, companion Reconciliation Act P.L. 111–152, Title III, Subtitle A, Sec. 3503, Public Health Services Act, 42 U.S.C. 201, 2010 Amendments to the P.H.S. Act, Sec. 935, (pp. 1055–1061). Accessed July 19, 2011 at http://www.healthcare.gov/center/authorities/title_iii_improving_the_quality_and_efficiency.pdf.

38. Fairview Health System—Medication Therapy Management Program. Accessed July 18, 2011 at http://www.fairview.org/Pharmacy/MedicationTherapyManagement/index.htm.

39. Rosser WW, Colwill JM, Kasperski J, Wilson L. Progress of Ontario's family health team model: a patient-centered medical home. *Ann Fam Med.* 2011;9:165–171.

40. Rosser WW, Colwill JM, Kasperski J, Wilson L. Patient-centered medical homes in Ontario. *N Engl J Med.* 2010; 362(3):e7.

41. Losinski VL. *Educating for Action: Understanding the Development of Pharmaceutical Care Practitioners.* A PhD dissertation presented to Faculty of the Graduate School of the University of Minnesota, May 23, 2011.

SUMMARY: FUTURE PROSPECTS

Medication management is a global concern. Over the past 30 years we have seen firsthand in a number of countries the evolution of services dedicated to meeting the needs of patients undergoing drug therapy. Indeed, we have been privileged to have participated in the development of pharmaceutical care practices, and its later incarnation-medication management services, in many countries. We have at one time or another encountered the obstacles and issues reported in the foregoing section.

Adverse drug events are global phenomena. The evidence for this is now vast. Moreover, there is increasing evidence that both human and economic costs are of a magnitude that are quite unacceptable. The two most vital questions of the day are: What can be done? And, who will do it? These are questions that must be addressed in all places where drug therapy exists.

This volume has sought to address the first question and offers a comprehensive, systematic, and rational approach to medication management. This volume also argues that the pharmacist is a central figure in the remediation of drug-related problems.

We have concluded that the pharmacy profession consists of individuals who have the knowledge base required to make a difference. But, will they? We strongly believe that they will, and recent developments, here and abroad, tend to support our optimism. Professional associations in many parts of the world are on record as supportive of major changes in this direction for the profession. Establishing the pharmacist as a legitimate health care provider, rather than merely a purveyor and distributor of products, is now a central part of any dialogue within the profession. Thus, while we will always find points of disagreement, we also find shared core values, goals, purpose, and roles. Pharmacists should and can serve as major participants in the comprehensive management of a patient's drug therapy. Where this has been tried it has been shown to be effective at saving lives, saving money, and improving the quality of patients' lives. We now have significant data to back up our claims and now is the time to move more proactively in new directions.

All of the above is essentially a preamble to our strongly held belief that pharmacy must develop a more pervasive presence in health care organizations. One essential step to accomplish this is to develop and actively promote an identity that is first and foremost clinical and patient-centered in nature. At present widespread acceptance of the pharmacist-as-clinician is not found either in the "collective consciousness" of other health practitioners or the general public. This is not to say that some pharmacists are not doing clinical work. On the contrary, there is considerable evidence that all pharmacists, at one time or another do make positive clinical interventions. Rather, we are saying that clinical "acts" are not presently defining pharmacy. We find that physicians and other health care practitioners recognize the nature and depth of pharmaceutical knowledge held by pharmacists. But, in the rough and tumble world of health care practices, individuals or groups are judged more by their actions rather than their articulated claim to expert knowledge. Outsiders want to see for themselves what the pharmacist can do with this complex knowledge. They are not impressed with abstract claims as they are by action and results. Positive outcomes traced directly to pharmacists' interventions are seen as credible evidence that their claims of expertise have validity. Thus, future developments must include more demonstration projects, research, and practice that can be evaluated by pharmacists, other practitioners, and patients alike. The central idea here is to continue to build practice-based evidence not only to demonstrate value, but also to create ongoing dynamic practices that are highly visible and open to professional and public scrutiny.

To achieve a truly legitimate professional presence requires a determined statement of collective purpose and action. Any professional identity must send a clear message that speaks to who we are, and defines the prevailing realities of our collective mission. Leaders, elected or otherwise, should be acutely aware of the importance of building a consensus as to the profession's goals and use these to move pharmacy from disparate sets of activities and roles to a more nuanced philosophical statement of collective engagement in important clinical practice. Simply listing numerous clinical activities that pharmacists may or may not do is failing to present a cohesive plan of action to reinvent and reinvigorate a profession with so much to offer. There must be a unified single purpose—to attend to the clinical therapeutic needs of patients. In sum, pharmacy, as a profession, has little or no choice but to cultivate an identity that is universally recognized as one committed to the science and art of healing. Such an identity where pharmacy is established as a practice profession, understood, respected, and legitimized by other health care professionals, and the general public, will provide the momentum necessary to increase the value of its services, and facilitate the growth and development of the profession.

Standards of Practice for Pharmaceutical Care

Standards of practice for pharmaceutical care are:

A. Standards of care:

A set of expectations of the performance of an *individual* practitioner

B. Professional standards:

A set of expectations for a *community* of practitioners

A. STANDARDS OF CARE FOR PHARMACEUTICAL CARE PRACTITIONERS

Standard of Care 1: Collection of Patient-specific Information

STANDARD 1: THE PRACTITIONER COLLECTS RELEVANT PATIENT-SPECIFIC INFORMATION TO USE IN DECISION MAKING CONCERNING ALL DRUG THERAPIES.

Measurement criteria
1. Pertinent data are collected using appropriate interview techniques.
2. Data collection involves the patient, family and caregivers, and other health care providers when appropriate.
3. The medication experience is elicited by the practitioner and incorporated as the context for decision making.
4. The data are used to develop a pharmacologically relevant description of the patient, the patient's health status, and the patient's drug-related needs.
5. The relevance and significance of the data collected are determined by the patient's present conditions, illnesses, wants, needs, and preferences.

6. The medication history is complete and accurate.
7. The current medication record is complete, accurate, and includes indication, drug product, dosage regimen, and result to date.
8. The data collection process is systematic, comprehensive, and ongoing.
9. Only data that are required and used by the practitioner are elicited from the patient.
10. Relevant data are documented in a retrievable form.
11. All data collection and documentation is conducted in a manner that ensures patient confidentiality.

Standard of Care 2: Assessment of Drug-related Needs

STANDARD 2: THE PRACTITIONER ANALYZES THE ASSESSMENT DATA TO DETERMINE IF THE PATIENT'S DRUG-RELATED NEEDS ARE BEING MET, THAT ALL THE PATIENT'S MEDICATIONS ARE APPROPRIATELY INDICATED, THE MOST EFFECTIVE AVAILABLE, THE SAFEST POSSIBLE, AND THE PATIENT IS ABLE AND WILLING TO TAKE THE MEDICATION AS INTENDED.

Measurement criteria

1. The patient-specific data collected in the assessment are used to decide if all of the patient's medications are appropriately indicated.
2. The data collected are used to decide if the patient needs additional medications that are not presently being taken.
3. The data collected are used to decide if all of the patient's medications are the most effective products available for the conditions.
4. The data collected are used to decide if all of the patient's medications are dosed appropriately to achieve the goals of therapy.
5. The data collected are used to decide if any of the patient's medications are causing adverse effects.
6. The data collected are used to decide if any of the patient's medications are dosed excessively and causing toxicities.
7. The patient's behavior is assessed to determine if all medications are being taken appropriately in order to achieve the established goals of therapy.

Standard of Care 3: Identification of Drug Therapy Problems

STANDARD 3: THE PRACTITIONER ANALYZES THE ASSESSMENT DATA TO DETERMINE IF ANY DRUG THERAPY PROBLEMS ARE PRESENT.

Measurement criteria

1. Drug therapy problems are identified from the assessment findings.
2. Drug therapy problems are validated with the patient, family, caregivers, and/or health care providers, when necessary.
3. Drug therapy problems are expressed so that the medical condition and the drug therapy involved are explicitly stated and the relationship or cause of the problem is described.
4. Drug therapy problems are prioritized, and those to be resolved first are addressed.
5. Drug therapy problems are documented in a manner that suggest the goals of therapy and desired outcomes within the care plan.

Standard of Care 4: Development of Goals of Therapy

STANDARD 4: THE PRACTITIONER IDENTIFIES GOALS OF THERAPY THAT ARE PATIENT-CENTERED.

Measurement criteria

1. Goals of therapy are established for each indication managed with drug therapy.
2. Desired goals of therapy are described in terms of the observable or measurable clinical and/or laboratory parameters to be used to evaluate effectiveness and safety of drug therapy.
3. Goals of therapy are mutually negotiated with the patient and other health care practitioners when appropriate.
4. Goals of therapy are realistic in relation to the patient's present and potential capabilities.
5. Goals of therapy include a time frame for achievement.

Standard of Care 5: Statement of Interventions

STANDARD 5: THE PRACTITIONER DEVELOPS A
CARE PLAN THAT INCLUDES INTERVENTIONS TO
RESOLVE DRUG THERAPY PROBLEMS, ACHIEVE
GOALS OF THERAPY, AND PREVENT DRUG THERAPY
PROBLEMS.

Measurement criteria

1. Each intervention is individualized to the patient's conditions, drug-related needs, and drug therapy problems.
2. All appropriate therapeutic alternatives to resolve drug therapy problems are considered, and the best are selected.
3. The plan is developed in collaboration with the patient, family and/or caregivers, and other health care practitioners, when appropriate.
4. All interventions are documented.
5. The plan provides for continuity of care by including a schedule for continuous follow-up evaluation.

Standard of Care 6: Establish a Schedule for Follow-up Evaluations

STANDARD 6: THE PRACTITIONER DEVELOPS A
SCHEDULE TO FOLLOW-UP AND EVALUATE THE
EFFECTIVENESS OF DRUG THERAPIES AND ANY ADVERSE
EVENTS EXPERIENCED BY THE PATIENT.

Measurement criteria

1. The clinical and laboratory parameters to evaluate effectiveness are established, and a time frame for collecting the relevant information is selected.
2. The clinical and laboratory parameters to evaluate the safety of the patient's medications are selected, and a time frame for collecting the relevant information is determined.
3. A schedule for the follow-up evaluation visits is established with the patient.
4. The schedule and plan for follow-up evaluation is documented.

Standard of Care 7: Follow-up Evaluation

STANDARD 7: THE PRACTITIONER EVALUATES THE PATIENT'S OUTCOMES AND DETERMINES THE PATIENT'S PROGRESS TOWARD THE ACHIEVEMENT OF THE GOALS OF THERAPY, DETERMINES IF ANY SAFETY OR ADHERENCE ISSUES ARE PRESENT, AND ASSESSES WHETHER ANY NEW DRUG THERAPY PROBLEMS HAVE DEVELOPED.

Measurement criteria

1. The patient's outcomes from drug therapies and other interventions are documented.
2. The effectiveness of drug therapies is evaluated, and the patient's status is determined by comparing the outcomes within the expected time frame to achieve the goals of therapy.
3. The safety of the drug therapy is evaluated.
4. Patient adherence is evaluated.
5. The care plan is revised, as needed.
6. Revisions in the care plan are documented.
7. Evaluation is systematic and ongoing until all goals of therapy are achieved.
8. The patient, family and/or caregivers, and other health care practitioners are involved in the evaluation process, when appropriate.

B. PROFESSIONAL STANDARDS FOR THE COMMUNITY OF PHARMACEUTICAL CARE PRACTITIONERS

Standard I: Quality of Care

Practitioners evaluate their own practice in relation to professional practice standards and relevant statutes and regulations.

Measurement criteria

1. The pharmaceutical care practitioner uses evidence from the literature to evaluate performance in practice.
2. The pharmaceutical care practitioner seeks peer review on a continual and frequent basis.
3. The pharmaceutical care practitioner utilizes data generated from practice to critically evaluate performance.

Standard II: Ethics

The practitioner's decisions and actions on behalf of patients are determined in an ethical manner.

Measurement criteria

1. The practitioner maintains patient confidentiality.
2. The practitioner acts as a patient advocate.
3. The practitioner delivers care in a nonjudgmental and nondiscriminatory manner that is sensitive to patient diversity.
4. The practitioner delivers care in a manner that preserves/protects patient autonomy, dignity, and rights.
5. The practitioner seeks available resources to help formulate ethical decisions.

Standard III: Collegiality

The pharmaceutical care practitioner contributes to the professional development of peers, colleagues, and others.

Measurement criteria

1. The practitioner offers professional assistance to other practitioners whenever asked.
2. The practitioner promotes supportive relationships with patients, physicians, nurses, and other health care providers.

Standard IV: Collaboration

The practitioner collaborates with the patient, family members, and health care providers in providing patient care.

Measurement criteria

1. The patient is seen as the ultimate decision maker, and the practitioner collaborates accordingly.
2. The practitioner collaborates with the patient's health care providers whenever it is in the best interest of the patient.

Standard V: Education

The practitioner acquires and maintains current knowledge in pharmacology, pharmacotherapy, and pharmaceutical care practice.

Measurement criteria

1. The practitioner uses the skills of reflecting on practice to identify areas where knowledge needs to be supplemented.
2. The practitioner continually updates knowledge with journal subscriptions, current texts, practitioner interactions, and continuing education programs.

Standard VI: Research

The practitioner routinely uses research findings in practice and contributes to research findings when appropriate.

Measurement criteria

1. The practitioner uses research results as the basis for practice decisions.
2. The pharmaceutical care practitioner systematically reviews the literature to identify knowledge, skills, techniques, and products that are helpful in practice and implements them in a timely manner.
3. The practitioner approaches practice with a perspective to conduct applied research in practice when appropriate.

Standard VII: Resource Allocation

The practitioner considers factors related to effectiveness, safety, and cost in planning and delivering patient care.

Measurement criteria

1. The pharmaceutical care practitioner is sensitive to the financial needs and resource limitations of the patient, the health care providers, and the institution.
2. Decisions are made by the pharmaceutical care practitioner to conserve resources and maximize the value of those resources consumed in practice.

Glossary

absolute risk reduction

- Difference in event rates for two groups, usually treatment and control groups

adherence

- The patient's ability or willingness to take a drug regimen that the practitioner has clinically judged to be appropriately indicated, effective, and, based on all available evidence, can produce the desired outcomes without any harmful effects
- The patient is able and willing to take the medication as intended.

advocacy (patient)

- The willingness to assume an active role in obtaining resources or resolving problems on behalf of a patient
- May require an intervention on the part of a health care professional for the benefit of a patient

assessment

- A systematic review and appraisal of the patient's drug-related needs
- Completed for the purpose of assuring that all the patient's drug therapy is appropriately indicated, the most effective available, and the safest possible assuring that the patient is able and willing to comply with the pharmacotherapeutic regimen, and identifying drug therapy problems
- Includes the decision-making processes of the Pharmacotherapy Workup
- One of three steps in the patient care process in the practice of pharmaceutical care (the care plan and the follow-up evaluation complete the process)

beneficence

- Doing what is best for the patient
- One of the primary ethical principles that underlies the practice of pharmaceutical care

care plan

- A detailed schedule outlining the practitioner's and the patient's activities and responsibilities; designed to achieve goals of therapy, and resolve and prevent drug therapy problems
- Organized according to medical condition or indication for drug therapy
- Includes (1) a statement of the goals of therapy; (2) the interventions by the practitioner and the actions to be taken by the patient to resolve any drug therapy problems, meet the goals of therapy, and prevent drug therapy problems; and (3) a schedule for the follow-up evaluation

caring

- A state of responsiveness to others that entails the willingness to become personally involved
- The commitment to alleviate another person's vulnerability and suffering
- Considered to be the cornerstone of the therapeutic relationship and a principal component of the philosophy of pharmaceutical care practice
- Consists of three activities that the practitioner must accomplish: (1) assess the patient's needs, (2) obtain the resources required to meet these needs, and (3) determine if the help provided has produced positive or negative outcomes

clinical pharmacy

- An emphasis in the profession of pharmacy from the mid-1960s to the present, which moved the focus from drug product to patient-oriented services including consultations
- Includes a number of different services such as individualized (pharmacokinetic) dosing services, and drug utilization review, which are primarily provided in the institutional setting
- The majority of the services are provided to/for physicians or at the request of physicians or are directed toward institutional policies and procedures
- ACCP Definition: A health science discipline that embodies the application and development, by pharmacists, of scientific principles of pharmacology, toxicology, therapeutics, clinical pharmacokinetics, pharmacoeconomics, pharmacogenomics, and other life science for the care of patients

clinically competent

- A practitioner who is legally and ethically informed and is able to draw upon appropriate pharmaceutical knowledge while problem solving to meet the patient's needs

compliance

- The ability and willingness of a patient to use a pharmacotherapeutic regimen agreed upon between patient and practitioner
- The terms adherence and concordance are also used
- The term is used here specifically to mean compliance with a dosage regimen, not compliance with the orders of a paternalistic or authoritarian figure

confidentiality (patient)

- The act of protecting a patient's personal information from public view
- Keeping private all aspects of a patient's care in the manner deemed acceptable to the patient and prescribed by law (see Health Insurance Portability and Accountability Act [HIPAA], April 14, 2003)
- One of the ethical principles that underlies the practice of pharmaceutical care

conflict of interest

- Personal, financial, or political interests that undermine an individual's ability to meet or fulfill primary professional, ethical, or legal obligations

contraindication

- A condition or factor that renders the use of a drug product in the care of a specific patient improper or undesirable
- A reason or explanation, such as a symptom or condition, that makes a particular treatment or procedure inadvisable

current medication record

- Organized information describing all of the drug therapies a patient is presently taking or receiving
- Includes the indication for the medication, the specific drug product, dosage regimen, duration of therapy, and clinical results to date
- Includes prescription products, nonprescription agents, alternative products, vitamins, nutritional supplements, herbal remedies, and any other product the patient is taking that is intended to have therapeutic effects

diagnosis

- The process of determining the nature of a medical disease and distinguishing one disease from another
- Identification of a disease by considering the patient's signs and symptoms, history, laboratory findings, and physical examination when necessary

disease

- Specific illness or medical disorder characterized by a recognizable set of signs and symptoms
- A pathological, objectified condition of the body that presents a group of physiologically and biologically defined symptoms
- Any abnormality or failure to function, except those that result directly from physical injury

dosage

- The total amount of active medication that a patient takes over a specified period of time
- Includes the dose of the medication, the method of administration, the frequency, and the duration of treatment

dose

- The amount of active ingredient that the patient takes each time he or she self-administers the drug product
- The amount of drug administered to the patient as a single event

dosing interval

- The amount of time between administered doses (e.g., every 8 hours)
- Frequency of doses over a specified period of time (e.g., three times a day)

drug

- Any substance or product used by or administered to a patient for therapeutic, preventive, or diagnostic purposes

drug-related morbidity

- The incidence and prevalence of disease and illness or harm associated with drug therapy
- One aspect of the social need addressed in the philosophy of pharmaceutical care practice

drug-related mortality

- The incidence and prevalence of death associated with drug therapy
- One aspect of the social need addressed in the philosophy of pharmaceutical care practice

drug-related need

- The health care needs of a patient related to drug therapy for which the pharmaceutical care practitioner can offer professional assistance

- Includes (1) the appropriate use of the medication for each medical condition, (2) the most effective product for each indication, (3) the safest drug regimen possible, and (4) the willingness and ability of the patient to comply with the instructions for taking a medication

drug therapy

- Includes the drug product and the dosage regimen being taken by a patient for a therapeutic indication
- Used synonymously with pharmacotherapy

drug therapy problem

- Any undesirable event experienced by a patient that involves, or is suspected to involve, drug therapy and that interferes with achieving the desired goals of therapy and requires clinical judgment to resolve or prevent
- Stated to include a description of the patient's condition or problem, the drug therapy involved, and the association between the two
- A problem that is categorized in the following way:

    A. inappropriate indication for use
       1. patient needs additional drug therapy
       2. patient is taking unnecessary drug therapy
    B. ineffective drug therapy
       3. patient is taking an ineffective drug product
       4. patient is taking too low of a dosage
    C. unsafe drug therapy
       5. patient is experiencing an adverse drug reaction
       6. patient is taking too high of a dosage
    D. inappropriate adherence (non-compliance)
       7. patient is unable or unwilling to take the drug therapy as intended

effectiveness (of drug therapy)

- Ability of the drug therapy to produce the desired or intended beneficial result (outcome) in a specific patient
- The effect of an intervention as applied to an individual patient in real practice

efficacy

- The evidence that a drug can produce a beneficial effect in a population of patients
- The effect of an intervention as measured under controlled circumstances, as in a clinical trial

ethical dilemma

- The conflict that results from two different resolutions to a situation, both of which are ethical
- Result of a clinical situation that involves two individuals with different values, different levels of knowledge, expectations, and desires
- Used synonymously with ethical problem and ethical issue

ethical principles

- Concepts that describe the moral standards applied in patient care
- Form the foundation of the philosophy of pharmaceutical care practice
- Include beneficence, nonmaleficence, veracity, justice, fidelity, autonomy, and confidentiality

ethics

- A set of moral principles or values that help to establish right from wrong encompassed in the standards of professional behavior for a practitioner
- Character or ideals governing an individual or profession

evaluation (follow-up)

- Patient encounters at planned intervals to determine outcomes of drug therapy
- Purpose is to record actual patient outcomes resulting from pharmacotherapy, evaluate progress of the patient toward achieving goals of therapy, determine if previous drug therapy problems have been resolved, and assess whether new drug therapy problems have developed
- The third component of the patient care process in the practice of pharmaceutical care (the other two are assessment and care plan)

expired

- One of the standard terms for describing the outcome status of a patient's medical condition being treated with pharmacotherapy
- Patient died while receiving drug therapy

failure

- One of the standard terms for describing the outcome status of a patient's medical condition being treated with pharmacotherapy
- The goals of therapy have not been achieved despite adequate dosages and adequate duration of therapy. Discontinuation of the present medication and initiation of new drug therapy is required

fidelity
- The act of being faithful and keeping promises
- One of the primary ethical principles that underlies the practice of pharmaceutical care

generalist
- A practitioner who provides continuing, comprehensive, and coordinated care to a population of patients undifferentiated by gender, disease, drug treatment, or organ system
- A practitioner who is the point of first medical contact within the health care system, providing open and unlimited access to its users, dealing with all health problems regardless of the age, sex, or any other characteristic of the person concerned.

goals of therapy
- The desired endpoint for pharmacotherapy
- Expressed as: prevention of a disease or illness, curing a disease, the reduction or elimination of signs and symptoms, slowing the progression of a disease, the normalization of laboratory values, or a way to facilitate the diagnostic process
- Includes clinical parameters (signs and symptoms) and/or laboratory values that are observable, measurable, and realistic, a desired value or observable change in the parameter, and a specific time frame

illness
- The patient's lived experience of a disease or condition
- May be considered as a "process," often occurring over a protracted period of time
- The experience of illness encompasses physical, social, psychological, and cultural factors

improved
- One of the standard terms for describing the outcome status of a patient's medical condition being treated with pharmacotherapy
- Adequate progress is being made toward achieving the goals of therapy at this point in time. The same drug therapy will be continued

incidence
- The number of new cases or occurrences of illness arising in a population over an established period of time

indication (for drug therapy)

- Reason for the use of drug therapy for the treatment, prevention, or diagnosis of a condition (illness, symptom) in a specific patient
- A sign or symptom to suggest the necessity or advisability to initiate pharmacotherapy

initial

- One of the standard terms used for describing the outcome status of a patient's medical condition being treated with pharmacotherapy
- Denotes the beginning of drug therapy for a medical indication

justice

- Fair, equitable, and appropriate treatment in light of what is due or owed to persons
- One of the primary ethical principles that underlies the practice of pharmaceutical care

medication

- A drug product being used for therapeutic, preventive, or diagnostic purposes by a patient

medication experience

- The sum of all the events in a patient's lifetime that relate to drug therapy
- The patient's personal experience with medications
- The lived experience that includes a patient's attitudes, beliefs, preferences, concerns, expectations, and medication taking behavior
- Includes the patient's expression of the experience, the patient's medication history, and the patient's current medication record

medication history

- A record of past uses of medications and preventive pharmacotherapies
- Includes prescription medications, nonprescription products, alternative therapies, nutritional supplements, and all other agents used by the patient for therapeutic purposes
- Includes immunizations, social drug use, medication allergies and adverse reactions, alerts, special needs, and a history of relevant medication use

medication management services

- Medication management services are the professional activities needed to meet the standard of care that ensures each patient's medications (whether they are prescription, nonprescription, alternative, traditional, vitamins, or nutritional supplements) are individually assessed to determine that each medication is appropriate for the medical condition being treated, that the medication is being effective and achieving the goals established, that the medication is safe for the patient in the presence of the comorbidities and other medications the patient may be taking, and the patient is able and willing to take the medications as intended. This assessment is completed in a systematic and comprehensive manner

- In addition to the comprehensive assessment of the patient's drug-related needs, medication management services include an individualized care plan that utilizes the patient's medication experience and preferences to determine desired goals of therapy with the patient, as well as appropriate follow-up to evaluate actual patient outcomes that result from the care plan. This all occurs because the patient understands, agrees with, and actively participates in the treatment regimen, thus optimizing each patient's medication experience and clinical outcomes. Medication management services must be delivered and documented in a manner that adds unique value to the care of the patient and integrates easily with the medical team caring for the patient
- Medication management services must be grounded in the philosophy and ethics of the professional practice of pharmaceutical care and delivered according to the standards of practice for the patient care process prescribed by the practice

medication taking behavior

- The decisions a patient makes and acts upon related to the use of drug products and dosage regimens observed as patient compliance or adherence
- Is influenced by the patient's beliefs, attitudes, preferences, wants, and experiences related to drug therapy

medication therapy management

- The term used by the U.S. Federal Government to describe the activities performed when eligible Medicare patients receive a service from the Part D drug benefit portion of the Medicare plan and described as patient-focused services aimed at improving therapeutic outcomes
- A term used for billing with Clinical Procedural Terminology codes (CPT) in the United States (established by the American Medical Association)
- Defined by the American Medical Association as face-to-face patient assessment and intervention as appropriate, by the pharmacist, upon request. Medication therapy management service is provided to optimize

the response to medications or to manage treatment-related medication interactions or complications. Includes the following documented elements: review of the pertinent patient history, medication profile (prescription and nonprescription) and recommendations for improving health outcomes and treatment compliance.

morality

- Used synonymously with ethics (see ethics)

nonmaleficence

- Above all, do no harm
- One of the primary ethical principles that underlies the practice of pharmaceutical care

number needed to treat

- Number of persons who must be treated for a given period to achieve an event (treatment) or to prevent an event (prophylaxis). Calculated as the reciprocal of the absolute risk reduction

onset of action

- Amount of time from the administration of the medication to the first evidence of its pharmacological effect

outcomes, patient

- The actual results of interventions involving drug therapies
- Can have characteristics that are economic (i.e., cost), social/behavioral (i.e., patient preferences), or physiological and clinical (i.e., laboratory values, signs and symptoms)

outcome status

- The primary clinical decision made at a follow-up evaluation for each medical condition being managed with drug therapy
- Characterizes the effectiveness of the patient's drug therapy over time
- Is described with a standard set of definitions for medical conditions that are resolved, stable, improved, partially improved, unimproved, worsened, failure, and expired

partially improved

- One of the standard terms for describing the outcome status of a patient's medical condition being treated with pharmacotherapy

- Some measurable progress is being made toward achieving the desired goals of therapy, but adjustments in drug therapy are required. Usually dosage changes or the addition of additive or synergistic therapies is required

paternalistic (approach to patient care)

- An approach in which an authority figure undertakes to regulate the conduct of those in his or her control in matters affecting them as individuals as well as in their relations to that authority and to each other
- Characterized by practitioners making decisions with little regard to the patient's wishes
- An authoritarian approach which is inconsistent with the practice of pharmaceutical care

patient

- An individual who receives or requires health care services
- A person who possesses a unique set of needs, values, and beliefs that are brought to an interaction with a health care practitioner
- Sometimes described as client, consumer, or customer

patient care process

- A standard set of activities undertaken by all patient care practitioners in the care of individual patients
- The systematic activities that occur when a practitioner provides pharmaceutical care to a patient, consisting of the assessment, care plan, and follow-up evaluation
- A process that allows the practitioner to make rational, well-reasoned, and evidence-based decisions

patient-centered

- Care that places the patient's needs as the focus of the clinician's work
- Care that maintains the patient as a "holistic" being and does not fragment the patient into disease groups, organ systems, or drug categories
- A cornerstone of the philosophy of pharmaceutical care practice

patient-centered adherence

- Patient-centered adherence is achieved once the pharmaceutical care practitioner ensures that only those medications, which are determined to be appropriate, effective, and safe for the individual patient being treated, are used and that the individualized care plan developed with the patient takes into account the unique medication experience of that patient. The patient is able to actively participate in the decisions made to treat medical conditions with medications, as well as participate in the development of the care plan to achieve the goals of therapy, and the patient is able to take responsibility for the actions needed to take to achieve optimal outcomes

pharmaceutical care

- A patient-centered practice in which the practitioner assumes responsibility for a patient's drug-related needs and is held accountable for this commitment
- A health care professional practice designed to meet the patient's drug-related needs by identifying, resolving, and preventing drug therapy problems
- The aim of pharmaceutical care practice is the provision of responsible drug therapy for the purpose of achieving positive patient outcomes.

pharmacotherapy

- The use of drugs to treat or prevent human disease
- Includes the drug product and the dosage regimen being taken by a patient for an indication
- Used synonymously with drug therapy

Pharmacotherapy Workup

- A rational decision-making process used in pharmaceutical care practice
- The practitioner's clinical decisions involved in assessing a patient's drug-related needs, identifying drug therapy problems, establishing goals of therapy, selecting interventions, and evaluating outcomes
- Description of the thought processes, hypotheses, established relationships, decisions, and resolved drug therapy problems in providing pharmaceutical care

practice

- The creative application of knowledge, guided by a common philosophy and patient care process, to the resolution of specific problems in a manner and at a standard accepted by society
- The experiences a practitioner encounters in the process of caring for patients
- The group (set) of patients being cared for by a practitioner

practice philosophy

- A set of values that guides behaviors associated with a professional practice

- Aids the practitioner in making clinical, ethical, and management decisions and is used by a practitioner to determine what is important and to set priorities.
- Indicates what should be done at all times, and applies to all practitioners in a professional practice
- Guides how a practitioner practices, day in and day out
- The philosophy of practice for pharmaceutical care includes meeting the social obligation to minimize drug-related morbidity and mortality, accepting direct responsibility to identify, resolve, and prevent drug therapy problems, and applying the caring paradigm in a patient-centered manner

practitioner

- An individual who possesses a unique body of knowledge, skills, and values and uses this to meet the health care needs of a patient
- Subscribes to a specific philosophy of practice and way of practicing (patient care process) that is consistent with other members of the practice community
- An individual who practices based upon specific standards of care and standards for professional behavior and holds colleagues, to these standards
- Used synonymously with clinician

prevalence

- The number of all cases or occurrences during a particular period of time

preventive

- Measures intended to thwart or ward off illness or disease, includes drug therapies and interventions to reduce the risk of drug therapy problems and/or medical conditions from developing

profession

- A vocation requiring training in the arts or sciences and advanced studies in a specialized field
- A body of qualified persons in a specific occupation or field
- Embodies the following attributes: (1) service above self-interest; (2) application of specialized knowledge; (3) skills in the service of humanity; (4) an ethical code; (5) a fiduciary practitioner–client relationship; (6) registration or state certification, which embodies standards of training and practice in some statutory form; (7) regulation of advertising services; and (8) independence from external control

professional ethics

- A set of moral principles and values defined by the philosophy of practice
- Prescriptive, appropriate behavior for practitioners

relative risk

- Risk for achieving an event or outcome with treatment in the treatment group relative to the control group. Can also describe preventing an event with prophylaxis
- In clinical trials used to compare the risk of developing a disease in people not receiving the new treatment (or placebo) versus people who are receiving an established (standard) treatment
- Also used to compare the risk of developing a side effect in people receiving a drug as compared to people who are not receiving the treatment (or placebo)

relative risk reduction

- Reduction in events with treatment compared with control. This number is often expressed as a percentage
- Calculated by dividing the absolute risk reduction by the control event rate
- Can be more useful than the absolute risk reduction in determining an appropriate treatment plan because it accounts not only for the effectiveness of a proposed treatment, but also for the relative likelihood of an incident (positive or negative) occurring in the absence of treatment

reflective practitioner

- The practitioner who engages in active, deliberate, and conscious activity to become aware, critically analyze, and learn from practice experiences in order to improve clinical competence and patient relationships

resolved

- One of the standard terms for describing the outcome status of a patient's medical condition being treated with pharmacotherapy
- Goals of therapy have been achieved. Drug therapy has been completed or can now be discontinued. Usually associated with successful therapy for an acute disorder

specialist

- A practitioner who identifies, resolves, and prevents problems that are more complex than those addressed by the generalist
- Uses the same patient care process as the generalist to facilitate communication between the two practitioners

- Usually sees patients on a referral or consulting basis
- In the medical fields, is associated with a specific area of practice such as nephrology, pulmonary medicine, cardiology, neurology, urology, gastroenterology and infectious diseases

safety (of the patient)

- Extent to which a patient is free from side effects, toxicity, or other undesirable pharmacological actions that a drug is known to exhibit at the doses used to treat patients

stable

- One of the standard terms for describing the outcome status of a patient's medical condition being treated with pharmacotherapy
- Goals of therapy have been achieved. The same drug therapy will be continued. Usually associated with therapy for chronic disorders

standards for professional behavior

- Authoritative statements in which a profession describes the responsibilities for which its practitioners are held accountable
- Practitioners' accountability to the public
- Includes guidelines for quality of care, ethics, collegiality, collaboration, education research, and resource allocation

standards of care

- The level at which a practitioner is expected to provide care to a patient
- The set of behaviors each patient has a right to expect from a practitioner claiming to provide care in a particular profession
- The set of behaviors that is subject to evaluation by peers, regulators, and the public
- Includes guidelines for assessment, drug therapy problem identification, care plan development, and follow-up evaluation

strength (of a product)

- The amount of active ingredient available in each dosage form (e.g., 750 mg per tablet)

therapeutic relationship

- A partnership or alliance between the practitioner and the patient formed for the purpose of optimizing the patient's medication experience
- Characterized by: trust, empathy, respect, authenticity, and responsiveness

unimproved

- One of the standard terms for describing the outcome status of a patient's medical condition being treated with pharmacotherapy
- No measurable progress in achieving goals of therapy can be demonstrated at this time. It is judged that more time is needed to produce adequate response.

  No changes will be made. The same drug therapy will be continued at this time

worsened

- One of the standard terms for describing the outcome status of a patient's medical condition being treated with pharmacotherapy
- There has been a decline in health status while receiving the current drug regimen. Some adjustments in drug product selection and/or drug dosage are required

Pharmacotherapy Workup Notes

Pharmacotherapy Workup© **NOTES**	**ASSESSMENT**			

CONTACT INFORMATION

Name				
Address	City		State	Postal Code
Telephone (h)	(w)	(cell)	e-mail	
Pharmacy Name		Clinic Name		
(tel)		(tel)		

DEMOGRAPHICS

Age	Date of Birth		Gender: M/F
Weight	Height	Lean Body Weight	
Pregnancy status: Y/N	Breast Feeding: Y/N	Due Date	
Occupation			
Living Arrangements/Family			
Health Insurance (coverage issues):			

REASON FOR THE ENCOUNTER

MEDICATION EXPERIENCE

Question	Needs attention in care plan	
	Y	N
What is the patient's general attitude toward taking medication?	Y	N
What does the patient want/expect from his/her drug therapy?	Y	N
What concerns does the patient have with his/her medications?	Y	N
To what extent does the patient understand his/her medications?	Y	N
Are there cultural, religious, or ethical issues that influence the patient's willingness to take medications?	Y	N
Describe the patient's medication taking behavior	Y	N

	Substance	History of Use	Substance	History of Use
SOCIAL DRUG USE	Tobacco □ No tobacco use	□ 0–1 packs per day □ >1 packs per day □ previous history of smoking □ attempts to quit	Alcohol □ No alcohol use	□ < 2 drinks per week □ 2–6 drinks per week □ > 6 drinks per week □ history of alcohol dependence
	Caffeine □ No caffeine use	□ < 2 cups per day □ 2–6 cups per day □ > 6 cups per day □ history of caffeine dependence	Other recreational drug use	

Recommended immunization schedule for persons aged 0 through 6 years–United States • 2011
For those who fall behind or start late, see the catch-up schedule

Vaccine ▼ Age ►	Birth	1 month	2 months	4 months	6 months	12 months	15 months	18 months	19–23 months	2–3 years	4–6 years
Hepatitis B[1]	HepB	HepB			HepB						
Rotavirus[2]			RV	RV	RV[2]						
Diphtheria, Tetanus, Pertussis[3]			DTaP	DTaP	DTaP	see footnote[3]	DTaP				DTaP
Haemophilus influenzae type b[4]			Hib	Hib	Hib[4]	Hib					
Pneumococcal[5]			PCV	PCV	PCV	PCV					PPSV
Inactivated Poliovirus[6]			IPV	IPV		IPV					IPV
Influenza[7]						Influenza (Yearly)					
Measles, Mumps, Rubella[8]						MMR		see footnote[8]			MMR
Varicella[9]						Varicella		see footnote[9]			Vari-cella
Hepatitis A[10]						HepA (2 doses)				HepA Series	
Meningococcal[11]										MCV4	

Range of recommended ages for certain high-risk groups

Range of recommended ages for all children

Recommended immunization schedule for persons aged 7 through 18 years—United States • 2011

For those who fall behind or start late, see the schedule below and the catch-up schedule

Vaccine ▼ Age ▶	7–10 years	11–12 years	13–18 years
Tetanus, Diphtheria, Pertussis[1]		Tdap	Tdap
Human Papillomavirus[2]	see footnote[2]	HPV (3 doses)(females)	HPV Series
Meningococcal[3]	MCV4	MCV4	MCV4
Influenza[4]	Influenza (Yearly)		
Pneumococcal[5]	Pneumococcal		
Hepatitis A[6]	HepA Series		
Hepatitis B[7]	HepB Series		
Inactivated Poliovirus[8]	IPV Series		
Measles, Mumps, Rubella[9]	MMR Series		
Vericella[10]	Vericella Series		

	Range of recommended ages for certain high-risk groups	Range of recommended ages for catch-up immunization	Range of recommended ages for all children

☐ **Current on all childhood immunizations**

Recommended adult immunization schedule, by vaccine and age group

Vaccine ▼ Age group ▶	19–26 years	27–49 years	50–59 years	60–64 years	≥65 years
Influenza[1,*]	1 dose annually				
Tetanus, Diphtheria, Pertussis (Td/Tdap)[2,*]	Substitute 1-time dose of Tdap for Td booster; then boost with Td every 10 yrs				Td booster every 10 yrs
Varicella[3,*]	2 doses				
Human Papillomavirus (HPV)[4,*]	3 doses (females)				
Zoster[5]				1 dose	
Measles, Mumps, Rubella (MMR)[6,*]	1 or 2 doses		1 dose		
Pneumococcal (polysaccharide)[7,8]	1 or 2 doses				1 dose
Meningococcal[9,*]	1 or more doses				
Hepatitis A[10,*]	2 doses				
Hepatitis B[11,*]	3 doses				

*Covered by the vaccine injury compensation program.

For all persons in this category who meet the age requirements and who lack evidence of immunity (e.g., lack documentation of vaccination or have no evidence of previous infection)

Recommended if some other risk factor is present (e.g., based on medical, occupational, lifestyle, or other indications)

No recommendation

☐ **Current on all adult immunizations**

*see http://www.cdc.gov/vaccines/ for more information, footnotes and references

(Copyright © 2003-2012 Cipolle RJ, Strand LM, Morley PC.)

ALLERGIES & ALERTS

Medication Allergies (drug, timing, reaction—rash, shock, asthma, nausea, anemia)
Adverse reactions to drugs in the past
Other Alerts/Health Aids/Special Needs (sight, hearing, mobility, literacy, disability)

CURRENT MEDICAL CONDITIONS AND MEDICATIONS

INDICATION	DRUG PRODUCT	DOSAGE REGIMEN dose, route, frequency, duration	START DATE	RESPONSE effectiveness/safety

PAST DRUG THERAPIES

INDICATION	DRUG THERAPY	RESPONSE	DATE

PAST MEDICAL HISTORY (RELEVANT ILLNESSES, HOSPITALIZATIONS, SURGICAL PROCEDURES, INJURIES, PREGNANCIES, DELIVERIES)

NUTRITIONAL STATUS (NOTE DAILY INTAKE OF CALORIES, CALCIUM, SODIUM, CHOLESTEROL, FIBER, POTASSIUM, VITAMIN K)			
calories	K$^+$	cholesterol	Vitamin K
calcium	Na$^+$	fiber	

OTHER FOOD OR DIETARY RESTRICTIONS / NEEDS

Vital signs: BP _____/_____   HR _____bpm   Resp Rate _____   Temp____

		y/n			y/n
REVIEW OF SYSTEMS	General Systems	Poor appetite	GU/Reproductive	Dysmenorrhea/ menstrual bleeding	
		Weight change		Incontinence	
		Pain		Impotence	
		Headache		Decreased sexual drive	
		Dizziness (vertigo)			
	EENT	Change in vision		Vaginal discharge or itching	
		Loss of hearing			
		Ringing in the ears (tinnitus)		Hot flashes	
		Bloody nose (epistaxis)	Kidney/Urinary	Urinary frequency	
				Bloody urine (hematuria)	
		Allergic rhinitis		Renal dysfunction	
		Glaucoma			
		Bloody sputum (hemoptysis)	Hematopoietic Symptoms	Excessive bruising	
				Bleeding	
	Cardiovascular	Chest pain		Anemia	
		Hyperlipidemia	Musculoskeletal	Back pain	
		Hypertension		Arthritis pain (osteo/rheumatoid)	
		Myocardial Infarction		Tendonitis	
		Orthostatic hypotension		Painful muscles	
	Pulmonary	Asthma	Neuropsychiatric	Numb, tingling sensation in extremities (parasthesia)	
		Shortness of breath			
		Wheezing			
	Gastrointestinal	Heartburn		Tremor	
		Abdominal pain		Loss of balance	
		Nausea		Depression	
		Vomiting		Suicidal	
		Diarrhea		Anxiety, nervousness	
		Constipation		Inability to concentrate	
	Skin	Eczema/Psoriasis			
		Itching (pruritis)		Seizure	
		Rash		Stroke/TIA	
	Endocrine Systems	Diabetes		Memory loss	
		Hypothyroidism	Infectious Disease	HIV/AIDS	
		Menopausal Symptoms		Malaria	
	Hepatic	Cirrhosis		Syphilis	
		Hepatitis		Gonorrhea	
	Nutrition/Fluid/ Electrolytes	Dehydration		Herpes	
		Edema		Chlamydia	
		Potassium deficiency		Tuberculosis	

DRUG THERAPY PROBLEMS TO BE RESOLVED

MEDICAL CONDITION AND DRUG THERAPY INVOLVED	INDICATION
	Unnecessary Drug Therapy __No medical indication __Duplicate therapy __Nondrug therapy indicated __Treating avoidable ADR __Addictive/recreational **Needs Additional Drug Therapy** __Untreated condition __Preventive/prophylactic __Synergistic/potentiating
MEDICAL CONDITION AND DRUG THERAPY INVOLVED	EFFECTIVENESS
	Needs Different Drug Product __More effective drug available __Condition refractory to drug __Dosage form inappropriate __Not effective for condition **Dosage Too Low** __Wrong dose __Frequency inappropriate __Drug interaction __Duration inappropriate
MEDICAL CONDITION AND DRUG THERAPY INVOLVED	SAFETY
	Adverse Drug Reaction __Undesirable effect __Unsafe drug for patient __Drug interaction __Dosage administered or changed too rapidly __Allergic reaction __Contraindications present **Dosage Too High** __Wrong dose __Frequency inappropriate __Duration inappropriate __Drug interaction __Incorrect administration
MEDICAL CONDITION AND DRUG THERAPY INVOLVED	COMPLIANCE
	Noncompliance __Directions not understood __Patient prefers not to take __Patient forgets to take __Drug product too expensive __Cannot swallow/administer __Drug product not available

(Side label: DRUG THERAPY PROBLEMS)

___No Drug Therapy Problem(s) at this time

Pharmacotherapy Workup© **NOTES**   **CARE PLAN**

INDICATION _____
(Description and history of the present illness or medical condition including previous approaches to treatment and responses)

GOALS OF THERAPY (improvement or normalization of signs/symptoms/laboratory tests or reduction of risk)
1.

2.

DRUG THERAPY PROBLEMS to be resolved

☐ None at this time

Therapeutic Alternatives (to resolve the drug therapy problem)
1.

2.

PHARMACOTHERAPY PLAN (Includes current drug therapies and changes)

MEDICATIONS (DRUG PRODUCTS)	DOSAGE INSTRUCTIONS (DOSE, ROUTE, FREQUENCY, DURATION)	NOTES CHANGES

Other interventions to optimize drug therapy

SCHEDULE FOR NEXT FOLLOW-UP EVALUATION:

Pharmacotherapy Workup© NOTES	EVALUATION

Medical Condition: _____

	Outcome Parameter	Pretreatment Baseline (Date)	First Follow-up (Date)	Second Follow-up (Date)
EFFECTIVENESS	Sign/symptom			
	Sign/symptom			
	Lab value			
	Lab value			
SAFETY	Sign/symptoms			
	Signs/symptoms			
	Lab value			
	Lab value			
	Other			
STATUS	STATUS **Initial:** goals being established, initiate new therapy **Resolved:** goals achieved, therapy completed **Stable:** goals achieved, continue same therapy **Improved:** adequate progress being made, continue same therapy **Partial Improvement:** progress being made, adjustments in therapy required **Unimproved:** no progress yet, continue same therapy **Worsened:** decline in health, adjust therapy **Failure:** goals not achieved, discontinue current therapy and replace with different therapy			
	New Drug Therapy Problems Identified		☐ none at this time ☐ documented	☐ none at this time ☐ documented

Date	Schedule for next follow-up	Comments

Signature_____ Date_____

Parameters Commonly Used to Evaluate Effectiveness and/or Safety of Drug Therapy

Parameter	Goals of therapy (Normal values)	Clinical use
Blood pressure	Goals of therapy include: systolic blood pressure of 110–140 mmHg diastolic blood pressure of 75–85 mmHg < 130/80 with diabetes or kidney disease	Used to evaluate effectiveness and safety of antihypertensive drug therapies such as diuretics, beta blockers, ACE inhibitors, angiotensin II receptors blockers, aldosterone antagonists, calcium blockers.
Total Cholesterol	Goal of therapy < 200 mg/dl (SI < 5.17 mmol/L)	Represents all of the different kinds of cholesterol in the blood and includes high-density lipids (HDL), low-density lipids (LDL), and triglycerides (TG).
LDL Low-density lipoprotein	Goal of therapy varies depending on other risk factors including cigarette smoking, hypertension, HDL< 40mg/dl, family history of CHD and male > 45 or female> 55. • without other risk factors <160 mg/dl (SI <4.1 mmol/L) • with 2 risk factors <130 mg/dl (SI <3.4 mmol/L) • with CHD and ≥2 risk factors < 100 mg/dl (SI < 2.6 mmol/L)	Used to evaluate the effectiveness of lipid lowering drug therapies including atorvastatin (Lipitor®), fluvastatin (Lescol®), lovastatin (Mevacor®), pravastatin (Pravachol®), simvastatin (Zocor®) nicotinic acid (Niacin®) gemfibrozil (Lopid®), clofibrate (Atromid-S®) colestipol (Colestid®), cholestyramine (Questran®)
HDL High-density lipoprotein	Goals of therapy > 40 mg/dl (SI > 1.04 mmol/L)	HDL removes excess cholesterol from peripheral tissues and is considered "good" cholesterol. Elevated HDL levels are associated with decreased risk for coronary heart disease.

(Continued)

(Continued) Parameters Commonly Used to Evaluate Effectiveness and/ or Safety of Drug Therapy

Parameter	Goals of therapy (Normal values)	Clinical use
Triglycerides	<160 mg/dl <1.8 mmol/L	Elevated triglycerides considered an independent risk factor for coronary heart disease.
Glucose	Goal of therapy includes: preprandial blood glucose of 80–120 mg/dL bedtime blood glucose of 100–140 mg/dL Fasting plasma glucose of >126 mg/dL on two occasions is consistent with the diagnosis of diabetes mellitus	Used to evaluate drug therapy to manage hyperglycemia associated with diabetes mellitus including insulin (Humulin®) (Novolin®), glipizide (Glutcotrol®), glyburide (Diabeta®) (Mircronase®), pioglitazone (Actos®), rosiglitazone (Avandia®)
HbA$_{1c}$ Hemoglobin A$_{1c}$	Goal of therapy <7% some <8% Normal range 4–6%	Used to evaluate the effectiveness of glucose control in patients with diabetes. Reflects the blood glucose control over the past 2 to 3 months.
TSH Thyroid Stimulating Hormone	Goals of therapy include the reduction of TSH levels to the normal range of 0.3–5 µU/ml (SI 0.3–5 mU/L)	Used to evaluate the effectiveness of thyroid replacement therapy to manage hypothyroidism. levothyroxine (Synthroid®). Elevated TSH levels are indicative of hypothyroidism.
INR International Normalized Ratio	Goal of therapy varies with the indication. INR 2.0–3.0 for atrial fibrillation, deep vein thrombosis, pulmonary emboli INR 2.5–3.5 for mechanical prosthetic values	Used to evaluate the effectiveness and safety of anticoagulant therapy. Used to determine dosage adjustments for warfarin (Coumadin®) therapy.

(Continued)

(Continued) Parameters Commonly Used to Evaluate Effectiveness and/ or Safety of Drug Therapy

Parameter	Goals of therapy (Normal values)	Clinical use
K+ Serum Potassium	Goal of therapy is to maintain serum potassium within the normal range of 3.5–5.0 mEq/L (SI 3.5–5.0 mmol/L)	Used to evaluate and prevent cardiac toxicity associated with hypokalemia caused by diuretics, diarrhea/ vomiting. Can aggravate digoxin (Lanoxin®) toxicity. Hyperkalemia associated with renal dysfunction, ACE inhibitors including captopril (Capoten®), enalapril (Vasotec®), lisinopril (Prinivil®) (Zestril®), ramipril (Altace®) and ARBs including: irbesartan (Avapro®), losartan (Cozaar®), valsartan (Diovan®).
Creatinine serum creatinine (SCr) creatinine clearance (CrCl)	Creatinine normal range 0.6–1.3 mg/dL (SI 53–115 µmol/L) Creatinine Clearance normal range 80–100 ml/min Drug dosage adjustments often required when CrCl is <30 ml/min	Used as a guideline to determine appropriate dosage of medications which are dependent on renal function for elimination. Used to determine if drug therapy is causing nephrotoxicity or if drugs are accumulating to unsafe levels due to decreasing renal function.
ALT Alanine aminotransferase	Normal values Males 10–40 Units/ml Females 8–35 Units/ml	Used to evaluate liver damage caused by medications such as simvastatin (Zocor®), pravastatin, lovastatin (Mevacor®), atorvastatin (Lipitor®), fluvastatin (Lescol®), carbamazepine, phenytoin, acetaminophen
AST Aspartate aminotransferase	Males 20–40 Units/ml Females 15–30 Units/ml	If elevated 2–3 times drug-induced hepatic damage to be suspected

Page numbers followed by *f* or *t* indicate figures or tables, respectively.